Advances in Veterinary Dermatology

Advances in Veterinary Dermatology

Volume 7

Proceedings of the Seventh World Congress of Veterinary Dermatology
Vancouver, Canada
July 24–28, 2012

Edited by

Sheila M. F. Torres

College of Veterinary Medicine, University of Minnesota, St Paul, Minnesota, USA

Co-editors

Linda A. Frank

College of Veterinary Medicine, University of Tennessee, Knoxville, Tennessee, USA

Ann M. Hargis

DermatoDiagnostics, Edmonds, Washington, and Department of Comparative Medicine, School of Medicine, University of Washington, Seattle, Washington, USA

WILEY-BLACKWELL

Blackwell Publishing was acquired by John Wiley & Sons in February 2007. Blackwell's publishing programme has been merged with Wiley's global Scientific, Technical, and Medical business to form Wiley-Blackwell.

Registered office
John Wiley & Sons Ltd, The Atrium, Southern Gate, Chichester, West Sussex, PO19 8SQ, United Kingdom

Editorial offices
9600 Garsington Road, Oxford, OX4 2DQ, United Kingdom
2121 State Avenue, Ames, Iowa 50014-8300, USA

For details of our global editorial offices, for customer services and for information about how to apply for permission to reuse the copyright material in this book please see our website at http://www.wiley.com/wiley-blackwell.

ISBN: 9781118644874
ISSN: 0959-4493 (Print)
ISSN: 1365-3164 (Online)

A catalogue record for this book is available from the British Library.

Wiley also publishes its books in a variety of electronic formats. Some content that appears in print may not be available in electronic books.

Cover Image credits: Canada Place Sails (courtesy of Canada Place and Port Metro Vancouver); Network pathways generated through the use of IPA (Ingenuity® Systems, www.ingenuity.com); Mycobacterial granuloma (*Mycobacterium* sp. strain Tarwin) on the nasal planum and adjacent skin of a cat from rural Victoria, Australia. (Photograph courtesy of Dr Robert Hilton, Yarrambat, Australia.)
Cover design by Andy Meaden

Set in Univers-Light 9/11.5 points by SPS

Printed in Singapore

Contents

*This study was not published in the special issue of the *Veterinary Dermatology* journal (VDE 2013; 24:1).

Sponsors of the Seventh World Congress of Veterinary Dermatology

Principal Sponsors

Science For A Better Life

Major Sponsors

Dechra Veterinary Products
Elanco
Sogeval Shared Solutions

Supporting Sponsors

Heska
Merck Animal Health
P&G Pet Care/Iams
Veterinary Allergy Reference Laboratory (VARL)

Sponsors

LDCA/Dermoscent
Nestle Purina PetCare
Rayne Clinical Nutrition
Vetoquinol

Officers and Organizing Committees of the Seventh World Congress of Veterinary Dermatology

Officers

President: Dr Manon Paradis
Secretary: Dr Stephen White
Treasurer: Dr Rosario Cerundolo

Executive Organizing Committee

The Officers and:
Dr Douglas DeBoer, Fundraising
Dr Alan Hoey, Local Organizing Committee
Dr Chiara Noli, Programme
Dr Rusty Muse, Publicity
Dr Sheila Torres, Publications
Prof. Richard Halliwell, WAVD Representative
Dr Masahiko Nagata, Asia Representative

Committees

Fundraising Committee

Dr Douglas DeBoer (Chairperson)
Dr Wayne Rosenkrantz (Co-chairperson)

Local Organizing Committee

Dr Alan Hoey (Chairperson)
Dr Vincent Defalque (Co-chairperson)

Programme Committee

Dr Chiara Noli (Chairperson)
Sonya Bettenay (Co-chairperson)
Mona Boord (Co-chairperson)
Kerstin Bergvall
Valerie Fadok
Andy Hillier
Koji Nishifuji
David Robson
Manolis Saridomichelakis
Anthony Yu

Publications Committee

Dr Sheila Torres (Chairperson)
Dr Linda Frank
Dr Ann Hargis

Publicity Committee

Dr Rusty Muse (Chairperson)
Dr Mandy Burrows (Co-chairperson)
Dr Kinga Gortel
Dr Ian Spiegel
Dr Claudia Nett
Dr Masahiko Nagata

WAVD Representatives

Prof. Richard Halliwell (UK)
Dr Masahiko Nagata (Asia)

Members of the Administrative Committee of the WAVD

Kenneth Kwochka (USA)	President WAVD, Representative of ACVD
Didier Noel Carlotti (France)	Past President WAVD, President WCVD8
Amanda Burrows (Australia)	Secretary WAVD, Representative DCACVS
David Lloyd (UK)	Treasurer WAVD, President WCVD5
Phil Roudebush (USA)	Representative of AAVD
Luc Beco (Belgium)	Representative of ESVD
Emmanuel Bensignor (France)	Representative of ECVD
Manon Paradis (Canada)	Representative of CAVD, President WCVD7
Carmel Taylor (Hong Kong)	Representative of AiSVD
Claudia Nett-Mettler (Switzerland)	Member-at-Large
Wayne Rosenkrantz (USA)	Member-at-Large
Richard Halliwell (UK)	President WCVD1, Past President WAVD
Hans Koch (Germany)	President WCVD3
Peter Ihrke (US)	President WCVD4

Preface

The Seventh World Congress of Veterinary Dermatology, held in Vancouver, Canada, from July 24 to 28, was unquestionably a success! The Congress was organized with the support of the World Association for Veterinary Dermatology (WAVD) and its affiliated societies. A record number of more than 1600 delegates from over 50 countries participated, reflecting the worldwide interest in the Veterinary Dermatology specialty.

The scientific programme was exceptional and covered a broad range of topics. Speakers of six state of the art, six supporting review and 20 supporting original studies presented cutting edge information in the areas of allergy, immunology, skin biology, therapy, infectious diseases and oncology. The 69 free communications and 121 posters provided diverse high-quality research and reports of clinical cases catering to the broad interest of the audience. Moreover, there was an extensive and well-attended advance and comprehensive continuing education programme for veterinary practitioners, not to mention the programmes exclusively focused in equine, feline and exotic dermatology. Last but not least, 14 workshops, where experts presented topics in various areas, provided a wonderful opportunity for colleagues to ask questions and exchange ideas in an informal atmosphere. This large number of scientific presentations and the high calibre of the material delivered by colleagues from across the globe reflect, unquestionably, the worldwide advancement of the Veterinary Dermatology field and, for this, we should all be proud.

This hardbound volume, *Advances in Veterinary Dermatology 7*, contains the manuscripts published in the special issue in addition to the workshop reports. The memory of the other scientific presentations is preserved in the abstract issue of *Veterinary Dermatology*, Volume 23 Supplement 1, July 2012, and in the Proceedings of the Continuing Education Programme.

The success of this Congress is largely a result of the hard work of the officers and members of the various organizing committees who unpretentiously donate countless hours of their time to make this a memorable event. Moreover, without the kind support of the corporate sponsors this Congress would not be possible. On behalf of all participants, I would like to take this opportunity to thank all the sponsors of the Seventh World Congress of Veterinary Dermatology.

I hope you are already making plans for the Eighth World Congress of Veterinary Dermatology which will take place in Bordeaux, France, and promises to be as outstanding as this one.

Sheila Torres
College of Veterinary Medicine, University of Minnesota, St Paul, Minnesota, USA

Part 1

ALLERGY

To cite this article, please use DOI: 10.1111/j.1365-3164.2012.01079.x

1.1

Epidemiology of human atopic dermatitis – seven areas of notable progress and seven areas of notable ignorance

Hywel C. Williams

Centre of Evidence-Based Dermatology, Room A103, Lenton Lane, University of Nottingham King's Meadow Campus, Nottingham NG7 2NR, UK

Correspondence: Hywel C. Williams, Centre of Evidence-Based Dermatology, Room A103, Lenton Lane, University of Nottingham King's Meadow Campus, Nottingham NG7 2NR, UK. E-mail: hywel.williams@nottingham.ac.uk

Background – This narrative review highlights areas within the epidemiology of human atopic dermatitis (AD) where significant progress has been made and where considerable ignorance still exists. The review is supported by systematic reviews wherever possible, with the purpose of stimulating fresh approaches to human and veterinary research into AD.

Progress – Areas of progress include valid and repeatable methods of disease definition, global documentation of disease prevalence and impact, clarification of the role of some genetic factors, such as filaggrin gene mutations, clear evidence that environmental factors are key, as demonstrated by the positive social class gradient and rising prevalence, a possible protective effect of infections in early life, documentation of comorbidities, such as a reduced risk of glioma, and mapping the evidence base through systematic reviews and an online global resource of clinical trials.

Ignorance – Areas where significant uncertainty still exists include the question of whether AD is more than one disease, the tendency for researchers to look at the same old risk factors, lack of specific environmental risk factors that are amenable to manipulation, inconsistencies in the hygiene hypothesis, sparse knowledge about adult AD, lack of evidence that eczema can be prevented, and little scientific work exploring what causes flares in people with established AD.

Introduction

Epidemiology is concerned with much more than simply documenting the prevalence of a disease such as atopic dermatitis.[1] By observing cases with atopic dermatitis (AD) and contrasting them with those who do not have AD in relation to various genetic and environmental factors, critical information about potential risk factors for determining disease expression can be gleaned. Identification of such risk factors brings us one step closer to the dream of disease prevention, an important concept in a society so preoccupied with disease treatment. The beauty of epidemiology is that knowledge of pathophysiology and scientific mechanism is not a prerequisite to identifying important risk factors that can be acted upon. By simply counting diseased cases in relation to population denominators served by different water supplies, John Snow was able to deduce that some 'morbid matter' transmitted by water was responsible for the terrible cholera epidemics in London in the 1850s, and was able to halt the epidemics by appropriate action. These discoveries were made long before germ theory had demonstrated the responsible bacteria.[2]

It is not possible to summarize all knowledge relating to the distribution and determinants of human AD in one review article without reducing everything to superficial and potentially uninteresting summary statements. The author edited an entire textbook of 250 pages on the epidemiology of AD over 10 years ago,[3] and inclusion of subsequent studies would now probably fill 500 pages. Instead, and with the readership of veterinary dermatologists in mind, who might be looking for ideas and parallels between human and animal AD, the author has chosen to highlight areas where significant progress has been made over the last 12 years, as well as to highlight some areas of notable ignorance, which may serve to stimulate new research. The selection of which seven areas of progress and seven areas of uncertainty to include is a personal choice of the author based upon 23 years researching the epidemiology of AD. The author has also become more aware of existing and missing evidence through evidence mapping in the form of systematic reviews in his previous work as dermatology lead for the UK National Electronic Library for Health, now called *NHS Evidence*.[4]

Seven areas of notable progress

Disease definition

In the 1970s, many synonyms for atopic dermatitis were in use over the world, and it is unclear whether they all referred to the same clinical concept. The Hanifin and Rajka consensus criteria marked an important development in listing the clinical features of AD, although their complexity and lack of validity and repeatability meant

Accepted 30 May 2012
Sources of Funding: University of Nottingham.
Conflict of Interest: No conflicts of interest have been declared.

that they were unsuitable for epidemiological studies.[5] This was the task of the UK Working Party, which refined the Hanifin and Rajka criteria to a minimum list of reliable discriminators that could be used in epidemiological studies (Table 1).[6] An independent systematic review of diagnostic criteria for AD found 19 validation studies of the UK diagnostic criteria, which showed sensitivity and specificity ranging from 10 to 100 and from 89.3 to 99.1%, respectively.[7] These criteria have now been used in many studies worldwide, although more validation in the very young and in adults is still needed. The criteria permit a more standardized approach towards defining the AD phenotype in a way that any researcher can understand and replicate. It is encouraging to note that a similar approach for developing diagnostic criteria for canine AD has been undertaken.[8]

Advances have also been made with disease nomenclature. It should be pointed out that the term 'atopic dermatitis' or its synonymous term 'atopic eczema' should only be used when denoting those with the phenotype of eczema who also have evidence of allergen-specific circulating immunoglobulin E (IgE) antibodies, as demonstrated by serum or skin prick tests.[9,10] Evidence from the International Study of Asthma and Allergies in Children (ISAAC) Phase Two, the largest sample of well-defined AD cases in the world, suggests that around 50% of examined AD cases in developed countries are, in fact, not atopic, and an even greater proportion in developing countries are not atopic.[11] The study has concluded that any association between atopy and examined flexural eczema is weak and more variable than previously suggested, and that the strength of this association is positively linked to gross national income.[11] Part of the misguided obsession with atopy resides in the fact that atopy is more common in people with more severe skin disease who typically characterize hospital-based populations that are easy to study.[10] Indeed, some have even argued that raised serum IgE could be an epiphenomenon of disease severity.[10] The World Allergy Organization (WAO) nomenclature committee has recommended that the term 'eczema' is used to denote what we typically refer to as the phenotype of atopic dermatitis, and that the prefix 'atopic' is used when defining a subset that is truly atopic.[9] The WAO proposition makes good sense and it obviates the need for yet more sets of diagnostic criteria, such as the 'millennium criteria', which look remarkably like the original Hanifin and Rajka criteria, with IgE reactivity stuck on top as a necessary criterion.[12] We will, however, continue to use the term atopic dermatitis (AD) throughout this article, simply for familiarity to the reader.

Table 1. The UK refinement of the Hanifin and Rajka diagnostic criteria for atopic dermatitis (reproduced with permission of John Wiley & Sons, Ltd).[6]

To qualify as a case, the child must have:
An itchy skin
Plus three or more of:
Onset under age 2 years
History of rash in skin creases
Personal history of asthma or hay fever
A history of a generally dry skin
Visible flexural dermatitis

Prevalence and impact

Although scores of *ad hoc* prevalence studies have documented the burden of AD to a variable extent, such studies are not truly comparable because of the different diagnostic criteria and sampling methods used and age groups studied. The advent of the ISAAC has opened up the global map of AD by using identical methods in over a million children in over 100 countries worldwide.[13] The latest ISAAC Phase Three world map of AD symptoms shows that for 385,853 children aged 6–7 years from 143 centres in 60 countries, the prevalence of AD ranged from 0.9% in India to 22.5% in Ecuador, with new data showing high values in Asia and Latin America.[14] For the 663,256 aged 13–14 years from 230 centres in 96 countries, AD prevalences ranged from 0.2% in China to 24.6% in Columbia, with the highest values in Africa and Latin America.[14] Current eczema was lower for boys than girls (odds ratio, 0.94 and 0.72 at ages 6–7 and 13–14 years, respectively). The ISAAC data have shown that AD is now a common problem in cities in developing countries that are undergoing rapid demographic transition, as well as in developed countries. Phase Two of the ISAAC study also included physical examination of 28,591 randomly selected children aged 8–12 years and skin prick testing, enabling much firmer exploration of the link between AD and atopy across the world.[11] Point prevalences of flexural eczema by skin examination ranged between 0.4% in Kintampo, Ghana to 14.2% in Östersund, Sweden.[11] The association between atopy and examined flexural eczema was weak, especially in nonaffluent countries.[11]

One limitation of the ISAAC study was low participation from the USA, for reasons that are unclear. That lack of information has been filled by a recent analysis of a nationally representative sample of 102,353 children aged 17 years and under who took part in the 2003 National Survey of Children's Health.[15,16] The survey showed that the prevalence of AD diagnosis ranged from 8.7 to 18.1% between states and districts, with the highest prevalence reported in East Coast states. Metropolitan living, black ethnicity and high educational level in the household were all associated with increased AD prevalence.[15,16]

Four systematic reviews have summarized the impact of AD.[17–20] Sleep loss seems to be the dominant problem, which affects the entire family as well as the child with AD.[19] Depression, anxiety and quality-of-life impairment may also occur, and morbidity is comparable to other 'important' noncommunicable diseases.[21,22] The direct and indirect financial costs of AD can be significant. A review of 59 US studies estimated that national annual AD costs in 2008 could be as large as $3.8 billion US dollars.[20]

Role of genetic factors

A strong familial component has always been a feature of AD, and twin studies pointed to a strong influence of genetic factors.[23] While earlier work on the genetics of AD focused on immunological phenomena with mixed findings,[24] significant breakthroughs into understanding the role of genetics in AD occurred following the discovery of filaggrin gene mutations responsible for the dry skin seen in eczema.[25] Filaggrin is a skin protein that appears to be essential for maintaining the integrity of skin barrier function, which is important in AD and other dry skin conditions, including ichthyosis vulgaris.[25] Profilaggrin gene mutations resulting in loss of function are present in around 10% of western European and North American populations.[26] In addition, such mutations predict AD severity, disease persistence and allergic sensitization and may be involved in the progression of AD to other allergic diseases, such as allergic rhinitis and asthma.[27,28] The chronology of the discovery of the filaggrin gene and its subsequent association has been documented in a recent review by Brown and McLean.[25] The remaining challenge in AD is to establish whether other genes responsible for barrier integrity are also important and to explore whether filaggrin mutations have important therapeutic applications, including disease prevention. The author's group is involved in developing a national study to see whether barrier enhancement of babies born to parents with atopic disease can reduce the incidence and severity of AD.[29] Many immunological and skin barrier similarities between human and canine AD have emerged, such as increased transepidermal water loss, abnormal lipid lamellae, decreased ceramides and reduced filaggrin protein expression, and these are summarized comprehensively by Marsella *et al.*[30]

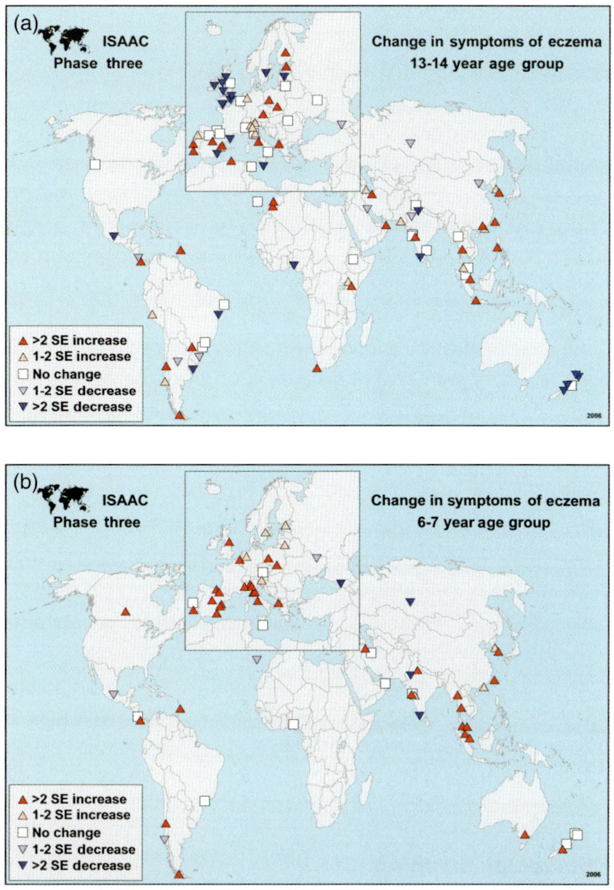

Figure 1. (a, b) World maps from the International Study of Asthma and Allergies in Childhood depicting flexural eczema symptoms in the last year, showing changes in the prevalence of eczema symptoms for 13–14 and 6–7 year olds in consecutive prevalence surveys conducted 5–10 years apart. SE, standard error (reproduced with permission of Elsevier).[35]

Key role for the environment

While the breakthroughs associated with filaggrin gene mutations have been illuminating and helpful in refocusing interest on the outside skin barrier rather than on immune cells within the body, the environment must also play a key role.[31] Thus, it is difficult to find a genetic explanation for the observation that AD is more common in wealthier and more educated families,[15,32] or in smaller families,[33] or in those ethnic groups migrating from a country of low prevalence to a country of high prevalence.[34] The ISAAC study has provided convincing evidence that eczema symptom prevalence has increased substantially over a 5–10 year time span (Figure 1), especially in younger children.[35] Such rapid increases in disease prevalence cannot be explained by genetics, nor can they be explained by our current knowledge of risk factors for AD, such as exposure to allergens. While there is little doubt that allergic factors are important in AD, especially in severe disease, their role has been overemphasized, perhaps because there has been little else, such as filaggrin gene mutations, to look at until recently. The concept that allergic sensitization is a risk factor for AD has been challenged,[10,11] and it is possible that increasing exposure to allergens at a critical time of immune development to induce tolerance may be more fruitful than trying to reduce ubiquitous allergens, such as house dust mite.[36]

Protective effect of infections in early life

The observation that AD is more common in smaller families and in younger rather than older siblings led to the hygiene hypothesis.[37] In other words, AD may become manifest when a developing immune system is deprived of the obligatory stimulation from certain microbial antigens. Such a protective effect on AD development that could be mediated by microbial stimulation is also observed with increased endotoxin exposure, infant day care attendance, consumption of unpasteurized farm milk,[38] and even being raised with a dog during early life.[39] In a recent updated systematic review of the hygiene hypothesis in relation to AD, Flohr and Yeo conclude that the protective effects seen with early day care, endotoxin, unpasteurized farm milk and animal exposure are likely to be due to a general increase in exposure to nonpathogenic microbes, a hypothesis which might also explain the increase in risk of AD by the use of broad-spectrum antibiotics.[40] Loss of exposure to gut helminths may also predispose to more atopy and AD,[41,42] suggesting that increased allergic disease may be one of the prices to pay for the benefits of deworming. The picture is far from clear, and research is now needed to improve understanding of the interaction between genetic factors, such as defective skin barrier, and environmental microbial stimulation at critical times of early life.

Comorbidities

Several studies have evaluated possible disease associations with AD, and most have been inconclusive. Three areas have progressed in the last 10 years. The first is quantifying the risk of subsequent asthma in a child who has AD. A systematic review of 13 cohort studies by van der Hulst and co-workers in 2007 confirmed that although there is an increased risk of developing asthma after AD in early childhood, only one in every three such children developed asthma.[27] This is much lower than previously assumed. Another cohort study, of 1314 German children followed from birth to age 7 years, found a clear association between early AD and asthma at school age.[43] Yet, in many of these asthmatic children, wheezing manifested itself before or with the onset of AD, suggesting a distinct phenotype of early wheezers rather than a progressive development from AD to asthma.[43] There is little doubt about the strong association between asthma and AD, but it may not be a straightforward progression of events, as the simplistic notion of an 'atopic march' suggests.[44]

One systematic review has suggested an inverse relationship between atopic disorders and childhood leukaemia.[45] Another systematic review, of 10 case–control and two cohort studies involving 61,090 patients, suggested that the risk of glioma was substantially reduced in those with asthma, AD and hay fever, with odds ratios of 0.70 (95% confidence interval 0.62–0.79, $P < 0.001$), 0.69 (95% confidence interval 0.62–0.78, $P < 0.001$), and 0.78 (95% confidence interval 0.70–0.87, $P < 0.001$), respectively.[46] Reasons for such a protective effect, although suspected for a long time,[47] remain unclear.

Finally, some interest has been shown in a possible association between attention deficit hyperactivity disorder and AD.[48] As most studies are cross-sectional, it is difficult to say which came first, but it is an area worthy of further study.

Knowledge mapping

Knowing what research has been done and collating reliable evidence in one place has been undertaken by the Centre of Evidence-Based Dermatology at Nottingham.[49] When the Centre was part of the National Electronic Library for Health, annual searches were conducted for new evidence regarding AD in the form of systematic reviews with accompanying detailed critical commentaries on the relevance and reliability of the evidence.[50,51] Every systematic review on AD identified through these annual updates has been mapped into a central resource at the Centre, which is freely available in the public domain.[49] Each systematic review is catalogued under epidemiology (27), prevention (44), topical treatments (68), systemic treatments (47), phototherapy (15), dietary approaches (15), psychological and educational interventions (8), physical therapies (10), complementary and alternative therapies (18) and other interventions (13). Each category is further subdivided into more specific topics; for example, epidemiology is divided into 'risk factors, definition, impact, et cetera', and each review is hyperlinked to the original abstract. The comprehensive mapping of AD systematic reviews is a useful resource for researchers, clinicians and the public, and is currently undergoing a further update, which will be available later in 2012.

For all randomized controlled trials of AD, the Centre has created an international collection called the GREAT (Global Resource of EczemA Trials) database, which is updated annually.[52] This mapping exercise of randomized controlled trials is also free in the public domain.[53]

The purpose behind these mapping exercises is to reduce research wastage, which is a significant problem in human medicine.[54] Research is often undertaken in a vacuum rather than being informed by a systematic review of all relevant studies to date. The creation of an international repository of systematic reviews and randomized controlled trials of AD will hopefully reduce efforts in locating essential evidence and unnecessary duplication of exhaustive searches.

Seven areas of notable ignorance

Is AD more than one disease?

Reference has already been made to the revised nomenclature for eczema, and of its division into 'atopic' (or extrinsic) and 'nonatopic' (or intrinsic or atopiform) eczema.[9] The author is sceptical of the utility of such a division, given that atopy may be a marker of disease severity rather than a distinct phenotype.[10] If true, then it means that studies making claim that intrinsic and extrinsic eczema behave in different ways should ideally measure IgE responsiveness repeatedly over time, or at least adjust for disease severity when making comparisons. Differentiating into those with enhanced barrier defects caused by filaggrin gene defects may make more sense in predicting the natural history of disease.[28] Other patterns of eczema associated with AD in children, such as the discoid (nummular) pattern, may represent aberrant responses to *Staphylococcus aureus* infections. Perhaps there is a distinct form of AD associated with respiratory disease,[43] and other suggestions may emerge as new discoveries are made. The division of AD into subtypes should not occur lightly, but should be preceded by studies that demonstrate that division into subtypes is clinically or scientifically worthwhile, for example by explaining or predicting responsiveness to treatment or suggesting that a particular strategy, such as allergen tolerance or reduction, will be worthwhile in that group.

Looking at the same old risk factors

A search on the epidemiology of AD in April 2012 revealed 2197 studies. While encouraging, many of the identified citations were found not to be true epidemiological studies and those that were tended to be rather similar, with a few notable exceptions. Two patterns seemed to emerge. The first is a 'fishing' expedition type of study that includes less than 1000 children, which finds yet more evidence that only family history of atopic disease is a strong risk factor for AD. The second type of study revisits a well-explored intervention, such as breastfeeding and AD, using the same design and limitations, such as inadequate consideration of confounding, as previous studies, which unsurprisingly comes to the same inconclusive results as others.[55] What is needed is a fresh approach that identifies new areas for research by exploring the interfaces between AD and other areas of medicine. This could entail learning from other chronic relapsing and remitting diseases, or by working with other branches of science that might, at first, appear to have little to do with AD. For example, our previous work with medical geographers showed that AD was more common in geographic regions with hard water.[56] The finding led to a randomized controlled trial of ion-exchange water softeners in AD.[57] Although the trial showed that water softeners were not helpful in AD, the study nevertheless visited a new and plausible hypothesis that may still turn out to be important.

Lack of risk factors that are amenable to manipulation

There is a need to progress from documenting how attributes such as age, sex and social class explain some of the differences in AD prevalence to drilling down into exploring the specific components of such attributes. It is difficult to act on the knowledge that AD seems to improve during adolescence in many children, but if such an observation opens up new insights, such as an association between hormonally induced sebum production in puberty with enhanced skin barrier function, more specific interventions can then be developed to prevent or ameliorate existing disease.

Inconsistencies in the hygiene hypothesis

The author has deliberately mentioned the hygiene hypothesis in the progress and ignorance section. While it has been an exciting hypothesis that has explained some of the epidemiological findings, such as decreased risk of AD in younger siblings, large family size and living on a farm, the topic is far more complex and is studded with inconsistent findings in different countries. The type of microbial or parasitic exposure, the timing of exposure, the intensity of exposure and whether specific or broad exposures are required for disease risk reduction are still unclear.[40]

Sparse knowledge about adult AD

It is not surprising that most epidemiological studies of AD have been done in children because AD is more common in childhood, the effects of the disease may be critical in early life and school children make an easily accessible population for research. However, as Herd *et al.* point out,[58] adults over 16 years still constitute around one-third of the total AD cases in a given community. Such adults often suffer from more severe and chronic disease than children, and the effects of AD on their employment and leisure activities may be considerable. Virtually nothing is known about the epidemiology of AD in adults except that it probably affects at least 3% of adults,[59] and it tends to be persistent.[60] We know little about the validity of diagnostic criteria in adults,[61] the natural history of disease, and whether risk factors for disease persistence are similar to those for childhood AD.

Not enough research on eczema prevention

Although at least 44 systematic reviews relating to AD prevention have been published,[49] a recent overview of seven systematic reviews (covering 39 relevant trials with 11,897 participants) of prevention strategies for AD failed to find any convincing evidence that any were effective in unselected infants.[62] There was some evidence to suggest that exclusive breastfeeding for at least 6 months and prebiotics might reduce eczema incidence in high-risk participants, although the studies supporting these assertions were scant and had methodological shortcomings. Such an absence of evidence cannot be equated as evidence of no effect due to the limitations in design, size and refinement of the intervention, and further studies that evaluate hydrolysed formulae, prebiotics and probiotics, as well as enhancement of the skin barrier are worthwhile.[62]

What causes atopic dermatitis to flare?

Much confusion can arise if those studying AD do not at least consider separating the risk factors for disease occurrence, risk factors for disease flares and risk factors for disease perpetuation, because they may not necessarily be the same. Although textbooks about AD typically cite a long list of factors that may exacerbate established AD, very few of these are based on scientific studies. A previous systematic review of studies that explored factors that may cause eczema flares showed that only four of 28 studies were of a longitudinal design, an arguably essential design in order to separate the temporal relationship between cause and effect.[63] One panel study from Germany suggested (*post hoc*) that there may be a summer and winter type of AD,[64] which was not confirmed in a larger subsequent study.[65] That later study by Langan *et al.* evaluated 60 children aged 1–15 years intensively for up to 9 months using electronic diaries and additional meteorological information. Autoregressive moving average models were used to study the impact of exposures on AD severity for individuals over time. Nylon clothing, dust, unfamiliar pets, sweating and shampoos were shown to play a role in worsening AD in children.[65] Interestingly, the study found that combinations of exposures may be acting in concert. In other words, a putative exacerbating factor, such as dust, may not cause a child's AD to worsen on one day, but it would on another day if that child was also tired and had been sweating. Further work in exploring such a multiple component hypothesis is worthwhile, although the length and intensity of follow-up is challenging. Even defining what is meant by a flare is not straightforward, because it is relative to each individual. Simple definitions, such as escalation of treatment or seeking additional healthcare, may be as good as more numerically exact sounding but clinically meaningless methods.[66]

Reflections

This review has illustrated the considerable progress that has been made over the last 12 years in understanding the epidemiology of human AD. The tree of AD research (Figure 2) is no longer as bent over by the imbalance of basic science as it has been, and basic scientists and epidemiologists are finally discovering the value of working together, as exemplified by the field of skin barrier genes,[26] and exploring the possible role of autoimmunity.[67] This review is not intended to condemn well-intentioned efforts of the past, but to stimulate more research in those areas that need it most, with the ultimate aim of reducing human (and animal) suffering from this common disease. More effort needs to be made into conducting much larger and well-designed studies that focus on testing new and existing clearly defined hypotheses, and such studies need to be much more clearly reported according to STROBE (STrengthening the Reporting of OBservational studies in Epidemiology) criteria so that others can understand exactly what was done and

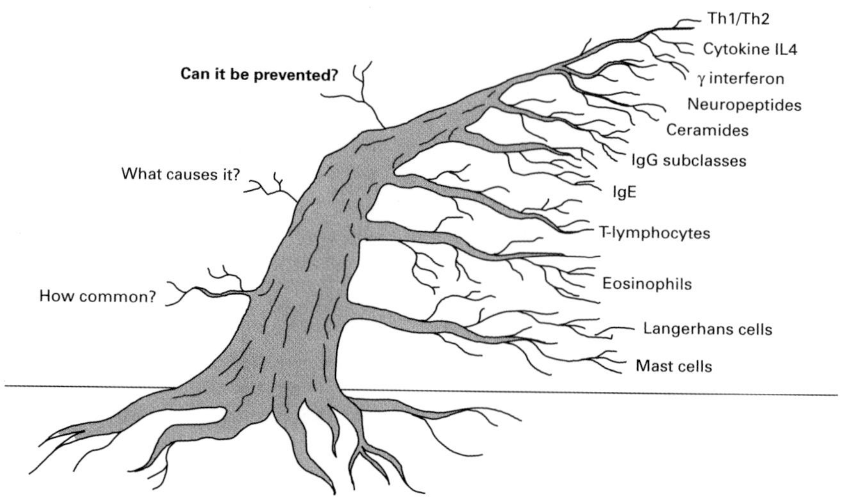

Figure 2. Depiction of how research into atopic dermatitis has been imbalanced by basic science in the past. Abbreviations: AD, atopic dermatitis; IgE, immunoglobulin E; and Th2, T helper 2 (reproduced with permission by Cambridge University Press).[3]

replicate the research if necessary.[68] More international research should be undertaken in order to explore new exposures and the intensity of those exposures that may vary within and across different countries, as has been exemplified by the ISAAC group.[69] Cross-disciplinary research, such as working across the human and small animal divide, may be key in eliciting new ideas about disease causes. Such research is a two-way process. Some ideas, such as skin barrier genes and the role of allergy and gut helminths, are worth exploring in more detail, for example, in canine AD. Some areas in veterinary dermatology, such as *Malassezia* sensitivity and the role of essential fatty acids in canine and feline AD, need revisiting for human AD. And so the constructive dialogue continues....

References

1. Williams HC. Beyond the year 2000: how may epidemiology influence future clinical practice in dermatology? *Clin Dermatol* 2001; 19: 55–58.
2. Williams HC. Epidemiology of atopic dermatitis. *Clin Exp Dermatol* 2000; 25: 522–529.
3. Williams HC. *Atopic Dermatitis. The Epidemiology, Causes and Prevention of Atopic Eczema.* Cambridge: Cambridge University Press, 2000; p. 251.
4. Evidence in Health and Social Care. NHS Evidence. Available at: https://www.evidence.nhs.uk/. Accessed April 11, 2012.
5. Langan S, Williams HC. Clinical features and diagnostic criteria of atopic dermatitis. In: Irvine A, Hoeger P, Yan A eds. *Textbook of Pediatric Dermatology.* 3rd edn. Oxford: Blackwell Publishing Ltd, 2011; 28.1–28.19.
6. Williams HC, Burney PGJ, Hay RJ *et al.* The U.K. Working Party's Diagnostic Criteria for Atopic Dermatitis. I. Derivation of a minimum set of discriminators for atopic dermatitis. *Br J Dermatol* 1994; 131: 383–396.
7. Brenninkmeijer EE, Schram ME, Leeflang MM *et al.* Diagnostic criteria for atopic dermatitis: a systematic review. *Br J Dermatol* 2008; 158: 754–765.
8. Olivry T, International Task Force of Canine Atopic Dermatitis. New diagnostic criteria for canine atopic dermatitis. *Vet Dermatol* 2010; 21: 123–126.
9. Johansson SG, Bieber T, Dahl R *et al.* Revised nomenclature for allergy for global use: Report of the Nomenclature Review Committee of the World Allergy Organization, October 2003. *J Allergy Clin Immunol* 2004; 113: 832–836.
10. Flohr C, Johansson SGO, Wahlgren CF *et al.* How atopic is atopic dermatitis? *J Allergy Clin Immunol* 2004; 114: 150–158.
11. Flohr C, Weiland SK, Weinmayr G *et al.* The role of atopic sensitization in flexural eczema: findings from the International Study of Asthma and Allergies in Childhood (ISAAC) Phase Two. *J Allergy Clin Immunol* 2008; 121: 141–147.
12. Bos JD, Brenninkmeijer EE, Schram ME *et al.* Atopic eczema or atopiform dermatitis. *Exp Dermatol* 2010; 19: 325–331.
13. Williams HC, Robertson CF, Stewart AW *et al.* Worldwide variations in the prevalence of atopic eczema symptoms. *J Allergy Clin Immunol* 1999; 103: 125–138.
14. Odhiambo J, Williams H, Clayton T *et al.* Global variations in prevalence of eczema symptoms in children from ISAAC Phase Three. *J Allergy Clin Immunol* 2009; 124: 1251–1258.
15. Shaw TE, Currie GP, Koudelka CW *et al.* Eczema prevalence in the United States: data from the 2003 National Survey of Children's Health. *J Invest Dermatol* 2011; 131: 67–73.
16. Williams HC. Eczema across the world: the missing piece of the jigsaw revealed. *J Invest Dermatol* 2011; 131: 12–14.
17. Schiffner R, Schiffner-Rohe J, Landthaler M *et al.* Treatment of atopic dermatitis and impact on quality of life: a review with emphasis on topical non-corticosteroids. *Pharmacoeconomics* 2003; 21: 159–179.
18. Chida Y, Hamer M, Steptoe A. A bidirectional relationship between psychosocial factors and atopic disorders: a systematic review and meta-analysis. *Psychosom Med* 2008; 70: 102–116.
19. Meltzer LJ, Moore M. Sleep disruptions in parents of children and adolescents with chronic illnesses: prevalence, causes, and consequences. *J Pediatr Psychol* 2008; 33: 279–291.
20. Mancini AJ, Kaulback K, Chamlin SL. The socioeconomic impact of atopic dermatitis in the United States: a systematic review. *Pediatr Dermatol* 2008; 25: 1–6.
21. Emerson RM, Williams HC, Allen BR *et al.* How much disability does atopic eczema cause compared with other common childhood health problems? *Br J Dermatol* 1997; 137(Suppl 50): 19.
22. Su JC, Kemp AS, Varigos GA *et al.* Atopic eczema: its impact on the family and financial cost. *Arch Dis Child* 1997; 76: 159–162.
23. Schultz Larsen F. The epidemiology of atopic dermatitis. *Monogr Allergy* 1993; 31: 9–28.
24. Cookson WO, Moffatt MF. The genetics of atopic dermatitis. *Curr Opin Allergy Clin Immunol* 2002; 2: 383–387.
25. Brown SJ, McLean WH. One remarkable molecule: filaggrin. *J Invest Dermatol* 2012; 132: 751–762.

26. Baurecht H, Irvine AD, Novak N *et al.* Toward a major risk factor for atopic eczema: meta-analysis of filaggrin polymorphism data. *J Allergy Clin Immunol* 2007; 120: 1406–1412.
27. van der Hulst AE, Klip H, Brand PL. Risk of developing asthma in young children with atopic eczema: a systematic review. *J Allergy Clin Immunol* 2007; 120: 565–569.
28. Rodríguez E, Baurecht H, Herberich E *et al.* Meta-analysis of filaggrin polymorphisms in eczema and asthma: robust risk factors in atopic disease. *J Allergy Clin Immunol* 2009; 123: 1361–1370.
29. Centre of Evidence-Based Dermatology Barrier Enhancement Eczema Prevention (BEEP) Pilot Study. Available at: http://www.nottingham.ac.uk/scs/divisions/evidencebaseddermatology/research/nihrprogrammegrant/barrierenhancementeczemaprevention(beep)feasibilitystudy.aspx. Accessed May 28, 2012.
30. Marsella R, Olivry T, Carlotti DN *et al.*Current evidence of skin barrier dysfunction in human and canine atopic dermatitis. *Vet Dermatol* 2011; 22: 239–248.
31. Williams HC. Atopic eczema. *BMJ* 1995; 311: 1241–1242.
32. Williams HC, Strachan DP, Hay RJ. Childhood eczema: disease of the advantaged? *BMJ* 1994; 308: 1132–1135.
33. Williams HC, Hay RH, Strachan D. Eczema and family size. *J Invest Dermatol* 1992; 98: 601.
34. Burrell-Morris C, Williams HC. Atopic dermatitis in migrant populations. In: Williams HC, ed. *Atopic Dermatitis.* Cambridge: Cambridge University Press, 2000; 169–182.
35. Williams H, Stewart A, von Mutius E *et al.* Is eczema really on the increase worldwide? *J Allergy Clin Immunol* 2008; 121: 947–954.
36. Williams HC. Perspective: acting on the evidence. *Nature* 2011; 479: S16.
37. Strachan DP. Hay fever, hygiene, and household size. *BMJ* 1989; 299: 1259–1260.
38. Flohr C, Pascoe D, Williams HC. Atopic dermatitis and the 'hygiene hypothesis': too clean to be true? *Br J Dermatol* 2005; 152: 202–216.
39. Langan S, Flohr C, Williams HC. The role of furry pets in eczema: a systematic review. *Arch Dermatol* 2007; 143: 1570–1577.
40. Flohr C, Yeo L. Atopic dermatitis and the hygiene hypothesis revisited. *Curr Probl Dermatol* 2011; 41: 1–34.
41. Flohr C, Tuyen LN, Quinnell RJ *et al.* Reduced helminth burden increases allergen skin sensitization but not clinical allergy: a randomized, double-blind, placebo-controlled trial in Vietnam. *Clin Exp Allergy* 2010; 40: 131–142.
42. Mpairwe H, Webb EL, Muhangi L *et al.* Anthelminthic treatment during pregnancy is associated with increased risk of infantile eczema: randomised-controlled trial results. *Pediatr Allergy Immunol* 2011; 22: 305–312.
43. Illi S, von Mutius E, Lau S *et al.* The natural course of atopic dermatitis from birth to age 7 years and the association with asthma. *J Allergy Clin Immunol* 2004; 113: 925–931.
44. Williams H, Flohr C. How epidemiology has challenged 3 prevailing concepts about atopic dermatitis. *J Allergy Clin Immunol* 2006; 118: 209–213.
45. Linabery AM, Jurek AM, Duval S *et al.* The association between atopy and childhood/adolescent leukemia: a meta-analysis. *Am J Epidemiol* 2010; 171: 749–764.
46. Chen C, Xu T, Chen J *et al.* Allergy and risk of glioma: a meta-analysis. *Eur J Neurol* 2011; 18: 387–395.
47. Wang H, Diepgen TL. Is atopy a protective or a risk factor for cancer? A review of epidemiological studies *Allergy* 2005; 60: 1098–1111.
48. Schmitt J, Buske-Kirschbaum A, Roessner V. Is atopic disease a risk factor for attention-deficit/hyperactivity disorder? A systematic review *Allergy* 2010; 65: 1506–1524.
49. Centre of Evidence-Based Dermatology website. Maps of systematic review on atopic eczema. Available at: http://www.nottingham.ac.uk/scs/documents/documentsdivisions/documentsdermatology/methodologicalresources/mapsofsystematicreview sonatopiceczema.pdf. Accessed April 16, 2012.
50. Centre of Evidence-Based Dermatology website, Batchelor J, Williams HC. "What's new?" — a tour of the 2009 Annual Evidence Update on Atopic Eczema with the busy clinician in mind. Available at: http://www.nottingham.ac.uk/scs/documents/documentsdivisions/documentsdermatology/methodologicalresources/2009-annual-evidence-update-on-atopic-eczema.pdf. Accessed April 16, 2012.
51. Centre of Evidence-Based Dermatology website, Shams K, Williams HC. "What's new?" — a tour of the 2010 Annual Evidence Update on Atopic Eczema with the busy clinician in mind. Available at: http://www.nottingham.ac.uk/scs/documents/documentsdivisions/documentsdermatology/methodologicalresources/2010-annual-evidence-update-on-atopic-eczema.pdf. Accessed April 17, 2012.
52. Nankervis H, Maplethorpe A, Williams HC. Mapping randomised controlled trials of treatments for eczema - The GREAT database (the Global Resource of EczemA Trials: a collection of key data on randomized controlled trials of treatments for eczema from 2000 to 2010). *BMC Dermatol* 2011; 11: 10.
53. Centre of Evidence-Based Dermatology website, Nankervis H, Williams HC. Global Resource of Eczema Trials. GREAT Database. 2000–2011.Centre of Evidence-Based Dermatology, University of Nottingham. Available at: http://www.greatdatabase.org.uk/. Accessed April 16, 2012.
54. Chalmers I, Glasziou P. Avoidable waste in the production and reporting of research evidence. *Lancet* 2009; 374: 86–89.
55. Yang YW, Tsai CL, Lu CY. Exclusive breastfeeding and incident atopic dermatitis in childhood: a systematic review and meta-analysis of prospective cohort studies. *Br J Dermatol* 2009; 161: 373–383.
56. McNally NJ, Williams HC, Phillips DR *et al.* Atopic eczema and domestic water hardness. *Lancet* 1998; 352: 527–531.
57. Thomas K, Koller K, Dean T *et al.* A multicentre randomised controlled trial and economic evaluation of ion-exchange water softeners for the treatment of eczema in children: the Softened Water Eczema Trial (SWET). *Health Technol Assess* 2011; 15: 1–156.
58. Herd RM, Tidman MJ, Prescott RJ *et al.* Prevalence of atopic eczema in the community: the Lothian atopic dermatitis study. *Br J Dermatol* 1996; 135: 18–19.
59. Muto T, Hsieh SD, Sakurai Y *et al.* Prevalence of atopic dermatitis in Japanese adults. *Br J Dermatol* 2003; 148: 117–121.
60. Sandström Falk MH, Faergemann J. Atopic dermatitis in adults: does it disappear with age? *Acta Derm Venereol* 2006; 86: 135–139.
61. Lan CC, Lee CH, Lu YW *et al.* Prevalence of adult atopic dermatitis among nursing staff in a Taiwanese medical center: a pilot study on validation of diagnostic questionnaires. *J Am Acad Dermatol* 2009; 61: 806–812.
62. Foisy M, Boyle RJ, Chalmers JR *et al.* The prevention of eczema in infants and children: an overview of Cochrane and non-Cochrane reviews. *Evid Based Child Health* 2011; 6: 1322–1339.
63. Langan SM, Williams HC. What causes worsening of eczema? A systematic review *Br J Dermatol* 2006; 155: 504–514.
64. Krämer U, Weidinger S, Darsow U *et al.* Seasonality in symptom severity influenced by temperature or grass pollen: results of a panel study in children with eczema. *J Invest Dermatol* 2005; 124: 514–523.
65. Langan S, Silcocks P, Williams HC. What causes flares of eczema in children? *Br J Dermatol* 2009; 161: 640–646.
66. Langan SM, Thomas K, Williams HC. What is meant by a "flare" in atopic dermatitis? A systematic review and proposal *Arch Dermatol* 2006; 142: 1190–1196.
67. Tang TS, Bieber T, Williams HC. Does "autoreactivity" play a role in eczema? - a systematic review *J Allergy Clin Immunol* 2012; 129: 1209–1215.
68. Langan SM, Schmitt J, Coenraads PJ *et al.* STROBE and reporting observational studies in dermatology. *Br J Dermatol* 2011; 164: 1–3.
69. Beasley R, Clayton T, Crane J *et al.* Association between paracetamol use in infancy and childhood, and risk of asthma, rhinoconjunctivitis, and eczema in children aged 6–7 years: analysis from Phase Three of the ISAAC programme. *Lancet* 2008; 372: 1039–1048.

To cite this article, please use DOI: 10.1111/j.1365-3164.2012.01094.x

1.2

The genomics revolution: will canine atopic dermatitis be predictable and preventable?

Tim Nuttall

The University of Liverpool School of Veterinary Science, Leahurst Campus, Neston, UK

Correspondence: Tim Nuttall, The University of Liverpool School of Veterinary Science, Leahurst Campus, Chester High Road, Neston, Cheshire CH64 7TE, UK. E-mail: timn@liv.ac.uk

Background – Heritability studies suggest that atopic dermatitis (AD) involves multiple genes and interactions with environmental factors. Advances in genomics have given us powerful techniques to study the genetics of AD.

Objective – To review the application of these techniques to canine AD.

Results – Candidate genes can be studied using quantitative PCR and genomic techniques, but these are hypothesis-dependent techniques and may miss novel genes. Hypothesis-free techniques avoid this limitation. Microarrays quantify expression of large numbers of genes, although false-positive associations are common. In the future, expression profiling could be used to produce a complete tissue transcriptome. Genome-wide linkage studies can detect AD-associated loci if enough affected dogs and unaffected relatives are recruited. Genome-wide association studies can be used to discover AD-associated single nucleotide polymorphisms without relying on related dogs. Genomic studies in dogs have implicated numerous genes in the pathogenesis of AD, including those involved in innate and adaptive immunity, inflammation, cell cycle, apoptosis, skin barrier formation and transcription regulation. These findings, however, have been inconsistent, and problems include low case numbers, inappropriate controls, inconsistent diagnosis, incomplete genome coverage, low-penetrance mutations and environmental factors.

Conclusions – Canine AD has a complex genotype that varies between breeds and gene pools. Breeding programmes to eliminate AD are therefore unlikely to succeed, but this complexity could explain variations in clinical phenotype and response to treatment. Genotyping of affected dogs will identify novel target molecules and enable better targeting of treatment and management options. However, we must avoid misuse of genomic data.

Introduction

Human and canine AD

Canine atopic dermatitis (AD) is very similar to human AD;[1–4] both are inflammatory dermatoses with characteristic clinical features. They are complex diseases involving immune dysregulation, allergic sensitization, skin barrier defects, microbial colonization and environmental factors. Human and canine AD are very common conditions, affecting up to one-third of children in Western societies and 10% of all dogs.[1,5–8]

It's in the genes

Both the human and canine conditions have a genetic component. Family history is a major risk factor for human AD.[1–3] Strong breed predispositions, with high prevalences in some dog breeds (e.g. up to 25% in West Highland white terrier dogs), suggest that this is also true in canine AD.[9–11] In British guide dogs (mostly Labrador and golden retriever cross-bred dogs) the mean heritability is 0.47 (range 0.13–0.81), suggesting that the genetic background accounts for almost 50% of the risk of developing AD.[12] Experimental laboratory colonies of dogs with conditions that mimic clinical AD have also been established.[4,13–15]

It's not all genetic – environmental factors in AD

The risk of developing AD, the severity and the response to treatment are highly variable. This may be explained by complex genotypes, but it is also likely that environmental influences are important.[8] Environmental factors that influence the development of canine AD are listed in Table 1.[10,16,17] These may be important in immunity, tolerance and skin barrier function. The environmental influence, however, appears to vary with breed; for example, these factors do not affect the prevalence of AD in West Highland white terrier dogs.

Genetic studies in AD

Historically, studies have been limited to observations of breed predispositions, as well as heritability and linkage studies. Advances in genomics now allow us to study the genetics of AD in more detail. The aim of this paper is to review these techniques, the current evidence for the genetic basis of canine AD and future opportunities.

Accepted 28 June 2012

Sources of Funding: This study was self-funded.

Conflict of Interest: No conflicts of interest have been declared.

Table 1. Environmental factors that influence the development of canine atopic dermatitis

Risk of developing atopic dermatitis	Environmental factor
Increased	Urban life
	High human population density
	Increased average annual rainfall
	Living in southern Sweden
	Adoption at the age of 8–12 weeks
	Regular bathing
Reduced	Rural life
	Living with other animals
	Walking in forests
	Feeding noncommercial foods to lactating bitches
No effect	Sex
	Season of birth
	Home environment
	Vaccination
	Deworming

Investigating AD-associated genotypes

Genome-wide linkage studies

Genome-wide linkage studies have been widely used to investigate human AD.[8] These are family-based approaches using affected individuals, their parents and nonaffected family members. The inheritance of the disease is compared with the inheritance of microsatellite markers.

This technique can evaluate the whole genome, avoiding the limitations of candidate gene approaches. Microsatellite markers have been used to identify chromosomal loci associated with human AD.[8] However, the usefulness of this approach has been questioned, because there has been little overlap in the results from these studies. The linked loci extend over large areas of each chromosome, spanning several genes and making it difficult to identify a candidate gene without either extensive chromosomal sequencing or further genotyping of additional microsatellite markers clustered around the loci of interest. It is difficult, furthermore, to amass enough affected individuals and unaffected relatives to perform genome-wide linkage studies in dogs.

Candidate gene association studies

It is possible to genotype markers specifically associated with candidate genes of interest. This allows the use of relatively simple markers, such as single nucleotide polymorphisms (SNPs), insertions, deletions and repeats. In addition, candidate gene approaches are not limited to families, making it easier to recruit large numbers of affected individuals and control subjects.[8] However, case–control studies can be confounded by population stratification effects, such as ethnicity or breed and geography. A major disadvantage of this approach is that it is hypothesis dependent in that the genetic analysis is restricted to genes that have been previously implicated in the pathogenesis of AD. Novel genes may therefore be missed.

Genome-wide association studies

Genome-wide association studies (GWASs) are a hypothesis-free way to discover disease-associated SNPs.[8] This avoids the limitations of using candidate genes, while retaining the advantages of the case–control approach. Genome sequencing has identified large numbers of genetic variants that can be read on SNP arrays. This allows identification of SNPs that are more frequent in affected individuals than control subjects. These disease-associated SNPs mark regions of the genome that may be involved in the pathogenesis of AD (Figure 1). Depending on the number and distribution of SNPs, GWASs can interrogate the entire genome. However, fine mapping relies on having many SNPs evenly distributed throughout the genome. In addition, disease-associated SNPs may be located in unknown areas of the genome. Further sequencing and functional studies are therefore required to confirm whether the disease association is causal. The functional effects, moreover, may depend on the specific combinations of SNPs within a gene and/or interactions with SNPs in other genes, or both. Another weakness of this approach is that GWASs are limited to identifying common SNPs with small effects. They cannot identify rare SNPs with large effects, untyped SNPs and some structural variations, e.g. microsatellites, variable number tandem repeats, insertions, deletions and duplications.

Genome-wide association studies in dogs can take advantage of their strong linkage disequilibrium (LD). In humans, LD is relatively weak (extending over about 10–100 kbp), necessitating high-density arrays (up to 1.6×10^6 SNPs) and large cohorts (at least 1000 cases and controls).[18] Dog breeds are of recent origin and are highly inbred, with LD over long distances (0.8–5 Mbp),[19,20] meaning that fewer genetic markers and smaller sample sizes can be used. For example, complete coverage of the canine genome requires only 5000 to 30,000 SNPs.[21] However, low numbers of SNPs can result in incomplete coverage that could miss important genes. For example, the first GWAS in canine AD[22] used the Illumina Canine SNP20 chip (San Diego, CA, USA). This includes 22,362 canine SNPs from the CanFam2.0 assembly based on the boxer dog, with the partial sequence of a standard poodle dog and 100,000 sequence reads from nine other breeds. Despite this, many genes of interest (e.g. filaggrin) were not included. These gaps should be covered by continued development of the Dog Genome Project.

Quantitative RT-PCR

Quantification of mRNA can be performed in any tissue to identify genes that are differentially regulated in affected individuals compared with control subjects. Microarrays can be used for hypothesis-free assessment of very large numbers of genes on single chips.[23] Gene transcription, however, does not necessarily imply causality; the change may be secondary to the disease process. Despite this, gene expression studies are useful to identify candidate genes and to confirm involvement of genes associated with AD in genomic studies. Genome-wide microarrays can produce a hypothesis-free transcriptome of all known genes in any tissue, but the high cost and complex results are barriers to widespread use at present.[8]

Bias and false results

Genomic studies are prone to bias and error that reduce the power of the analyses and affect replication of the

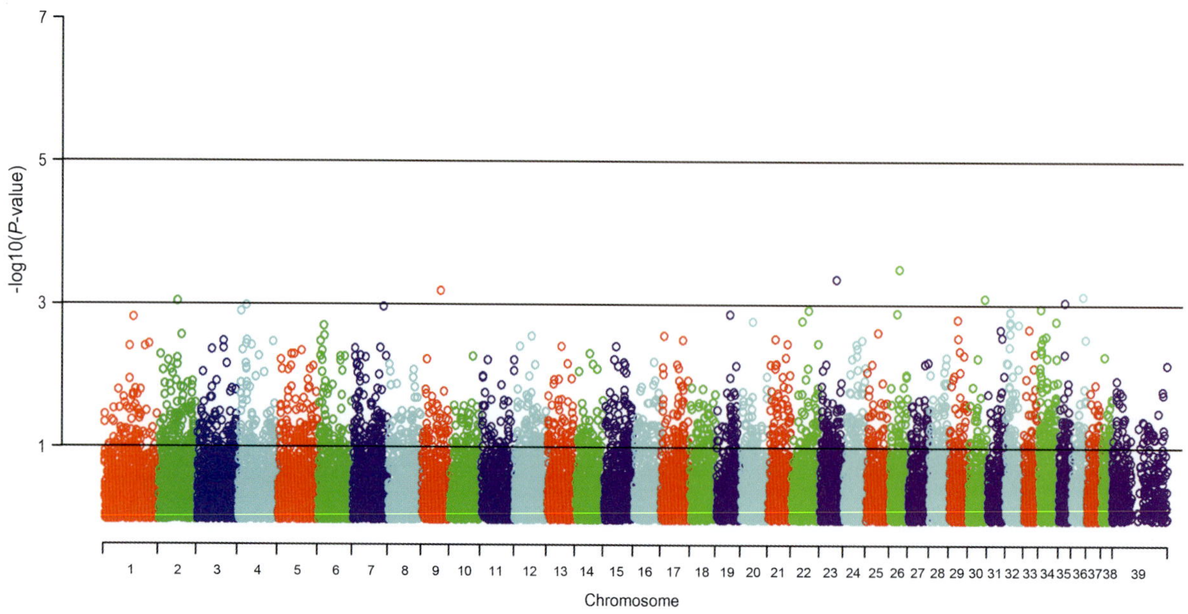

Figure 1. Whole-genome association plot of significance for canine atopic dermatitis (AD) (after Wood *et al.* with permission of Springer Science+Business Media).[22] This study used a chip with approximately 22,000 single nucleotide polymorphisms (SNPs) to study SNP frequency in atopic dogs and healthy control dogs. The SNPs are plotted on the *x*-axis according to their position on each chromosome, with their association with AD on the *y*-axis shown as $\log_{10}$ *P*-value. The circles represent individual SNPs, which are grouped by chromosome. The SNPs that are statistically more frequent in the atopic population identify potentially AD-associated genes or loci for further studies.

results. Accurate phenotyping is critical, because any variation will have a profound impact on determining associations with AD. Other issues include failing to account for population stratification in case–control studies. Studies with relatively low numbers of cases are vulnerable to type II (i.e. false-negative) errors. Type I (i.e. false-positive) errors can occur following multiple testing unless corrections are used to reduce the false discovery rate. In addition, the effects of nonrandom mating, mutations, selection, small population effects, genetic drift etc. mean that canine populations may not be in be Hardy–Weinberg equilibrium (i.e. allele and genotype frequencies in a population remain in equilibrium).

Genomic studies in canine AD

Atopic dermatitis is a complex disease

Observations of atopic West Highland white terriers indicated that the inheritance patterns were consistent with a common fully penetrant dominant or recessive major locus.[24–26] However, studies in other breeds suggest that canine AD is a multifactorial and polygenic condition with a complex mode of inheritance.[4,12,15,27] Genomic studies in dogs have now implicated numerous genes in the pathogenesis of canine AD (Table 2), although whether these are associated with cause or effect is not always clear. These include genes involved in innate and adaptive immunity, inflammation, cell cycle, apoptosis, skin barrier formation and transcription regulation, many of which have also been implicated in human AD.

Microarray studies

An initial paper reported that 54 of 22,000 genes (Agilent 22K oligonucleotide canine array; Agilent Technologies, Palo Alto, CA, USA) showed significantly different transcription in canine AD compared with control dogs (Table 2).[23] The genes were broadly grouped into inflammation/immunity, cell cycle/apoptosis/repair, barrier formation, transport/regulation and transcription pathways. Most of the inflammation or immunology markers were upregulated in atopic, particularly lesional, skin. Other genes were generally underexpressed, especially in nonlesional atopic skin. A large number of these downregulated genes are involved in the transport of calcium, potassium and other ions which may affect expression and function of other mediators involved in inflammation and barrier function. The most dysregulated gene was S100 calcium binding protein A8 (S100A8). This is an important pro-inflammatory molecule located on the epidermal differentiation complex. Interestingly, a recent paper correlated S100A8 expression with the clinical severity of canine AD.[28] Release is stimulated by tumour necrosis factor-α, the levels of which also correlate with clinical severity.[29] The epidermal differentiation complex comprises genes for proteins such as profilaggrin, loricrin, involucrin and S100, which are essential for keratinocyte and epidermal barrier differentiation.[30] These genes were not available on the canine microarray and GWAS chips used in earlier studies,[22,23] and since these studies canine and human AD have been associated with loss-of-function filaggrin mutations and altered filaggrin expression.[31–34]

This microarray study[23] provided a rapid, wide-ranging assessment of many genes and identified novel targets and pathways for further investigation; however, it was limited by the omission of key epidermal barrier and inflammatory cytokine genes. In addition, the study used a relative low number of dogs, which reduced its power to detect small changes. Using multiple breeds may have also confounded the results and reduced the power of the study.

Table 2. Genes that have been implicated in canine atopic dermatitis by candidate gene quantitative PCR (qPCR), microarray, genome-wide linkage studies (GWLS), candidate gene single nucleotide polymorphism (SNP) studies or genome-wide association studies (GWAS)

Gene	Study	Potential relevance to canine atopic dermatitis
Inflammation or immunology		
S100A8	Microarray[23] GWLS[26] qPCR[35]	Pro-inflammatory; correlated with clinical severity
INPPL1	Microarray[23] qPCR[35] SNP[38]	Affects allergen-specific IgE responses, allergen presentation and uptake, T-cell activation and inflammatory responses
SCCA-2	Microarray[23]	Serine protease inhibitor; marker for squamous cell carcinoma
SAA	Microarray[23]	Expressed in response to inflammatory stimuli
SAA3	Microarray[23]	
Serum amyloid A protein (*Canis familiaris*)	Microarray[23]	
TIMP1	Microarray[23] qPCR[35]	Tissue inhibitor of metalloproteinase 1; promotes cell proliferation; anti-apoptosis
ARTS-1	Microarray[23]	Cytokine receptor regulation; antigen presentation
C10orf118	Microarray[23]	Unknown
IL1RAPL1	Microarray[23]	Synthesis of pro-inflammatory proteins
DPP4	qPCR[35] SNP[38]	Regulation of inflammation; interacts with tumour necrosis factor-α and tissue inhibitor of metalloproteases 1 (TIMP1)
PKP2	qPCR[35]	Upregulates T-cell activity and survival
TNF	qPCR[35]	Pro-inflammatory; tumour necrosis factor-α correlates with clinical severity
PTPN22	GWAS[25]	Regulation of B- and T-cell receptor signalling; regulation of innate immune response; regulation of natural killer cell proliferation; associated with immune-mediated disorders
TSLP-receptor	SNP[38]	Cytokine gene transcription; implicated in allergic inflammation
MS4A2	SNP[38]	High-affinity IgE receptor β subunit
CD83	GWAS[40]	Antigen presentation and humoral immunity
CMA1	GWAS[22]	Mast cell chymase
NOD1	GWAS[22]	Intracellular microbial pattern recognition receptor; innate and adaptive immunity
SELP (P-selectin)	GWAS[22]	Leukocyte recruitment
Cell cycle, apoptosis, repair or lesion formation		
RAD50 homologue isoform 1	Microarray[23]	Unknown
POSTN	Microarray[23]	Epithelial cell adhesion and migration
POSTN	qPCR[35]	
CIDE-3	Microarray[23]	Apoptosis and cell proliferation
SDC1 (syndecan 1)	Microarray[23]	Integral membrane protein; involved in cell binding, cell signalling, cytoskeleton organization, cell proliferation, cell migration and cell–matrix interaction
Cadherin-13	Microarray[23]	Cell signalling; cell migration and differentiation
Cullin 4A	Microarray[23] qPCR[35]	Cell cycle regulation and development; DNA repair
DCLRE1B	GWAS[25]	Unknown
BCL2L15 (BCL2-like 15)	GWAS[25]	Regulation of apoptosis and tolerance
ANGPTL4	GWAS[22]	Skin wound healing; keratinocyte migration, endothelial apoptosis survival factor
Transport or regulation		
Kinectin 1	Microarray[23]	Unknown
Myosin Va	Microarray[23]	Unknown
A-kinase anchor protein 9 isoform 2	Microarray[23]	Unknown
Sperm-associated antigen 5	Microarray[23]	Unknown
Canis familiaris ret proto-oncogene	Microarray[23]	Unknown
Nucleoprotein TPR	Microarray[23]	Unknown
Phospholipase C, zeta 1	Microarray[23]	Unknown
Potassium channel tetramerization	Microarray[23]	Unknown
FERM, RhoGEF, pleckstrin domain protein 2	Microarray[23]	Unknown
ATP-binding cassette C12e	Microarray[23]	Unknown
SFXN5 sideroflexin 5	GWAS[25]	Unknown
EXOC6B exocyst complex component 6B	GWAS[25]	Exocytosis
AP4B1	GWAS[25]	Endocytosis and secretion
ABCC3	GWAS[22]	Protein transport; drug efflux
Barrier formation		
GOLGA4 subfamily a5 **GOLGA4 subfamily a4**	Microarray[23]	Golgi body function; glycosylation and transport of proteins and lipids
SPINK5	qPCR[35]	Regulates proteolysis and keratinocyte differentiation; filaggrin function; T helper-2 polarization

Table 2. *(continued)*

Gene	Study	Potential relevance to canine atopic dermatitis
SGPL1	qPCR[35]	Skin barrier regulation; antimicrobial activity; keratinocyte proliferation and differentiation
Mucin-15	Microarray[23]	Cell adhesion to matrix
Mucin-2	Microarray[23]	Mucosal mucin protection
Tight junction protein 3	Microarray[23]	Signal transduction; cell adhesion
PPAR gamma	qPCR[35]	Reduced lamellar body formation and lipid processing; anti-inflammatory
FLG (Filaggrin)	SNP[38]	Alterations in filaggrin expression and function associated with human and canine atopic dermatitis
RAB3C	GWAS[22]	Implicated in epidermal lipid layer and skin barrier formation
Transcription and translation regulation		
eIF-5B	Microarray[23]	Unknown
STAT2	Microarray[23]	Cell growth, survival and differentiation; inflammation and immunity; interferon-γ regulation; tolerance
CGGBP1 (CGG repeat binding protein 1)	Microarray[23]	Unknown
FUSE binding protein 2	Microarray[23]	Unknown
FOXO4 (foxhead box)	Microarray[23]	Cell metabolism and proliferation; tolerance
Empty spiracles homologue 1	GWAS[25]	Unknown
ZNF638 zinc finger protein 638	GWAS[25]	Unknown
PAIP2B	GWAS[25]	Unknown
PHTF1	GWAS[25]	Unknown
HIPK1	GWAS[25]	Unknown
TRIM33	GWAS[25]	Regulation of transforming growth factor-β receptor signalling
Miscellaneous		
EEA1	Microarray[23]	Unknown
CG15747-PA	Microarray[23]	Unknown
HIF1a (Hypoxia-induced gene 1a)	Microarray[23]	Unknown
C6orf142	Microarray[23]	Unknown
Sushi-repeat-containing protein SRPX	Microarray[23]	Antioxidant; cytokine regulation
RING-H2 protein	Microarray[23]	Unknown
ATRX1	Microarray[23]	Unknown
C1orf163	Microarray[23]	Unknown
FBXL10	Microarray[23]	Unknown
FOLH1	Microarray[23]	Unknown
S6K-alpha 6	Microarray[23]	Serine kinase; cell growth and differentiation
mSin3A-associated protein 130	Microarray[23]	Unknown
PH domain leucine-rich repeat protein phosphatase-like	Microarray[23]	Inhibitor of kinases and growth factor-induced signalling
Spag6	Microarray[23]	Unknown
Ecotropic viral integration site 1	Microarray[23]	Unknown
SPR sepiapterin reductase	GWAS[25]	Unknown
Cytochrome P450 26B1	GWAS[25]	Lipid metabolism and barrier function; cytochrome P450 activity
DYSF dysferlin	GWAS[25]	Unknown
NAGK *N*-acetylglucosamine kinase	GWAS[25]	Unknown
RSBN1L	GWAS[25]	Unknown
OLFML3	GWAS[25]	Unknown
SYT6 synaptotagmin VI	GWAS[25]	Endocytosis; cell adhesion
PROM1	GWAS[22]	Unknown
RAB7A	GWAS[22]	Melanocyte function and melanogenesis
SORCS2	GWAS[22]	Neuropeptide receptor activity

The bold and italic refers to genes that were differentially expressed in atopic skin compared with healthy control dogs; bold, upregulated and italic, downregulated.

Candidate gene studies

One study using atopic and healthy skin quantified mRNA for 20 genes identified from the microarray study[23] and/or earlier literature.[35] Significant differences were seen for 11 genes, involving immune responses, regulation and skin barrier function. Seven of these have been associated with human AD. S100A8 was again the most dysregulated gene. Three genes correlated with Canine Atopic Dermatitis Extent and Severity Index (CADESI)-03 scores (S100A8, SAA-1 and PKP2), and four genes correlated with intradermal test results (CMA1, SAA-1, SPINK5 and S100A8); these have been associated with inflammation, T-cell survival and skin barrier function.[28,36,37] Weaknesses of this study included the relatively small sample size, use of multiple dog breeds and the variable time scale of the lesions at presentation.

Analysis of 97 SNPs in 25 candidate genes in 659 dogs of eight breeds from the UK, USA and Japan found that six were significantly associated with canine AD.[38] A SNP in the thymic stromal lymphopoietin (TSLP)-receptor, which has been implicated in allergic inflammation,[39] was seen in all eight breeds. Other canine AD-associated

SNPs, however, were restricted to certain dog breeds and locations (e.g. filaggrin with UK Labrador retriever, and INPPL1 and MS4A2 with Japanese shiba inu).

A linkage study in West Highland white terrier dogs[24] used specific microsatellite markers for fine mapping of the *FLG* locus. There were, however, no haplotypes that associated significantly with canine AD. This makes a primary role for filaggrin defects in AD in these dogs unlikely, although this has been implicated in other breeds.[31–33]

Genome-wide linkage studies

A genome-wide family-based linkage approach using microsatellites [256 markers from the Minimal Screening Set 2 (MSS-2) that covered the genome with an average intermarker distance of 8.59 cM] in 90 West Highland white terrier dogs from families with AD did not detect any chromosomal regions that were significantly linked to canine AD.[26] However, some chromosomal regions were not covered at high density, reducing the power of this study. The highest linkage score was for a region on CFA7 that contains the S100A8 gene, which has been associated with canine AD.[23,28,35] This study excluded linkage to the *FLG* locus, corroborating the results of other reports.[24,38,40] This suggests that primary defects in filaggrin expression are not important in the pathogenesis of canine AD in West Highland white terrier dogs.

Genome-wide association studies

The first GWAS in canine AD[22] evaluated DNA from 242 atopic and 417 control dogs of eight breeds from the UK, US and Japan. The top 40 SNPs were selected for validation (Figure 2). Nine chromosomes expressed multiple SNPs, suggesting a haplotype effect. Subsequent quantitative PCR with quality assurance testing and corrections for the false discovery rate and population structure revealed that 13 SNPs had a significant association with canine AD; however, a number were intergenic, with unknown functions and interactions.

Two independent intergenic SNPs were linked with canine AD in all eight breeds; rs22114085 (CFA10) was associated with susceptibility, while rs23472497 (CFA29) was protective. These may represent novel loci for sequencing and fine mapping.[22] There was a lack of interbreed correspondence between the AD-associated SNPs, suggesting that the atopic genotype varies among breeds. However, the numbers of each individual breed in this study were relatively low, which reduced the statistical power. Furthermore, the relevance of the intergenic SNPs is unclear, and fine mapping of these areas on the genome is required.

Some breed-specific gene-associated SNPs were identified. AD in golden retriever dogs was associated with SNPs in RAB3C (rs22859255) and PROM1 (rs23602938). This RAB3C SNP also formed a significant haplotype with another RAB3C SNP (rs22784610). Atopic Labrador retriever dogs and West Highland white terrier dogs from the UK showed associations with a SNP within RAB7A (rs22915894), as well as the intergenic SNP rs8806978, which is downstream of RAB7A. German Shepherd dogs from the UK showed an association with SORCS2. Significant associations were, however, variable between breeds and within breeds from different geographical locations. However, the fact that a SNP is associated with AD in one breed, but not another, does not necessarily mean that the SNP is not a risk factor for canine AD, because a SNP may have different levels of penetrance in different breeds.[41] However, breed variation in genotype may explain breed-specific phenotypes in canine AD.[9]

A further GWAS was performed on 35 atopic and 25 nonatopic West Highland white terrier dogs using an Affymetrix Canine SNP V2 array with approximately 42,800 SNPs.[25] This reported significant association with a locus on CFA17. Nineteen genes less than 0.5 Mbp from this region were identified. Two other main linkage peaks for canine AD were also found on CFA6 and CFA9. These candidate genes covered a range of functions, including innate and adaptive immunity, skin barrier function, and transcription and regulation. Another GWAS using this array found a significant association between serum *Dermatophagoides farinae*-specific IgE levels in West Highland white terriers and a 2.3 Mbp area on CFA35.[40] CD83, a gene closely associated with this region, is important in antigen presentation and humoral immunity. Sequencing detected an intronic polymorphic repeat sequence, but this did not explain the GWAS association in these dogs.

Finally, a very recent GWAS used allergen-specific immunoglobulin levels (IgE, IgG1 and IgG4 specific for *D. farinae*, and IgE specific for *Dermatophagoides pteronyssinus*, *Tyrophagus putrescentiae*, *Lepidoglyphus destructor*, *Acarus siro*, *Alternaria alternata*, *Cladosporium herbarum*, *Aspergillus fumigatus*, *Penicillinum*, cat epithelium, flea saliva and *Blatella germanica*) as phenotypic markers for AD in Labrador retriever dogs.[42] The GWAS analysed 113,021 SNPs in 135 affected dogs and 24 control animals, with correction for false discovery rate, population stratification and relatedness. The 27 most associated SNPs were clustered on CFA5 from 79.0 to 82.5 Mbp, with the 28th SNP on CFA37. However, only two of the SNPs on CFA5 were significantly associated with *A. siro*-specific serum IgE levels (BICF2S2297212 and BICF2P1022237). A further SNP on CFA5 (BICF2G630182288) was significantly associated with *T. putrescentiae*-specific serum IgE levels. No genes involved in IgE regulation are known to reside in this area on CFA5 or its human equivalent. These results may therefore indicate the presence of a novel gene, and these loci warrant further investigation and fine mapping. However, the relevance of *Acarus*- and *Tyrophagus*-specific serum IgE in the pathogenesis of canine AD is unclear,[43,44] and the use of surrogate markers such as serum IgE levels will identify only a subset of atopic dogs.

Conclusions

These studies have greatly improved our understanding of canine AD. Despite this, the genetic background for canine AD is still far from clear. There has been little correlation between the studies published so far. This variation could be due to the complexity of the genotype, although it is also likely to reflect environmental factors, phenotypic differences between dogs in the studies, different study techniques, mutations with low pene-

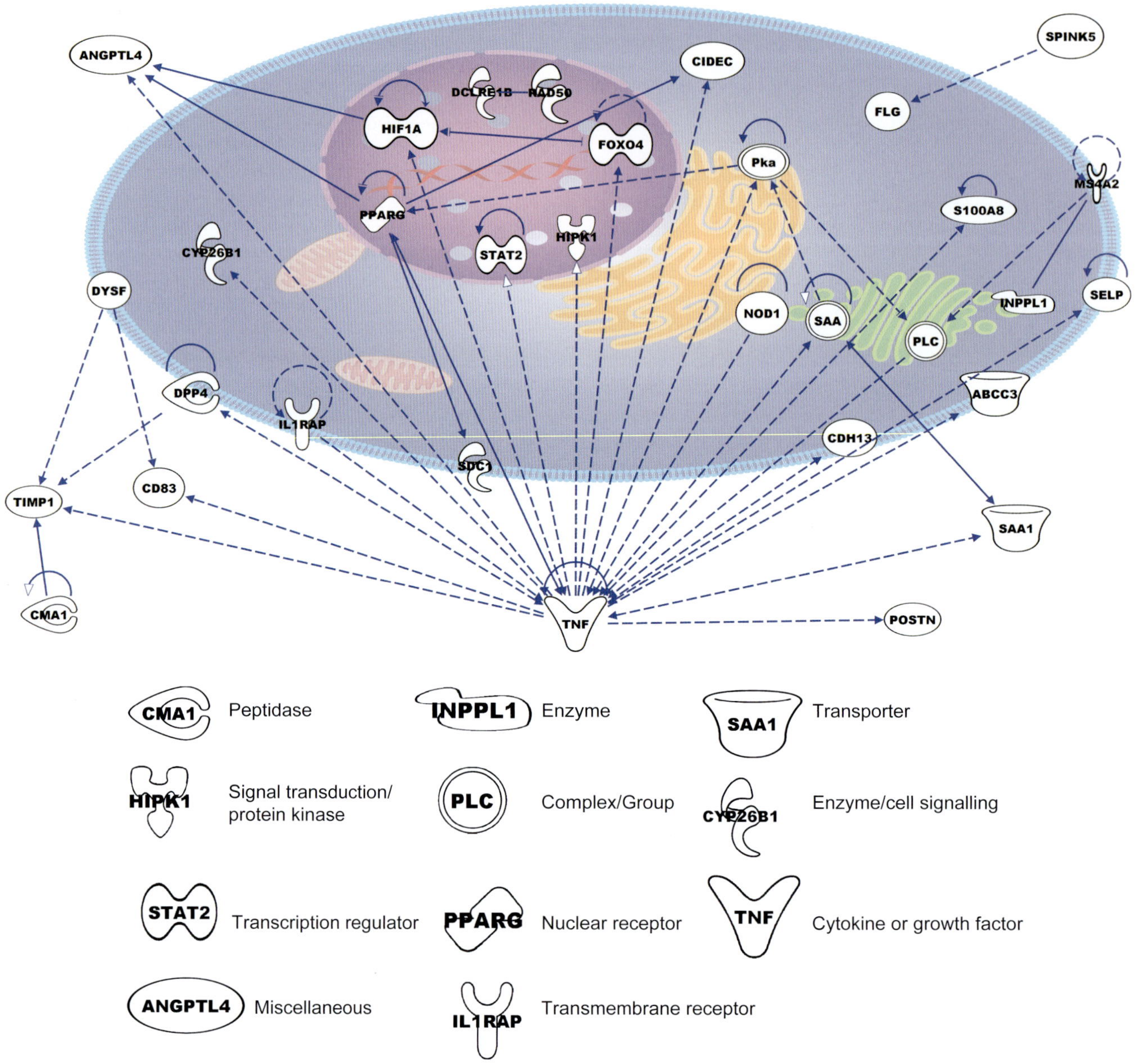

Figure 2. Network pathway of genes associated with canine atopic dermatitis supported by at least one reference from the literature or from canonical information stored in the Ingenuity® Knowledge Base (IPA; Ingenuity Systems, http://www.ingenuity.com). Nodes are displayed using various shapes that represent the functional class of the gene product.

trance, and incomplete genome coverage. Genome-wide association studies appear to be the most powerful technique to study the genotype of canine AD, but future studies will require larger cohorts of individual breeds from defined geographical areas.

Atopic dermatitis involves a complex network of many genes, with multiple variants affecting gene function and expression (Figure 2). The effect of any one polymorphism is likely to be relatively small, and the final phenotype will depend on their interactions across the genome. These findings also suggest that the genetic background to canine AD varies between breeds and geographical gene pools. This could explain variations in clinical phenotype and response to treatment between individuals and breeds.

This complexity, and the high prevalence of canine AD, means that a screening and breeding programme to eliminate the condition is unlikely to succeed. Despite this, the genomics revolution has huge potential. These techniques will allow identification of target molecules for novel treatments. In addition, we should be able to genotype atopic dogs and relate this to their phenotype. Understanding of the genotype will enable better targeting of treatment options; for example, some dogs may respond well to skin barrier therapy, whereas others would benefit more from allergen-specific immunotherapy. We should also be able to identify dogs that may have a poor response or have an increased risk of adverse effects to certain anti-inflammatory drugs. Finally, it may be possible to discover atopic genotypes in young dogs and manage environmental and other factors to minimize their risk of developing clinical AD. However, we must be careful to avoid misuse of genomic data in diagnosis and by breeders or insurance companies.

Glossary

Allele	One of two or more forms of a gene or DNA sequence on a chromosome that may be associated with a phenotypic trait. Diploid organisms can be homozygous (i.e. two copies of the same allele) or heterozygous (i.e. two different alleles).
Exon	DNA sequences within a gene that make up the final RNA transcript. Exons are usually separated by one or more introns in a gene.
Genotype	The specific genetic makeup of an individual. The genotype, epigenetic factors (i.e. changes in gene expression not associated with the DNA sequence) and environmental influences determine the phenotype.
Haplotype	A combination of alleles at adjacent loci on the chromosome that are inherited together. Haplotype also refers to a set of single nucleotide polymorphisms on a single chromosome that are statistically associated.
Intron	DNA sequence within a gene that is removed during transcription to produce the final RNA sequence.
Linkage disequilibrium	Nonrandom association of alleles at two or more loci, which may be on the same or different chromosomes.
Locus	The specific location of a gene or DNA sequence on a chromosome.
Microsatellite markers [simple sequence repeats (SSRs) or short tandem repeats (STRs)]	Highly polymorphic repeating sequences of two to six base pairs (bp) throughout the genome used in inheritance studies.
Penetrance	The proportion of individuals with a particular genotype that develop the associated phenotype.

Glossary (*Continued*)

Phenotype	An individual's observable characteristics or traits. These may include morphology, development, physiology, behaviour and/or disease states.
Population stratification	Differences in allele frequencies between groups in a study population that are associated with ancestry (e.g. race, breed, geography) rather than a disease condition.
Single nucleotide polymorphisms (SNPs)	A difference in single nucleotide (A, T, C or G) in a DNA sequence; for example, AGC**C**TA and AGC**T**TA.

References

1. Bieber T. Atopic dermatitis. *Ann Dermatol* 2010; 22: 125–137.
2. Bieber T, Novak N. Pathogenesis of atopic dermatitis: new developments. *Curr Allergy Asthma Rep* 2009; 9: 291–294.
3. Bieber T. Mechanisms of disease: atopic dermatitis. *New Eng J Med* 2008; 358: 1483–1494.
4. Marsella R, Girolomoni G. Canine models of atopic dermatitis: a useful tool with untapped potential. *J Invest Dermatol* 2009; 129: 2351–2357.
5. Lund EM, Armstrong PJ, Kirk CA *et al.* Health status and population characteristics of dogs and cats examined at private veterinary practices in the United States. *J Am Vet Med Assoc* 1999; 214: 1336–1341.
6. Hillier A, Griffin CE. The ACVD task force on canine atopic dermatitis (I): incidence and prevalence. *Vet Immunol Immunopathol* 2001; 81: 147–151.
7. Scott DW, Miller WH Jr, Griffin CE. Skin immune system and allergic skin disease. In: *Muller and Kirk's Small Animal Dermatology*, 6th edition. Philadelphia, PA: W.B. Saunders Co., 2001; 543–666.
8. Barnes KC. An update on the genetics of atopic dermatitis: scratching the surface in 2009. *J Allergy Clin Immunol* 2010; 125: 16–29.
9. Wilhem S, Kovalik M, Favrot C. Breed-associated phenotypes in canine atopic dermatitis. *Vet Dermatol* 2011; 22: 143–149.
10. Picco F, Zini E, Nett C *et al.* A prospective study on canine atopic dermatitis and food-induced allergic dermatitis in Switzerland. *Vet Dermatol* 2008; 19: 150–155.
11. DeBoer DJ, Hill PB. Serum immunoglobulin concentrations in West Highland White Terriers do not predict development of atopic dermatitis. *Vet Dermatol* 2000; 10: 275–281.
12. Shaw SC, Wood JLN, Freeman J *et al.* Estimation of heritability of atopic dermatitis in Labrador and Golden Retrievers. *Am J Vet Res* 2004; 65: 1014–1020.
13. Marsella R, Olivry T, Nicklin CF *et al.* Pilot investigation of a model for canine atopic dermatitis: environmental house dust mite challenge of high-IgE-producing beagles, mite hypersensitive dogs with atopic dermatitis and normal dogs. *Vet Dermatol* 2006; 17: 24–35.
14. Olivry T, Deangelo KB, Dunston SM *et al.* Patch testing of experimentally sensitized beagle dogs: development of a model for skin lesions of atopic dermatitis. *Vet Dermatol* 2006; 17: 95–102.
15. Schiessl B, Zemann B, Hodgkin-Pickart LA *et al.* Importance of early allergen contact for the development of a sustained immunoglobulin E response in a dog model. *Int Arch Allergy Immunol* 2003; 130: 125–134.
16. Nodtvedt A, Guitian J, Egenvall A *et al.* The spatial distribution of atopic dermatitis cases in a population of insured Swedish dogs. *Prev Vet Med* 2007; 78: 210–222.
17. Nødtvedt A, Bergvall K, Sallander M *et al.* A case–control study of risk factors for canine atopic dermatitis among boxer, bullterrier and West Highland white terrier dogs in Sweden. *Vet Dermatol* 2007; 18: 309–315.
18. Esparza-Gordillo J, Weidinger S, Fölster-Holst R *et al.* A common variant on chromosome 11q13 is associated with atopic dermatitis. *Nat Genet* 2009; 41: 596–601.
19. Lindblad-Toh K, Wade CM, Mikkelsen TS *et al.* Genome sequence, comparative analysis and haplotype structure of the domestic dog. *Nature* 2005; 438: 803–819.
20. Sutter NB, Ostrander EA. Dog star rising: the canine genetic system. *Nat Rev Genet* 2004; 5: 900–910.
21. Starkey MP, Scase TJ, Mellersh CS *et al.* Dogs really are man's best friend – Canine genomics has applications in veterinary and human medicine! *Brief Funct Genomic Proteomic* 2005; 4: 112–128.
22. Wood SH, Ke XY, Nuttall T *et al.* Genome-wide association analysis of canine atopic dermatitis and identification of disease related SNPs. *Immunogenetics* 2009; 61: 765–772.
23. Merryman-Simpson AE, Wood SH, Fretwell N *et al.* Gene (mRNA) expression in canine atopic dermatitis: microarray analysis. *Vet Dermatol* 2008; 19: 59–66.
24. Barros Roque J, O'Leary CA, Kyaw-Tanner M *et al.* Haplotype sharing excludes canine orthologous *Filaggrin* locus in atopy in West Highland White Terriers. *Anim Genet* 2009; 40: 793–794.
25. Roque JB, O'Leary CA, Duffy DL *et al.* Atopic dermatitis in West Highland white terriers is associated with a 1.3-Mb region on CFA 17. *Immunogenetics* 2012; 64: 209–217.
26. Salzmann CA, Olivry TJ, Nielsen DM *et al.* Genome-wide linkage study of atopic dermatitis in West Highland White Terriers. *BMC Genet* 2011; 12: 37.
27. Schwartzman RM. Immunologic studies of progeny of atopic dogs. *Am J Vet Res* 1984; 45: 375–378.

28. Chung T-H, Oh J-S, Lee Y-S *et al.* Elevated serum levels of s100 calcium binding protein a8 (s100a8) reflect disease severity in canine atopic dermatitis. *J Vet Med Sci* 2010; 72: 693–700.
29. Nuttall TJ, Knight PA, McAleese SM *et al.* Expression of T-helper 1 cytokine mRNA in canine atopic dermatitis correlates with clinical severity. In: Hillier A, Foster AP, Kwochka KW eds. *Advances in Veterinary Dermatology*, volume 5. Oxford: Blackwell Publishing Ltd, 2004: 17–27.
30. Candi E, Schmidt R, Melino G. The cornified envelope: a model of cell death in the skin. *Nat Rev Mol Cell Biol* 2005; 6: 328–340.
31. Chervet L, Galichet A, McLean WHI *et al.* Missing C-terminal filaggrin expression, NFkappaB activation and hyperproliferation identify the dog as a putative model to study epidermal dysfunction in atopic dermatitis. *Exp Dermatol* 2010; 19: e343–e346.
32. Marsella R, Olivry T, Carlotti D-N *et al.* Current evidence of skin barrier dysfunction in human and canine atopic dermatitis. *Vet Dermatol* 2011; 22: 239–248.
33. Marsella R, Samuelson D, Harrington L. Immunohistochemical evaluation of filaggrin polyclonal antibody in atopic and normal beagles. *Vet Dermatol* 2009; 20: 547–554.
34. O'Regan GM, Sandilands A, McLean WH, Irvine AD. Filaggrin in atopic dermatitis. *J Allergy Clin Immunol* 2008; 122: 689–693.
35. Wood SH, Clements DN, Ollier WE *et al.* Gene expression in canine atopic dermatitis and correlation with clinical severity scores. *J Dermatol Sci* 2009; 55: 27–33.
36. Moffatt MF. *SPINK5*: a gene for atopic dermatitis and asthma. *Clin Exp Allergy* 2004; 34: 325–327.
37. Ding Y, Shen S, Lino AC *et al.* Beta-catenin stabilization extends regulatory T cell survival and induces anergy in nonregulatory T cells. *Nat Med* 2008; 14: 162–169.
38. Wood SH, Ollier WE, Nuttall T *et al.* Despite identifying some shared gene associations with human atopic dermatitis the use of multiple dog breeds from various locations limits detection of gene associations in canine atopic dermatitis. *Vet Immunol Immunopathol* 2010; 138: 193–197.
39. Liu YJ. Thymic stromal lymphopoietin: master switch for allergic inflammation. *J Exp Med* 2006; 203: 269–273.
40. Roque JB, O'Leary CA, Duffy DL *et al.* IgE Responsiveness to *Dermatophagoides farinae* in West Highland white terrier dogs is associated with region on CFA35. *J Hered* 2011; 102: S74–S80.
41. McCarthy MI, Hirschhorn JN. Genome-wide association studies: potential next steps on a genetic journey. *Hum Mol Genet* 2008; 17: R156–R165.
42. Owczarek-Lipska M, Lauber B, Molitor V *et al.* Two loci on chromosome 5 are associated with serum IgE levels in Labrador retrievers. *PLoS One* 2012; 7: e39176.
43. Nuttall TJ, Hill PB, Bensignor E *et al.* House dust and forage mite allergens and their role in human and canine atopic dermatitis. *Vet Dermatol* 2006; 17: 223–235.
44. Gill C, McEwan N, McGarry J *et al.* House dust and storage mite contamination of dry dog food stored in open bags and sealed boxes in 10 domestic households. *Vet Dermatol* 2011; 22: 162–172.

To cite this article, please use DOI: 10.1111/j.1365-3164.2012.01109.x

1.3

Serum anti-*Staphylococcus pseudintermedius* IgE and IgG antibodies in dogs with atopic dermatitis and nonatopic dogs

Jennifer Bexley*, Timothy J. Nuttall†, Bruce Hammerberg‡, J. Ross Fitzgerald§ and Richard E. Halliwell¶

*Avacta Animal Health, Unit 651, Street 5, Thorp Arch Estate, Wetherby, Leeds LS23 7FZ, UK
†School of Veterinary Science, The University of Liverpool, Leahurst Campus, Chester High Road, Neston, Cheshire CH64 7TE, UK
‡College of Veterinary Medicine, Center for Comparative Medicine and Translational Research, North Carolina State University, 1060 William Moore Drive, Raleigh, NC 27607, USA
§The Roslin Institute and Edinburgh Infectious Diseases, University of Edinburgh, Easter Bush, Midlothian, Edinburgh EH25 9RG, UK
¶Royal (Dick) School of Veterinary Studies, University of Edinburgh, Easter Bush, Midlothian, Edinburgh EH25 9RG, UK

Correspondence: Jennifer Bexley, Avacta Animal Health, Unit 651, Street 5, Thorp Arch Estate, Wetherby, Leeds LS23 7FZ, UK.
E-mail: jennifer.bexley@avacta.com

Background – Dogs and humans with atopic dermatitis (AD) are predisposed to colonization and recurrent infection with *Staphylococcus* spp. Studies in humans suggest that staphylococcus-specific immunoglobulin E (IgE) plays a key role in disease pathogenesis. Few such studies have been undertaken in dogs.

Hypothesis/Objectives – The aim of this study was to compare levels of staphylococcus-specific IgE and immunoglobulin G (IgG) in dogs with AD, nonatopic dogs with staphylococcal pyoderma, and nonatopic and non-infected control dogs.

Animals – Sera were collected from 108 dogs with AD, 39 nonatopic dogs with staphylococcal pyoderma secondary to different underlying conditions, 67 age-matched nonatopic control dogs, and nine control dogs reared in minimal disease conditions.

Methods – Serum *Staphylococcus pseudintermedius*-specific IgE and IgG antibodies were measured by enzyme-linked immunosorbent assay.

Results – Dogs with AD had significantly higher levels of anti-staphylococcal IgE than nonatopic dogs with staphylococcal pyoderma and the two groups of control dogs. Levels of anti-staphylococcal IgG were significantly higher in atopic dogs and nonatopic dogs with pyoderma compared with nonatopic control dogs and control dogs reared in minimal disease conditions, but there was no significant difference in levels of anti-staphylococcal IgG between dogs with AD and nonatopic dogs with pyoderma.

Conclusions and clinical importance – A significantly increased IgE response to *S. pseudintermedius* antigens in atopic dogs suggests an immunopathogenic role for anti-staphylococcal IgE. The finding of elevated IgE and IgG in atopic dogs is also important as a prelude to studies on antigenic specificity and possible correlations with disease phenotype.

Introduction

Staphylococcal infection is a major complicating factor in both canine and human atopic dermatitis (AD).[1,2] Furthermore, it is increasingly recognized that the immunoglobulin E (IgE) response to staphylococcal antigens in humans plays an important role in the pathogenesis of the disease.[3] There are, in fact, two conditions in humans associated with anti-staphylococcal IgE and recurrent staphylococcal skin infections, namely AD and hyper-IgE syndrome.[1] However, no condition analogous to the latter has yet been reported in dogs.

Numerous studies have investigated the IgE response to *Staphylococcus aureus* antigens in human AD.[1,4–6] Amongst the atopic diseases, the production of IgE directed against microbial antigens appears to be limited to AD, and there is no such response in patients suffering from atopic respiratory diseases.[6,7] In most studies, allergen-specific IgE levels correlate with disease severity, which is suggestive of a significant immunopathogenic role.[5,6] More recently, attention has focused on soluble staphylococcal toxins, particularly superantigens, which are documented in >50% of cases.[6,8] Not only are

Accepted 17 July 2012
Sources of Funding: This study was funded by Avacta Animal Health, Wetherby, UK.
Conflict of Interest: J.B. is an employee of Avacta Animal Health. T.J.N. and R.E.H, are consultants for Avacta Animal Health. B.H. has a license agreement with Avacta Animal Health.

superantigens capable of inducing inflammation through polyclonal B and T cell activation, but they also provide a rich source of allergen to the skin immune system.[8,9] It is suggested that the combination of superantigen-producing staphylococci and the subsequent IgE response may be very important factors in determining the severity of AD.[6,8,9]

The major canine skin pathogen is *Staphylococcus pseudintermedius*,[10] and its complete genomic sequence has been recently published.[11] It is known that dogs suffering from canine AD have a higher rate of carriage of *S. pseudintermedius* than do normal dogs, and that lesional skin of affected dogs is frequently colonized by this organism.[12] *Staphylococcus pseudintermedius* produces a range of exotoxins, including superantigens. In one study, 25 of 96 isolates from cases of canine pyoderma in the UK were shown to produce multiple superantigens, usually staphylococcal enterotoxin A (SEA) and C (SEC).[13] In another study, a novel enterotoxin-related gene, *se-int*, found in all 44 isolates examined, shared >50% homology with both SEC and staphylococcal enterotoxin B (SEB).[14]

There are few published studies on the immune response to staphylococcal antigens in canine AD and other canine skin conditions. One study examined the IgE and IgG response to staphylococcal antigens in 31 dogs with pyoderma secondary to AD, 34 cases of recurrent idiopathic pyoderma, 14 cases of idiopathic deep recurrent pyoderma, 15 cases of single-episode pyoderma, and 39 healthy control dogs that were not age matched.[15] Both dogs with AD and those with recurrent superficial pyoderma had significantly higher levels of anti-staphylococcal IgE than did the healthy dogs. Levels of IgG antibody appeared to be much higher than those of IgE, and were found to increase with increasing chronicity of the infection. A later study examined the IgG and IgA response to staphylococcal antigens in dogs suffering from AD with and without concomitant pyoderma, as well as cases of idiopathic deep pyoderma, pustular demodicosis, flea-allergy dermatitis with pyoderma and anal furunculosis, and in healthy control dogs (albeit not age matched).[16] All affected animals had significantly higher levels of IgG antibody than the healthy control animals, but no significant differences were found between the affected groups. However, the significance of this study, which did not assess IgE levels, for the pathogenesis of AD is unclear.

Canine AD and human AD share many common features.[17] The most recent research in human AD has emphasized the very important role of staphylococcal infection and the subsequent immune response; thus, there is a need to revisit this in canine AD, employing age-matched control animals and more refined methods of antigen extraction. The aim of this study was to measure levels of staphylococcus-specific IgE and IgG in a large population of dogs suffering from AD and compare them with levels in dogs suffering from staphylococcal infection secondary to other causes and in two control groups with no history of skin disease or infection. We hypothesized that if an immunopathogenic role for anti-staphylococcal IgE in canine AD exists, anti-staphylococcal IgE levels would be greater in atopic dogs than in age-matched nonatopic dogs, irrespective of their pyoderma status.

Materials and methods

Serum samples

Sera were assayed from the following groups.

1. Group 1, AD dogs, comprising 108 dogs including 43 dogs with a clinical diagnosis[18] of canine AD and secondary pyoderma (confirmed by cytology and isolation of *S. pseudintermedius*) seen at the Small Animal Teaching Hospital, University of Liverpool, UK over a 4 month period and 65 dogs suffering from chronic dermatitis whose sera had been submitted to Avacta Animal Health UK over a 1 year period for serological testing for environmental allergen-specific IgE, and that subsequently underwent immunotherapy. The latter were diagnosed with canine AD after exclusion of other causes of pruritus by the submitting veterinarian, and sera selected for the study showed positive reactions to one or more relevant allergens following confirmation by one of the authors (REH) that the history, clinical signs and investigation detailed on the submission form were compatible with a diagnosis of canine AD using appropriate criteria.[18,19] Dogs with any present or past history of flea-allergy dermatitis or that had shown any response to ectoparasiticidal therapy were excluded. The presence and type of pyoderma in the latter dogs was, however, not always documented.
2. Group 2, nonatopic dogs with pyoderma, comprising 39 dogs with pyoderma (confirmed by cytology and isolation of *S. pseudintermedius*) seen at the Small Animal Teaching Hospital, University of Liverpool UK over a 4 month period. Of these, 11 had atopic-like dermatitis, 11 had demodicosis, seven had a seborrhoeic disorder, three had recurrent idiopathic pyoderma, two had hypothyroidism, three had an adverse food reaction, and two had nonrecurrent idiopathic pyoderma.
3. Group 3, nonatopic control dogs, comprising 67 age-matched control dogs with no history or clinical signs of skin disease at time of sampling. These sera were submitted by veterinarians over a 1 year period for investigation of gastrointestinal problems (chronic vomiting and/or diarrhoea).
4. Group 4, minimal disease (MD) control dogs, comprising nine laboratory-bred dogs that were reared in minimal disease conditions at Charles River Laboratories (Ballina, Co. Mayo, Ireland).

The number, sex and ages of dogs in each group are shown in Table 1. The study was approved by The University of Liverpool School of Veterinary Science Ethics Committee. In the case of Groups 1–3, all sera were derived from excess serum that was drawn for diagnostic purposes. In the case of Group 4, sera were obtained and supplied under the appropriate licence (Charles River Laboratories via the Minister of Health and Children, Ireland).

Antisera

An alkaline phosphatase-conjugated monoclonal antibody (mAb, clone 5.91; North Carolina State University, Raleigh, NC, USA) was used to detect staphylococcus-specific IgE. This antibody has been shown to be specific for canine IgE with no cross-reactivity to IgG.[20] Staphylococcus-specific IgG was detected using alkaline phosphatase-conjugated goat anti-dog IgG (γ-chain specific; Kirkegaard and Perry Laboratories, Gaithersburg, MD, USA).

Preparation of *Staphylococcus pseudintermedius* antigen extract

Fifteen *S. pseudintermedius* isolates from cases of canine pyoderma were used in initial studies. Soluble and cell wall-associated antigens from both stationary and exponential growth phases were prepared as previously described.[21] The extracted proteins were assessed for protein A content by PAGE and western blotting using a chicken anti-protein A (IgY; Gallus Immunotech, Fergus, ON, Canada). The specificity of the chicken anti-protein A was shown using *S. aureus* Newman SpA (protein A-producing) and *S. aureus* Newman Δ SpA

Table 1. Number, sex and age of dogs in the study

Group*	Number of dogs	Sex ratio, males:females (no. neutered, N)	Median age (months)	Mean age (months)	Age range (months)
1	108	70 (29 N):38 (19 N)	53	58†	8–147
2	39	28 (5 N):11 (3 N)	58	63†	7–132
3	67	37 (19 N):30 (16 N)	42	53†	4–144
4	9	2:7	5	5	4–5

*Group 1, dogs with atopic dermatitis; Group 2, nonatopic dogs with staphylococcal pyoderma; Group 3, nonatopic control dogs; and Group 4, control dogs reared in minimal disease conditions.
† Significantly different from Group 4, $P < 0.001$.

(nonprotein A-producing) positive and negative controls, respectively. Three strains that were protein A negative using this criterion were further assessed for IgG binding. The preparation derived from a strain (8012) that showed minimal binding to serum from a MD dog was selected for use in the study.

Assessment of *Staphylococcus pseudintermedius* strain 8012 for *se-int* gene

Strain 8012 was assessed for the presence of the superantigen *se-int* gene by PCR. Genomic DNA was extracted from 500 μL of stationary-phase culture grown in tryptic soy broth at 37°C using the Edge Biosystems PurElute Bacterial Genomic kit (Edge Biosystems, Gaithersburg, MD, USA) following the manufacturer's instructions, with the addition of 250 μg/mL (final concentration) of lysostaphin (Ambi Products, Lawrence, NY, USA) prior to incubation. The PCR was performed using Promega GoTaq DNA Polymerase (M8301) with the Promega dNTP mix (U1511; Promega UK Ltd, Southampton, UK), employing the following primers (Invitrogen, Life Technologies Ltd, Paisley, UK): *se-int* forward 5′-TATAGGTACCCTTGGACTTTTGGATG-3′; and *se-int* reverse 5′-TGGCGAGCTCCAAATCCATTAGCC-3′. Appropriate positive (genomic DNA from *S. pseudintermedius* strain ED99) and negative controls (no template) were included.

Enzyme-linked immunosorbent assay (ELISA)

Serum staphylococcus-specific antibodies were assayed by ELISA using protocols modified from previous studies.[20,22] Briefly, microtitre plates (Greiner Labortechnik, Frickenhausen, Germany) were coated with *S. pseudintermedius* extract diluted 1:1000 (IgE ELISA) and 1:3000 (IgG ELISA) in 0.05 M carbonate/bicarbonate buffer, pH 9.6, and blocked with phosphate-buffered saline containing 0.5% polyvinylpyrrolidone (average molecular weight 10,000) and 0.5% sucrose. All dilutions of serum and secondary antibodies were in Tris-buffered saline containing 0.05% Tween-20 (TBST) and 0.5% human serum albumin. Samples were assayed in duplicate at dilutions of 1:10 (IgE) and 1:400 (IgG). Immunoglobulin E was detected with 1 μg/mL phosphatase-conjugated mAb (clone 5.91); IgG was detected with 0.125 μg/mL phosphatase-conjugated goat anti-dog IgG (γ-chain specific). Between incubation steps, plates were washed three times with TBST using an automated plate washer (Bio-Tek, Winooski, VT, USA). Colour was developed using AP Yellow One Component Microwell Substrate (pNPP; BioFx Laboratories, Owings Mills, MD, USA) for 30 min at room temperature before the reaction was stopped by the addition of 1 M NaOH. Absorbances were determined at 405 nm using a microplate reader (Tecan, Männedorf, Switzerland). Results were expressed as optical density (OD) units at 405 nm, determined as an average of duplicate results after correction by subtracting the mean OD value of duplicate blank wells.

Statistical analysis

All data were analysed using SPSS 20.0 (IBM UK Ltd, Portsmouth, UK). Differences were considered statistically significant when the *P*-value was <0.05. After testing for normality, differences in age and levels of antibodies between groups were tested by one-way ANOVA followed by Dunnett's *post hoc* test for multiple comparisons, assuming unequal variance between groups. Linear regression was used to assess whether there was any statistically significant association between duration of staphylococcal infection and levels of anti-staphylococcal antibodies.

Results

PCR results for strain 8012

The PCR results were positive for the superantigen gene *se-int*.

Reproducibility

From the assay controls, the mean intra-assay variations were 6.3 and 9.7% for IgE and IgG ELISAs, respectively. Mean interassay variations were 11.6 and 12.2% for IgE and IgG ELISAs, respectively.

Serum anti-*Staphylococcus pseudintermedius* IgE

There was a highly significant difference in anti-staphylococcal IgE levels between the four groups ($P < 0.009$, ANOVA; Figure 1). Group 1 atopic dogs had significantly higher levels of anti-staphylococcal IgE than Group 2 nonatopic dogs with pyoderma ($P < 0.05$, Dunnett's *post hoc* test) and both the age-matched Group 3 nonatopic control dogs and Group 4 MD control dogs (both $P < 0.05$, Dunnett's *post hoc* test). Significantly higher levels of anti-staphylococcal IgE were also seen in the Group 2 nonatopic dogs with pyoderma and Group 3 nonatopic dogs compared with the Group 4 MD dogs (both $P < 0.05$, Dunnett's *post hoc* test). There was no significant difference in IgE levels between the Group 2 nonatopic dogs with pyoderma and the Group 3 nonatopic dogs without pyoderma.

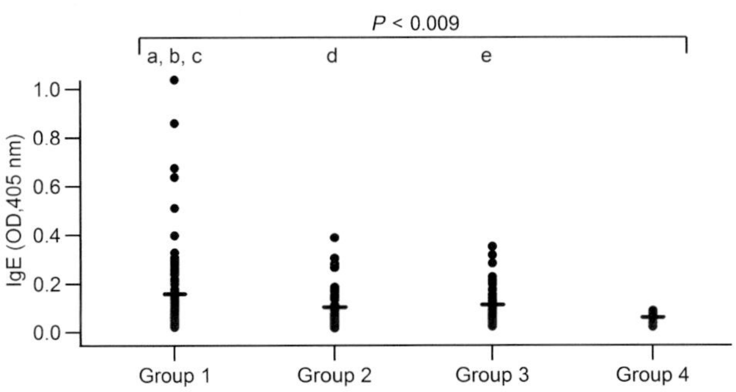

Figure 1. Anti-staphylococcal IgE in Group 1 dogs with atopic dermatitis, Group 2 nonatopic dogs with pyoderma, Group 3 nonatopic control dogs, and Group 4 minimal disease control dogs. Bars indicate the mean of each group. [a] Significantly different from Group 2, $P < 0.05$; [b] significantly different from Group 3, $P < 0.05$; and [c,d,e] significantly different from Group 4, $P < 0.05$.

Serum anti-*Staphylococcus pseudintermedius* IgG

There was a highly significant difference in anti-staphylococcal IgG levels between the four groups ($P < 0.0001$, ANOVA Figure 2). Group 1 atopic dogs had significantly higher levels of serum staphylococcus-specific IgG than Group 3 nonatopic control dogs and Group 4 MD control dogs (both $P < 0.05$, Dunnett's *post hoc* test). In addition, Group 2 nonatopic dogs with pyoderma and Group 3 nonatopic control dogs had significantly higher levels of serum staphylococcus-specific IgG than Group 4 MD control dogs (both $P < 0.05$, Dunnett's *post hoc* test). There was no significant difference in IgG levels between the Group 1 atopic dogs and the Group 2 nonatopic dogs with pyoderma, or between the Group 2 dogs and the Group 3 nonatopic dogs without pyoderma.

Duration of infection

The duration of infection was not correlated with levels of either anti-staphylococcal IgE or IgG antibodies in dogs with clinically diagnosed pyoderma (R^2 = 0.178 and 0.032 for IgE and IgG, respectively).

Discussion

This study compared levels of staphylococcus-specific IgE and IgG in dogs with AD and those suffering from staphylococcal pyoderma secondary to other causes with levels in two groups of control dogs. Some Group 1 dogs with AD were not seen by the authors, but all were suffering from chronic pruritic dermatitis, had IgE to one or more relevant environmental IgE allergens, were diagnosed as suffering from canine AD by the submitting veterinarian, and subsequently underwent immunotherapy. Compatibility with a diagnosis of canine AD was confirmed by one of the authors by perusal of the clinical and historical data on the submission forms. The Group 3 nonatopic control dogs were also not seen by the authors, but were age-matched dogs reported as suffering from gastrointestinal problems manifested by chronic and recurrent diarrhoea and/or vomiting. These dogs had no known history or clinical signs of skin disease. The MD control dogs (Group 4) were of a young age and reared in minimal disease conditions and thus likely to have had limited exposure to staphylococci. Group 1 atopic dogs, Group 2 nonatopic dogs suffering from staphylococcal pyoderma, and Group 3 nonatopic control dogs were age matched, with no significant differences between the means, but the Group 4 MD control dogs were significantly younger (Table 1). These were nevertheless included as negative controls because they were likely to have low to undetectable levels of serum anti-staphylococcal antibody. The pyoderma status of the 65 atopic dogs in Group 1, whose sera were submitted to Avacta Animal Health, was not always known. It is, however, well established that staphylococci colonize lesional skin and mucosal sites in >90% of atopic dogs,[12] and in one study 74% of dogs with AD undergoing allergen-specific immunotherapy required treatment for pyoderma when followed over a 9 month period.[23] Furthermore, levels of anti-staphylococcal IgG were significantly higher in the Group 1 atopic dogs than the two groups of control dogs, suggesting that staphylococcal infection may have been recurrent in these atopic dogs for a number of years. It can thus be assumed that most, if not all, of these dogs were exposed to antigens of *S. pseudintermedius* at some point during the course of their disease.

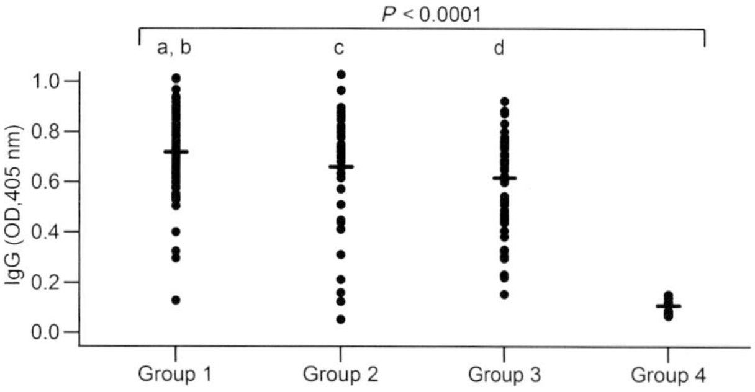

Figure 2. Anti-staphylococcal IgG in Group 1 dogs with atopic dermatitis, Group 2 nonatopic dogs with pyoderma, Group 3 nonatopic control dogs, and Group 4 minimal disease control dogs. Bars indicate the mean of each group. [a] Significantly different from Group 3, $P < 0.05$; and [b,c,d] significantly different from Group 4, $P < 0.05$.

Similar to studies in human AD,[1,4,24] significantly higher levels of staphylococcus-specific IgE were found in dogs with AD than in nonatopic, noninfected control dogs. Moreover, IgE levels were significantly higher in dogs with AD than in dogs with staphylococcal infection secondary to other causes. In contrast, the level of anti-staphylococcal IgG in the two groups was not significantly different. This suggests that anti-staphylococcal IgE may have an important role in the pathogenesis of canine AD. As will be discussed later, it is possible that it is a reflection of superantigen production by the strain involved and a resultant T-helper 2 (Th2) skewing of the immune response.[25] In a previous study, higher levels of staphylococcus-specific IgE were found not only in dogs with AD, but also in dogs with recurrent idiopathic pyoderma, although the dogs were not age matched.[15] It was concluded that hypersensitivity reactions to staphylococcal antigens could be contributing to the inflammatory process in those dogs. In the same study, there was also some evidence that chronicity led to increased levels of anti-staphylococcal antibody, although this apparent trend was not subjected to statistical evaluation. There was no evidence of a relationship between staphylococcal antibody levels and duration of infection in our study (although duration in our study refers to the overall history of pyoderma, not the duration of each occurrence). The presence of high levels of staphylococcus-specific IgE in some nonatopic dogs with pyoderma in this and other studies[15] emphasizes that anti-staphylococcal IgE is not restricted to dogs suffering from canine AD. It is, of course, possible that some of these dogs were subclinically atopic dogs, although intradermal and serological allergen tests were negative at presentation.

Microbial colonization aggravates the clinical signs of AD in humans and dogs. The role of superantigens is of particular interest, because their presence is associated with particularly severe AD in humans.[6] Superantigens induce polyclonal T cell and B cell activation, and topical application to both mice[25] and humans[26,27] induces inflammation. Furthermore, they may favour a Th2-skewed immune response, facilitating an IgE response to staphylococcal antigens and possibly other environmental allergens. Simultaneous cutaneous application of SEB together with house dust mite antigen lowers the threshold for a positive reaction in humans.[28] Epicutaneous application of SEB to mice increases expression of the Th2 cytokine interleukin-4, with no detectable interferon-γ.[25] A later study using the same model yielded evidence of a mixed T-helper 1 (Th1) and Th2 response, but application of SEB led to a heightened IgE response to ovalbumin that was attributable to the superantigen.[29] Finally, addition of toxic shock syndrome toxin-1 to peripheral blood mononuclear cells (PBMC) cultures from atopic patients significantly increased pollen-specific IgE production.[30] Similar superantigens are produced by canine staphylococcal isolates, and further studies to show whether they influence IgE responses in canine AD are required.

As with humans,[31] no particular strain of *S. pseudintermedius* is associated with colonization of the skin of atopic dogs.[12] Although the superantigen profile of canine isolates has been the subject of a number of recent studies, the differing methodologies employed make conclusions difficult to interpret. A study in which SEA, SEB, SEC, SED and toxic shock syndrome toxin-1 were reported in canine isolates was undertaken using a commercial reversed passive latex agglutination toxin detection kit;[13] most of the other reports, in contrast, employed PCR. As *se-int* shares >50% homology with SEC and SEB, and this enterotoxin-related gene is present in all isolates according to one study[14] (and, indeed, was present in the strain used for the studies reported herein), this could raise questions regarding studies employing less specific methodology. Recently, a novel exfoliative toxin (EX1), which selectively digests canine desmoglein 1, was reported from an isolate from a dog with impetigo.[32] This is distinct from the previously described *S. intermedius* exfoliative toxin (SIET) that is reportedly produced by all canine strains.[33] It is clear that much more work is necessary to identify all of the superantigens present in canine isolates of *S. pseudintermedius* precisely, to document their prevalence and to assess their biological activity and possible correlates with disease phenotype.

In conclusion, this study has shown that dogs suffering from canine AD show a significantly increased IgE response to staphylococcal antigens. It is likely that this response plays an important role in the pathogenesis of canine AD. Further studies are, however, required to define the immune response to specific staphylococcal antigens and superantigens involved in canine AD.

Acknowledgements

The authors are grateful to The University of Liverpool Small Animal Teaching Hospital for the provision of sera from dogs with bacterial pyoderma; and to Robyn Cartwright, The Roslin Institute and Edinburgh Infectious Diseases, University of Edinburgh, for the PCR studies.

References

1. Abramson JS, Dahl MV, Walsh G *et al.* Antistaphylococcal IgE in patients with atopic dermatitis. *J Am Acad Dermatol* 1982; 7: 105–110.
2. Picco F, Zini E, Nett C *et al.* A prospective study on canine atopic dermatitis and food-induced allergic dermatitis in Switzerland. *Vet Dermatol* 2008; 19: 150–155.
3. Ong PY, Leung DY. Immune dysregulation in atopic dermatitis. *Curr Allergy Asthma Rep* 2006; 6: 384–389.
4. Walsh GA, Richards KL, Douglas SD *et al.* Immunoglobulin E anti-*Staphylococcus aureus* antibodies in atopic patients. *J Clin Microbiol* 1981; 13: 1046–1048.
5. Motala C, Potter PC, Weinberg EG *et al.* Anti-*Staphylococcus aureus*-specific IgE in atopic dermatitis. *J Allergy Clin Immunol* 1986; 78: 583–589.
6. Zollner TM, Wichelhaus TA, Hartung A *et al.* Colonization with superantigen-producing *Staphylococcus aureus* is associated with increasing severity of atopic dermatitis. *Clin Exp Allergy* 2000; 30: 994–1000.
7. Reginald K, Westritschnig K, Werfel T *et al.* Immunoglobulin E antibody reactivity to bacterial antigens in atopic dermatitis patients. *Clin Exp Allergy* 2011; 41: 357–369.
8. Ong PY, Patel M, Ferdman RM *et al.* Association of staphylococcal superantigen-specific IgE with mild and moderate atopic dermatitis. *J Pediatr* 2008; 153: 803–806.
9. Leung DY, Harbeck R, Bina P *et al.* Presence of IgE antibodies to staphylococcal exotoxins on the skin of patients with atopic dermatitis. Evidence for a new group of allergens. *J Clin Invest* 1993; 92: 1374–1380.
10. Fitzgerald JR. The *Staphylococcus intermedius* group of bacterial pathogens: species re-classification, pathogenesis and the emergence of meticillin resistance. *Vet Dermatol* 2009; 20: 490–495.
11. Ben Zakour NL, Bannoehr J, Van den Broek AH *et al.* Complete genome sequence of the canine pathogen *Staphylococcus pseudintermedius*. *J Bacteriol* 2011; 193: 2363–2364.
12. Fazakerley J, Nuttall T, Sales D *et al.* Staphylococcal colonization of mucosal and lesional skin sites in atopic and healthy dogs. *Vet Dermatol* 2009; 20: 179–184.
13. Hendricks A, Schuberth HJ, Schueler K *et al.* Frequency of superantigen-producing *Staphylococcus intermedius* isolates from canine pyoderma and proliferation-inducing potential of superantigens in dogs. *Res Vet Sci* 2002; 73: 273–277.
14. Futagawa-Saito K, Suzuki M, Ohsawa M *et al.* Identification and prevalence of an enterotoxin-related gene, *se-int*, in *Staphylococcus intermedius* isolates from dogs and pigeons. *J Appl Microbiol* 2004; 96: 1361–1366.
15. Morales CA, Schultz KT, DeBoer DJ. Antistaphylococcal antibodies in dogs with recurrent staphylococcal pyoderma. *Vet Immunol Immunopathol* 1994; 42: 137–147.
16. Shearer DH, Day MJ. Aspects of the humoral immune response to *Staphylococcus intermedius* in dogs with superficial pyoderma, deep pyoderma and anal furunculosis. *Vet Immunol Immunopathol* 1997; 58: 107–120.
17. Marsella R, Girolomoni G. Canine models of atopic dermatitis: a useful tool with untapped potential. *J Invest Dermatol* 2009; 129: 2351–2357.
18. Favrot C, Steffan J, Seewald W *et al.* A prospective study on the clinical features of chronic canine atopic dermatitis and its diagnosis. *Vet Dermatol* 2010; 21: 23–31.
19. Willemse T. Atopic skin disease: a review and a reconsideration of diagnostic criteria. *J Small Anim Pract* 1986; 27: 771–778.
20. Bexley J, Hogg JE, Hammerberg B *et al.* Levels of house dust mite-specific serum immunoglobulin E (IgE) in different cat populations using a monoclonal based anti-IgE enzyme-linked immunosorbent assay. *Vet Dermatol* 2009; 20: 562–568.
21. Roche FM, Massey R, Peacock SJ *et al.* Characterization of novel LPXTG-containing proteins of *Staphylococcus aureus* identified from genome sequences. *Microbiology* 2003; 149: 643–654.

22. Foster AP, Knowles TG, Moore AH *et al.* Serum IgE and IgG responses to food antigens in normal and atopic dogs, and dogs with gastrointestinal disease. *Vet Immunol Immunopathol* 2003; 92: 113–124.
23. Colombo S, Hill PB, Shaw DJ *et al.* Requirement for additional treatment for dogs with atopic dermatitis undergoing allergen-specific immunotherapy. *Vet Rec* 2007; 160: 861–864.
24. Schopfer K, Baerlocher K, Price P *et al.* Staphylococcal Ig E antibodies, hyperimmunoglobulinemia E and *Staphylococcus aureus* infections. *N Engl J Med* 1979; 300: 835–838.
25. Laouini D, Kawamoto S, Yalcindag A *et al.* Epicutaneous sensitization with superantigen induces allergic skin inflammation. *J Allergy Clin Immunol* 2003; 112: 981–987.
26. Strange P, Skov L, Lisby S *et al.* *Staphylococcus* enterotoxin B applied on intact normal and intact atopic skin induces dermatitis. *Arch Dermatol* 1996; 132: 27–33.
27. Skov L, Olsen JV, Giorno R *et al.* Application of staphylococcal enterotoxin B on normal and atopic skin induces up-regulation of T cells by a superantigen-mediated mechanism. *J Allergy Clin Immunol* 2000; 105: 820–826.
28. Langer K, Breuer K, Kapp A *et al.* *Staphylococcus aureus*-derived enterotoxins enhance house dust mite-induced patch test reactions in atopic dermatitis. *Exp Dermatol* 2007; 16: 124–129.
29. Savinko T, Lauerma A, Lehtimaki S *et al.* Topical superantigen exposure induces epidermal accumulation of CD8$^+$ T cells, a mixed Th1/Th2-type dermatitis and vigorous production of IgE antibodies in the murine model of atopic dermatitis. *J Immunol* 2005; 175: 8320–8326.
30. Hofer MF, Harbeck RJ, Schlievert PM *et al.* Staphylococcal toxins augment specific IgE responses by atopic patients exposed to allergen. *J Invest Dermatol* 1999; 112: 171–176.
31. Kim DW, Park JY, Park KD *et al.* Are there predominant strains and toxins of *Staphylococcus aureus* in atopic dermatitis patients? Genotypic characterization and toxin determination of *S. aureus* isolated in adolescent and adult patients with atopic dermatitis. *J Dermatol* 2009; 36: 75–81.
32. Iyori K, Futagawa-Saito K, Hisatsune J *et al.* *Staphylococcus pseudintermedius* exfoliative toxin EXI selectively digests canine desmoglein 1 and causes subcorneal clefts in canine epidermis. *Vet Dermatol* 2011; 22: 319–326.
33. Yoon JW, Lee GJ, Lee SY *et al.* Prevalence of genes for enterotoxins, toxic shock syndrome toxin 1 and exfoliative toxin among clinical isolates of *Staphylococcus pseudintermedius* from canine origin. *Vet Dermatol* 2010; 21: 484–489.

To cite this article, please use DOI: 10.1111/j.1365-3164.2012.01105.x

1.4

Characterization of canine filaggrin: gene structure and protein expression in dog skin

Satoko Kanda*†, Takashi Sasaki‡§, Aiko Shiohama†, Koji Nishifuji*, Masayuki Amagai‡, Toshiroh Iwasaki* and Jun Kudoh†

*Laboratory of Veterinary Internal Medicine, Tokyo University of Agriculture and Technology, Tokyo, Japan
†Laboratory of Gene Medicine, ‡Department of Dermatology and §Centre for Integrated Medical Research, Keio University School of Medicine, Tokyo, Japan

Correspondene: Jun Kudoh, Laboratory of Gene Medicine, Keio University School of Medicine, 35 Shinanomachi, Shinjuku-ku, Tokyo 160-8582, Japan. E-mail: jkudoh@a8.keio.jp

Background – Filaggrin (FLG) is a key protein for skin barrier formation and hydration of the stratum corneum. In humans, a strong association between *FLG* gene mutations and atopic dermatitis has been reported. Although similar pathogenesis and clinical manifestation have been argued in canine atopic dermatitis, our understanding of canine FLG is limited.

Hypothesis/Objectives – The aim of this study was to determine the structure of the canine *FLG* gene and to raise anti-dog FLG antibodies, which will be useful to detect FLG protein in dog skin.

Methods – The structure of the canine *FLG* gene was determined by analysing the publicly available canine genome DNA sequence. Polyclonal anti-dog FLG antibodies were raised based on the canine FLG sequence analysis and used for defining the FLG expression pattern in dog skin by western blotting and immunohistochemistry.

Results – Genomic DNA sequence analysis revealed that canine *FLG* contained four units of repeated sequences corresponding to FLG monomer protein. Western blots probed with anti-dog FLG monomer detected two bands at 59 and 54 kDa, which were estimated sizes. The results of immunohistochemistry showed that canine FLG was expressed in the stratum granulosum of the epidermis as a granular staining pattern in the cytoplasmic region.

Conclusions and clinical importance – This study revealed the unique gene structure of canine *FLG* that results in production of FLG monomers larger than those of humans or mice. The anti-dog FLG antibodies raised in this study identified FLG in dog skin. These antibodies will enable us to screen FLG-deficient dogs with canine atopic dermatitis or ichthyosis.

Introduction

Filaggrin (FLG) is known to be a key protein for skin barrier formation. Filaggrin is translated as a large precursor protein, proFLG, which consists of tandem FLG monomer repeats. Each FLG monomer repeat is then processed to generate the FLG monomer in keratohyalin granules in the stratum granulosum of the epidermis. Filaggrin monomer proteins function in keratin filament aggregation in the stratum corneum (SC)[1] and are degraded to natural moisturizing factors during SC differentiation, which play an important role in skin hydration.[2]

Recently, it was reported that *FLG* gene mutations cause ichthyosis vulgaris in humans, which is characterized as a 'dry and scaly' phenotypic keratinization disorder.[3] A strong association between *FLG* gene mutations and atopic dermatitis (AD) has been reported in Irish and other human populations, indicating that skin barrier dysfunction caused by *FLG* mutations represents a strong predisposing factor for AD.[4]

Similarity in the pathogenesis and clinical manifestation between human and canine AD (cAD) has been reported.[5,6] Furthermore, genetic inheritance of AD was also reported in both species.[7] It is important to validate whether skin barrier impairment caused by a *FLG* gene mutation is associated with cAD, as shown in human AD.

The gene structure and protein architecture of FLG has been reported in humans and mice.[8,9] These studies showed that N-terminal and C-terminal regions of proFLG were conserved but the number and length of the FLG monomers differed between humans and mice. [8,9] It has been suggested that amino acid sequences of FLG monomers are highly variable in mammals. The aim of this study was to determine the FLG repeat structure of the canine *FLG* gene and to evaluate whether the deduced proFLG sequence differs from the human and mouse FLG sequence. Moreover, we raised anti-dog FLG antibodies

Accepted 12 July 2012
Sources of Funding: This work was supported in part by a grant from the Ministry of Health, Labour and Welfare of Japan (Research for Intractable Diseases) and the Global COE Program for *in vivo* Human Metabolomic Systems Biology from the Ministry of Education, Culture, Sports, Science and Technology (MEXT) of Japan.
Conflict of Interest: No conflicts of interest have been declared.

against a synthetic peptide design based on the canine FLG monomer sequence predicted in this study. These novel anti-dog FLG antibodies were used to examine the expression pattern of FLG proteins in dog skin.

Materials and methods

Canine *FLG* genomic DNA sequence

The DNA sequence of the canine *FLG* gene was obtained from the database (http://asia.ensembl.org/index.html) that is based on the whole genome shotgun assembly CanFam2.0.[10] Dot-matrix analysis by the dotter program[11] was used to find repeated *FLG* sequences in the canine *FLG* gene sequence. The multiple sequence alignment program Clustalx[12] was used for FLG comparison analysis. Sequence data of human *FLG* gene (NM_002016) and mouse *Flg* gene[13] were used for comparison with the canine *FLG* gene sequence.

Animals

Three healthy laboratory beagle dogs were used for skin biopsy, two for histopathology and one for protein extract, and a healthy laboratory beagle dog was used for tape stripping (TS) in this study. A neonatal mouse (C57BL/6J strain) was used for protein extraction from skin. All animal experiments performed were approved by Keio University Ethics Committee for Animal Experiments and the animal research committee at Tokyo University of Agriculture and Technology.

Antibodies

Rabbit anti-dog FLG sera were prepared by immunizing New Zealand white rabbits with a synthetic peptide with amino acid sequence SRHSRTGHGSGNSKHR, which is located in the FLG monomer and corresponds to amino acid residues 998–1013, 1547–1562, 2096–2111 and 2603–2618 in canine proFLG. For western blotting, the IgG fraction was affinity purified using HiTrap™ Protein G HP (GE Healthcare, Uppsala, Sweden). For immunohistochemistry (IHC), the anti-dog FLG antibodies were affinity purified using antigen peptide and HiTrap™ NHS-activated HP (GE Healthcare).

Skin biopsy for histopathology and protein extraction

Six-millimetre-diameter punch biopsy specimens were obtained from the footpad, dorsal neck and axillae of healthy beagle dogs for histopathological examination and protein extraction. Samples for histopathology were fixed in 10% neutral buffered formalin and embedded in paraffin.

The protein samples for western blotting were extracted from the skin of a healthy beagle dog and a neonatal mouse (C57BL/6J strain). Skin extracts from the dog and the mouse were chopped and sonicated in sodium dodecyl sulfate (SDS) sample buffer [2% SDS, 0.125 mol/L Tris–HCl (pH 6.8), 10% glycerol, 0.005% bromophenol blue and 5% 2-mercaptoethanol], boiled at 95°C for 5–10 min, and then centrifuged at 20,400***g*** for 10 min to collect the supernatant.

Western blotting

The extracted proteins were separated on 5–12% SDS–polyacrylamide gels and then transferred to Immobilon-P (Millipore, Billerica, MA, USA). Blots were probed with polyclonal rabbit anti-mouse FLG antibodies (Covance, Berkeley, CA, USA) diluted 1:6000 with phosphate-buffered saline (PBS; 137 mmol/L NaCl, 8.1 mmol/L Na_2HPO_4, 2.7 mmol/L KCl and 1.47 mmol/L KH_2PO_4) or polyclonal rabbit anti-dog FLG antibodies diluted 1:1000 with PBS and incubated overnight at 4°C. Immunoreactive proteins were detected in a second reaction using horseradish peroxidase-conjugated anti-rabbit immunoglobulin antibodies (Dako, Glostrup, Denmark) diluted 1:10,000 with PBS, incubated for 1 h at 25°C and visualized with ECL Plus western blotting detection reagents (GE Healthcare, Little Chalfont, UK).

Immunohistochemistry

Formalin-fixed and paraffin-embedded specimens were deparaffinized and then the antigen was retrieved by microwaving for 20 min in HistoVT One (Nacalai tesque, Kyoto, Japan). The slides were blocked with 10% goat serum and incubated with polyclonal anti-dog FLG rabbit antibodies diluted 1:200 with PBS overnight at 4°C. Incubation with secondary antibodies using Histofine SAB-PO (MULTI) (Nichirei Biosciences, Tokyo, Japan) was performed for 1 h at 25°C. The Histofine DAB (3,3′-Diaminobenzoide) substrate (Nichirei Biosciences) was used for the visualization of the immunolabelling, and slides were counterstained with haematoxylin.

Tape stripping and sample extraction

Skin biopsy samples were collected before and after 20 consecutive TS using PPS 625-25 (Nichiban, Tokyo, Japan) to collect the SC from a healthy beagle dog. The protein was extracted from each of 1–5, 6–10, 11–15 and 16–20 consecutive stripped tapes. Tapes were washed and boiled with SDS sample buffer, and then centrifuged as described above. Haematoxylin and eosin staining of skin biopsy specimens from samples collected before and after TS were performed to confirm the remaining amount of SC.

The extracted proteins from TS were separated on 10% SDS–polyacrylamide gels and transferred as described above. The blots were probed with polyclonal rabbit anti-dog FLG antibodies diluted 1:1000 with PBS or monoclonal mouse anti-pancytokeratin (clone AE1/AE3) antibodies (Thermo Fisher Scientific, Rockford, IL, USA) diluted 1:6000 with PBS. Immunoreactive proteins were detected using secondary antibodies and visualized as described above.

Results

Canine *FLG* sequence analysis

The canine *FLG* genomic DNA sequence in whole genome shotgun assembly (CamFam2.0)[10] indicated that the epidermal differential complex (EDC) containing *FLG* was located on chromosome 17 in the canine genome. To distinguish the *FLG* gene from a *FLG*-like gene in EDC, we compared the order and direction of canine EDC genes with human and mouse genes. These analyses indicated that the order and direction of EDC genes are mostly conserved among humans, mice and dogs;[14,15] therefore, we considered the canine *FLG* gene found in whole genome shotgun (CanFam2.0) to be a canine orthologue of the *FLG* gene (Figure 1a) and used this sequence for further analysis.

In order to analyse the canine *FLG* repeat structure, an open reading frame sequence of proFLG from exon 2 and exon 3 was self-compared using the dot-matrix analysis. A repeated structure in the FLG coding sequence emerged from this analysis (see Figure S1). For detailed analysis, one of the FLG repeats was compared with the open reading frame by dot-matrix analysis. Four units of FLG repeat, which consisted of three 1647 bp FLG repeats and one 1521 bp FLG repeat, flanked by two incomplete repeats, were found (Figure 1b). The predicted canine proFLG consisted of 2882 amino acids, including three full near-identical repeats of a 549 amino acid FLG monomer and one shorter repeat of a 507 amino acid FLG monomer, flanked by two incomplete, truncated FLG sequences (Figure 1c).

The whole architecture of the canine proFLG was similar to that of humans and mice. We then compared the canine proFLG protein sequence with those of humans and mice. The N-terminal 92 amino acid sequence showed high similarity among humans, mice and dogs, although the rest of the N-terminal region showed lower similarity and a difference in length (Table 1 and Figure 2a).

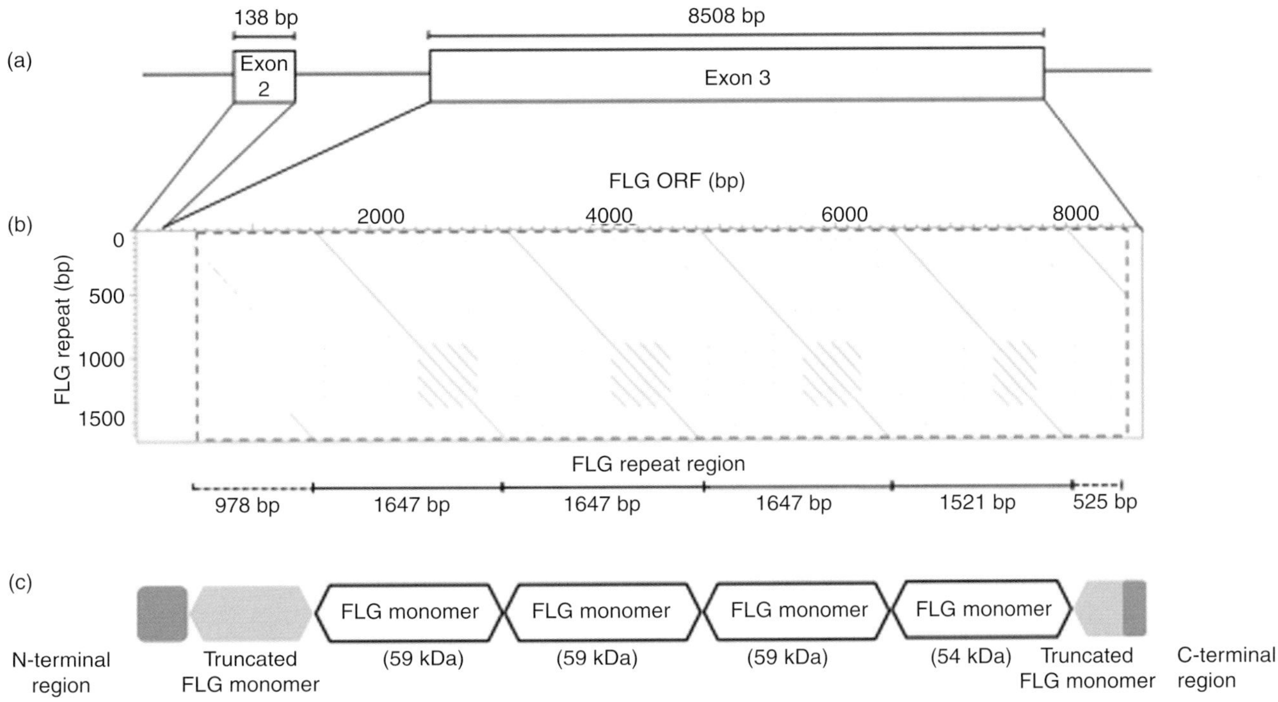

Figure 1. Features of canine filaggrin (*FLG*) gene and protein. (a) Deduced structure of canine *FLG* gene. The *FLG* gene consists of three exons in humans and mice. Unidentified exon 1 of canine FLG was assumed to be a noncoding exon, similar to the human and mouse genes. (b) The dot-matrix analysis between the canine proFLG coding sequence and the FLG repeat 1 sequence. Canine proFLG has four FLG repeats flanked by two truncated FLG repeats. (c) Structure of proFLG protein. Profilaggrin consists of an N-terminal region, four units of FLG monomers flanked by two truncated FLGs, and a C-terminal region. Abbreviation: ORF, open reading frame.

Comparison of the amino acid sequence of the canine FLG monomer with mouse and human FLG showed differences in length and limited similarity between humans, mice and dogs (Table 1 and Figure 2b).

The putative canine linker sequence that undergoes proteolytic cleavage during the processing of proFLG to FLG and extends over both ends of the FLG monomer sequence also showed low but significant similarity with those of humans[16] and mice[17] (Figure 2b). This linker sequence, preserved in the dog, divided the canine proFLG into four FLG monomers, which was consistent with the number of FLG monomers predicted by self dot-matrix analysis (see Figure S1). Alignment of the C-terminal region of proFLG revealed that the sequence was conserved between humans and mice, but was not conserved in dogs (Figure 2c). Although we identified a canine DNA sequence that showed partial similarity to the mouse DNA sequence encoding the conserved C-terminal sequence, this sequence was located downstream of the open reading frame in the canine *FLG* gene (Figure 2d,e).

Expression pattern and localization of canine FLG by western blot and IHC

Based on the canine FLG sequence analysis, we raised polyclonal anti-dog FLG antibodies that recognized peptides within the canine FLG monomer, with the goal of evaluating the expression and localization of FLG in dog skin. Proteins extracted from healthy beagle dog skin were analysed by western blot using anti-dog FLG antibodies. Two distinct bands of 59 and 54 kDa in size were detected, which corresponded to the predicted size of FLG monomers (Figure 3a). Western blot using anti-mouse FLG antibodies detected mouse FLG of 30 kDa in size (Figure 3b; lane 1), but did not detect canine FLG with the estimated size (Figure 3b; lane 2).

The localization and expression pattern of the FLG protein in dog skin obtained from the footpad, dorsal neck and axilla of healthy beagle dogs was analysed by IHC using the anti-dog FLG antibodies. The IHC showed a granular, cytoplasmic staining pattern in the stratum granulosum of the footpad (Figure 4a), dorsal neck (Figure 4b) and axilla (Figure 4c) skin of a healthy

Table 1. Comparison of profilaggrin protein structure among humans, mice and dogs

Species	N-Terminal region (aa)	FLG repeat unit (aa)	Number of FLG repeat units	C-Terminal region (aa)	ProFLG (aa)
Human	292	324–325	10–12	157	4062*
Dog	188	507–549	4	39	2882
Mouse†	283	246–255	17†	26	4658

Abbreviations: aa, amino acid; and FLG, filaggrin.
*Allele with 10 units of FLG repeats.
†C57BL/6J mouse.

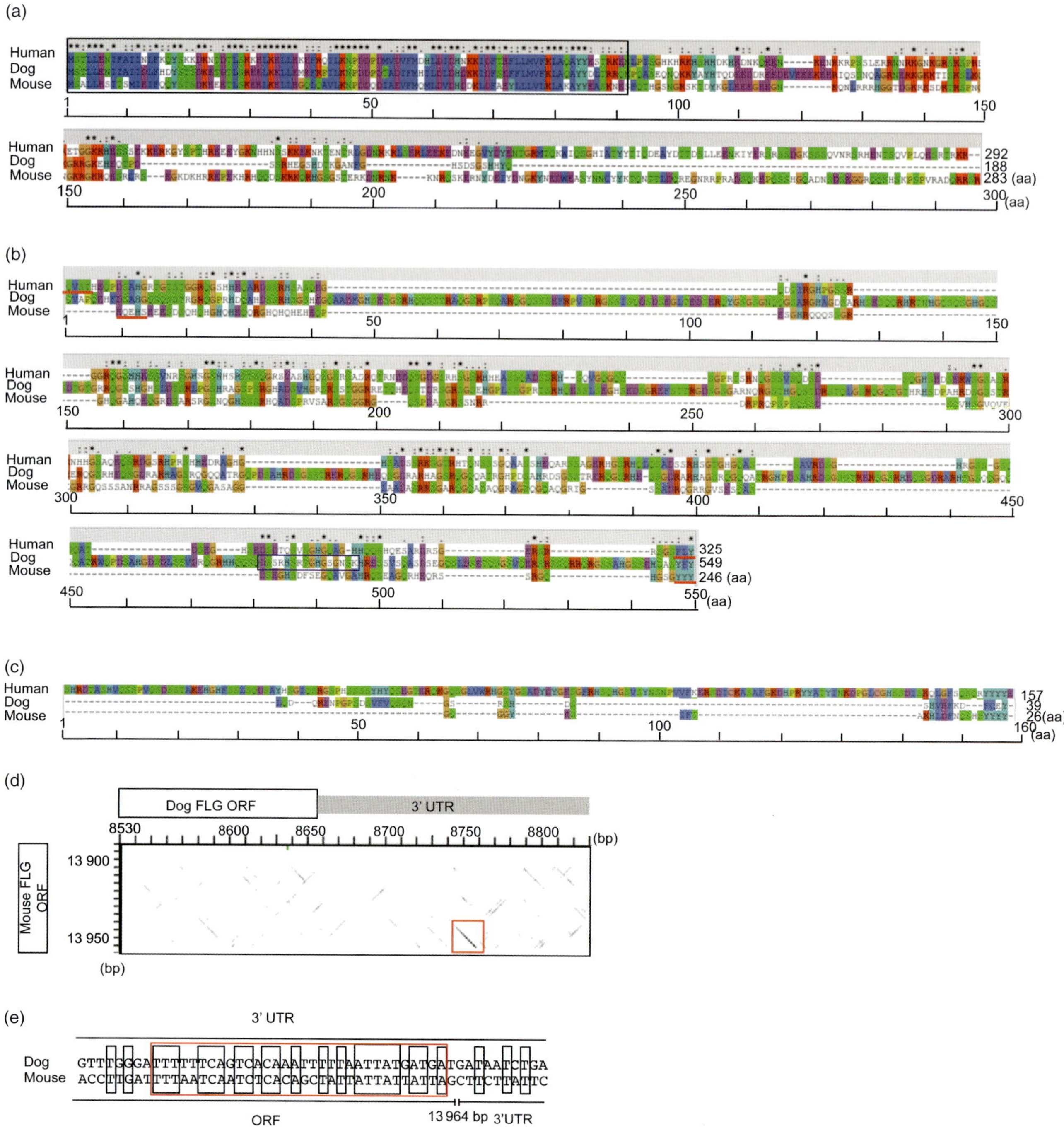

Figure 2. Similarity of amino acid (aa) and nucleotide sequences of profilaggrin (proFLG) among humans, mice and dogs. (a) Alignment of the N-terminal region of proFLG protein among humans, mice and dogs. The 92 amino acid residues in the box are highly conserved. (b) Alignment of FLG monomer among humans, mice and dogs. The antigen peptide for anti-dog FLG antibodies is boxed. The linker sequences of humans and mice are underlined in red. (c) Alignment of FLG C-terminal region among humans, mice and dogs. The amino acid sequence at the end of the C-terminal region is conserved between humans and mice, but few amino acids are conserved between dogs and humans or mice. (d) Dot-matrix analysis comparing the DNA sequence of the mouse and dog FLG C-terminal region. A short DNA sequence conserved between mice and dogs is shown in the red box. (e) Alignment of the dog and mouse DNA sequences that showed similarity in (d). Identical bases are boxed, and the most similar sequences (21 of 32 bases are identical) are in the red box.

dog, which is equivalent to keratohyalin granules. Anti-dog FLG antibodies stained SC in the dorsal neck (Figure 4b) and axilla (Figure 4c) skin but not in the footpad (Figure 4a) by IHC.

Localization of FLG in the SC was further confirmed by western blotting. Tape stripping (TS) was performed to obtain proteins from the SC, and proteins were analysed by western blotting using anti-dog FLG antibodies. Western blot revealed bands of same size as those of FLG in the epidermis shown in Figure 3a (Figure 5a). Skin samples stained with haematoxylin and eosin taken before and after TS confirmed that the SC layer was removed by TS and that the remainder of the epidermal layer cells seemed normal (Figure 5b,c).

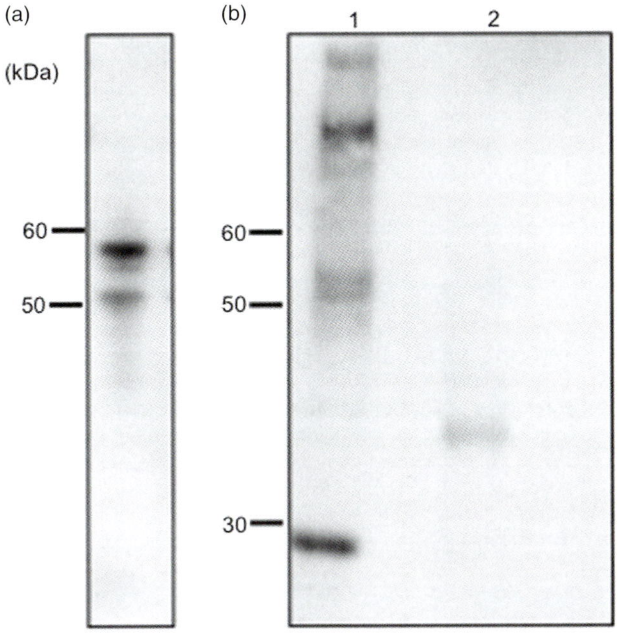

Figure 3. Western blot using anti-dog filaggrin (FLG) antibodies or anti-mouse FLG antibodies. (a) Western blotting probed with anti-dog FLG antibodies. Bands of 59 and 54 kDa in size were detected in protein extracted from dog skin. (b) Western blotting probed with polyclonal anti-mouse FLG antibodies. A band of 30 kDa in size was detected in protein extracted from mouse epidermis (lane 1). A weak, fuzzy band between the 30 and 50 kDa markers was detected in protein extracted from dog skin (lane 2); however, it was considered to be a nonspecific band because the size of the band was not consistent with those of canine FLG bands (59 and 54 kDa; a).

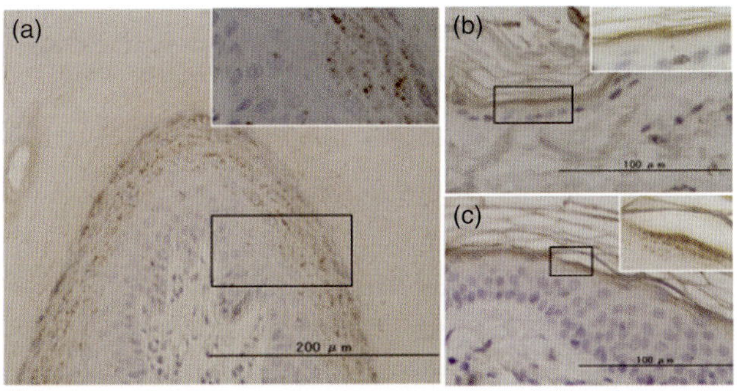

Figure 4. Localization of filaggrin (FLG) in the dog epidermis by immunohistochemistry. Anti-dog FLG antibodies stained the stratum granulosum of the footpad (a), dorsal neck (b) and axilla (c) skin in a granular, cytoplasmic staining pattern. The stratum corneum is stained in the dorsal neck (b) and axillae (c).

Discussion

The *FLG* gene structure and proFLG architecture has been reported in humans and mice. Those reports described its unique structure, containing multiple FLG repeat units.[8,9] In the present study, we found that canine proFLG was composed of four units of FLG, which are repeated and flanked by two partial FLG repeats. The number and size of the canine FLG monomers differed from those of humans and mice.

We were surprised that the canine proFLG consisted of only four FLG monomers, in comparison with the human FLG, which contains 10–12,[16,18,19] and mouse FLG,

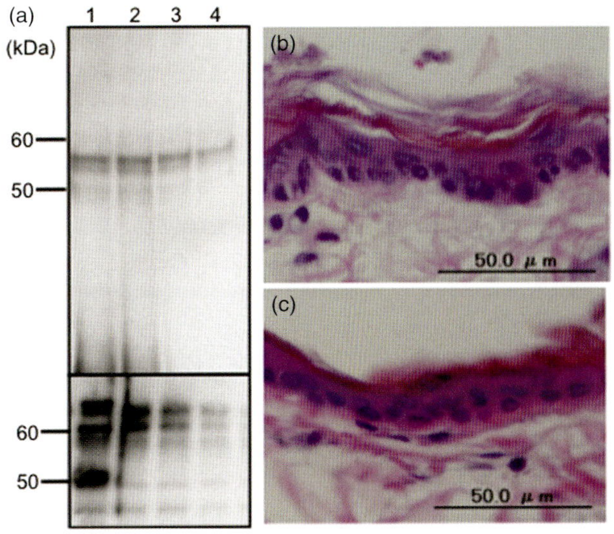

Figure 5. Western blotting analysis of filaggrin (FLG) monomers in protein extracts from stratum corneum (SC) collected by tape stripping (TS). (a) Protein extracts from 20 consecutive TSs (TS 1–5, lane 1; TS 6–10, lane 2; TS 11–15, lane 3; and TS 16–20, lane 4) were analysed by western blotting (top panel). Anti-dog FLG antibodies detected bands of the same size as the ones detected in the dog skin (Figure 3a). Keratin1/10 staining of a duplicate blot was performed as a loading control (bottom panel). A skin biopsy was obtained before TS (b) and after 20 consecutive TSs (c). Haematoxylin and eosin staining.

which has 16 or 17 repeats.[13] Although the relation between the skin barrier function and the number of FLG monomers in different species is not certain, it has been reported that the number of FLG monomers contributes to the risk of AD in humans;[19] therefore, research on the possible variation in the number of FLG monomers in the canine *FLG* gene and its correlation with cAD will be interesting.

We also analysed the similarity in the amino acid sequence of the FLG monomer of humans, mice and dogs, which might reflect the common function of FLG in these three species. The composition of amino acids in the canine FLG monomer was compared with those of humans and mice and revealed that the percentages of major amino acids, such as serine, glycine, arginine, glutamine and histidine, were conserved among these species (Table S1). With this result, we hypothesized that the composition, rather than the sequence, of amino acids of FLG might be important for the function of the FLG monomer.

The sequence analysis of proFLG identified a highly conserved N-terminal region. In previous studies, the function of the N-terminal region has been analysed, and it has been determined to possess a calcium-binding domain, known as EF-hands, that is associated with the proteolytic process.[9,20]

It has been hypothesized that the C-terminal region of proFLG plays an important role in proper processing of proFLG to FLG because a patient with a nonsense mutation (Lys4021Ter) in the truncated FLG repeat near the C-terminal end had reduced FLG and keratohyalin granules in the epidermis.[21] In the present study, although the length of the C-terminal region of human, dog and mouse were different from each other, the

C-terminal sequence was conserved between human and mouse; however, this conserved sequence was not found in the C-terminal region of the dog. Interestingly, we found a short canine DNA sequence downstream of the open reading frame, which showed similarity to the mouse DNA sequence encoding the conserved C-terminal sequence (Figure 2d,e). These results suggest that dogs have lost this conserved C-terminal sequence in an evolutionary process. It is unlikely that the conserved C-terminal sequence is essential for the proper processing of proFLG in mammals, because we found FLG monomers that were generated through proper processing of canine proFLG in dog skin. Although we could not identify any sequence conserved among the three species in the C-terminal region of proFLG, it is possible to assume that a motif which consists of only a few amino acids is essential for processing of proFLG or a processing signal is located in the truncated FLG domain that was disrupted by the Lys4021Ter mutation.

Based on the data from the detailed sequence analysis of proFLG, we raised polyclonal antibodies against the canine FLG monomer. Western blotting using these novel anti-dog FLG antibodies detected two bands at 59 and 54 kDa, which correspond to the size of the FLG monomer predicted by the sequence analysis. Anti-dog FLG antibodies stained the stratum granulosum with a granular pattern by IHC. This finding is in keeping with the location of the FLG protein reported in humans[3] and mice.[13] We therefore assumed that the antibodies successfully detected keratohyalin granules that contained FLG. The antibodies also stained SC in dorsal neck and axilla, but not in footpad, by IHC. We hypothesize that keratin filaments are tightly packed with FLG monomers in the thick SC of the footpad and that these attributes change the conformation of SC, making it unlike that of the epidermis of the dorsal neck or axilla. This could explain the inability of the antibodies to detect the FLG monomers in the footpad SC.

The expression pattern of FLG in canine skin and cAD had previously been evaluated by IHC with commercial polyclonal anti-mouse FLG antibodies.[22,23] Although these data imply a correlation between FLG deficiency and cAD, the implied mutation of the *FLG* gene has not yet been detected.

We raised antibodies that recognize the amino acid sequence of the canine FLG monomer to evaluate the canine FLG expression pattern in dog skin. The results of this study support that these anti-dog FLG antibodies detect canine FLG correctly by IHC and western blotting. The antibodies raised in this study will be useful for screening FLG-deficient dogs with cAD or ichthyosis by IHC and western blotting.

Acknowledgements

The authors thank Mie Furuhashi for excellent technical assistance.

References

1. Manabe M, Sanchez M, Sun TT *et al.* Interaction of filaggrin with keratin filaments during advanced stages of normal human epidermal differentiation and in ichthyosis vulgaris. *Differentiation* 1991; 48: 43–50.
2. Rawlings AV, Harding CR. Moisturization and skin barrier function. *Dermatol Ther* 2004; 17(Suppl 1): 43–48.
3. Smith FJ, Irvine AD, Terron-Kwiatkowski A *et al.* Loss-of-function mutations in the gene encoding filaggrin cause ichthyosis vulgaris. *Nat Genet* 2006; 38: 337–342.
4. Sandilands A, Terron-Kwiatkowski A, Hull PR *et al.* Comprehensive analysis of the gene encoding filaggrin uncovers prevalent and rare mutations in ichthyosis vulgaris and atopic eczema. *Nat Genet* 2007; 39: 650–654.
5. Marsella R, Girolomoni G. Canine models of atopic dermatitis: a useful tool with untapped potential. *J Invest Dermatol* 2009; 129: 2351–2357.
6. Terada Y, Nagata M, Murayama N *et al.* Clinical comparison of human and canine atopic dermatitis using human diagnostic criteria (Japanese Dermatological Association, 2009): proposal of provisional diagnostic criteria for canine atopic dermatitis. *J Dermatol* 2011; 38: 784–790.
7. Sousa CA, Marsella R. The ACVD task force on canine atopic dermatitis (II): genetic factors. *Vet Immunol Immunopathol* 2001; 81: 153–157.
8. Presland RB, Haydock PV, Fleckman P *et al.* Characterization of the human epidermal profilaggrin gene. Genomic organization and identification of an S-100-like calcium binding domain at the amino terminus. *J Biol Chem* 1992; 267: 23772–23781.
9. Zhang D, Karunaratne S, Kessler M *et al.* Characterization of mouse profilaggrin: evidence for nuclear enlargement and translocation of the profilaggrin B-domain during epidermal differentiation. *J Invest Dermatol* 2002; 119: 905–912.
10. Lindblad-Toh K, Wade CM, Mikkelsen TS *et al.* Genome sequence, comparative analysis and haplotype structure of the domestic dog. *Nature* 2005; 438: 803–819.
11. Sonnhammer EL, Durbin R. A dot-matrix program with dynamic threshold control suited for genomic DNA and protein sequence analysis. *Gene* 1995; 167: GC1–GC10.
12. Thompson JD, Gibson TJ, Plewniak F *et al.* The CLUSTAL_X windows interface: flexible strategies for multiple sequence alignment aided by quality analysis tools. *Nucleic Acids Res* 1997; 25: 4876–4882.
13. Fallon PG, Sasaki T, Sandilands A *et al.* A homozygous frameshift mutation in the mouse *Flg* gene facilitates enhanced percutaneous allergen priming. *Nat Genet* 2009; 41: 602–608.
14. Mischke D, Korge BP, Marenholz I *et al.* Genes encoding structural proteins of epidermal cornification and S100 calcium-binding proteins form a gene complex ('epidermal differentiation complex') on human chromosome 1q21. *J Invest Dermatol* 1996; 106: 989–992.
15. Rothnagel JA, Longley MA, Bundman DS *et al.* Characterization of the mouse loricrin gene: linkage with profilaggrin and the flaky tail and soft coat mutant loci on chromosome 3. *Genomics* 1994; 23: 450–456.
16. Gan SQ, McBride OW, Idler WW *et al.* Organization, structure, and polymorphisms of the human profilaggrin gene. *Biochemistry* 1990; 29: 9432–9440.
17. Resing KA, Walsh KA, Haugen-Scofield J *et al.* Identification of proteolytic cleavage sites in the conversion of profilaggrin to filaggrin in mammalian epidermis. *J Biol Chem* 1989; 264: 1837–1845.
18. Sasaki T, Kudoh J, Ebihara T *et al.* Sequence analysis of filaggrin gene by novel shotgun method in Japanese atopic dermatitis. *J Dermatol Sci* 2008; 51: 113–120.
19. Brown SJ, Kroboth K, Sandilands A *et al.* Intragenic copy number variation within filaggrin contributes to the risk of atopic dermatitis with a dose-dependent effect. *J Invest Dermatol* 2012; 132: 98–104.
20. Pearton DJ, Dale BA, Presland RB. Functional analysis of the profilaggrin N-terminal peptide: identification of domains that regulate nuclear and cytoplasmic distribution. *J Invest Dermatol* 2002; 119: 661–669.

21. Nemoto-Hasebe I, Akiyama M, Nomura T *et al.* *FLG* mutation p.Lys4021X in the C-terminal imperfect filaggrin repeat in Japanese patients with atopic eczema. *Br J Dermatol* 2009; 161: 1387–1390.
22. Marsella R, Samuelson D, Harrington L. Immunohistochemical evaluation of filaggrin polyclonal antibodies in atopic and normal beagles. *Vet Dermatol* 2009; 20: 547–554.
23. Chervet L, Galichet A, McLean WH *et al.* Missing C-terminal filaggrin expression, NFkappaB activation and hyperproliferation identify the dog as a putative model to study epidermal dysfunction in atopic dermatitis. *Exp Dermatol* 2010; 19: e343–e346.

Supporting Information

Additional Supporting Information may be found in the online version of this article:

Figure S1. Self dot-matrix analysis of canine *FLG* gene.

Table S1. Amino acid compositions of FLG monomer.

Part 2

Immunology

To cite this article, please use DOI: 10.1111/j.1365-3164.2012.01082.x

2.1

Innate immune defense system of the skin

Maryam Afshar and Richard L. Gallo

Division of Dermatology, Department of Medicine, University of California, San Diego, 8899 University Center Lane, San Diego, CA 92122, USA

Correspondence: Richard L. Gallo, Division of Dermatology, Department of Medicine, University of California, San Diego, CA 92126, USA.
E-mail: rgallo@ucsd.edu

Background – Antimicrobial peptides (AMPs) have a pivotal role in cutaneous innate immunity. They are present in the skin of many animals, including mammals, and are both constitutively present and inducible by infection and injury.

Functions – Antimicrobial peptides exhibit antimicrobial activity against bacteria, viruses, fungi and parasites, with different potencies depending on their peptide structure. They also act as multifunctional effector molecules that influence diverse cellular processes, including cell migration, proliferation and differentiation, cytokine production, angiogenesis and wound healing. Suppressed AMP production has been associated with increased susceptibility to microbial insults and the pathogenesis of atopic dermatitis.

This review highlights recent observations on the expression and role of AMPs, particularly the AMPs cathelicidin and β-defensin, in healthy and diseased skin.

Introduction

Skin is the largest organ of the body and provides an effective immune barrier between the internal and external environment. The cutaneous immune system can be arbitrarily divided into innate and adaptive components.[1] The innate immune system of the skin is the first-line, fast, nonspecific and active mechanism against environmental toxins and invading microbes. The innate immune response is followed by acquired immune responses, particularly T- and B-cell activation and proliferation against specific antigens.[1–3]

The innate immune system of the skin is comprised of both a physical and a chemical shield. The uppermost layer of the epidermis, the stratum corneum, consists of keratinocytes tightly linked by desmosomes in a hydrophobic cellular matrix, thereby creating an anatomical barrier against irritants, allergens and shear force.[4–6] In addition to an immediate physical barrier, this intrinsic resistance system functions through chemical mediators (cytokines), specialized signalling pathways, the complement cascade, leukocytes and host defense peptides [antimicrobial peptides (AMPs)]. In particular, AMP production is a critical mechanism for immune response of the skin to cutaneous infection and injury. This review discusses the seminal role of AMPs in skin innate immunity.

Accepted 30 May 2012

Sources of Funding: M.A. is supported by a fellowship grant from the National Psoriasis Foundation. R.L.G. is supported by NIH grants R01 AR052728, R01 AI052453, R01 AI0833358, HHSN272201000020C and a Merit Award from the Veterans Administration.

Conflict of Interest: No conflicts of interest have been declared.

Antimicrobial peptides

Antimicrobial peptides are evolutionarily conserved major contributors to host innate immune defense against bacteria, viruses, fungi, parasites and tumour cells.[3,7,8] Over 1700 AMPs are currently known.[9] They have been described in plants, insects, invertebrates and vertebrates;[10] however, great variability among species exists in AMP tissue distribution, genetic make-up and regulation of expression.[11] These differences suggest that AMPs are of varying significance for each species' antimicrobial or innate immune response.[12]

Skin expression of AMPs has been demonstrated in humans[13] and many animals, including primates,[14] pigs,[15] cows,[14] sheep,[16] chickens,[17] rats,[18] horses[19] and dogs.[12] Cutaneous AMPs are constitutively present and further induced by infection or injury or both (Figure 1).[4]

In normal human skin, the main source of AMPs is the keratinocyte.[20] Synthesis of AMPs primarily occurs in the stratum granulosum; AMPs are then packaged into lamellar bodies and transported to the stratum corneum.[21] Sebocytes, mast cells and neutrophils are also important sources of AMPs in normal human skin.[20] Antimicrobial peptides are also present in skin secretions, such as saliva and sweat.[4]

Upon skin infection or injury or both, recruited neutrophils, mast cells and other leukocytes contribute to the majority of AMP production.[20] Production is triggered by activation of pattern recognition receptors, such as Toll-like receptors (TLRs), mannose receptors and helicases.[4] These receptors are activated by lipopolysaccharides from Gram-negative bacteria, lipoteichoic acid and peptidoglycans from Gram-positive bacteria, mannans from yeast and fungi, and nucleic acids from pathogens and self.[4,22] Antimicrobial peptide upregulation is a secondary response, which limits the severity of infection or injury when the primary line of defense (constitutive AMP expression) fails.[20]

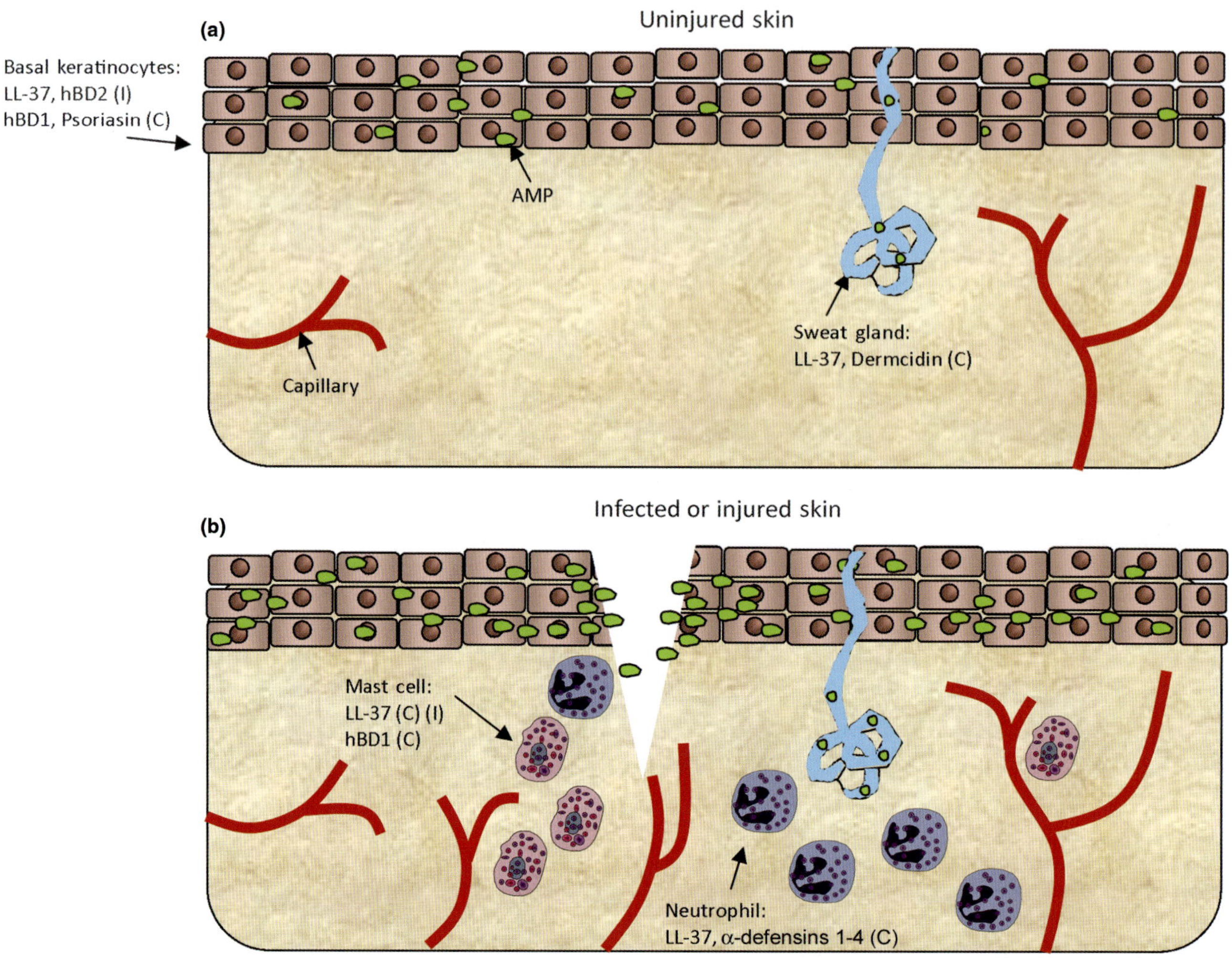

Figure 1. Antimicrobial peptide (AMP) expression in normal and infected or injured skin. (a) Normal skin is composed of an epidermal layer (keratinocytes) and a dermis containing capillaries. Keratinocytes and sweat glands produce low levels of AMPs to minimize microbial colonization. (b) Upon infection or injury, keratinocytes increase AMP production, which initiates neutrophil and mast cell recruitment to the site of injury via chemotaxis. These infiltrating leukocytes also make AMPs, and the consequent robust increase of AMPs at the injured site stimulates angiogenesis and keratinocyte proliferation to regenerate the damaged tissue. Abbreviations: C, constitutive expression; and I, inducible. (Adapted from Radek and Gallo,[26] with permission of Springer Science+Business Media.)

A major role of AMPs in innate immunity is their direct antibiotic-like inhibition of microbial pathogens. Most AMPs carry an overall net positive charge; this ensures their interaction with the negatively charged phospholipids in the cell membranes of both Gram-positive and Gram-negative bacteria, as well as the anionic components of fungi and viruses.[23,24] The peptides attach to, align with, and then insert into the microbial phospholipid bilayer.[25] As the peptides associate with the lipid head groups of the phospholipid bilayer, transmembrane 'pores' form.[25,26] The 'pores' disrupt and destabilize the bacterial cell membrane, ultimately leading to bacterial lysis.[25,26] Antimicrobial peptides preferentially target replicating bacteria, especially at the site of cell division.[27]

There are many AMPs expressed in human and animal skin. Together, they carry out a variety of functions in cutaneous host defense, ranging from influencing cell signalling to inhibiting the growth of a wide spectrum of pathogens. The expression, structures, processing, induction and antimicrobial and immunomodulatory properties vary between the peptides.[19] Cathelicidins and β-defensins are the well-characterized AMPs.[11,28,29] Key features of human cathelicidin and β-defensins are summarized in Table 1.

Table 1. Key features of human antimicrobial peptides (adapted from Izadpanah and Gallo,[40] with permission of Elsevier)

	Cathelicidins	β-Defensins
Structure	α-Helix Cathelin prodomain 37 Amino-acid peptides, other processed forms	β-Sheet Six cysteine motifs Disulfide bridges
Source	Keratinocytes, neutrophils, mast cells, lymphocytes, sweat glands	Keratinocytes, sebocytes, sweat glands
Regulation	Constitutive and inducible	Constitutive and inducible
Antimicrobial properties	Broad spectrum	Broad spectrum

Cathelicidins

Cutaneous expression

Cathelicidins were the first AMPs found in mammalian skin.[30] Since their discovery, cathelicidins have been identified in the skin of humans,[31] marsupials,[32] dogs[33] and cats.[34]

In humans, cathelicidin predominantly resides in granules of the superficial epidermis and in the extracellular spaces in the stratum corneum.[35] Likewise, in dogs, it resides in the stratum granulosum and less so in the stratum corneum.[33,36]

Structure

Only one cathelicidin is encoded by humans (LL-37), mice (CRAMP) and dogs (cCath), while multiple cathelicidins have been discovered in pigs, horses, cattle and chickens.[11,37]

The human cathelicidin gene (*CAMP*) encodes an 18 kDa α-helical precursor protein [human cathelicidin antimicrobial protein (hCAP-18)][4] that consists of an N-terminal prodomain region, cathelin, the amino-acid sequence of which is highly conserved across species.[38–40] In contrast, the C-terminal domain of hCAP-18 varies between 20 and 40 amino acids among different species; this variability contributes significantly to the broad-spectrum antimicrobial activity of cathelicidins.[26] The hCAP-18 has a 68% mRNA sequence similarity and a 57% protein sequence similarity to cCath.[36]

Peptide processing is essential for providing both the regulation and diverse biological activity of cathelicidin.[29] The full-length precursor, hCAP-18, is thought to be inactive in its immature form.[29] The hCAP-18 is commonly cleaved by serine proteases, such as kallikrein 5 and 7 in keratinocytes, and by neutrophil proteases, such as serine protease 3, to release the mature 37-amino-acid peptide that begins with two leucine residues, LL-37.[37,41–43] In sweat, LL-37 is further processed, generating KR-20, a 20-amino-acid derivative, KS-30, a 30-amino-acid derivative, and RK-31, a 31-amino-acid derivative.[44,45]

Unlike hCAP-18, processed cathelicidins demonstrate fast, potent, broad-spectrum antimicrobial activity.[26] The expression of cathelicidin as a full-length precursor that requires proteolysis for its activation allows for the stable control of its antimicrobial and proinflammatory action in the presence of particular stimuli.[26]

Induction

Infection, cutaneous injury and vitamin D_3 are all potent inducers of cathelicidin expression. LL-37 is induced by both bacterial components, such as lipopolysaccharide, and proinflammatory mediators, such as interleukin-6 and retinoic acid.[46,47] Cathelicidin expression levels are upregulated in the presence of Gram-positive bacteria.[48,49] LL-37 is induced within the epidermis during the development of verruca vulgaris.[50] Cutaneous injury induces the release of cathelicidin active against group A *Streptococcus*.[31] Vitamin D_3 can also induce hCAP-18/LL-37 expression in keratinocytes.[42]

Antimicrobial functions

Cathelicidins are potent antimicrobial agents. Cathelicidins possess an intrinsic ability to kill Gram-negative and Gram-positive bacteria, fungi and viruses.[44,46] Cathelicidin expression levels correlate with resistance to cutaneous infections.[51] The CRAMP knockout mice show increased susceptibility to skin infections with group A *Streptococcus* and vaccinia.[52] LL-37 has been shown to neutralize lipopolysaccharide endotoxin.[53]

Immunomodulatory functions

Antimicrobial peptide LL-37 interacts with mammalian cells to induce a host response by triggering inflammatory cell recruitment and cytokine release (Figure 2). LL-37 acts as a chemoattractant through binding of formyl peptide receptor-like 1, which belongs to the G_i protein-coupled receptor family.[54] LL-37 promotes the recruitment of neutrophils, T cells, mast cells and monocytes to sites of injury and infection, and stimulates angiogenesis.[54–56] LL-37 also induces histamine release from mast cells and intracellular Ca^{2+} mobilization.[57] Cathelicidin may help repair skin wounds by inducing keratinocyte migration via transactivation of the epidermal growth factor receptor.[58] LL-37 significantly inhibits the lipopolysaccharide-induced release of proinflammatory cytokines by macrophages.[59] LL-37 influences TLR signalling in immune cells, specifically by inhibiting TLR4- but not TLR2-mediated induction of dendritic cell maturation and cytokine release.[60] LL-37 also binds extracellular self-DNA fragments, enabling them to enter plasmacytoid dendritic cells, which initiates TLR9 activation to produce type I interferons.[28] LL-37 changes the expression of phagocytic receptors, significantly enhancing the ability of dendritic cells to undergo phagocytosis.[61] The immunomodulatory mechanisms of cathelicidin complements its antimicrobial properties and reinforce its role as an integral defense molecule in innate immune responses.

β-Defensins

Cutaneous expression

β-Defensins (BDs) identified in mammalian skin include human BD (hBD) 1, 2 and 3, chicken gallinacin-3, bovine lingual AMP, porcine BD2, 3, 4 and 129, equine BD2 and canine BD (cBD) 1, 2, 3, 102, 103, 122 and 127.[12,15,17,62–64] Of the cBDs, only cBD1 and cBD103 have readily detectable cutaneous expression, with cBD103 having the highest expression.[65] The cCath has a higher mRNA expression in canine skin than cBD1, 2 and 3, with a more than 358-fold expression compared with cBD2.[33] cCath mRNA expression level was followed by cBD3 and cBD1, while cBD2 was the least expressed.[33]

Canine BD1, cBD2, cBD3 and cCath fluorescence show cytoplasmic expression.[33] Canine BD2 and cBD3 are diffusely distributed throughout the epidermis.[33,36] Immunohistochemistry demonstrated cBD103 peptide in the epidermis, hair follicles and sebaceous glands comparable to hBD3 expression in human skin.[62] Equine BD2 was detected in the apocrine glands of the equine scrotal skin.[63] Skin specimens from the ventrum and dorsum of six dogs of different breeds and ages showed essentially the same cBD103 mRNA expression level when comparing skin from the different dogs, and also when comparing the dorsal or ventral surface.[65]

Structure

Defensins are low molecular weight (3–5 kDa) AMPs.[10,66] They have arginine residues and six conserved cysteine residues that form intramolecular disulfide bridges, which stabilize their triple-stranded β-sheet structure.[4] A major defensin family produced in the skin is the BD.[4]

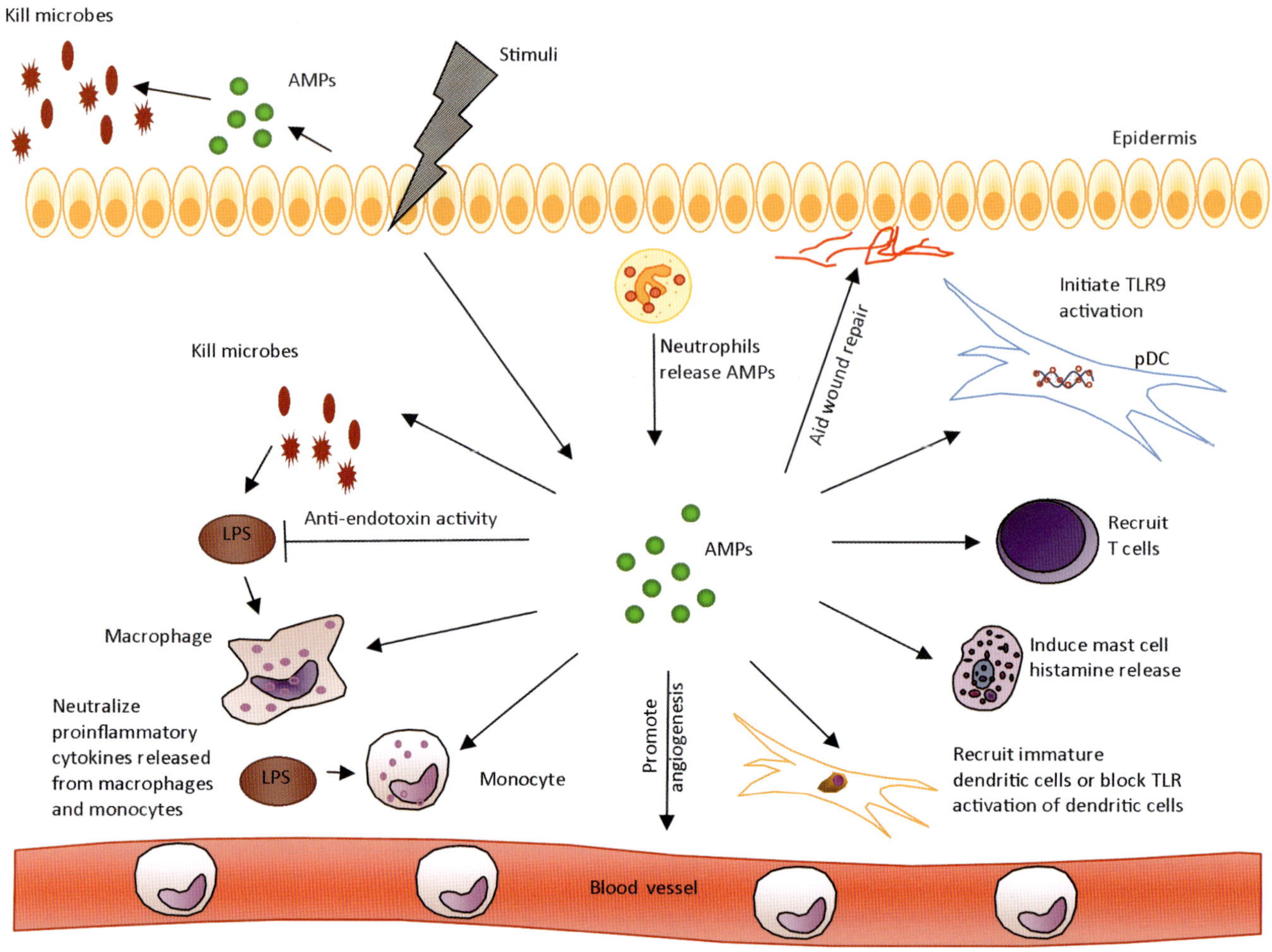

Figure 2. Several of the functions of AMPs in host defense. Antimicrobial peptides recruit leukocytes to the infection site, block or activate TLR signalling, protect against infection, control inflammation and promote wound healing. Abbreviations: AMP, antimicrobial peptide; LPS, lipopolysaccharide; pDC, plasmacytoid dendritic cell; and TLR, Toll-like receptor (adapted from Lai and Gallo,[28] with permission of Elsevier).

Human BDs have a homology of about 51–71% with the first three cBDs.[67] Based on sequence comparisons, it appears that cBD1 is an orthologue of hBD1, cBD103 of hBD3, and that cBD102 and hBD2 have no equivalent orthologues.[65] The gene encoding cBD103 demonstrates two polymorphisms: a common 3 bp deletion allele and a gene copy-number variation.[65] Golden retriever and Labrador retriever dogs encode the variant cBD103 allele, cBD103ΔG23, and the cBD103 gene copy-number polymorphism.[65]

Induction

β-Defensins are produced by keratinocytes, sebocytes and sweat glands.[68] Keratinocytes constitutively express hBD1.[4] Keratinocyte hBD2, 3 and 4 expression levels are very low at the steady state and typically are upregulated by infection, proinflammatory cytokines (e.g. tumour necrosis factor-α, interferon-γ) and injury; they then accumulate in the skin.[69–72] *Staphylococcus epidermidis*, a skin commensal bacterium, upregulates hBD2 and hBD3 expression via TLR2-induced p38 mitogen-activated protein kinase signalling.[73] Chronic wounds have a higher baseline expression of hBD2, probably maintained by ongoing tissue damage and bacterial exposure.[74] Middle- to long-chain sebum free fatty acids lauric acid, palmitic acid and oleic acid enhance the innate immune defense of the skin by inducing hBD2 in human sebocytes.[75]

Antimicrobial functions

Human BD1 exhibits minor antimicrobial activity compared with other defensins.[76,77] While hBD1 and hBD2 demonstrate strong activity against Gram-negative bacteria, such as *Escherichia coli* and *Pseudomonas aeruginosa*, neither is particularly active against Gram-positive bacteria, including *Staphylococcus aureus*.[69] Human BD3, however, has broad-spectrum activity against Gram-negative and Gram-positive bacteria, particularly *S. aureus*, and fungi.[78,79]

The activity of β-defensins against infections has also been studied in canine skin. Recombinant cBD103 and cBD103ΔG23 exhibited potent and similar antimicrobial killing of both meticillin-susceptible and meticillin-resistant *Staphyococcus pseudintermedius*.[65] Both sets of canine BDs showed potent antimicrobial activity against endogenous bacteria found on canine skin (*Bacillus licheniformis*, *Micrococcus* spp. and *Bacillus cereus*), in addition to a laboratory strain of *Escherichia coli* D31.[65]

Immunomodulatory functions

In addition to antimicrobial defense, BDs also exhibit diverse immunomodulatory roles (Figure 2). hBD2 promotes histamine secretion from mast cells, suggesting a role for hBD2 in the allergic pathway.[80] Human BD2 is chemotactic for immature dendritic cells and memory T cells.[81] Human BD2, hBD3 and hBD4 stimulate keratinocytes to increase their gene expression of many proinflammatory cytokines, chemokines and proteins, including interleukin-6, interleukin-10, monocyte chemoattractant protein-1 and macrophage chemoattractant protein-1.[82] Human BDs also elicit intracellular Ca^{2+} mobilization and participate in wound repair by increasing keratinocyte migration and proliferation.[82] Of note, a mutation of a BD in dogs has been associated with coat colour.[83] This observation underscores the pleiotropic and sometimes unexpected functions of AMPs.

Dermcidin

The AMP dermcidin is constitutively expressed as a small precursor protein in eccrine sweat glands.[84] Dermcidin is secreted into sweat, where it is activated through proteolysis.[84] In contrast to most AMPs, dermcidin-derived AMPs do not induce pore formation on the bacterial cell membrane;[85] however, they do bind to unidentified targets on the bacterial cell envelope, leading to decreased RNA and protein synthesis.[85] Dermcidin exhibits antimicrobial activity against *S. aureus*, *E. coli* and *Candida albicans*.[84]

Psoriasin

Psoriasin is an AMP in the skin of humans, cows and horses.[19,86] It is the most hydrophobic epidermal AMP.[87] Psoriasin may be secreted with sebum lipids; large amounts accumulate in sebaceous glands and the epidermis of sebaceous skin.[87] Psoriasin expression is upregulated in keratinocytes *in vivo* and *in vitro* after *E. coli* challenge.[87]

Antimicrobial peptide production in atopic dermatitis

Atopic dermatitis, an inflammatory pruritic skin disease, occurs in humans, horses,[88] cats[89] and dogs.[90] Canine atopic dermatitis, which affects approximately 10% of all dogs, has an immunopathogenesis comparable to that of human atopic dermatitis.[62] Similar to their human atopic counterparts, who have high rates of secondary recurrent *S. aureus* and *Malassezia* spp. infections,[91] there are high rates of *S. pseudintermedius* and *M. pachydermatis* superinfections in canine atopic skin.[90] These cutaneous superinfections complicate management and further compromise the integrity of the skin barrier, and may be due in part to abnormally low AMP levels.

In humans, atopic dermatitis skin has significantly lower AMP expression than psoriatic skin, even though both disorders are associated with inflammation and a defective cutaneous barrier.[51] This defect has been attributed to AMP suppression by elevated levels of T-helper 2 cytokines interleukin-4 and interleukin-13 in atopic dermatitis.[69,70] Lower AMP levels create a diminished antimicrobial barrier, and consequently, an increased susceptibility to *S. aureus* and other microbial superinfections in atopic dermatitis patients.[51,92,93] A history of eczema herpeticum is associated with the inability to induce hBD2, hBD3 and cathelicidin in the skin of patients with atopic dermatitis.[94] A hBD1 polymorphism is associated with the atopic dermatitis phenotype.[95]

The expression levels of cBD1, cBD2, cBD3 and cCath are increased in canine lesional and nonlesional atopic skin compared with the skin of healthy dogs.[36,62] Canine lesional skin cBD1 expression was 12-fold higher, and nonlesional skin cBD1 expression fivefold higher, than cBD1 expression in the skin of healthy control dogs.[62] No comparison between expression in atopic lesional skin and lesional skin of normal dogs with inflammation by scratch or wound injury was made; therefore, it is unclear whether the atopic milieu also suppressed induction of these AMPs in dogs. Furthermore, data on cBD103 expression are conflicting. Expression of cBD103 has been found to be both twofold downregulated[62] and similar [65] in atopic dogs compared with healthy dogs. Expression of cBD103 was comparable at lesional and nonlesional sites.[65] The increased cBD1, cBD2, cBD3 and cCath expression and similar or decreased cBD103 expression in the skin of atopic dogs suggests that their canine cutaneous innate immune system may be altered.[36,62] Whether this partly explains the recurrent secondary bacterial infections in dogs with atopic dermatitis requires additional study. The investigation of the involvement of AMPs in the pathogenesis of atopic dermatitis in animals is complicated by multiple confounding factors, such as different breeds, living conditions and diet.[36] The functional role of AMPs in atopic dermatitis, especially with regard to susceptibility to recurrent superinfections, requires further analysis.

Conclusion

Antimicrobial peptides constitute an evolutionarily conserved defense system that is an important component of cutaneous innate immunity. These peptides have antimicrobial and immunomodulatory effects, many of which have only recently been defined, and which influence both the immediate defense response and the slower adaptive and repair processes. As these peptides continue to be investigated, their precise function and relevance in skin and its pathology will be better defined. The multiple roles of AMPs as 'natural antibiotics' and 'immune regulators' suggest that they may be promising therapeutic agents. Thus, a greater understanding of the protective properties of AMPs yields great promise for new strategies in the control of cutaneous disease.

References

1. Medzhitov R, Janeway C. Innate immunity. *N Engl J Med* 2000; 343: 338–344.
2. Fearon DT, Locksley RM. The instructive role of innate immunity in the acquired immune response. *Science* 1996; 272: 50–54.
3. Bals R. Epithelial antimicrobial peptides in host defense against infection. *Respir Res* 2000; 1: 141–150.
4. Bernard J, Gallo R. Protecting the boundary: the sentinel role of host defense peptides in the skin. *Cell Mol Life Sci* 2011; 68: 2189–2199.

5. Cork MJ, Danby SG, Vasilopoulos Y *et al.* Epidermal barrier dysfunction in atopic dermatitis. *J Invest Dermatol* 2009; 129: 1892–1908.
6. Proksch E, Brandner JM, Jensen J-M. The skin: an indispensable barrier. *Exp Dermatol* 2008; 17: 1063–1072.
7. Williams S, Brown T, Roghanian A *et al.* SLPI and elafin: one glove, many fingers. *Clin Sci (Lond)* 2006; 110: 21–35.
8. Zasloff M. Antimicrobial peptides in health and disease. *N Engl J Med* 2002; 347: 1199–1200.
9. Wang G, Epand RF, Mishra B *et al.* Decoding the functional roles of cationic side chains of the major antimicrobial region of human cathelicidin LL-37. *Antimicrob Agents Chemother* 2012; 56: 845–856.
10. Ganz T. Defensins: antimicrobial peptides of innate immunity. *Nat Rev Immunol* 2003; 3: 710–720.
11. Linde A, Ross CR, Davis EG *et al.* Innate immunity and host defense peptides in veterinary medicine. *J Vet Intern Med* 2008; 22: 247–265.
12. Wingate KV, Torres SM, Silverstein KAT *et al.* Expression of endogenous antimicrobial peptides in normal canine skin. *Vet Dermatol* 2009; 20: 19–26.
13. Ali RS, Falconer A, Ikram M *et al.* Expression of the peptide antibiotics human β defensin-1 and human β defensin-2 in normal human skin. *J Invest Dermatol* 2001; 117: 106–111.
14. Zeeuwen PLJM, Hendriks W, de Jong WW *et al.* Identification and sequence analysis of two new members of the SKALP/elafin and SPAI-2 gene family. *J Biol Chem* 1997; 272: 20471–20478.
15. Sang Y, Patil A, Zhang G *et al.* Bioinformatic and expression analysis of novel porcine β-defensins. *Mamm Genome* 2006; 17: 332–339.
16. Brown T, Mistry R, Gray R *et al.* Characterization of the ovine ortholog of secretory leukoprotease inhibitor. *Mamm Genome* 2005; 16: 621–630.
17. Zhao C, Nguyen T, Liu L *et al.* Gallinacin-3, an inducible epithelial β-defensin in the chicken. *Infect Immun* 2001; 69: 2684–2691.
18. Patil AA, Cai Y, Sang Y *et al.* Cross-species analysis of the mammalian β-defensin gene family: presence of syntenic gene clusters and preferential expression in the male reproductive tract. *Physiol Genomics* 2005; 23: 5–17.
19. Bruhn O, Grötzinger J, Cascorbi I *et al.* Antimicrobial peptides and proteins of the horse - insights into a well-armed organism. *Vet Res* 2011; 42: 98.
20. Gallo RL, Nakatsuji T. Microbial symbiosis with the innate immune defense system of the skin. *J Invest Dermatol* 2011; 131: 1974–1980.
21. Aberg KM, Man M-Q, Gallo RL *et al.* Co-regulation and interdependence of the mammalian epidermal permeability and antimicrobial barriers. *J Invest Dermatol* 2007; 128: 917–925.
22. Janeway CA, Medzhitov R. Innate immune recognition. *Annu Rev Immunol* 2002; 20: 197–216.
23. Jenssen H, Hamill P, Hancock R. Peptide antimicrobial agents. *Clin Microbiol Rev* 2006; 19: 491–511.
24. Yeaman M, Yount N. Mechanisms of antimicrobial peptide action and resistance. *Pharmacol Rev* 2003; 55: 27–55.
25. Henzler-Wildman KA, Martinez GV, Brown MF *et al.* Perturbation of the hydrophobic core of lipid bilayers by the human antimicrobial peptide LL-37. *Biochemistry* 2004; 43: 8459–8469.
26. Radek K, Gallo R. Antimicrobial peptides: natural effectors of the innate immune system. *Semin Immunopathol* 2007; 29: 27–43.
27. Kristian SA, Timmer AM, Liu GY *et al.* Impairment of innate immune killing mechanisms by bacteriostatic antibiotics. *FASEB J* 2007; 21: 1107–1116.
28. Lai Y, Gallo RL. AMPed up immunity: how antimicrobial peptides have multiple roles in immune defense. *Trends Immunol* 2009; 30: 131–141.
29. Schauber J, Gallo RL. Antimicrobial peptides and the skin immune defense system. *J Allergy Clin Immunol* 2008; 122: 261–266.
30. Gallo RL, Ono M, Povsic T *et al.* Syndecans, cell surface heparan sulfate proteoglycans, are induced by a proline-rich antimicrobial peptide from wounds. *Proc Natl Acad Sci U S A* 1994; 8: 11035–11039.
31. Dorschner RA, Pestonjamasp VK, Tamakuwala S *et al.* Cutaneous injury induces the release of cathelicidin anti-microbial peptides active against group A *Streptococcus. J Invest Dermatol* 2001; 117: 91–97.
32. Carman RL, Old JM, Baker M *et al.* Identification and expression of a novel marsupial cathelicidin from the tammar wallaby (*Macropus eugenii*). *Vet Immunol Immunopathol* 2009; 127: 269–276.
33. Santoro D, Bunick D, Graves TK *et al.* Expression and distribution of antimicrobial peptides in the skin of healthy beagles. *Vet Dermatol* 2011; 22: 61–67.
34. Leonard BC, Chu H, Johns JL *et al.* Expression and activity of a novel cathelicidin from domestic cats. *PLoS One* 2011; 6: e18756.
35. Braff MH, Nardo AD, Gallo RL. Keratinocytes store the antimicrobial peptide cathelicidin in lamellar bodies. *J Invest Dermatol* 2005; 124: 394–400.
36. Santoro D, Marsella R, Bunick D *et al.* Expression and distribution of canine antimicrobial peptides in the skin of healthy and atopic beagles. *Vet Immunol Immunopathol* 2011; 144: 382–388.
37. Zanetti M, Gennaro R, Romeo D. Cathelicidins: a novel protein family with a common proregion and a variable C-terminal antimicrobial domain. *FEBS Lett* 1995; 374: 1–5.
38. Zaiou M, Nizet V, Gallo R. Antimicrobial and protease inhibitory functions of the human cathelicidin (hCAP18/LL-37) prosequence. *J Invest Dermatol* 2003; 120: 810–816.
39. Verbanac D, Zanetti M, Romeo D. Chemotactic and protease-inhibiting activities of antibiotic peptide precursors. *FEBS Lett* 1993; 317: 255–258.
40. Izadpanah A, Gallo RL. Antimicrobial peptides. *J Am Acad Dermatol* 2005; 52: 381–390.
41. Durr U, Sudheendra U, Ramamoorthy A. LL-37, the only human member of the cathelicidin family of antimicrobial peptides. *Biochim Biophys Acta* 2006; 1758: 1408–1425.
42. Schauber J, Dorschner RA, Yamasaki K *et al.* Control of the innate epithelial antimicrobial response is cell-type specific and dependent on relevant microenvironmental stimuli. *Immunology* 2006; 118: 509–519.
43. Dorschner RA, Lin KH, Murakami M *et al.* Neonatal skin in mice and humans expresses increased levels of antimicrobial peptides: innate immunity during development of the adaptive response. *Pediatr Res* 2003; 53: 566–572.
44. Braff MH, Hawkins MiA, Di Nardo A *et al.* Structure-function relationships among human cathelicidin peptides: dissociation of antimicrobial properties from host immunostimulatory activities. *J Immunol* 2005; 174: 4271–4278.
45. Murakami M, Lopez-Garcia B, Braff M *et al.* Postsecretory processing generates multiple cathelicidins for enhanced topical antimicrobial defense. *J Immunol* 2004; 172: 3070–3077.
46. Dorschner RA, Lopez-Garcia B, Peschel A *et al.* The mammalian ionic environment dictates microbial susceptibility to antimicrobial defense peptides. *FASEB J* 2006; 20: 35–42.
47. Frohm M, Agerberth B, Ahangari G *et al.* The expression of the gene coding for the antibacterial peptide LL-37 is induced in human keratinocytes during inflammatory disorders. *J Biol Chem* 1997; 272: 15258–15263.
48. Nagy I, Pivarcsi A, Kis K *et al. Propionibacterium acnes* and lipopolysaccharide induce the expression of antimicrobial peptides and proinflammatory cytokines/chemokines in human sebocytes. *Microbes Infect* 2006; 8: 2195–2205.
49. Lee D-Y, Yamasaki K, Rudsil J *et al.* Sebocytes express functional cathelicidin antimicrobial peptides and can act to kill *Propionibacterium acnes. J Invest Dermatol* 2008; 128: 1863–1866.
50. Conner K, Nern K, Rudisill J *et al.* The antimicrobial peptide LL-37 is expressed by keratinocytes in condyloma acuminatum and verruca vulgaris. *J Am Acad Dermatol* 2002; 47: 347–350.
51. Ong PY, Ohtake T, Brandt C *et al.* Endogenous antimicrobial peptides and skin infections in atopic dermatitis. *N Engl J Med* 2002; 347: 1151–1160.
52. Howell MD, Jones JF, Kisich KO *et al.* Selective killing of vaccinia virus by LL-37: implications for eczema vaccinatum. *J Immunol* 2004; 172: 1763–1767.

53. Rosenfeld Y, Papo N, Shai Y. Endotoxin (lipopolysaccharide) neutralization by innate immunity host-defense peptides. *J Biol Chem* 2006; 281: 1636–1643.
54. Yang D, Chen Q, Schmidt AP *et al.* LL-37, the neutrophil granule- and epithelial cell-derived cathelicidin, utilizes formyl peptide receptor-like 1 (FPRL1) as a receptor to chemoattract human peripheral blood neutrophils, monocytes, and T cells. *J Exp Med* 2000; 192: 1069–1074.
55. Di Nardo A, Vitiello A, Gallo RL. Cutting edge: mast cell antimicrobial activity is mediated by expression of cathelicidin antimicrobial peptide. *J Immunol* 2003; 170: 2274–2278.
56. Koczulla R, von Degenfeld G, Kupatt C *et al.* An angiogenic role for the human peptide antibiotic LL-37/hCAP-18. *J Clin Invest* 2003; 111: 1665–1672.
57. Niyonsaba F, Someya A, Hirata M *et al.* Evaluation of the effects of peptide antibiotics human β-defensins-1/-2 and LL-37 on histamine release and prostaglandin D_2 production from mast cells. *Eur J Immunol* 2001; 31: 1066–1075.
58. Tokumaru S, Sayama K, Shirakata Y *et al.* Induction of keratinocyte migration via transactivation of the epidermal growth factor receptor by the antimicrobial peptide LL-37. *J Immunol* 2005; 175: 4662–4668.
59. Scott MG, Rosenberger CM, Gold MR *et al.* An α-helical cationic antimicrobial peptide selectively modulates macrophage responses to lipopolysaccharide and directly alters macrophage gene expression. *J Immunol* 2000; 165: 3358–3365.
60. Di Nardo A, Braff MH, Taylor KR *et al.* Cathelicidin antimicrobial peptides block dendritic cell TLR4 activation and allergic contact sensitization. *J Immunol* 2007; 178: 1829–1834.
61. Davidson DJ, Currie AJ, Reid GSD *et al.* The cationic antimicrobial peptide LL-37 modulates dendritic cell differentiation and dendritic cell-induced T cell polarization. *J Immunol* 2004; 172: 1146–1156.
62. van Damme CMM, Willemse T, van Dijk A *et al.* Altered cutaneous expression of β-defensins in dogs with atopic dermatitis. *Mol Immunol* 2009; 46: 2449–2455.
63. Yasui T, Fukui K, Nara T *et al.* Immunocytochemical localization of lysozyme and β-defensin in the apocrine glands of the equine scrotum. *Arch Dermatol Res* 2007; 299: 393–397.
64. Bagnicka E, Strzałkowska N, Jóźwik A *et al.* Expression and polymorphism of defensins in farm animals. *Acta Biochim Pol* 2010; 57: 487–497.
65. Leonard BC, Marks SL, Outerbridge CA *et al.* Activity, expression and genetic variation of canine β-defensin 103: a multifunctional antimicrobial peptide in the skin of domestic dogs. *J Innate Immun* 2012; 4: 248–259.
66. Selsted ME, Harwig SS, Ganz T *et al.* Primary structures of three human neutrophil defensins. *J Clin Invest* 1985; 76: 1436–1439.
67. Sang Y, Ortega MT, Blecha F *et al.* Molecular cloning and characterization of three β-defensins from canine testes. *Infect Immun* 2005; 73: 2611–2620.
68. Koczulla AR, Bals R. Antimicrobial peptides: current status and therapeutic potential. *Drugs* 2003; 63: 389–406.
69. Harder J, Bartels J, Christophers E *et al.* A peptide antibiotic from human skin. *Nature* 1997; 387: 861.
70. Nomura I, Goleva E, Howell MD *et al.* Cytokine milieu of atopic dermatitis, as compared to psoriasis, skin prevents induction of innate immune response genes. *J Immunol* 2003; 171: 3262–3269.
71. Gallo RL, Murakami M, Ohtake T *et al.* Biology and clinical relevance of naturally occurring antimicrobial peptides. *J Allergy Clin Immunol* 2002; 110: 823–831.
72. Froy O. Regulation of mammalian defensin expression by Toll-like receptor-dependent and independent signalling pathways. *Cell Microbiol* 2005; 7: 1387–1397.
73. Lai Y, Cogen AL, Radek KA *et al.* Activation of TLR2 by a small molecule produced by *Staphylococcus epidermidis* increases antimicrobial defense against bacterial skin infections. *J Invest Dermatol* 2010; 130: 2211–2221.
74. Butmarc J, Yufit T, Carson P *et al.* Human β-defensin-2 expression is increased in chronic wounds. *Wound Repair Regen* 2004; 12: 439–443.
75. Nakatsuji T, Kao MC, Zhang L *et al.* Sebum free fatty acids enhance the innate immune defense of human sebocytes by upregulating β-defensin-2 expression. *J Invest Dermatol* 2010; 130: 985–994.
76. Zaalouk TK, Bajaj-Elliott M, George JT *et al.* Differential regulation of β-defensin gene expression during *Cryptosporidium parvum* infection. *Infect Immun* 2004; 72: 2772–2779.
77. Yadava P, Zhang C, Sun J *et al.* Antimicrobial activities of human β-defensins against *Bacillus* species. *Int J Antimicrob Agents* 2006; 28: 132–137.
78. Kisich K, Howell M, Boguniewicz M *et al.* The constitutive capacity of human keratinocytes to kill *Staphylococcus aureus* is dependent on β-defensin 3. *J Invest Dermatol* 2007; 127: 2368–2380.
79. García J-R, Jaumann F, Schulz S *et al.* Identification of a novel, multifunctional β-defensin (human β-defensin 3) with specific antimicrobial activity. *Cell Tissue Res* 2001; 306: 257–264.
80. Befus AD, Mowat C, Gilchrist M *et al.* Neutrophil defensins induce histamine secretion from mast cells: mechanisms of action. *J Immunol* 1999; 163: 947–953.
81. Yang D, Chertov O, Bykovskaia SN *et al.* Beta-defensins: linking innate and adaptive immunity through dendritic and T cell CCR6. *Science* 1999; 286: 525–528.
82. Niyonsaba F, Ushio H, Nakano N *et al.* Antimicrobial peptides human β-defensins stimulate epidermal keratinocyte migration, proliferation and production of proinflammatory cytokines and chemokines. *J Invest Dermatol* 2007; 127: 594–604.
83. Candille SI, Kaelin CB, Cattanach BM *et al.* A β-defensin mutation causes black coat color in domestic dogs. *Science* 2007; 318: 1418–1423.
84. Schittek B, Hipfel R, Sauer B *et al.* Dermcidin: a novel human antibiotic peptide secreted by sweat glands. *Nat Immunol* 2001; 2: 1133–1137.
85. Senyurek I, Paulmann M, Sinnberg T *et al.* Dermcidin-derived peptides show a different mode of action than the cathelicidin LL-37 against *Staphylococcus aureus*. *Antimicrob Agents Chemother* 2009; 53: 2499–2509.
86. Regenhard P, Petzl W, Zerbe H *et al.* The antibacterial psoriasin is induced by *E. coli* infection in the bovine udder. *Vet Microbiol* 2010; 143: 293–298.
87. Glaser R, Harder J, Lange H *et al.* Antimicrobial psoriasin (S100A7) protects human skin from *Escherichia coli* infection. *Nat Immunol* 2004; 6: 57–64.
88. White SD. Advances in equine atopic dermatitis, serologic and intradermal allergy testing. *Clin Tech Equine Pract* 2005; 4: 311–313.
89. Reedy LM. Results of allergy testing and hyposensitization in selected feline skin diseases. *J Am Anim Hosp Assoc* 1982; 18: 618–623.
90. Olivry T, Sousa CA. The ACVD task force on canine atopic dermatitis (XIX): general principles of therapy. *Vet Immunol Immunopathol* 2001; 81: 311–316.
91. Leung DYM, Boguniewicz M, Howell MD *et al.* New insights into atopic dermatitis. *J Clin Invest* 2004; 113: 651–657.
92. Howell MD, Gallo RL, Boguniewicz M *et al.* Cytokine milieu of atopic dermatitis skin subverts the innate immune response to vaccinia virus. *Immunity* 2006; 24: 341–348.
93. Howell MD, Wollenberg A, Gallo RL *et al.* Cathelicidin deficiency predisposes to eczema herpeticum. *J Allergy Clin Immunol* 2006; 117: 836–841.
94. Hata TR, Kotol P, Boguniewicz M *et al.* History of eczema herpeticum is associated with the inability to induce human β-defensin (HBD)-2, HBD-3 and cathelicidin in the skin of patients with atopic dermatitis. *Br J Dermatol* 2010; 163: 659–661.
95. Prado-Montes de Oca E, García-Vargas A, Lozano-Inocencio R *et al.* Association of β-defensin 1 single nucleotide polymorphisms with atopic dermatitis. *Int Arch Allergy Immunol* 2007; 142: 211–218.

To cite this article, please use DOI: 10.1111/j.1365-3164.2012.01091.x

2.2

Evaluation of canine antimicrobial peptides in infected and noninfected chronic atopic skin

Domenico Santoro*, David Bunick†, Thomas K. Graves* and Mariangela Segre‡

*Departments of Veterinary Clinical Medicine, †Comparative Biosciences and ‡Pathobiology, University of Illinois at Urbana-Champaign, Urbana, IL, USA

Correspondence: Domenico Santoro, Department of Veterinary Clinical Medicine, College of Veterinary Medicine, University of Illinois at Urbana-Champaign, Urbana, IL 61802, USA. E-mail: dsantor2@illinois.edu

Background – Antimicrobial peptides (AMPs) are small immunomodulatory peptides produced by epithelial and immune cells. β-Defensins (BDs) and cathelicidins (Caths) are the most studied AMPs. Recently, increased cutaneous expression of AMPs was reported in atopic humans and in beagles with experimentally induced atopy.

Hypothesis/Objectives – Our goal was to analyse mRNA expression and protein levels of canine (c)BD1-like, cBD2-like/122, cBD3-like, cBD103 and cCath in healthy and naturally affected atopic dogs, with and without active skin infection, along with their distribution in the epidermis using indirect immunofluorescence.

Animals – Skin biopsies were taken from 14 healthy and 11 atopic privately owned dogs.

Methods – The mRNA levels of *cBD1-like, cBD2-like/122, cBD3-like, cBD103* and *cCath* were quantified using quantitative real-time PCR. The protein levels of cBD3-like and cCath were analysed by relative competitive inhibition enzyme-linked immunosorbent assay, while the distributions of cBD2-like/122, cBD3-like and cCath were detected by indirect immunofluorescence.

Results – Dogs with atopic dermatitis had significantly greater mRNA expression of *cBD103* (P = 0.04) than control dogs. Furthermore, atopic skin with active infection had a higher *cBD103* mRNA expression (P = 0.01) and a lower *cBD1-like* mRNA expression (P = 0.04) than atopic skin without infection. No significant differences in protein levels (cBD3-like and cCath) or epidermal distribution of AMPs (cBD2-like/122, cBD3-like and cCath) were seen between healthy and atopic dogs.

Conclusions and clinical importance – Expression of *cBD103* mRNA was greater, while expression of *cBD1-like* mRNA was lower in dogs with atopic dermatitis that had active infections. Work is needed to clarify the biological mechanisms and possible therapeutic options to maintain a healthy canine skin.

Introduction

Atopic dermatitis (AD) has recently been redefined by the International Task Force on Canine Atopic Dermatitis as 'genetically predisposed inflammatory and pruritic allergic skin disease with characteristic clinical features associated with IgE antibodies most commonly directed against environmental allergens'.[1] In both humans and dogs, AD is extremely common, affecting up to 30 and 10% of the respective populations.[2,3] Recently, in both human and veterinary medicine, researchers have shown altered skin barrier integrity to be the main factor involved in the pathogenesis and predisposition to AD.[4–18] As part of the skin barrier, antimicrobial peptides (AMPs) have been studied in different species, including humans.[19–22] To date, over 1000 AMPs, subclassified based on their molecular structure, have been identified in diverse species (e.g. peptides, lipids, histones).[19,20] Of these peptides, β-defensins (BDs) and cathelicidins (Caths) have received the most research attention. Such peptides have many functions; they have antimicrobial activity against a variety of micro-organisms, are potent angioactive and chemotactic molecules, are involved in wound healing, act as potent 'host defense peptides' able to chemoattract immune cells and respond to danger signals by alerting the adaptive immune system, and they also modulate the innate and adaptive immune responses in higher organisms.[20,23–25] An increased expression of AMPs (e.g. BDs, LL-37, psoriasin and ribonuclease 7) in some human inflammatory conditions, such as AD and psoriasis, has demonstrated an involvement of such AMPs in inflammatory skin conditions.[2,26–30]

Few studies have been published on the possible involvement of AMPs in the pathogenesis of AD in dogs. In fact, only two studies have investigated the association of canine AMPs with canine AD. The first used chronically

Accepted 20 June 2012
Sources of Funding: American College of Veterinary Dermatology.
Conflict of Interest: No conflicts of interest have been declared.

naturally affected atopic dogs and the second used experimentally affected atopic beagles.[31,32] Results were similar to human studies, showing increased mRNA expression of some canine peptides (*cBD1*, *cBD1-like*, *cBD3-like* and *cCath*) in lesional and nonlesional skin of dogs with AD when compared with healthy control dogs;[31,32] however, decreased mRNA expression of *cBD103* was detected only in naturally affected atopic dogs.[31]

In the above-mentioned study,[32] particular care was taken to avoid cutaneous infections in order to reduce confounding factors. Although AMPs are known for their antimicrobial effects, their behaviour in actively infected atopic skin has not been reported. However, the presence of cutaneous infections (bacteria and yeast) is extremely common in AD compared with other skin diseases,[33–36] and a decreased production of AMPs or production of nonfunctional AMPs has been hypothesized as a possible cause of the higher susceptibility to skin infection in AD.[30]

To gain more insight into the role of AMPs in canine AD, we analysed the mRNA expression of four cBDs (*cBD1-like*, *cBD2-like/122*, *cBD3-like* and *cBD103*) and *cCath* in healthy and atopic dogs, with and without active skin infection, using a quantitative reverse transcriptase PCR (qRT-PCR). The cBDs and cCath used were selected based on previously demonstrated antimicrobial properties and presence in canine skin.[37–40] In addition, we evaluated their distribution in the epidermis using indirect immunofluorescence (IIF) and their skin protein levels using competitive inhibition enzyme-linked immunosorbent assay (ciELISA).

Material and methods

The study was approved by the Institutional Animal Care and Use Committee. All dogs entered the study with the owners' written informed consent.

Inclusion criteria

Atopic dogs.
The diagnosis of canine AD was based on compatible history, clinical findings and the exclusion of possible differential diagnoses for pruritus (e.g. scabies, demodicosis, food allergy, flea allergy) as previously reported.[41,42] In particular, for dogs with nonseasonal pruritus a strict food trial with a novel protein source for at least 10 weeks was done. When required, multiple skin scrapings were performed to rule out *Demodex* spp., and a miticidal drug trial was performed to rule out scabies. Dogs included in this group were divided in two subgroups based on the evidence of active skin infection (bacterial, *Malassezia* spp., or both). The diagnosis of infections by bacteria or yeast was based on clinical signs, history and skin cytology with evidence of inflammatory cells and bacteria, yeasts, or both. All the dogs were on commercially available diets at the time of enrolment in this study.

Healthy dogs.
Healthy control dogs were recruited from dogs presented to the Veterinary Teaching Hospital for annual vaccination or were dogs that belonged to the hospital staff. To be included in the study, the dogs had to have no history or presence of any cutaneous or systemic disease.

Exclusion criteria

All dogs.
Dogs were excluded if topical, systemic and depot glucocorticoids had been used for at least 2, 4 and 8 weeks, respectively, or if systemic or topical calcineurin inhibitors had been used for at least 4 weeks. Dogs were also excluded from the study if systemic or topical antibiotic or antifungal medications had been used for at least 2 weeks.

Atopic dogs.
Dogs with AD were excluded from the study if there was a history of administration of allergen-specific immunotherapy, or if there were other allergic conditions (e.g. food and flea allergy) or any other skin (e.g. endocrinopathies or neoplasia) or other systemic disease (e.g. parasitic, metabolic or neoplastic disease).

Healthy dogs.
Control dogs were excluded from the study if there was evidence of superficial or deep bacterial or *Malassezia* spp. infection.

Skin sample collection

Two 8 mm skin biopsy samples were obtained from abdominal skin using local anaesthesia [subcutaneous injection of 1 mL of lidocaine hydrochloride 2% (Hospira Inc., Lake Forest, IL, USA).] It was not necessary to sedate dogs for this procedure. One skin biopsy sample was immediately divided into quarters and placed in 1.5 mL microfuge tubes, quickly flash frozen in liquid nitrogen, and then stored at −80°C until processed for molecular evaluation (qRT-PCR). The other skin biopsy sample was immediately fixed in 10% neutral buffered formalin for IIF evaluation. The abdominal region was chosen for the skin biopsy site because it is an easily accessible area with low hair density and a common area involved in canine AD.

Quantitative RT-PCR

One quarter of the 8 mm skin biopsy sample was homogenized using a PowerGen 125 (Fisher Scientific, Pittsburgh, PA, USA) using the AllPrep® RNA/protein kit (Qiagen, Valencia, CA, USA) reagents and then processed into RNA according to manufacturer's protocol as described.[40] Total RNA concentrations were determined at 260 nm using UV NanoDrop1000® spectrophotometry (Thermo Scientific, Wilmington, DE, USA), and integrity and quality of the RNA was checked using an Agilent 2100 Bioanalyzer (Agilent Biotechnologies Inc., Santa Clara, CA, USA). After DNAse treatment using a Turbo DNA-free™ kit (Invitrogen, Carlsbad, CA, USA), total RNA (0.5 μg) was converted to complementary DNA (cDNA) by reverse transcription of mRNA using SuperScript First-Strand Synthesis System (Invitrogen). Sense and antisense primers for each AMP (Table 1) were generated using Primer Designer software (Scientific and Educational Software Inc., Palo Alto, CA, USA) as reported.[40] Each primer was designed to cross an exon–exon boundary, maximizing the amplification specificity of the mRNA transcript target and minimizing amplification of any residual contaminating genomic DNA. The primers were generated from previously published GenBank AMP sequences.[37–39] All primer sequences were subjected to Basic Local Alignment Search Tool (BLAST) comparison to the canine genome build 2.0 for unintended homologies. The relative mRNA expression levels were quantified using SYBR® Green (Qiagen) and ABI (Applied Biosystems Inc., Foster City, CA, USA) quantitative RT-PCR methodology. All samples were tested in triplicate 25 μL reactions in an ABI 7500 Real Time PCR System (Applied Biosystems Inc). The PCR amplifications were carried out as follows: 50°C for 2 min; 95°C for 10 min; and 40 cycles of 95°C for 15 s and 60°C for 60 s. Amplifications were followed by dissociation (melting) curves to ensure specificity of the primers. The results were analysed using the comparative C_T (cycle threshold) method, and the relative mRNA expression of each AMP was compared using the $\Delta\Delta C_T$ method. This method is effective when the amplification efficiencies of the housekeeping gene and target gene are close to 100%. When this criterion is fulfilled the formula is: $2^{-[\Delta C_T \text{ experimental sample} - \Delta C_T \text{ control sample}]}$, where ΔC_T is the difference between the target gene and the normalizer gene expression.[43] All samples were normalized against the gene for canine ribosomal protein L15 (RPLO). This gene was chosen due to the highly stable and consistent expression previously shown for ribosomal genes in canine skin.[44]

Table 1. Primers used

Canine gene	Primer sequences	Amplicon length
cBD1-like	Forward: CGAGTGGAAAACTATGCTGT Reverse: GGAATCTGCTGAGATCAGAC	129
cBD2-like/122	Forward: AGTGGGAAACTATGCTGTCT Reverse: GTGCTAAGTGTCAGAATTGC	79
cBD3-like	Forward: CAGACATAAAAACAGACACA Reverse: AGTTGACCATATAGGTGTAG	78
cCath	Forward: CACTGTTGCTACTGCTGCTG Reverse: GTTGAAGCCATTCACAGCAC	98
cBD103	Forward: ACCTTGCCATCCAGTCTCAG Reverse: GGAACAGGCATCAAGAACAG	98
RPLO	Forward: TTGTGGCTGCTGCTCCTGTG Reverse: ATCCTCGTCCGATTCCTCCG	107

Antibody preparation

Polyclonal anti-canine-AMPs were synthesized by the Immunological Resource Center at the authors' Institution.[40] Briefly, the canine anti-AMP antibodies were generated from previously published GenBank AMP sequences.[36–38] All amino acid sequences were subjected to BLAST comparison to the canine genome build 2.0 for unintended homologies. Based on the aforementioned genetic and amino acid sequences, the most immunogenic epitopes were chosen for each protein, and synthetic peptides were created. As the amino acid sequence of cBD1-like overlaps with part of both cBD2-like/122 and cBD3-like sequences, it was not possible to generate an appropriate polyclonal antibody against it. Antibody production was carried out using three female New Zealand white rabbits, 3.2–3.6 kg in weight (about 2–3 months old), purchased from Harlan Laboratories, Inc. (Indianapolis, IN, USA). The peptide conjugates were mixed with an adjuvant and subcutaneously injected into the three rabbits. Titermax (Sigma, St Louis, MO, USA) was used for the primary immunization and incomplete Freund's adjuvant for all subsequent immunizations. Rabbits were immunized four times, and their blood was tested for an immune response using an ELISA technique with pre-immune serum as the control. When a satisfactory immune response (positive up to 1:51,200 dilution) had been achieved, animals were exsanguinated and the crude sera were used. The antibodies were tested by Immunodot blotting using the synthetic peptide as antigen, resulting in a positive signal in up to a 1:10,000 dilution. In addition, to verify the specificity of the primary antibodies, the anti-cBD2-like/122, anti-cBD3-like and anti-cCath were tested by immunoabsorption, incubating each antibody with a high concentration (20 μg/μL) of the respective and other synthetic peptides overnight at 4°C before being applied to the tissue sections. An ELISA technique was also used to test possible cross-reactions with each of the peptides synthetized. Multiple attempts to generate anti-canine-cBD103 resulted in unsuitable antibodies for ELISA or IIF technique because only part of the amino acidic sequence is predicted.

Indirect immunofluorescence

One half of the 8 mm skin biopsy sample was fixed in 10% neutral buffered formalin solution for no more than 48 h and then placed in phosphate buffer solution (PBS) until processed for IIF.[40] Briefly, 3 μm sections were processed using the immunohistochemical polymer procedure. The sections were blocked using a casein solution (Power Block®; BioGenex, San Ramon, CA, USA) followed by an extra wash using normal goat serum (BioGenex) as a blocking solution. Epitope retrieval was not necessary for cBD2-like/122 and cBD3-like, whereas it was required for cCath. In the latter case, the method consisted of using boiled sections, performed at 125–130°C under 7.7–10.4 kg pressure for 30 s followed by a 10 s treatment at 90°C. The sections were then stained for 1 h at room temperature using primary polyclonal rabbit antibodies specific for cBD2-like/122, cBD3-like and cCath.[39] The primary antibodies were used at 1:200 dilution. Negative controls were established using the pre-immune serum at 1:200 dilution. The sections were washed with a blocking solution (Power Block®; BioGenex) and then incubated for 30 min at room temperature with a polyclonal goat anti-rabbit antibody bound with a green fluorochrome (Alexa Fluor® 488; Invitrogen) at 1:1000 dilution, according to the manufacturer's recommendations. Finally, DAPI (4',6-diamidino-2-phenylindole; Invitrogen) was used as a counterstain for nuclear detection. Specimens were mounted on glass slides using Vectashield® Mounting Medium (Vector laboratories; Burlingame, CA, USA). The skin sections were examined using an inverted fluorescence microscope (Nikon Eclipse TE 2000-S®; Nikon Inc., Shelton, CT, USA). The images were analysed using MetaMorph® software (version 63r1; Molecular Devices, Sunnyvale, CA, USA). Five representative fields at ×400 magnification were examined for each section, and digital images were recorded.

Relative competitive inhibition enzyme-linked immunosorbent assay

One quarter of the 8 mm skin biopsy specimen was homogenized using a PowerGen 125 (Fisher Scientific) and then the proteins were extracted using the AllPrep® RNA/protein kit (Qiagen) reagents, according to the manufacturer's protocol. The protein concentration was determined at 280 nm using UV NanoDrop1000® spectrophotometry (Thermo Scientific). The ciELISA was then performed as previously described, with some modifications.[45] The 96-well flat-bottommed microtiter plates (Immunlon II® HB; Fischer, Pittsburgh, PA, USA) were coated with 50 μL per well of 50 ng/mL synthetic cBD3-like or 10 ng/mL synthetic cCath in coating PBS (Bio-Rad, Hercules, CA, USA; pH 7.4) and left overnight at 4°C. After discarding the coating buffer, the plates were blocked with 100 μL per well of 10% fetal bovine serum (Midwest Scientific, St Louis, MO, USA) in PBS for 2 h at room temperature. The plates were then washed three times using a blocking solution containing 10% fetal bovine serum and 0.05% Tween-20 (PBS-T; BioRad). A typical assay consisted of three sets of triplicate wells and three duplicate wells, as follows: (i) triplicate wells (positive controls) receiving 50 μL of specific anti-canine AMP polyclonal serum (1:8000 dilution for anti-cBD3-like and 1:16,000 dilution for anti-cCath) that would give the maximal optical density (OD); (ii) three duplicate wells (negative controls) receiving 50 μL of PBS-T only or 50 μL of secondary antibody only or 50 μL of each specific pre-immune serum that would give the minimal OD; (iii) triplicate wells receiving 50 μL per well of mixtures containing 25 μL (50 μg) of total protein extract (sample) and 25 μL of serum dilution (final protein dilution of 2 μg/μL); and (iv) a series of triplicate wells receiving a mixture of the serum dilution and 10-fold serial dilutions (from 1000 to 0.1 ng/mL) of the appropriate synthetic peptide, used to generate the inhibition standard curves.

The sera dilutions were chosen among those that gave OD values on the linear portion of the curve obtained from a twofold serial titration of each serum on plates coated with the appropriate peptide. The protein extract served as a competitive inhibitor for the binding of the antibodies to the synthetic peptides coating the plates. The plates were incubated for 90 min at room temperature, washed five times using the blocking solution, and 50 μL of a secondary antibody (horseradish peroxidase-conjugated goat anti-rabbit IgG at 1:4000 dilution; BioRad) was added and incubated in the dark for 1 h at room temperature. The plates were then washed seven times with blocking solution and 100 μL per well of ABTS (Kirkegaard and Perry Laboratories, Fischer, Pittsburgh, PA, USA), a colorimetric substrate, was added. The developed plates were read with an automated MR 500 ELISA reader (Dynatech, Chantilly, VA, USA). The percentage of inhibition obtained from each concentration of peptide was calculated using the average of the absorbance values of each set of triplicate wells and the average of the absorbance values of the positive control wells. To calculate the relative amount of peptide in the 'unknown' wells, the increasing percentage inhibition values were plotted versus the corresponding log concentration of the synthetic peptide used to generate the standard curves. Complete inhibition was obtained using 1000 ng/mL of each synthetic peptide. The cBD2-like/122 and cBD103 protein levels were not quantified owing to a lack of antibodies suitable for ELISA-based quantification. The relative amount of AMPs in the tissue extracts was expressed as the concentration (in nanograms per millilitre) of its synthetic peptide giving the same percentage of inhibition. This was then transformed into nanograms per square millimetre by dividing the concentration (in nanograms per millilitre) by the surface area of the skin used for the extraction (one quarter of the 8 mm biopsy sample), as follows: ng/mL/[3.14(r^2)].

Statistical analysis

Mean values and 95% confidence intervals were calculated for all results. The Kolmogorov–Smirnov test of normality was used (α = 0.05). Differences between ΔC_T (C_TAMP – C_TRPLO) of each AMP were compared using Student's unpaired *t*-test. Differences between ΔC_T (C_TAMP – C_TRPLO) of cCath were compared using the Mann–Whitney *U*-test because they did not follow a normal distribution. Differences between ODs of each AMP were compared using Student's unpaired *t*-test. In the expectation of higher AMP levels for atopic dogs and atopic dogs with active skin infections, we used a one-tailed test, and *P*-values of ≤0.05 were considered significant. Statistical analysis was done using GraphPad Prism software (GraphPad Software, Inc., San Diego, CA, USA).

Results

Dogs

A total of 25 dogs were enrolled in this study. Skin biopsy samples were taken from 14 healthy dogs [nine males (three intact) and five spayed females] with a mean age of 4 ± 2.9 years (range, 1–10 years; median, 3 years) and 11 atopic dogs [four males (one intact) and six females (two intact)] with an average age of 5.6 ± 4.1 years (range, 1–15 years; median, 5 years). Of the atopic dogs, four of 11 had active skin infection (three of four bacterial and one of four mixed bacterial and yeast). The majority of dogs were of mixed breed (n = 9), five were Labrador retrievers, and one each of the following dog breeds was included: pug, wirehaired dachshund, Australian shepherd dog, Siberian husky, Samoyed, bull terrier, Jack Russell terrier, miniature pinscher, mastiff, beagle and English setter (Table 2). No significant age or sex differences were seen between groups.

Expression of mRNA

When we compared mRNA expression of each AMP between the dogs with AD and healthy control animals, a statistically significant higher expression (1.9 times) of *cBD103* (P = 0.04), but not any other AMP, was shown in atopic dogs (Figure 1a). Likewise, *cBD103* mRNA expression was significantly higher (3.8 times) in dogs with AD that had active skin infection when compared with atopic dogs without skin infection (P = 0.01; Figure 1b). This difference was 4.4 times higher when compared with dogs with AD that had active skin infection and healthy control dogs (P = 0.001; Figure 1c). In contrast, the *cBD1-like* mRNA expression level was significantly lower (0.48 times) in dogs with AD that had active skin infection compared with dogs with AD without skin infection (P = 0.04; Figure 1b).

Expression of protein

Indirect immunofluorescence.

No differences were noted in the distribution of AMPs in the skin of healthy dogs and in dogs with AD demonstrated by IIF. The proteins were homogeneously distributed in skin samples from both groups of dogs. The cBD2-like/122 and cBD3-like were detectable in all layers of the epidermis, whereas cCath was detected predominantly in the stratum granulosum and stratum corneum, as previously reported (Figure 2).[32,40]

Table 2. Details of the 25 dogs enrolled in the study and the presence of active skin infection

Number	Sex	Age (years)	Breed	Atopic dermatitis	Infection
1	Mc	1	Mixed breed	No	
2	Mc	5	Labrador	Yes	No
3	Mc	10	Mixed breed	No	
4	Mc	6	Mixed breed	Yes	Yes
5	Mc	2	Pug	No	
6	M	1	Labrador	Yes	No
7	M	7	Wirehaired dachshund	No	
8	Fs	4	Mixed breed	Yes	No
9	Fs	4	Mixed breed	No	
10	Fs	1	Labrador	Yes	Yes
11	Fs	2	Australian shepherd	No	
12	F	2	Miniature pinscher	Yes	No
13	F	8	English setter	Yes	Yes
14	Fs	9	Labrador	Yes	Yes
15	M	1	Mixed breed	No	
16	M	8	Mixed breed	No	
17	Mc	4	Mastiff	Yes	No
18	Fs	3	Siberian husky	No	
19	Fs	3	Mixed breed	No	
20	Mc	6	Samoyed	No	
21	Fs	15	Beagle	Yes	No
22	Mc	6	Mixed breed	No	
23	Mc	1	Bull terrier	No	
24	Fs	7	Labrador	Yes	No
25	Fs	3	Jack Russell terrier	No	

Abbreviations: F, female intact; Fs, female spayed; M, male intact; and Mc, male castrated.

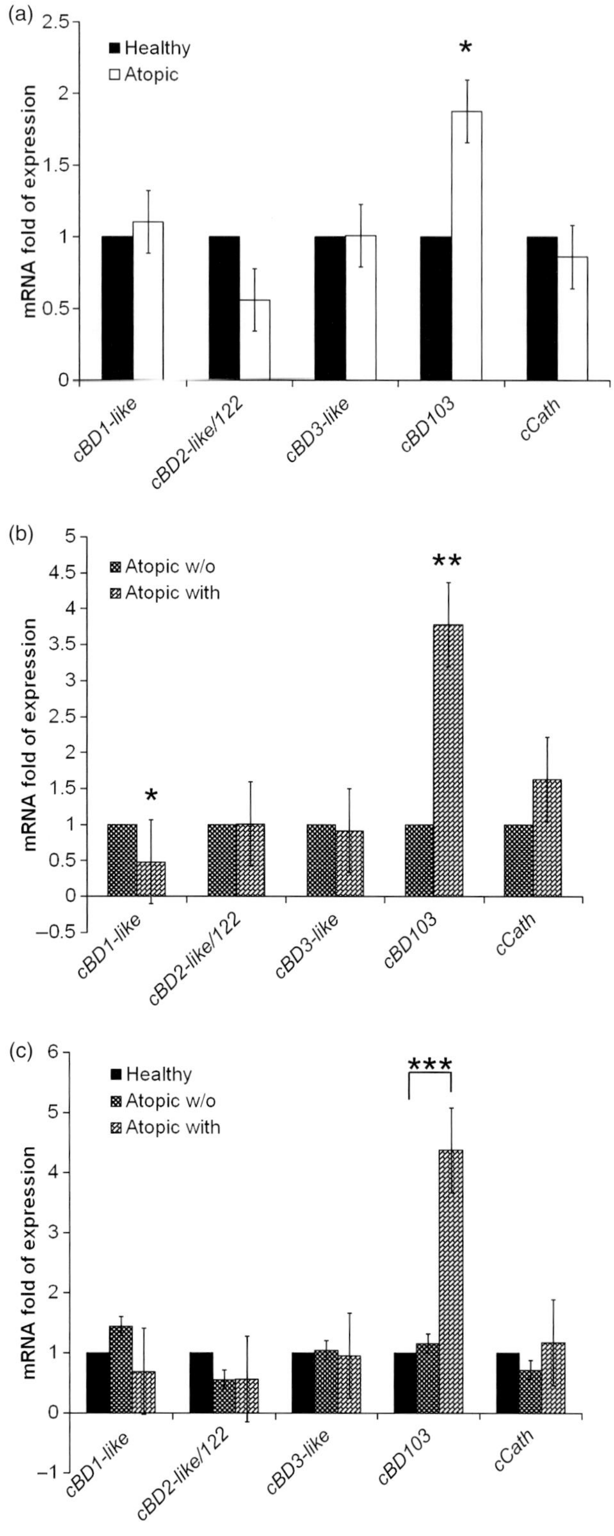

Figure 1. Relative mRNA expression for each antimicrobial peptide [canine β-defensin (*cBD*)*1-like*, *cBD2-like/122*, *cBD3-like*, cBD103 and canine cathelicidin (*cCath*)] in atopic dogs with and without (w/o) skin infection compared with normal control dogs. (a) Comparison between healthy dogs and dogs with atopic dermatitis (AD). (b) Comparison between dogs with AD, with and without active skin infection. (c) Comparison of healthy dogs and dogs with AD, with and without active skin infection. Groups were compared using Tukey's multiple comparison test (*$P \leq 0.05$, **$P \leq 0.01$ and ***$P \leq 0.001$; bars indicate SEM).

Relative competitive inhibition enzyme-linked immunosorbent assay.

Using the ciELISA, we were able to calculate the relative amount of cBD3-like and cCath per square millimetre of skin. The abdominal skin of healthy dogs had an amount of BD3-like corresponding to 1.1 ± 0.95 ng/mm^2 of synthetic cBD3-like and 1.4 ± 0.99 ng/mm^2 of synthetic cCath (Figure 3a). Abdominal skin of atopic dogs had an amount corresponding to 1.8 ± 1.8 and 4.7 ± 8.6 ng/mm^2 of synthetic cBD3-like and synthetic cCath, respectively (Figure 3a). The corresponding amounts of cBD3-like in atopic skin with and without active skin infection were 2.5 ± 1.5 and 1.4 ± 1.9 ng/mm^2, respectively (Figure 3b). The corresponding amounts of cCath were 5.15 ± 10.54 ng/mm^2 in dogs without infection and 4 ± 4.9 ng/mm^2 in dogs with active infection, respectively (Figure 3b). When we compared the amount of cBD3-like and cCath between the AD and healthy control groups, no statistically significant differences were seen (Figure 3a,b). However, a significant increase in cBD3-like and cCath was present when we compared dogs with AD that had active skin infection and healthy control dogs ($P = 0.04$ and $P = 0.05$, respectively; Figure 3c). A trend towards a significant increase of AD without skin infection versus healthy control was also seen ($P = 0.08$; Figure 3c).

Discussion

Our data showed a significant increase of *cBD103* mRNA expression levels in skin of dogs naturally affected with AD when compared with healthy control dogs. These results are in accordance with recent studies by Bellardini *et al.*[28] and Harder *et al.*,[30] in which a clear increase in mRNA expression and protein level of some AMPs, namely *LL-37*, *hBD2* and *hBD3/103A* (orthologue of *cBD103*), were demonstrated in the skin of atopic human patients when compared with healthy individuals. The results of the present study are also in accordance with the results of previous study in which we demonstrated increased mRNA expression levels of some AMPs in the skin of beagles with experimentally induced AD.[32]

The reason for higher expression and production of AMPs in atopic skin compared with healthy controls is not completely understood. Many hypotheses have been proposed, including the effects of the local immunological milieu, the disruption of the cutaneous barrier, differing rates of protein degradation and the presence of inflammatory cells.[24–26,46–50] The involvement of cytokines in the regulation of local AMPs is a subject of controversy. Although a strong inverse correlation between human AMPs and the expression of T helper 2 cytokines, such as interleukin-4, interleukin-10 and interleukin-13, has been shown *in vitro*,[46,48–50] an *in vivo* model has demonstrated higher expression of some AMPs in acute T helper 2-dominant AD lesions.[30] In addition, a strong correlation between alterations of the skin barrier, naturally present in AD skin, and production of AMPs has been demonstrated in both mouse and human models.[50,51] Increased degradation of active AMPs in atopic disease due to hyperactivation of several endogenous as well as exogenous proteases[52,53] has also been

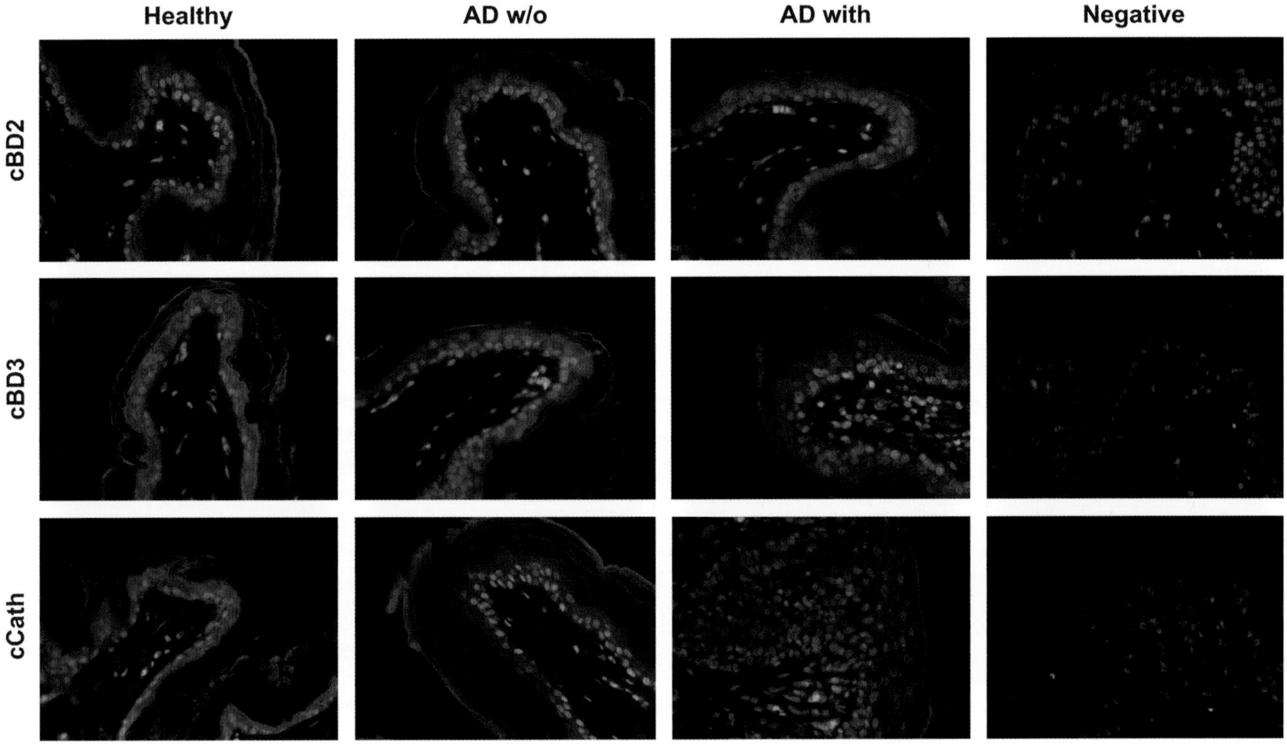

Figure 2. Photomicrographs of canine skin showing indirect immunofluorescence of cBD2-like/122, cBD3-like and cCath. The cBD2-like/122 and cBD3-like fluorescence is diffusely distributed throughout the epidermis, and scattered positive cells are also present in the superficial dermis; cCath is mainly detectable in the stratum granulosum and corneum along with few positive cells in the superficial dermis. The pictures are representative of all samples.

hypothesized in AD skin. In this latter case, the increased mRNA expression could be due to a 'feedback mechanism', in which the keratinocyte increases the genetic signal in an effort to repair the lack of protein expression. The increase in *cBD103* mRNA expression shown in the present study is in disagreement with van Damme *et al.*,[31] who reported a twofold decrease in mRNA expression of *cBD103* in the skin of dogs naturally affected with AD. Possible explanations for this discrepancy could be differences in skin biopsy location, the different ages of the dogs enrolled in the two studies (older in our study), the treatment with antimicrobials prior to enrolment in the study (avoided in our study), and the potential use of different shampoos and topicals (antimicrobial versus moisturizing products) used before enrolment in the two studies. Different AMP expression has been demonstrated in different body sites in people, with areas more subject to friction and environmental challenge having a higher AMP expression.[54] Increased AMP expression has also been reported in older versus younger human patients.[55]

We were not able to detect any significant differences in mRNA expression levels of the other AMPs (*cBD1-like*, *cBD2-like/122*, *cBD3-like* and *cCath*) between the two groups. These results are in contrast with a previous study showing an increase of such AMPs in the skin of beagles with experimentally induced AD.[32] One explanation for this discord could be the higher variability of mRNA expression found in the present study compared with the previous one. In fact, the use of a canine animal model allowed more efficient control of environmental and intrinsic variables, such as a shared environment (e.g. indoors versus outdoors), other pets in the household, age and breed.[56]

Atopic dogs, like atopic humans, are more susceptible to bacterial and *Malassezia* skin infection, but only recently has there been an increased interest in the role of AMPs in this predisposition.[23,31,32,37,38,56] However, no studies have reported expression patterns of AMPs in the skin of atopic dogs with or without active skin infection. The present study is the first to demonstrate higher mRNA expression for *cBD103* and lower expression of *cBD1-like*, but not the other *cBDs* and *cCath*, in the skin of naturally affected atopic dogs with active infections. We showed that the mRNA expression of *cBD103* was 3.8 times higher in infected skin when compared with noninfected skin. This difference increased to 4.4 times when comparing infected AD skin with the skin of healthy control dogs. This increased expression could be the direct effect of the bacterial stimulation, as demonstrated *in vitro*.[57,58] The significant decrease in *cBD1-like* mRNA expression level in dogs with AD that had active skin infection when compared with dogs with AD without skin infection could be due to less important antimicrobial effects of cBD1-like compared with other defensins; for this reason, cBD1-like might not be actively involved in skin infections.

We designed a semi-quantitative ciELISA for cBD3-like and cCath to detect the relative amounts of AMPs in canine abdominal skin. Although no significant differences were found between AD (total or without skin infection) and healthy skin, or between AD skin with and

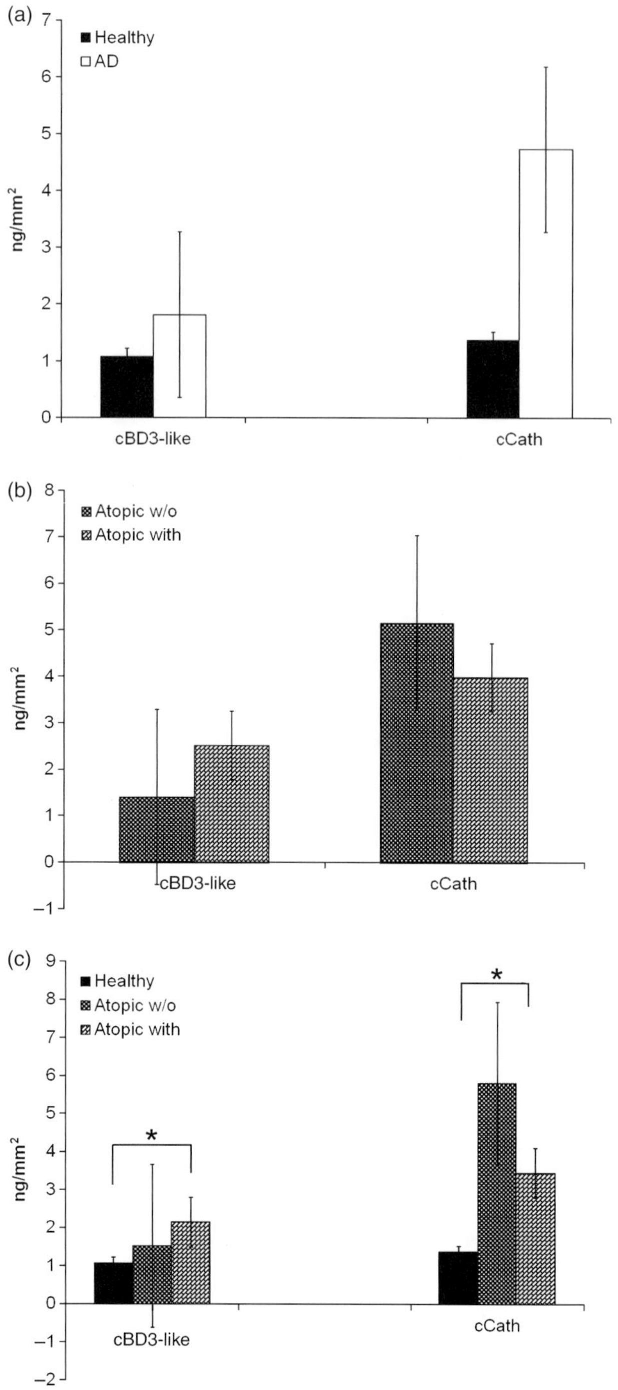

Figure 3. Protein levels for each antimicrobial peptide (cBD3-like and cCath) in atopic dogs with and without (w/o) skin infection compared with normal control dogs. (a) Comparison between healthy dogs and dogs with AD. (b) Comparison between dogs with AD, with and without active skin infection. (c) Comparison of healthy dogs and dogs with AD, with and without active skin infection. Groups were compared using Tukey's multiple comparison test (*$P \leq 0.05$; bars indicate SEM).

without skin infection, a significantly increased amount of cBD3-like and cCath was seen when infected AD skin was compared with healthy control skin. These results may suggest an active stimulation of some AMPs by bacteria and/or yeasts in AD skin, as previously demonstrated.[27,30,57,58] Unfortunately, at this point in time antibodies to detect cBD103 protein expression are not available. It would have been interesting to have a comparison between mRNA expression and protein production to confirm the possible major involvement of this AMP in the skin of dogs with AD. Finally, our study showed that there was no difference in cutaneous distribution of the tested AMPs between AD skin, with or without active infection, and healthy skin.

In conclusion, we have demonstrated that, as in people, a higher mRNA expression of *cBD103* (orthologue of *hBD3/103A*) is present in atopic dogs than in healthy control dogs. This difference was more striking when comparing the skin of normal dogs with skin of dogs with AD that had active infection, showing a potentially active role of *cBD103* in cutaneous infection in atopic dogs. In contrast, we showed a lower mRNA expression of *cBD1-like* in AD skin affected by active skin infection when compared with nonactively infected AD skin. These data may indicate that many AMPs may be involved in the cutaneous innate immunity as defense against external micro-organisms. In addition, it is possible that an alteration of the ratio between AMPs is the cause of increased infections in atopic patients. The present study and previous studies have yielded mixed results, raising questions concerning the regulation and the production of AMPs in cutaneous infections, and which AMP ratio is more important in controlling bacterial and yeast infections. Which AMPs are sufficient to control skin infection in healthy and atopic dogs, at what concentrations and what is the action of topicals (e.g. shampoos, foams and sprays) on cutaneous AMP production? More work is needed to clarify the biological mechanisms and the possible therapeutic treatments to maintain a healthy canine skin.

Acknowledgements

The authors thank Liping Wang and Rachel Breitenfeld for assistance in the production of antibodies, Sandy Grable for assistance during the collection of the skin samples, and Karen Campbell for her critical comments.

References

1. Halliwell R. Revised nomenclature for veterinary allergy. *Vet Immunol Immunopathol* 2006; 114: 207–208.
2. Bieber T. Atopic dermatitis. *Ann Dermatol* 2010; 22: 125–137.
3. Hillier A, Griffin CE. The ACVD task force on canine atopic dermatitis (I): incidence and prevalence. *Vet Immunol Immunopathol* 2001; 81: 147–151.
4. Proksch E, Brandner JM, Jensen JM. The skin: an indispensable barrier. *Exp Dermatol* 2008; 17: 1063–1072.
5. De Benedetto A, Rafaels NM, McGirt LY *et al.* Tight junction defects in patients with atopic dermatitis. *J Allergy Clin Immunol* 2011; 127: 773–786.
6. Irvine AD, McLean I, Leung DYM. Filaggrin mutations associated with skin and allergic diseases. *N Engl J Med* 2011; 365: 1315–1327.
7. De Benedetto A, Kubo A, Beck LA. Skin barrier disruption: a requirement for allergen sensitization? *J Invest Dermatol* 2012; 132: 949–963.
8. Inman AO, Olivry T, Dunston SM *et al.* Electron microscopic observations of stratum corneum intercellular lipids in normal and atopic dogs. *Vet Pathol* 2001; 38: 720–723.

9. Shimada K, Yoon JS, Yoshibara T *et al.* Increased transepidermal water loss and decreased ceramide content in lesional and non-lesional skin of dogs with atopic dermatitis. *Vet Dermatol* 2009; 20: 541–546.
10. Reiter LV, Torres SM, Wertz PW. Characterization and quantification of ceramides in the lesional and nonlesional skin of canine patients with atopic dermatitis compared with controls. *Vet Dermatol* 2009; 20: 260–266.
11. Marsella R, Samuelson D, Doerr K. Transmission electron microscopy studies in an experimental model of canine atopic dermatitis. *Vet Dermatol* 2010; 21: 81–88.
12. Santoro D, Marsella R, Bunick D *et al.* Expression and distribution of canine filaggrin in the skin of healthy and atopic beagles. *Vet Dermatol* 2010; 21: 323 (abstract).
13. Olivry T, Wofford J, Paps JS *et al.* Stratum corneum removal facilitates experimental sensitization to mite allergens in atopic dogs. *Vet Dermatol* 2011; 22: 188–196.
14. Marsella R, Ahrens K, Thomas AL *et al.* Evaluation of a polyclonal antibody against canine filaggrin in immunohistochemical studies in atopic and normal beagle dogs. *Vet Dermatol* 2011; 22: 289 (abstract).
15. Yoon JS, Nishifuji K, Sasaki A *et al.* Alteration of stratum corneum ceramide profiles in spontaneous canine model of atopic dermatitis. *Exp Dermatol* 2011; 20: 732–736.
16. Marsella R, Olivry T, Carlotti DN *et al.* Current evidence of skin barrier dysfunction in human and canine atopic dermatitis. *Vet Dermatol* 2011; 22: 239–248.
17. Olivry T. Is the skin barrier abnormal in dogs with atopic dermatitis? *Vet Immunol Immunopathol* 2011; 144: 11–16.
18. Cornegliani L, Vercelli A, Sala E *et al.* Transepidermal water loss in healthy and atopic dogs, treated and untreated: a comparative preliminary study. *Vet Dermatol* 2012; 23: 41–44, e9–e10.
19. Marshall SH, Arenas G. Antimicrobial peptides: a natural alternative to chemical antibiotics and a potential for applied biotechnology. *J Biotechnol* 2003; 6: 271–284.
20. Jenssen H, Hamill P, Hancock REW. Peptide antimicrobial agents. *Clin Microbiol Rev* 2006; 19: 491–511.
21. Linde A, Ross CR, Davis EG *et al.* Innate immunity and host defense peptides in veterinary medicine. *J Vet Intern Med* 2008; 22: 247–265.
22. Leonard BC, Affolter VK, Bevins CL. Antimicrobial peptides: agents of border protection for companion animals. *Vet Dermatol* 2012; 23: 177–187.
23. Schauber J, Gallo RL. Antimicrobial peptides and the skin immune defense system. *J Allergy Clin Immunol* 2008; 122: 261–266.
24. Lai Y, Gallo RL. AMPed up immunity: how antimicrobial peptides have multiple roles in immune defense. *Trends Immunol* 2009; 30: 131–141.
25. Nakatsuji T, Gallo RL. Antimicrobial peptides: old molecules with new ideas. *J Invest Dermatol* 2012; 132: 887–895.
26. Schittek B. The antimicrobial skin barrier in patients with atopic dermatitis. *Curr Probl Dermatol* 2011; 41: 54–67.
27. Asano S, Ichikawa Y, Kumagai T *et al.* Microanalysis of an antimicrobial peptide, β-defensin-2, in the stratum corneum from patients with atopic dermatitis. *Br J Dermatol* 2008; 159: 97–104.
28. Bellardini N, Johansson C, Lilja G *et al.* Enhanced expression of the antimicrobial peptide LL-37 in lesional skin of adults with atopic eczema. *Br J Dermatol* 2009; 161: 40–47.
29. Glaser R, Meyer-Hoffert U, Harder J *et al.* The antimicrobial protein psoriasin (S100A7) is upregulated in atopic dermatitis and after experimental skin barrier disruption. *J Invest Dermatol* 2009; 129: 641–649.
30. Harder J, Dressel S, Wittersheim M *et al.* Enhanced expression and secretion of antimicrobial peptides in atopic dermatitis and after superficial skin injury. *J Invest Dermatol* 2010; 130: 1355–1364.
31. van Damme CM, Willemse T, van Dijk A *et al.* Altered cutaneous expression of β-defensins in dogs with atopic dermatitis. *Mol Immunol* 2009; 46: 2449–2455.
32. Santoro D, Marsella R, Bunick D *et al.* Expression and distribution of canine antimicrobial peptides in the skin of healthy and atopic beagles. *Vet Immunol Immunopathol* 2011; 144: 382–388.
33. Howell MD. The role of beta defensins and cathelicidins in atopic dermatitis. *Curr Opin Allergy Clin Immunol* 2007; 7: 413–417.
34. Niyonsaba F, Ushio H, Nakano N *et al.* Antimicrobial peptides human β-defensins stimulate epidermal keratinocyte migration, proliferation and production of proinflammatory cytokines and chemokines. *J Invest Dermatol* 2007; 127: 594–604.
35. Wollenberg A, Rawer HC, Schauber J. Innate immunity in atopic dermatitis. *Clin Rev Allergy Immunol* 2011; 41: 272–281.
36. DeBoer D, Marsella R. The ACVD task force on canine atopic dermatitis (XII): the relationship of cutaneous infections to pathogenesis and clinical course of canine atopic dermatitis. *Vet Immunol Immunopathol* 2001; 81: 239–249.
37. Sang Y, Ortega T, Blecha F *et al.* Molecular cloning and characterization of three β-defensins from canine testes. *Infect Immun* 2005; 73: 2611–2620.
38. Sang Y, Ortegab T, Rune K *et al.* Canine cathelicidin (K9CATH): gene cloning, expression, and biochemical activity of a novel pro-myeloid antimicrobial peptide. *Dev Comp Immunol* 2007; 31: 1278–1296.
39. Erles K, Brownlie J. Expression of β-defensins in the canine respiratory tract and antimicrobial activity against *Bordetella bronchiseptica*. *Vet Immunol Immunopathol* 2010; 135: 12–19.
40. Santoro D, Bunick D, Graves TK *et al.* Expression and distribution of antimicrobial peptides in the skin of healthy beagles. *Vet Dermatol* 2011; 22: 61–67.
41. DeBoer D, Hillier A. The ACVD task force on canine atopic dermatitis (XV): fundamental concepts in clinical diagnosis. *Vet Immunol Immunopathol* 2001; 81: 271–276.
42. Favrot C, Steffan J, Seewald W *et al.* A prospective study on the clinical features of chronic canine atopic dermatitis and its diagnosis. *Vet Dermatol* 2010; 21: 23–31.
43. Pfaffl MW. A new mathematical model for relative quantification in real-time RT-PCR. *Nucleic Acids Res* 2001; 29: 2002–2007.
44. Wood SH, Clements DN, McEwan NA *et al.* Reference genes for canine skin when using quantitative real-time PCR. *Vet Immunol Immunopathol* 2008; 126: 392–395.
45. Muhumuza L, Segre D, Segre M. Antibodies with idiotypic and anti-idiotypic reactivity (epibodies) in conventional immune responses to dinitrophenylated carriers. *Immunology* 1998; 93: 572–580.
46. Nomura I, Goleva E, Howell MD *et al.* Cytokine milieu of atopic dermatitis, as compared to psoriasis, skin prevents induction of innate immune response genes. *J Immunol* 2003; 171: 3262–3269.
47. Liu L, Roberts AA, Ganz T. By IL-1 signaling, monocyte-derived cells dramatically enhance the epidermal antimicrobial responses to lipopolysaccharides. *J Immunol* 2003; 170: 575–580.
48. Howell MD, Novak N, Bieber T *et al.* IL-10 down-regulates antimicrobial peptide expression in atopic dermatitis. *J Invest Dermatol* 2005; 125: 738–745.
49. Howell MD, Boguniewicz M, Pastore S *et al.* Mechanism of HBD-3 deficiency in atopic dermatitis. *Clin Immunol* 2006; 121: 332–338.
50. Ahrens K, Schunck M, Podda GF *et al.* Mechanical and metabolic injury to the skin barrier leads to increased expression of murine β-defensin-1, -3, and -14. *J Invest Dermatol* 2011; 131: 443–452.
51. De Benedetto A, Agnihothri R, McGirt LY *et al.* Atopic dermatitis: a disease caused by innate immune defects? *J Invest Dermatol* 2009; 129: 14–30.
52. Elias PM. Stratum corneum defensive functions: an integrated view. *J Invest Dermatol* 2005; 125: 183–200.
53. Takai T, Ikeda S. Barrier dysfunction caused by environmental proteases in the pathogenesis of allergic diseases. *Allergol Int* 2011; 60: 25–35.

54. Ali RS, Falconer A, Ikram M *et al.* Expression of the peptide antibiotics human β-defensin 1 and human β-defensin 2 in normal skin. *J Invest Dermatol* 2001; 117: 106–111.
55. Matsuzaka K, Sato D, Ishihara K *et al.* Age-related differences in localization of beta-defensin-2 in human gingival epithelia. *Bull Tokyo Dent Coll* 2006; 47: 167–170.
56. Wingate KV, Torres SM, Silverstein KAT *et al.* Expression of endogenous antimicrobial peptides in normal canine skin. *Vet Dermatol* 2009; 20: 19–26.
57. Sørensen OE, Thapa DR, Rosenthal A *et al.* Differential regulation of β-defensin expression in human skin by microbial stimuli. *J Immunol* 2005; 174: 4870–4879.
58. Schauber J, Dorschner RA, Yamasaki K *et al.* Control of the innate epithelial antimicrobial response is cell-type specific and dependent on relevant microenvironmental stimuli. *Immunology* 2006; 118: 509–519.

To cite this article, please use DOI: 10.1111/j.1365-3164.2012.01098.x

2.3

Interleukin-31: its role in canine pruritus and naturally occurring canine atopic dermatitis

Andrea J. Gonzales, William R. Humphrey, James E. Messamore, Timothy J. Fleck, Gregory J. Fici, John A. Shelly, Janet F. Teel, Gary F. Bammert, Steven A. Dunham, Troy E. Fuller and Robert B. McCall

Global Therapeutics Research, Pfizer Animal Health, Kalamazoo, MI 49001, USA

Correspondence: Andrea J. Gonzales, Global Therapeutics Research, Pfizer Animal Health, 7000 Portage Road, Kalamazoo, MI 49001, USA. E-mail: andrea.gonzales@pfizer.com

Background – Interleukin-31 (IL-31) is a member of the gp130/interleukin-6 cytokine family that is produced by cell types such as T helper 2 lymphocytes and cutaneous lymphocyte antigen positive skin homing T cells. When overexpressed in transgenic mice, IL-31 induces severe pruritus, alopecia and skin lesions. In humans, IL-31 serum levels correlate with the severity of atopic dermatitis in adults and children.

Hypothesis/Objective – To determine the role of IL-31 in canine pruritus and naturally occurring canine atopic dermatitis (AD).

Animals – Purpose-bred beagle dogs were used for laboratory studies. Serum samples were obtained from laboratory animals, nondiseased client-owned dogs and client-owned dogs diagnosed with naturally occurring AD.

Methods – Purpose-bred beagle dogs were administered canine interleukin-31 (cIL-31) via several routes (intravenous, subcutaneous or intradermal), and pruritic behaviour was observed/quantified via video monitoring. Quantitative immunoassay techniques were employed to measure serum levels of cIL-31 in dogs.

Results – Injection of cIL-31 into laboratory beagle dogs caused transient episodes of pruritic behaviour regardless of the route of administration. When evaluated over a 2 h period, dogs receiving cIL-31 exhibited a significant increase in pruritic behaviour compared with dogs that received placebo. In addition, cIL-31 levels were detectable in 57% of dogs with naturally occurring AD (≥13 pg/mL) but were below limits of quantification (<13 pg/mL) in normal, nondiseased laboratory or client-owned animals.

Conclusions – Canine IL-31 induced pruritic behaviours in dogs. Canine IL-31 was detected in the majority of dogs with naturally occurring AD, suggesting that this cytokine may play an important role in pruritic allergic skin conditions, such as atopic dermatitis, in this species.

Introduction

Canine atopic dermatitis (AD) is a genetically predisposed inflammatory and pruritic allergic skin disease with characteristic clinical features.[1] One clinical feature that dogs with AD commonly display is pruritus, which can have a significant impact on the quality of life for the pet as well as for the owner. However, the underlying pathways and mechanisms involved in triggering pruritic behaviours are not clear, hampering the development of effective anti-pruritic therapies.

Interleukin-31 (IL-31) is a recently identified cytokine implicated in pruritic skin conditions such as human AD. When initially characterized in transgenic mice, overexpression of IL-31 led to the development of several hallmark signs of AD, which included increased inflammatory cell infiltration into the skin, severe pruritus, alopecia and skin lesions.[2] Interleukin-31 has been shown to be produced by activated T helper type 2 lymphocytes and by cutaneous lymphocyte antigen positive (CLA+) skin homing T cells from human AD patients, suggesting that these cells may represent a major source of this cytokine. Interleukin-31 has been found to be elevated preferentially in pruritic versus nonpruritic human skin conditions, and serum levels of IL-31 correlate with disease severity in human adults as well as children with AD.[2–8]

Interleukin-31 binds to a heterodimeric receptor consisting of IL-31 receptor A and oncostatin M receptor β. Upon ligand binding to this receptor complex, signal transduction cascades such as the Janus kinase–signal transducer and activator of transcription (JAK–STAT), mitogen-activated protein kinase (MAPK) and phosphatidylinositol 3-kinase (PI3K) pathways are activated.[9] Receptors for IL-31 are found on a variety of cells, such as keratinocytes, macrophages and eosinophils, and par-

Accepted 4 July 2012
Sources of Funding: This study was self-funded.
Conflict of Interest: All authors are Pfizer Inc. shareholders.

ticipate in regulating immune responses in these cell types.[9–11] Of great interest is the finding that these receptors are present on a subset of small-sized nociceptive neurons of mouse and human dorsal root ganglia, suggesting that this cytokine may directly activate pruritogenic signals in peripheral nerves.[4,12]

The cloning of canine interleukin-31 (cIL-31) has been previously reported.[13] These investigators were able to detect cIL-31 mRNA in freshly isolated canine peripheral blood mononuclear cells after concanavalin A treatment, suggesting that IL-31 may be produced by canine T cells; however, they were not able to detect cIL-31 mRNA in skin biopsy specimens from dogs diagnosed with AD, which calls into question the role of IL-31 in canine AD. To extend investigations of canine IL-31 to assessments of biological activity and protein levels in disease, the present study was conducted to evaluate the role of IL-31 in canine pruritus using purpose-bred beagle dogs and to evaluate whether IL-31 is present in the serum of animals with naturally occurring AD.

Materials and methods

Cloning and expression of cIL-31

Using total RNA isolated from canine testicular tissue and oligo-$(dT)_{20}$ primers, complementary DNA was synthesized with the SuperScript® III First-Strand Synthesis System for RT-PCR (Invitrogen, Carlsbad, CA, USA.) according to the manufacturer's protocol. Polymerase chain reactions were performed to amplify the cIL-31 gene from complementary DNA using primers TEF-1237 (5′- AGATCTGCCACCATGCTCTCCCACACAGGACCATCCAG-3′) and TEF-1240 (5′-GGTACCCTACTGAGGTCCAGAGTTTAGTGAC-3′). The PCR product was cloned into pCR®-Blunt II-TOPO® according to the manufacturer's protocols (Life Technologies, Grand Island, NY, USA) and further subcloned into the expression construct pSO0524. The cIL-31 expression construct was either transiently transfected into FreeStyle™ 293 suspension culture cells following the manufacturers' protocol (Life Technologies) or stably transfected into CHO cells using a site-specific integration system.[14]

Protein purification and analysis of recombinant cIL-31

Canine interleukin-31 was produced by cultured FreeStyle™ 293 cells or CHO cells. Conditioned media from these cells was collected, dialysed with buffer (20 mmol/L Tris, pH 8.0, and 40 mmol/L NaCl) and purified by anion exchange chromatography (Q Sepharose). Protein identity was confirmed by N-terminal sequencing and by liquid chromatography–mass spectrometry (LC-MS) analysis of a tryptic digest of the protein.

Cell culture

The DH82 canine monocytic cell line (American Type Culture Collection, Manassas, VA, USA) was used to evaluate cIL-31 cytokine function. DH82 cells were plated into CoStar 96-well flat-bottomed cell culture plates (Corning, Tewksbury, MA, USA) at a density of 1×10^5 cells per well in MEM growth media (Life Technologies) containing 15% heat-inactivated fetal bovine serum, 2 mmol/L GlutaMax, 1 mmol/L sodium pyruvate, 50 μg/L gentamicin and 10 ng/mL canine interferon-γ (R&D Systems, Minneapolis, MN, USA) for 24 h at 37°C in humidified air supplemented with 5% CO_2. The following day, cells were exposed to MEM growth media without serum or interferon-γ for 2 h. Following serum deprivation, cells were treated with cIL-31 for 5 min. Cytokine treatment was terminated by removing medium and then adding AlphaScreen SureFire™ lysis buffer (Perkin Elmer, Waltham, MA, USA) and freezing samples at −20°C.

Signal transduction pathway activation

Cell lysates were used to evaluate phosphorylation of signal transducer and activator of transcription 3 (STAT3) and extracellular signal-regulated kinase 1/2 (ERK1/2). Activation of STAT3 was detected using the Perkin Elmer AlphaScreen SureFire™ STAT3 p-Y705 kit, and activation of ERK1/2 was detected using the Perkin Elmer AlphaScreen SureFire™ MAPK p-T202/Y204 kit, following the manufacturer's protocol. Specifically, 4 μL of cIL-31-treated cell lysates was sequentially incubated with streptavidin-coated donor beads bound with biotinylated capture antibody, then with protein A-coated acceptor beads bound with antibody that recognized the phophorylation site on the target protein. Assay plates were placed on a Perkin Elmer Envision plate reader to cause excitation of the donor beads at 680 nm. Upon excitation of a donor bead, a singlet oxygen transfer occurs from the donor to an acceptor bead. Any acceptor bead in close proximity to a donor bead (due to the binding of capture and detection antibodies to the desired target protein) emits light at 520–620 nm as a result of a cascade of energy transfer triggered by the singlet oxygen. Light emission was detected by the Envision plate reader. Data were expressed as mean relative signal units, and the EC_{50} for induction of phosphorylated STAT3 (pSTAT3) and phosphorylated MAPK (pMAPK) was determined by a nonlinear fit model in GraphPad Prism 5.0 (GraphPad Software, San Diego, CA, USA).

Assessment of pruritus in animals

All animal procedures were approved by the Institutional Animal Care and Use Committee (Pfizer Animal Health, Kalamazoo, MI, USA) and were performed in compliance with the Animal Welfare Act, Regulations, 9 CFR Parts 1, 2 and 3, and with the *Guide for the Care and Use of Laboratory Animals*, issued by the US Institute for Laboratory Animal Research Commission of Life Sciences (National Academy Press, Washington, DC, 1996).

Purpose-bred beagle dogs (Marshall BioResources, North Rose, NY, USA) were used in these experiments. Dogs were acclimated for at least 1 h to single-housed runs equipped with ceiling cameras. To evaluate the effects of cIL-31 administration via various routes on pruritic behaviour, cIL-31 (10 μg) or vehicle control [phosphate-buffered saline (PBS) containing equivalent amounts of mammalian host cell proteins to those present in the cIL-31 preparation] was administered intradermally (i.d.), subcutaneously (s.c.) or intravenously (i.v.). Pruritic behaviours (e.g. scratching, licking, chewing, scooting, head shaking and body rubbing) were monitored using video surveillance. Pruritic behaviours were measured as the time (in seconds) over a 4 h baseline period or 4 h after cIL-31 administration by one or more observers who were blinded to the treatment.

To evaluate the pruritic effects of cIL-31 in a statistically powered study, vehicle control-treated animals were compared with cIL-31-treated animals. Pruritic behaviour was evaluated for 2 h starting approximately 30 min after vehicle control or cIL-31 injection (1.75 μg/kg, i.v.) by one or more observers who were blinded to the treatment. Observed pruritic behaviour was measured using a categorical scoring system. 'Yes/no' determinations of displayed pruritic behaviour were made during consecutive, discrete 1 min intervals. The number of minutes categorized as 'yes' for displayed pruritic behaviours for an animal was then summed. The maximal achievable score for a 2 h (120 min) observation period was 120.

Canine serum samples

Blood was collected in 5 mL plastic BD Vacutainer™ SST™ tubes (Beckton Dickinson & Co., Franklin Lakes, NJ, USA) with owners' signed informed consent when required, allowed to clot then separated according to the manufacturer's protocol. Serum was collected from the following populations of dogs and frozen prior to measurements of serum cIL-31.

1. Experimentally sensitized dogs. Twenty-four purpose-bred beagle dogs (Marshall BioResources) prior to and 1 week after the last exposure to house dust mite (HDM) allergen. Animals were sensitized to *Dermatophagoides farinae* by receiving a series of three 0.5 mL injections containing 10 μg of allergen (Greer

Laboratories, Inc., Lenoir, NC, USA), 2.0 mg Rehydragel (Reheis, Inc., Berkeley Heights, NJ, USA) and 0.4 mL sterile PBS. The injections were administered 2 weeks apart. All animals were approximately 9 months of age, and 12 neutered males and 12 spayed females were evaluated.

2. Flea-allergic dogs. Thirty research dogs with established flea allergy (Youngs Veterinary Research Services, Turlock, CA, USA) prior to flea infestation or approximately 1 week after infestation with adult cat fleas *(Ctenocephalides felis)* began. The majority of the dogs in this colony were of mixed breed. The mean age was 10.5 years. This colony consisted of 14 intact females, two spayed females, 11 intact males and three neutered males.
3. Pet dogs without allergic disease. Eighty-seven client-owned dogs with subclinical periodontal disease but otherwise determined to be in good health. Samples were collected across 18 veterinary clinics in the USA to perform serum chemistries and titre assessments as part of a screening protocol for entry into a study. All owners had provided written consent for remaining serum to be used in research. No additional samples were collected for this portion of the study. Approximately 86% of the dogs were purebred and approximately 18% of the total population were retrievers [Labrador (13%) and golden (5%)]. The mean age was 3.2 years. The population consisted of 9% intact females, 47% spayed females, 13% intact males and 31% neutered males.
4. Pet dogs with nonseasonal atopic dermatitis. Two hundred and twenty-three client-owned animals diagnosed with chronic, nonseasonal AD of at least 1 year duration diagnosed by a board-certified dermatologist [based on modified criteria of Willemse[15] and Prélaud *et al.*,[16] with a minimum of 'moderate itching' as assessed by the owner and a minimal skin lesion score of 25 on the Canine Atopic Dermatitis Extent and Severity Index (CADESI)-02]. All dogs underwent a diagnostic regimen sufficient to eliminate food allergy, flea allergy dermatitis, bacterial or fungal dermatitis, primary otitis, internal and external parasitism and metabolic disease as the cause of the pruritus. Samples were collected from 14 US specialty dermatology practices to perform serum chemistries as part of a screening protocol for entry into a study. All owners had provided written consent for remaining serum to be used in research. No additional samples were collected for this portion of the study. Approximately 75% of the dogs were purebred and approximately 25% of the total population were retrievers [Labrador (17.3%) and golden (8.2%)]. The mean age was 5.8 years. This population of dogs consisted of 3% intact females, 51% spayed females, 3% intact males and 43% neutered males.

Anti-IL-31 monoclonal antibody production

Anti-canine IL-31 monoclonal antibodies were produced at Maine Biotechnology Services (Portland, ME, USA). CF-1 mice were immunized on a biweekly schedule with cIL-31. Postimmunization, mouse sera and primary fusion products were screened for reactivity to cIL-31 by ELISA. Hybridomas were generated and subcloned by limiting dilution to ensure monoclonal cultures.

Anti-canine IL-31 hybridomas were grown in RPMI 1640 base medium supplemented with 10% ultra-low IgG fetal bovine serum, 2 mmol/L GlutaMAX, 100 U/mL penicillin, 100 μg/mL streptomycin and 55 μmol/L 2-mercaptoethanol. Antibodies were purified from the culture supernatants by protein A or protein G affinity chromatography.

Canine interleukin-31 immunoassays

A GyroLab sandwich immunoassay was used to quantify cIL-31 levels in canine serum. Serum samples were diluted 1:2 in Rexxip buffer (Gyrolab, Warren, NJ, USA) and run on Bioaffy 1000 nL CDs (Gyrolab) using the Gyrolab xP workstation. Canine interleukin-31 was captured with a biotin-labelled anti-IL-31 monoclonal antibody and detected with an Alexaflour 647-labelled anti-IL-31 monoclonal antibody. Sample concentrations of cIL-31 were extrapolated from an eight-point standard curve with a dynamic range of 0.013–250 ng/mL using a five-parameter fit equation with Gyrolab Evaluator software. The lower limit of quantification was determined to be 13 pg/mL based on the performance of quality control standards at this concentration. Specifically, the 13 pg/mL standards gave values at least two standard deviations above background, accuracy measurements consistently within 20% of intended concentrations, and precision or the percentage coefficient of variance (%CV) within 20%.

Statistical analysis

Data generated from the evaluation of pruritic effects of cIL-31 administered i.v. in beagle dogs were analysed using SAS software version 9.2 (SAS Institute Inc., Cary, NC, USA). PROC MIXED for mixed linear models was used to analyse pruritic score. The model included a fixed effect of treatment and random effects for room, block within room and error. Least squares means were used as estimates of treatment means. Standard errors for treatment means were calculated at 90% confidence intervals for treatment means constructed. All tests (significance of effects and treatment comparisons) were conducted at the two-sided 10% level of significance.

Results

Identification and functional assessment of canine IL-31

Canine interleukin-31 was cloned by RT-PCR from total RNA isolated from canine testicular tissue, a tissue shown to express IL-31 mRNA by other investigators.[2,13] The nucleotide sequence generated for cIL-31 was identical to the one independently determined and reported (GenBank AB455159).[13] Protein produced from the generated cIL-31 mammalian expression systems was confirmed to be cIL-31 by N-terminal sequencing and tryptic mapping (see Supporting information Figure S1). To confirm biological activity of the expressed and purified protein, cIL-31 was evaluated for its ability to activate the JAK-STAT, MAPK and PI3K pathways, because these signal transduction pathways have been reported to be involved in the signalling of human and mouse IL-31.[9] Specifically, cIL-31 treatment led to STAT3 and ERK1/2 phosphorylation in DH82 cells with EC_{50} values of 53.2 and 84.5 ng/mL, respectively (Figure 1a,b). Phosphorylation of these proteins is indicative of JAK/STAT and MAPK pathway activation, respectively. The phosphorylation of Akt, a marker of PI3K activity, was constitutively turned on in this cell line, so induction of this pathway (PI3K/Akt) by cIL-31 could not be evaluated adequately (see Supporting information Figure S2).

Administration of cIL-31 *in vivo* to purpose-bred beagle dogs caused transient episodes of pruritic behaviour ranging from two- to 10-fold increases above baseline measurements, regardless of the route of administration (Table 1). Behaviours varied among animals. For example, some animals primarily exhibited behaviours such as scratching or head shaking (e.g. dog no. 4807448), whereas others spent most of their time licking (e.g. dog no. 4746538). One animal did not appear to respond to IL-31 injections at all (dog no. 4802098). When pruritic behaviours were displayed, they were readily seen within 4 h after cIL-31 administration and tended to return to baseline levels within 24 h (data not shown). No other obvious clinical signs were observed in the animals. Phosphate-buffered saline vehicle containing residual host cell

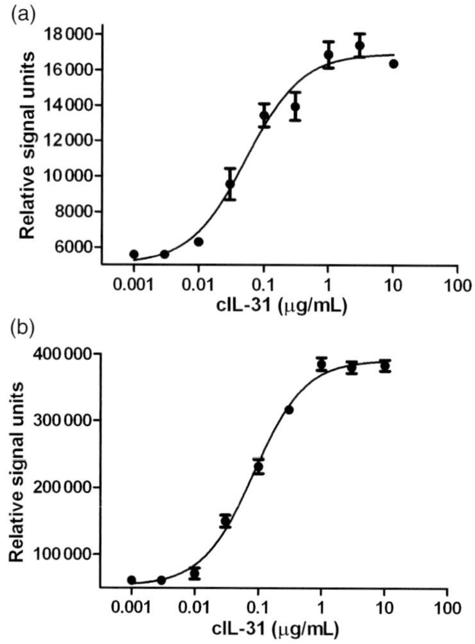

Figure 1. Canine interleukin-31 (cIL-31) induces phosphorylation of STAT3 (pSTAT3) and ERK1/2 (pERK1/2) in DH82 cells. pSTAT3 and pERK1/2 (b) were induced by cIL-31 in a dose-dependent manner. Data are expressed as mean relative signal units ± SEM (*n* = 3).

proteins at equivalent concentrations to those present in the cIL-31 preparations (mock protein) did not induce pruritic behaviours above baseline levels (e.g dog no. 3770044). When evaluated over a 2 h period using a categorical scoring system, dogs receiving cIL-31 (i.v.) exhibited a statistically significant increase in mean pruritic score when compared with the vehicle control treatment groups (Figure 2).

Detection of cIL-31 cytokine in dogs with naturally occurring atopic dermatitis

A variety of canine populations were evaluated for the presence of cIL-31 in serum. Levels were not detectable (<13 pg/mL) in the serum from purpose-bred beagle dogs prior to and after sensitization to HDM (*n* = 24 dogs), mixed breed dogs prior to and after flea infestation (*n* = 30 dogs) or client-owned dogs with periodontal disease but otherwise considered to be in good health, regardless of breed (*n* = 87 dogs). In the dogs with naturally occurring AD, cIL-31 was detectable (≥13 pg/mL) in 57% (127 of 223) of the animals, with 52% (117 of 223) of the samples showing serum cIL-31 levels between 13 and 1000 pg/mL, and 4% (10 of 223) showing levels above 1000 pg/mL (Table 2 and Supporting information Table S1).

Discussion

This report describes the generation of canine interleukin-31 protein and the biological function of this cytokine in canine systems. Canine IL-31 was found to activate the JAK-STAT pathway as well as the MAPK pathway in canine cells. Upon administration of cIL-31 to dogs, a significant increase in pruritic behaviours was observed. This study is the first to describe the biological function of IL-31 in canine models. These study results also corroborate the findings from others who have shown the same signalling cascades activated by mouse and human IL-31[9,17] and have observed pruritic phenotypes in mice infused with or engineered to overexpress IL-31.[2] Interleukin-31 may therefore play a role in inducing pruritus across a variety of species.

The types of pruritic behaviours observed in dogs after IL-31 injection included scratching, licking, chewing, scooting, head shaking and body rubbing; however, not all behaviours were seen in each animal. Instead, the types of behaviours displayed by each animal varied. One animal (dog no. 4802098) displayed as much pruritic behaviour during baseline monitoring as most dogs did after IL-31 injection, and IL-31 injection in this dog did not appear to increase the amount of pruritus displayed by this animal as determined by video monitoring and quantification of time spent scratching over a 4 h observation period. This dog could have been nonresponsive to IL-31 or may have already had endogenously circulating levels

Table 1. Effects of canine interleukin-31 (cIL-31) administration via different routes on pruritic behaviour in dogs

Dog no.	Total cIL-31 dose (μg)	Delivery route*	Observed pruritus (s) over 4 h intervals (mean ± SD): Baseline (*n* = 2–3)†	After cIL-31 Delivery (*n* = 1)‡	Fold increase in pruritus after cIL-31 (versus baseline)
4340761	10	i.d.	28 ± 26	162	5.8
4807448	10	i.d.	263 ± 59	862	3.3
4746538	10	i.d.	124 ± 67	1096	8.8
4701488	10	i.d.	417 ± 80	916	2.2
3770044	0 (mock protein)	i.d.	348 ± 111	254	0
4802098	10	s.c.	988 ± 223	782	0
4814975	10	s.c.	312 ± 37	885	2.8
4477138	10	s.c.	31 ± 15	201	6.5
4711921	10	s.c.	232 ± 84	1547	6.7
4340761	10	i.v.	103 ± 125	996	9.7
4701488	10	i.v.	480 ± 235	989	2.1
4477138	10	i.v.	163 ± 123	1147	7
3770044	0 (mock protein)	i.v.	359 ± 78	137	0

Observed pruritus (in seconds) over 4 h intervals is listed for baseline observations (means ± SD) and observations taken after cIL-31 treatment. Fold increase in pruritus from baseline is also calculated.

*i.d., intradermal injection (0.2 mL volume); s.c., subcutaneous injection (0.2 mL volume); or i.v., intravenous injection (1 mL volume).

†Replicate baseline observations were made on separate days but at the same time of day. Data represent means ± SD.

‡Administration of cIL-31 was performed on a different day from baseline observations, but at the same time of day.

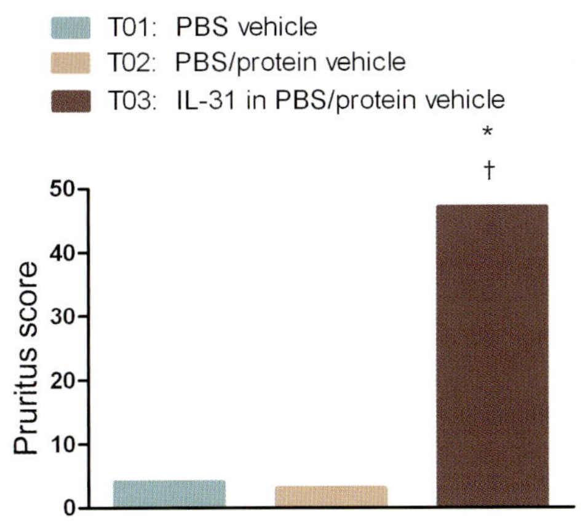

Figure 2. Canine interleukin-31 (cIL-31) administered intravenously induced pruritus in dogs. Pruritic scores from phosphate-buffered saline (PBS) vehicle-treated (T01), PBS/protein vehicle-treated (T02) and 1.75 μg/kg cIL-31 in PBS/protein vehicle-treated (T03) animals were compared. Pruritic behaviour was evaluated for 2 h starting approximately 30 min after cIL-31 injection. Mean pruritic scores (back transformed least square means) are shown. Canine IL-31 significantly induces pruritic behaviour in dogs compared with the vehicle control-treated groups (*T01 versus T03, $P = 0.0004$; †T02 versus T03, $P = 0.0003$. No significant difference was observed between T01 versus T02).

of IL-31. This animal was a neutered male 4 years of age and the heaviest dog in the study, weighing 26.8 kg. The correlation between body weight and IL-31 serum levels was not evaluated in this study but will be an important factor to consider in the future.

Evaluating the relevance of IL-31 in naturally occurring pruritic skin diseases, such as AD, was of interest in the present study, because observations from laboratory models do not always accurately reflect pathways or mediators involved in naturally occurring, chronic disease conditions. When serum samples from a variety of canine populations were analysed for IL-31 protein levels, IL-31 was detected in 57% of dogs diagnosed with naturally occurring AD. Interleukin-31 was not detected in normal dogs, in pruritic, flea-allergic dogs or in dogs sensitized to the HDM allergen *D. farinae*. These findings suggest that IL-31 may be dysregulated in dogs with AD and may contribute to the pathobiology of this chronic allergic skin disease. It is not surprising that IL-31 was not detected in HDM-sensitized dogs, because these dogs were not pruritic after the sensitization protocol. However, IL-31 levels were also not detected in the serum from flea-allergic dogs, even though these animals displayed pruritic behaviours. One explanation could be that this cytokine is not a key mediator of pruritus in flea allergy dermatitis. Alternatively, IL-31 could be acting locally within the skin and not readily detected in the serum. The length of flea infestation may also play a role. These animals were exposed to fleas for only 1 week prior to sampling. Interleukin-31 levels were not assessed in animals with prolonged infestation with fleas.

Table 2. Number of animals with detectable serum IL-31 in various canine populations

Canine population	Number of animals evaluated	Number of animals with detectable cIL-31 in serum*
Purpose-bred beagle dogs	24	0
Purpose-bred beagle dogs sensitized to house dust mite	24	0
Mixed breed dogs with no fleas	30	0
Mixed breed dogs infested with fleas	30	0
Healthy client-owned dogs of multiple breeds	87	0
Naturally occurring atopic dermatitis in client-owned dogs of multiple breeds	223	127

*Protein levels of cIL-31 were measured in canine populations using immunoassay techniques. The number of animals evaluated and the number of animals in which cIL-31 was detected (≥13 pg/mL) are listed for each population. A value <13 pg/mL is below the limit of quantification.

lAlthough IL-31 was detected in 57% of dogs with AD, a large percentage of animals with AD (43%) did not display detectable levels of IL-31 (<13 pg/mL). These animals may have had circulating levels of IL-31 that were below our assay limits of detection, or possibly IL-31 levels were acting locally within target tissues and not released into the circulation. Alternatively, IL-31 dysregulation may not play a significant role in the aetiology of AD in these animals with undetectable IL-31 levels. The latter interpretation is consistent with the concept that canine AD is a multifactorial disease that involves complex interactions between susceptibility genes, skin barrier dysfunction, immune dysregulation and neuroimmune interactions that collectively produce a hypersensitivity to environmental allergens and a pruritic allergic skin condition in dogs. Owing to the complexity of the disease, it is not surprising that not all dogs exhibit the same molecular or cellular changes.

Continued investigations of IL-31 in the canine AD population to determine whether serum levels correlate with a variety of parameters, such as age, breed, weight, sex and disease severity, will be important to improve our understanding of the role of IL-31 in this disease. Several investigators interested in the role of IL-31 in human AD have already extended their evaluations to the protein level and have generated data correlating serum levels of IL-31 to disease severity.[3,7] Specifically, studies have shown IL-31 to be elevated in the serum of human AD patients compared with healthy control subjects and that serum IL-31 levels correlate with disease severity in adults as well as children with AD.

Interleukin-31 in canine AD has been a topic of interest to other groups. Mizuno *et al.*[13] used RT-PCR techniques to evaluate IL-31 mRNA levels in a variety of canine tissues and in the skin of dogs with AD. This group was able to detect canine IL-31 mRNA in a variety of tissues; however, they were not able to detect IL-31 mRNA in the skin of dogs with naturally occurring AD ($n = 9$). They hypothesized that the biological function of IL-31 may be different in dogs versus other species or that evaluations of IL-31 protein could be more informative than looking at mRNA levels, given that mRNA levels do not always mimic changes that can be seen at the protein level. In our study, we were able to extend assessments of IL-31 to the protein level using quantitative immunoassay techniques and were able to detect elevated levels in the serum of dogs with AD. We were also able to evaluate a large population of dogs with naturally occurring AD (n = 224), which may have improved our chances of detecting IL-31 alterations in the canine AD population. Future studies should extend assessments of IL-31 protein levels to the skin of dogs with AD. Investigators have begun to perform these types of assessments in human AD patients and have found that IL-31 protein is elevated in the inflammatory infiltrates of skin biopsy specimens taken from AD subjects compared with skin biopsy specimens from patients with other types of skin diseases, suggesting that IL-31 dysregulation could be unique to AD.[8]

In summary, we demonstrated that canine IL-31 injected systemically or locally can induce pruritic behaviours in dogs and that this cytokine is elevated in a significant number of dogs with AD. We believe this pathway may play a role in the pathobiology of pruritic allergic skin conditions, such as canine AD, and may represent a novel pathway for therapeutic intervention.

Acknowledgements

The authors would like to thank Paul Aeed, Michelle Aleo, Larry Alward, Christopher Chio, Paula Clare, Eileen Coscarelli, Sallie Cosgrove, Betsy Galvan, James Curry, Antwain Howard, Dave Lowery, Donald Mann and Thomas Wilson for their technical contributions, Sean Mahabir for statistical assessments of data, and Olivier Martinon and Karen Greenwood for critical review of the manuscript.

References

1. Halliwell R. Revised nomenclature for veterinary allergy. *Vet Immunol Immunopathol* 2006; 114: 207–208.
2. Dillon SR, Sprecher C, Hammond A *et al.* Interleukin 31, a cytokine produced by activated T cells, induces dermatitis in mice. *Nat Immunol* 2004; 5: 752–760.
3. Raap U, Wichmann K, Bruder M *et al.* Correlation of IL-31 serum levels with severity of atopic dermatitis. *J Allergy Clin Immunol* 2008; 122: 421–423.
4. Sonkoly E, Muller A, Lauerma AI *et al.* IL-31: a new link between T cells and pruritus in atopic skin inflammation. *J Allergy Clin Immunol* 2006; 117: 411–417.
5. Bilsborough J, Leung DY, Maurer M *et al.* IL-31 is associated with cutaneous lymphocyte antigen-positive skin homing T cells in patients with atopic dermatitis. *J Allergy Clin Immunol* 2006; 117: 418–425.
6. Kim S, Kim HJ, Yang HS *et al.* IL-31 serum protein and tissue mRNA levels in patients with atopic dermatitis. *Ann Dermatol* 2011; 23: 468–473.
7. Ezzat MH, Hasan ZE, Shaheen KY. Serum measurement of interleukin-31 (IL-31) in paediatric atopic dermatitis: elevated levels correlate with severity scoring. *J Eur Acad Dermatol Venereol* 2011; 25: 334–339.
8. Nobbe S, Dziunycz P, Mühleisen B *et al.* IL-31 expression by inflammatory cells is preferentially elevated in atopic dermatitis. *Acta Derm Venereol* 2012; 92: 24–28.
9. Zhang Q, Putheti P, Zhou Q *et al.* Structures and biological functions of IL-31 and IL-31 receptors. *Cytokine Growth Factor Rev* 2008; 19: 347–356.
10. Kasraie S, Niebuhr M, Baumert K *et al.* Functional effects of interleukin 31 in human primary keratinocytes. *Allergy* 2011; 66: 845–852.
11. Kasraie S, Niebuhr M, Werfel T. Interleukin (IL)-31 induces proinflammatory cytokines in human monocytes and macrophages following stimulation with staphylococcal exotoxins. *Allergy* 2010; 65: 712–721.
12. Bando T, Morikawa Y, Komori T *et al.* Complete overlap of interleukin-31 receptor A and oncostatin M receptor β in the adult dorsal root ganglia with distinct developmental expression patterns. *Neuroscience* 2006; 142: 1263–1271.
13. Mizuno T, Kanbayashi S, Okawa T *et al.* Molecular cloning of canine interleukin-31 and its expression in various tissues. *Vet Immunol Immunopathol* 2009; 131: 140–143.
14. Lindenbaum M, Perkins E, Csonka E *et al.* A mammalian artificial chromosome engineering system (ACE System) applicable to biopharmaceutical protein production, transgenesis and gene-based cell therapy. *Nucleic Acids Res* 2004; 32: e172.
15. Willemse T. Atopic skin disease: a review and a reconsideration of diagnostic criteria. *J Small Anim Pract* 1986; 27: 771–778.
16. Prélaud P, Guaguère E, Alhaidari Z *et al.* Reevaluation of diagnostic criteria of canine atopic dermatitis. *Rev Med Vet (Toulouse)* 1998; 149: 1057–1064.
17. Diveu C, Lelievre E, Perret D *et al.* GPL, a novel cytokine receptor related to GP130 and leukemia inhibitory factor receptor. *J Biol Chem* 2003; 278: 49850–49859.

Supporting Information

Additional Supporting Information may be found in the online version of this article:

Figure S1. Amino acid sequence of the canine IL-31 construct. The identity of purified canine IL-31 protein was confirmed using mass spectrometry to analyse a tryptic digest of the protein and also by N-terminal sequencing.

Figure S2. Detection of phospho-Akt in cIL-31-treated DH82 cells. Using western blotting techniques, phospho-Akt levels were evaluated in DH82 cells treated with varying concentrations of IL-31 (0–10 μg/mL).

Table S1. Individual cIL-31 serum levels in dogs with atopic dermatitis. Protein levels of cIL-31 were measured in serum using immunoassay techniques in client-owned animals diagnosed with atopic dermatitis. Quantitative levels of cIL-31 in serum are listed for each dog evaluated.

To cite this article, please use DOI: 10.1111/j.1365-3164.2012.01096.x

2.4

Expression of thymic stromal lymphopoietin in canine atopic dermatitis

Jolanta Klukowska-Rötzler*, Ludovic Chervet†‡, Eliane J. Müller†§, Petra Roosje‡§, Eliane Marti*§ and Jozef Janda*

*Department of Clinical Research-VPH, Vetsuisse Faculty, University of Bern, Länggassstrasse 124, CH-3012 Bern, Switzerland
†Molecular Dermatology, Institute for Animal Pathology, Vetsuisse Faculty, University of Bern, Länggassstrasse 122, CH-3012 Bern, Switzerland
‡Division of Clinical Dermatology, Department of Clinical Veterinary Medicine, Vetsuisse Faculty, University of Bern, Länggassstrasse 128, CH-3012 Bern, Switzerland
§DermFocus, Vetsuisse Faculty, University of Bern, Länggassstrasse 122, CH-3012 Bern, Switzerland

Correspondence: Jozef Janda, Department of Clinical Research-VPH, Vetsuisse Faculty, University of Bern, Länggassstrasse 124, CH-3012 Bern, Switzerland. E-mail: jozef.janda@vetsuisse.unibe.ch

Background – In humans, thymic stromal lymphopoietin (TSLP) plays a central role in the development of allergic inflammation, such as atopic dermatitis (AD), but it is unknown whether it is involved in the pathogenesis of canine AD (CAD).

Hypothesis/Objectives – Our aim was to characterize canine *TSLP* and to assess its expression in CAD.

Methods – Canine *TSLP* was identified based on sequence homology with human *TSLP* and the complementary DNA (cDNA) cloned by RT-PCR. Real-time quantitative RT-PCR was established to assess the expression of canine *TSLP* in cultured canine keratinocytes and in skin biopsy specimens from lesional and nonlesional skin of 12 dogs with CAD and eight healthy control dogs.

Results – Partial canine *TSLP* cDNA was cloned and characterized. It contained four exons that shared 70 and 73% nucleotide identity with human and equine *TSLP*, respectively, encoding the signal peptide and full-length secreted protein. We found significantly increased *TSLP* expression in lesional and nonlesional skin of dogs with CAD compared with healthy control dogs ($P < 0.05$), whereas no difference was measured between lesional and nonlesional samples. In cultured primary canine keratinocytes, we found increased *TSLP* expression after stimulation with house dust mite allergen extract or Toll-like receptor ligands lipopolysaccharide and poly I:C.

Conclusions and clinical importance – Increased *TSLP* expression in the skin of dogs with CAD supports an involvement of TSLP in the pathogenesis of CAD similar to that in humans. Further studies should elucidate the function and therapeutic potential of TSLP in CAD.

Introduction

Thymic stromal lymphopoietin (TSLP) is an epithelial cell-derived cytokine, which plays a key role in differentiation of T-helper 2 (Th2) cells and development of allergic inflammation.[1] The expression of TSLP is increased in the skin of human patients with atopic dermatitis[2] and in the lungs of human asthma patients.[3] Results from mouse models support the central role of TSLP in allergic diseases, because tissue-specific overexpression of *TSLP* leads to the development of local allergic inflammation accompanied by a systemic Th2 response.[4,5] Conversely, mice lacking the TSLP receptor are more resistant to sensitization to inhaled allergens.[5] Thymic stromal lymphopoietin acts on dendritic cells (DCs), which then undergo maturation, express co-stimulatory molecules and efficiently present antigens.[2] In contrast to DCs stimulated by pathogens, human DCs stimulated by TSLP do not produce interleukin (IL)-12, which is the major T-helper 2 (Th1)-polarizing cytokine. Instead, TSLP-stimulated DCs induce differentiation of naive T cells into inflammatory Th2 cells, which produce IL-13, IL-4 and tumour necrosis factor-α.[2] Thus, TSLP may act as a master switch in allergic inflammation.[1]

Canine atopic dermatitis (CAD) is a common inflammatory skin disease of dogs, which shares several features with human atopic dermatitis (HAD), including predilection sites, genetic predisposition, age of onset, epidermal alterations[6] and immunopathological mechanisms.[7] Both HAD and CAD are characterized by imbalances in lymphocyte populations and their cytokines. Increased activities of both Th1 and Th2 cytokines have been observed in CAD, although results for individual cytokines differ among the studies. Nuttall *et al.*[8] observed overexpression of IL-4, interferon-γ, tumour necrosis factor-α and IL-2 and reduced expression of transforming growth factor-β1 in lesional skin of dogs with CAD. Another study[9] extended the analysis to include cytokines and transcription factors involved in

Accepted 29 June 2012
Sources of Funding: This study was self-funded.
Conflict of Interest: No conflicts of interest have been declared.

T-helper polarization and showed increased expression of signal transducer and activator of transcription 4 (STAT4), IL-13, suppressor of cytokine signaling 3 (SOCS3) and IL-10 and decreased expression of IL-12p40 and GATA-3 in lesional skin. The Th2 cytokines, such as IL-4 and IL-13, drive production of allergen-specific IgE antibodies,[10] which are a central feature in the pathogenesis of CAD.[11] Epicutaneous allergen challenge of sensitized dogs leads to an early increase in the expression of IL-6 and IL-13.[12] In analogy to humans and mice, TSLP could play an important role in Th2 polarization in CAD. However, canine *TSLP* has not been characterized and its role in CAD is not known.

The aim of this study, therefore, was to identify and characterize the canine *TSLP* gene and to establish real-time quantitative RT-PCR (RT-qPCR) protocols to assess the expression of *TSLP* in lesional and nonlesional skin of dogs with CAD and in cultured canine keratinocytes.

Materials and methods

Animals

This study was performed using 12 dogs diagnosed with CAD (five females and seven males; age range 3–12 years, mean 6.25 years and median 6 years) and eight healthy control dogs (five females and three males; age range 1.5–10 years, mean 6.7 years and median 6 years) of the following breeds: Labrador retriever, golden retriever, beagle, boxer, Jack Russell terrier, German shepherd, Hovawart, bull terrier, German Wachtelhund, American cocker spaniel and Newfoundland. These dogs were used and characterized in a previous study.[6] The diagnosis of CAD was based on a combination of history and clinical signs,[13] with exclusion of other pruritic differential diagnoses. Skin biopsy specimens (8 mm) were obtained from both lesional and nonlesional skin in the dogs with CAD. Normal skin tissue was obtained from eight age-matched and, if possible, breed-matched dogs with no known history or clinical signs of CAD. These dogs were euthanized for reasons unrelated to our study, and samples were taken immediately after euthanasia. The study protocol was approved by the local ethical committee on the use of animals, Canton Bern, Switzerland (BVET 84/05).

Isolation and culture of primary canine keratinocytes

Canine footpad keratinocytes were isolated from 10-week-old beagle dogs and cultured in monolayers as described.[14,15] Cells were maintained in William's E medium (BioConcept, Allschwill, Switzerland) including antibiotics (Gibco Antibiotic-Antimycotic 100X liquid; Gibco, Invitrogen, Carlsbad, CA, USA), 10% fetal calf serum (Gibco), 2 mmol/L L-glutamine (Gibco), 10^{-10} mol/L cholera toxin (Sigma-Aldrich, St Louis, MO, USA) and 10 ng/mL of human epidermal growth factor (EGF, E9644; Sigma-Aldrich). Monolayer culture cells were incubated at 34°C in air supplemented with 5% CO_2, passaged after trypsin digestion (5x Trypsin/EDTA PBS; BioConcept) and subcultured before they reached confluence. Cells between passages 12 and 20 were used for these experiments. For stimulation experiments, keratinocytes were incubated in complete medium lacking cholera toxin. Keratinocytes were stimulated for 4 h with phorbol 12-myristate 13-acetate (PMA, 50 ng/mL; Sigma-Aldrich) and ionomycin (1 μmol/L; Sigma-Aldrich) and for 18 h with concanavalin A (ConA, 5 μg/mL; Sigma-Aldrich), the Toll-like receptor (TLR)-4 ligand lipopolycaccharide (LPS, 1 μg/mL, derived from *Esherichia coli* 0128:B12; Sigma-Aldrich), the TLR-3 ligand polyinosinic:polycytidylic acid (poly I:C, 5 μg/mL; Sigma-Aldrich), the TLR-7 ligand imiquimod (5 μg/mL; Invivogen, San Diego, CA, USA), the TLR-2 ligand Pam3Cys (10 μg/mL; EMC microcollections, Tübingen, Germany), house dust mite extract (HDM, *Dermatophagoides farinae*, 5 μg/mL; Heska, Fribourg, Switzerland) and heat-inactivated HDM (5 μg/mL). Heat inactivation was performed at 99°C for 10 min in order to inhibit enzymatic activity of HDM. The TLR ligands were used at concentrations previously shown to induce activation of canine dendritic cells.[16] Cells were lysed in RLT buffer (Qiagen, Basel, Switzerland), and RNA was isolated as described in the next subsection.

Isolation of RNA and synthesis of cDNA

Total RNA was isolated from cultured keratinocytes using RNeasy Mini Kit (Qiagen) and from skin biopsy specimens using RNeasy Fibrous Tissue Kit (Qiagen) according to the manufacturer's instructions. Contaminating genomic DNA was removed by on-column DNase treatment. Total RNA was quantified spectrophotometrically at 260 nm (NanoDrop 1000; Thermo Scientific, Reinach, Switzerland), and samples were stored at −80°C until used.

Reverse transcription of total RNA was performed using Superscript III RT (Invitrogen) to generate complementary DNA (cDNA), which was used as a template for PCR. The cDNA synthesis reaction consisted of 500 ng RNA and 1 mmol/L random primers (Promega, Dübendorf, Switzerland), 0.5 mmol/L of each dNTP, 40 U RNase inhibitor (Promega) and 100 U SuperScript III reverse transcriptase (Invitrogen), in a total reaction volume of 40 μL. The RNA samples, random primers and dNTPs were incubated at 65°C for 5 min. Reverse transcriptase was added and the incubation continued at 25°C for 5 min followed by 50°C for 50 min. The reaction was terminated by heating at 70°C for 15 min. The cDNA samples were stored at −20°C until further processing.

Cloning of canine *TSLP*

To clone the canine *TSLP* cDNA, sequences homologous to human *TSLP* (GenBank accession NM_033035.4) were identified in *Canis familiaris* genome build 3.2 using BLASTN (blast.ncbi.nih.gov). From a skin biopsy specimen obtained from a dog affected with CAD, RNA was isolated and cDNA produced. Primers were designed using Primer3[17] based on homologies with human and equine[18] (Genbank NM_001164063) *TSLP*. The cloned primary sequence was determined by direct sequencing. Alignment of human and canine *TSLP* nucleotide and deduced amino acid sequences was performed using ClustalW.[19]

Real-time quantitative RT-PCR

Expression of *TSLP* mRNA was assessed by RT-qPCR with primers designed to span the exon 1 and 2 junction using Primer3 online software[16] (forward, 5′-AGT ACA CGG GGT GGC TGA-3′; reverse, 5′-GTC ATT TAC CAA GCC CTG GA-3′; and probe, 5′-FAM-TCC GTG CTC CTG GTC CCA TCC ATG TAT T-TAMRA-3′). The PCR consisted of 2 μL cDNA, primers (300 nmol/L each), fluorescence-labelled probe (200 nmol/L) and TaqMan Universal PCR Mastermix (Applied Biosystems, Austin, TX, USA). The PCRs were performed in a total volume of 25 μL and carried out in a 7300 Real-Time PCR System (Applied Biosystems). The PCR consisted of an initial 2 min at 50°C, 10 min denaturation at 95°C, followed by 45 cycles of 15 s denaturation at 95°C and 1 min annealing and elongation at 60°C. Reactions were performed in duplicates, and no-template and RT-negative controls were included in each run. Efficiencies of the PCRs were calculated using a relative standard curve derived from a cDNA pool. Gene expression was quantified using the $\Delta\Delta Ct$ method.[20] Expression of *TSLP* was normalized to the expression of the housekeeping gene 18S ribosomal RNA (18S rRNA; Applied Biosystems).

Statistical analysis

Statistical analyses were carried out with the software package NCSS 2001 (NCSS, Kaysville, UT, USA). The Mann–Whitney *U*-test was used to compare dogs withCAD with healthy control dogs. The Wilcoxon signed rank test was used for comparison of paired data (lesional versus nonlesional). Student's two-sample *t* test (unpaired) was used to compare stimulated and nonstimulated keratinocytes.

Results

Characterization of canine *TSLP*

A partial cDNA of canine *TSLP* was generated by RT-PCR from an RNA sample of lesional skin from a dog with CAD, cloned and sequenced and the sequence deposited in GenBank (accession JQ698664). The cDNA sequence contained 465 nucleotides and was organized in four exons (Figure 1). The exon–intron boundaries were in accord with the splicing scheme for human *TSLP* gene reported previously by Quentmeier *et al.*,[21] whose numbering scheme was followed by the investigators. The splice donor and acceptor sites were consistent with the GT/AG rule. The canine *TSLP* gene was located on chromosome 3 (1.503–1.507 Mbp), which corresponds to human chromosome 5 and equine chromosome 14. When the coding sequence of canine *TSLP* cDNA was aligned with the orthologous human and equine sequences (GenBank accession numbers NM_033035.4 and NM_001164063.1), the nucleotide identity was 70 and 73%, respectively, and covered the sequence encoding the signal peptide and full-length mature protein of human and equine *TSLP*. Alignment of canine and human nucleotide sequences is shown in Figure 2a.

The predicted amino acid sequence deduced from the canine *TSLP* cDNA shares 60.8 and 59.9% identity with human (NP_149024.1) and equine TSLP protein (NP_001157535.1), respectively. Alignment between canine and human TSLP proteins is shown in Figure 2b. Although the N-terminal part of the protein was not determined, it was possible to predict the cleavage site of the putative signal peptide and the N-terminus of the mature protein (Figure 1; SignalP, http://www.cbs.dtu.dk/services/SignalP), which are analogous to human and equine TSLP proteins. Furthermore, the deduced amino acid sequence ended with a stop codon, suggesting that the partial cDNA encodes the signal peptide and mature canine TSLP protein (Figure 1).

Increased expression of *TSLP* in the skin of dogs with atopic dermatitis

The expression of *TSLP* mRNA was determined by RT-qPCR in lesional and nonlesional skin of the 12 dogs with CAD and compared with skin from the eight healthy control dogs. The expression of *TSLP* was significantly higher in both lesional and nonlesional skin of dogs with CAD compared with the control dogs ($P < 0.05$; Figure 3), but there was no significant difference between lesional and nonlesional samples.

Expression of *TSLP* in primary canine keratinocytes

The primary canine keratinocyte cell line generated from canine footpad was stimulated with PMA + ionomycin, TLR ligands (LPS, polyI:C, Pam3Cys and imiquimod) and HDM, and the expression of *TSLP* was measured by RT-qPCR (Figure 4). The PMA + ionomycin induced the strongest upregulation of *TSLP* expression (262-fold increase; $P < 0.05$).

Lipopolysaccharide and poly I:C also upregulated *TSLP* expression in canine keratinocytes (15.9- and 18.1-fold increase, respectively; $P < 0.05$), whereas the other TLR ligands had no significant effect on *TSLP* expression. Concanavalin A also failed to induce *TSLP* expression in canine keratinocytes. Keratinocytes stimulated with HDM responded with upregulated *TSLP* expression (27-fold increase; $P < 0.05$). The effect of HDM was inhibited by heat inactivation of HDM at 99°C, i.e. the expression of TSLP was significantly lower after stimulation with heat-inactivated HDM than with intact HDM ($P < 0.05$; Figure 4, indicated by #).

Discussion

In the present study, we identified and characterized canine *TSLP* and assessed the expression of *TSLP* in the skin of dogs with CAD and in cultured primary canine keratinocytes. We found that *TSLP* expression was increased in both lesional and nonlesional skin samples from dogs with CAD compared with healthy control dogs (Figure 3). Moreover, we observed that primary canine keratinocytes upregulated *TSLP* expression when stimulated with HDM allergen extract (Figure 4). These findings suggest that TSLP may play an important role in the pathogenesis of CAD.

We identified and amplified a partial *TSLP* sequence analogous to human and equine *TSLP* that covers the signal peptide and full-length mature protein. There is a predicted canine *TSLP* sequence in GenBank (accession XM_844431.2), but when we designed primers based on this sequence we were not able to amplify it by RT-PCR. A possible explanation is that this sequence might be faulty, or it encodes a different gene or splicing variant that is not expressed in the tissue examined. Although our *TSLP* sequence does not cover the entire

```
ttgcctgatgccttattatctgttctgtcagtgtttttcaggaagatcttcgtcttgcag    Exon1
 L  P  D  A  L  L  S  V  L  S  V  F  F  R  K  I  F  V  L  Q
ctggtagggctggtgctaacc‖tacaatttcattgactgtgactttgagaagattagatgg
 L  V  G  L  V  L  T ‖ Y  N  F  I  D  C  D  F  E  K  I  R  W
aagtatcaggaagtcatttaccaagccctggagaaatacatggatgggac█caggagcacg    Exon2
 K  Y  Q  E  V  I  Y  Q  A  L  E  K  Y  M  D  G  T   R  S  T
cgagttcagccaccccgtgtactgcgcggacccg█ccgactgcctggccaggatcgagcgg    Exon3
 E  F  S  H  P  V  Y  C  A  D  P   P  D  C  L  A  R  I  E  R
ctcaccctgcaccgcatccgcggctgcgcgtcgggcgcccgggaggccttcgccgagggg
 L  T  L  H  R  I  R  G  C  A  S  G  A  R  E  A  F  A  E  G
acggtcgccgcgctcgccgccgagtgcccgggctacgccgcagcgccg█ataaataatacc    Exon4
 T  V  A  A  L  A  A  E  C  P  G  Y  A  A  A  P   I  N  N  T
caggcaaagaagaaaagaaaaaaaagaggagtcacaacaaataaatgccgggaacaagtc
 Q  A  K  K  K  R  K  K  R  G  V  T  T  N  K  C  R  E  Q  V
gcacacttaatagggctgtggcgtcgtttcagtcgcatttcatag
 A  H  L  I  G  L  W  R  R  F  S  R  I  S  -
```

Figure 1. Canine thymic stromal lymphopoietin (*TSLP*) nucleotide sequence and the deduced amino acid sequence. Exon–exon boundaries are marked by filled squares. The predicted signal peptide cleavage site is marked by ‖.

(a)

```
CanineTSLP      ---TTGCCTGATGCCTTATTATCTGTTCTGTCAGTGTTTTTCAGGAAGATCTTCGTCTTG 57
HumanTSLP       ATGTTCCCTTTTGCCTTACTATATGTTCTGTCAGTTTCTTTCAGGAAAATCTTCATCTTA 60
                   ** ***  ******* *** ************ * ********* ****** ****

CanineTSLP      CAGCTGGTAGGGCTGGTGCTAACCTACAATTTCATTGACTGTGACTTTGAGAAGATTAGA 117
HumanTSLP       CAACTTGTAGGGCTGGTGTTAACTTACGACTTCACTAACTGTGACTTTGAGAAGATTAAA 120
                ** ** ************ **** *** * **** * ********************* *

CanineTSLP      TGGAAGTATCAGGAAGTCATTTACCAAGCCCTGGAGAAATACATGGATGGGACCAGGAGC 177
HumanTSLP       GCAGCCTATCTCAGTACTATTTCTAAAGACCTGATTACATATATGAGTGGGACCAAAAGT 180
                      ****        ****   *** ****   * *** ***  ********  **

CanineTSLP      ACGGAGTTCAGCCACCCCGTGTACTGCGCGGACCCGCCCGACTGCCTGGCCAGGATCGAG 237
HumanTSLP       ACCGAGTTCAACAACACCGTCTCTTGTAGCAATCGGCCACATTGCCTTACTGAAATCCAG 240
                ** ******* * ** **** *  **     * * ***  * *****  *    *** **

CanineTSLP      CGGCTCACCCTGCACCGCATCCGCGGCTGCGCGTCGGGCGCCCGGGAGGCCTTCGCCGAG 297
HumanTSLP       AGCCTAACCTTCAATCCCACCGCCGGCTGCGCGTCGCTCGCCAAAGAAATGTTCGCCATG 300
                 * ** *** *  * * ** *  *************  ****   **    ******  *

CanineTSLP      GGGACGGTCGCCGCGCTCGCCGCCGAGTGCCCGGGCTACGCCGCAGCGCCGATAAATAAT 357
HumanTSLP       AAAACTAAGGCTGCCTTAGCTATCTGGTGCCCAGGCTATTCGGAAACTCAGATAAATGCT 360
                   **    ** **  * **   *  ****** *****  * * * * * *******  *

CanineTSLP      ACCCAGGCAAAGAAGAAAAGAAAAAAAAGAGGAGTCACAACAAATAAATGCCGGGAACAA 417
HumanTSLP       ACTCAGGCAATGAAGAAGAGGAGAAAAAGGAAAGTCACAACCAATAAATGTCTGGAACAA 420
                ** ******* ****** ** * ******   ********* ******** * *******

CanineTSLP      GTCGCACACTTAATAGGGCTGTGGCGTCGTTTCAGTCGCATTTCATAG------------ 465
HumanTSLP       GTGTCACAATTACAAGGATTGTGGCGTCGCTTCAATCGACCTTTACTGAAACAACAGTAA 480
                **  **** ***  ***  ********** **** ***   ** *  *
```

(b)

```
HumanTSLP       MFPFALLYVLSVSFRKIFILQLVGLVLTYDFTNCDFEKIKAAYLSTISKDLITYMSGTKS 60
CanineTSLP      -LPDALLSVLSVFFRKIFVLQLVGLVLTYNFIDCDFEKIRWKYQEVIYQALEKYMDGTRS 59
                 :* *** **** *****:**********:* :******:  * ..* : * .**.**:*

HumanTSLP       TEFNNTVSCSNRPHCLTEIQSLTFNPTAGCASLAKEMFAMKTKAALAIWCPGYSETQINA 120
CanineTSLP      TEFSHPVYCADPPDCLARIERLTLHRIRGCASGAREAFAEGTVAALAAECPGYAAAPINN 119
                ***.:.* *:: *.**:.*: **::   **** *:* **  * ****  ****: : **

HumanTSLP       TQAMKKRRKRKVTTNKCLEQVSQLQGLWRRFNRPLLKQQ 159
CanineTSLP      TQAKKKRKKRGVTTNKCREQVAHLIGLWRRFSRIS---- 154
                *** ***:** ****** ***::* ******.*
```

Figure 2. Alignment of canine and human *TSLP* nucleotide (a) and amino acid sequences (b) performed by ClustalW. Identities are shown by '*' and similarities by ':' and '.'. Start and stop codons are underlined.

coding sequence of canine *TSLP* (the 5′-terminal part is missing), it is possible to predict the signal peptide cleavage site, which is well conserved among species. Therefore, the sequence coding for the full-length mature TSLP protein is included in our sequence and it will be sufficient for cloning and expressing of recombinant canine TSLP protein, which will be needed for further functional studies and for production of canine TSLP-specific antibodies.

We established RT-qPCR and used it to assess the expression of *TSLP* in skin biopsy samples and in cultured keratinocytes. While RT-qPCR is a very sensitive and accurate method, its major limitation is that it does not allow identification of cellular sources of TSLP in tissue samples and does not assess the presence or biological activity of TSLP protein. In order to address these important questions, tools need to be developed, such as antibodies for immunohistochemistry or enzyme-linked immunosorbent assay.

The *TSLP* expression was measured in a small group of healthy dogs and CAD-affected dogs of various breeds. To confirm our findings, a larger study involving more dogs needs to be completed and expression of other genes assessed. A larger group of dogs would allow the association between *TSLP* expression and severity of lesions to be assessed. To gain more insight into the mechanisms of action of TSLP, the expression of TSLP target genes, such as *IL-4*, *IL-13*, *OX40L*, macrophage-derived chemokine (MDC) and thymus and activation-regulated chemokine (TARC)[2] needs to be measured.

A previous study using the same population of dogs has shown an aberrant expression of filaggrin in the skin of some dogs with CAD.[6] An epidermal barrier defect, aberrant filaggrin expression and increased TSLP expression may all play an important role in the pathogenesis of CAD, because a similar mechanism has been proposed in human AD.[22]

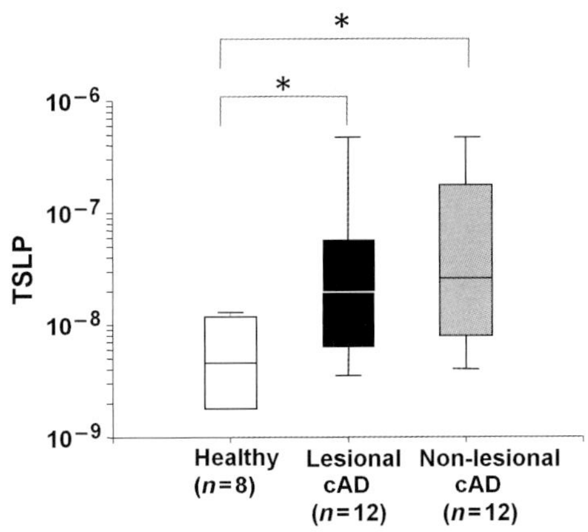

Figure 3. Expression of *TSLP* in canine atopic dermatitis (CAD). Relative expression of canine *TSLP* in lesional and nonlesional skin of 12 dogs with CAD and eight healthy control dogs. Values are normalized to the expression of a housekeeping gene, 18S rRNA. Statistical analysis was performed using the Mann–Whitney *U*-test (*$P < 0.05$).

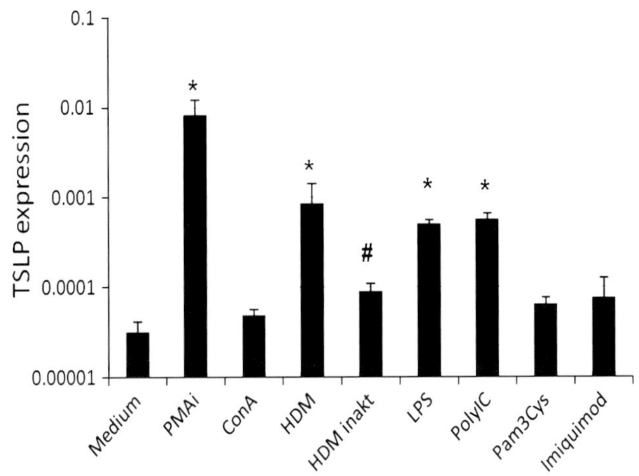

Figure 4. Expression of *TSLP* in canine keratinocytes. Relative expression of canine *TSLP* in cultured primary canine keratinocytes incubated with medium alone, or stimulated with phorbol 12-myristate 13-acetate (PMA, 50 ng/mL) + ionomycin (1 μmol/L; PMAi), concanavalin A (ConA, 5 μg/mL), lipopolysaccharide (LPS, 1 μg/mL), polyinosinic:polycytidylic acid (poly I:C, 5 μg/mL), imiquimod (5 μg/mL), Pam3Cys (10 μg/mL), house dust mite extract (HDM, 5 μg/mL) or heat-inactivated HDM (HDM inact, 5 μg/mL). Statistical analysis was performed by Student's two-sample *t*-test (unpaired). Significant differences between stimulants and medium are shown by * ($P < 0.05$); difference between HDM and heat-inactivated HDM is indicated by # ($P < 0.05$).

Stimulation of canine keratinocytes with HDM resulted in increased expression of *TSLP*. This finding highlights the role of TSLP in CAD, because HDM contains major allergens involved in the pathogenesis of CAD. Heat inactivation of HDM abrogated the induction of *TSLP* (Figure 4), suggesting that proteases or other heat-labile components are responsible for the induction of *TSLP* expression. Protease allergens have been shown to induce *TSLP* expression in human epithelial cells through the activation of protease-activated receptor-2.[23] Several mechanisms have been proposed by which proteases may facilitate sensitization and priming of Th2 responses.[24] Through the disruption of tight junctions, proteases may facilitate the transepithelial transfer of allergens. Proteases may also change the activity of DCs by cleaving of the co-stimulatory molecules CD40[25] or DC-SIGN,[26] as has been shown for Der p 1 allergen. Allergen proteases may also directly influence adaptive immune responses by cleaving of CD25 on T cells or CD23 on B cells. Cleavage of CD25 (IL-2 receptor α-chain) by Der p 1 resulted in reduced Th1 and enhanced Th2 cytokine expression in cultured T cells.[27] Der p 1 can also cleave CD23, the low-affinity receptor for IgE, which normally acts as a negative regulator of IgE synthesis.[28] More detailed studies will be needed to dissect the potential role of allergen proteases in CAD.

We used whole-body HDM extract for the stimulation of canine keratinocytes in our study. As this also includes mite gut content, it is likely to contain microbial molecules (TLR ligands) in addition to allergens. Therefore, the effect of HDM on *TSLP* expression measured in our study may be mediated, at least in part, by TLR ligands. We also included stimulation with purified TLR ligands and found that LPS and poly I:C, but not Pam3Cys or imiquimod, induced *TSLP* expression in cultured canine keratinocytes (Figure 4). It has been shown previously that keratinocytes express functional TLRs and can respond to TLR stimulation by production of cytokines,[29] including TSLP.[30] However, it is still unclear how TLR stimulation contributes to allergic responses.

Genetic analysis provides additional evidence of the involvement of TSLP in CAD. Genotyping of single nucleotide polymorphisms in 25 candidate genes in dogs of various breeds revealed an association between a single nucleotide polymorphism in the TSLP receptor gene and CAD in all studied breeds.[31] In human patients, associations between allergic diseases and polymorphisms of the *TSLP* gene have been described.[32,33]

In conclusion, we characterized the canine *TSLP* gene and found increased expression of *TSLP* in the skin of dogs with atopic dermatitis. These preliminary findings indicate an involvement of TSLP in the pathogenesis of atopic dermatitis in dogs. Further studies should elucidate the function of TSLP in CAD and explore its potential as a therapeutic target.

References

1. Liu Y-J. Thymic stromal lymphopoietin: master switch for allergic inflammation. *J Exp Med* 2006; 203: 269–273.
2. Soumelis V, Reche PA, Kanzler H *et al.* Human epithelial cells trigger dendritic cell mediated allergic inflammation by producing TSLP. *Nat Immunol* 2002; 3: 673–680.
3. Ying S, O'Connor B, Ratoff J *et al.* Thymic stromal lymphopoietin expression is increased in asthmatic airways and correlates with expression of Th2-attracting chemokines and disease severity. *J Immunol* 2005; 174: 8183–8190.
4. Yoo J, Omori M, Gyarmati D *et al.* Spontaneous atopic dermatitis in mice expressing an inducible thymic stromal lymphopoietin transgene specifically in the skin. *J Exp Med* 2005; 202: 541–549.
5. Zhou B, Comeau MR, De Smedt T *et al.* Thymic stromal lymphopoietin as a key initiator of allergic airway inflammation in mice. *Nat Immunol* 2005; 6: 1047–1053.
6. Chervet L, Galichet A, McLean WHI *et al.* Missing C-terminal filaggrin expression, NFkappaB activation and hyperproliferation identify the dog as a putative model to study epidermal

dysfunction in atopic dermatitis. *Exp Dermatol* 2010; 19: e343–e346.

7. Marsella R, Girolomoni G. Canine models of atopic dermatitis: a useful tool with untapped potential. *J Invest Dermatol* 2009; 129: 2351–2357.
8. Nuttall TJ, Knight PA, McAleese SM *et al.* T-helper 1, T-helper 2 and immunosuppressive cytokines in canine atopic dermatitis. *Clin Exp Allergy* 2002; 32: 789–795.
9. Schlotter YM, Rutten VPMG, Riemers FM *et al.* Lesional skin in atopic dogs shows a mixed Type-1 and Type-2 immune responsiveness. *Vet Immunol Immunopathol* 2011; 143: 20–26.
10. Poulsen LK, Hummelshoj L. Triggers of IgE class switching and allergy development. *Ann Med* 2007; 39: 440–456.
11. Halliwell RE, DeBoer DJ. The ACVD task force on canine atopic dermatitis (III): the role of antibodies in canine atopic dermatitis. *Vet Immunol Immunopathol* 2001; 8: 159–167.
12. Marsella R, Olivry T, Maeda S. Cellular and cytokine kinetics after epicutaneous allergen challenge (atopy patch testing) with house dust mites in high-IgE beagles. *Vet Dermatol* 2006; 17: 111–120.
13. DeBoer DJ, Hillier A. The ACVD task force on canine atopic dermatitis (XV): fundamental concepts in clinical diagnosis. *Vet Immunol Immunopathol* 2001; 81: 271–276.
14. Langedijk JPM, Janda J, Origgi FC *et al.* Canine distemper virus infects canine keratinocytes and immune cells by using overlapping and distinct regions located on one side of the attachment protein. *J Virol* 2011; 85: 11242–11254.
15. Engelhardt P, Wyder M, Zurbriggen A *et al.* Canine distemper virus associated proliferation of canine footpad keratinocytes in vitro. *Vet Microbiol* 2005; 107: 1–12.
16. Ricklin Gutzwiller ME, Moulin HR, Zurbriggen A *et al.* Comparative analysis of canine monocyte- and bone-marrow-derived dendritic cells. *Vet Res* 2010; 41: 40–52.
17. Rozen S, Skaletsky H. Primer3 on the WWW for general users and for biologist programmers. *Methods Mol Biol* 2000; 132: 365–386.
18. Klukowska-Rötzler J, Marti E, Bugno M *et al.* Molecular cloning and characterization of equine thymic stromal lymphopoietin. *Vet Immunol Immunopathol* 2010; 136: 346–349.
19. Larkin MA, Blackshields G, Brown NP *et al.* Clustal W and Clustal X version 2.0. *Bioinformatics* 2007; 23: 2947–2948.
20. Livak KJ, Schmittgen TD. Analysis of relative gene expression data using real-time quantitative PCR and the $2^{-\Delta\Delta CT}$ method. *Methods* 2001; 25: 402–408.
21. Quentmeier H, Drexler HG, Fleckenstein D *et al.* Cloning of human thymic stromal lymphopoietin (TSLP) and signaling mechanisms leading to proliferation. *Leukemia* 2001; 15: 1286–1292.
22. Lee KH, Cho KA, Kim JY *et al.* Filaggrin knockdown and Toll-like receptor 3 (TLR3) stimulation enhanced the production of thymic stromal lymphopoietin (TSLP) from epidermal layers. *Exp Dermatol* 2011; 20: 149–151.
23. Kouzaki H, O'Grady SM, Lawrence CB *et al.* Proteases induce production of thymic stromal lymphopoietin by airway epithelial cells through protease-activated receptor-2. *J Immunol* 2009; 183: 1427–1434.
24. Wills-Karp M, Nathan A, Page K *et al.* New insights into innate immune mechanisms underlying allergenicity. *Mucosal Immunol* 2010; 3: 104–110.
25. Ghaemmaghami AM, Gough L, Sewell HF *et al.* The proteolytic activity of the major dust mite allergen Der p 1 conditions dendritic cells to produce less interleukin-12: allergen-induced Th2 bias determined at the dendritic cell level. *Clin Exp Allergy* 2002; 32: 1468–1475.
26. Furmonaviciene R, Ghaemmaghami AM, Boyd SE *et al.* The protease allergen Der p 1 cleaves cell surface DC-SIGN and DC-SIGNR: experimental analysis of *in silico* substrate identification and implications in allergic responses. *Clin Exp Allergy* 2007; 37: 231–242.
27. Schulz O, Sewell HF, Shakib F. Proteolytic cleavage of CD25, the α subunit of the human T cell interleukin 2 receptor, by Der p 1, a major mite allergen with cysteine protease activity. *J Exp Med* 1998; 187: 271–275.
28. Schulz O, Laing P, Sewell HF *et al.* *Der p* I, a major allergen of the house dust mite, proteolytically cleaves the low-affinity receptor for human IgE (CD23). *Eur J Immunol* 1995; 25: 3191–3194.
29. Begon E, Michel L, Flageul B *et al.* Expression, subcellular localization and cytokinic modulation of Toll-like receptors (TLRs) in normal human keratinocytes: TLR2 up-regulation in psoriatic skin. *Eur J Dermatol* 2007; 17: 497–506.
30. Kinoshita H, Takai T, Le TA *et al.* Cytokine milieu modulates release of thymic stromal lymphopoietin from human keratinocytes stimulated with double-stranded RNA. *J Allergy Clin Immunol* 2009; 123: 179–186.
31. Wood SH, Ollier WE, Nuttall T *et al.* Despite identifying some shared gene associations with human atopic dermatitis the use of multiple dog breeds from various locations limits detection of gene associations in canine atopic dermatitis. *Vet Immunol Immunopathol* 2010; 138: 193–197.
32. Harada M, Hirota T, Jodo AI *et al.* Thymic stromal lymphopoietin gene promoter polymorphisms are associated with susceptibility to bronchial asthma. *Am J Respir Cell Mol Biol* 2011; 44: 787–793.
33. Hirota T, Takahashi A, Kubo M *et al.* Genome-wide association study identifies three new susceptibility loci for adult asthma in the Japanese population. *Nat Genet* 2011; 43: 893–896.

Part 3

Skin Biology

To cite this article, please use DOI: 10.1111/j.1365-3164.2012.01090.x

3.1

The stratum corneum: the rampart of the mammalian body

Koji Nishifuji* and Ji Seon Yoon†

*Department of Veterinary Medicine, Faculty of Agriculture, Tokyo University of Agriculture and Technology, Tokyo, Japan
†Department of Dermatology, College of Medicine, Seoul National University, Seoul, South Korea

Correspondence: Koji Nishifuji, Department of Veterinary Medicine, Faculty of Agriculture, Tokyo University of Agriculture and Technology, 3-5-8 Saiwai-cho, Fuchu, Tokyo 183-8509, Japan. E-mail: kojimail@cc.tuat.ac.jp

Background – The stratum corneum (SC) is the outermost region of the epidermis and plays key roles in cutaneous barrier function in mammals. The SC is composed of 'bricks', represented by flattened, protein-enriched corneocytes, and 'mortar', represented by intercellular lipid-enriched layers. As a result of this 'bricks and mortar' structure, the SC can be considered as a 'rampart' that encloses water and solutes essential for physiological homeostasis and that protects mammals from physical, chemical and biological assaults.

Structures and functions – The corneocyte cytoskeleton contains tight bundles of keratin intermediate filaments aggregated with filaggrin monomers, which are subsequently degraded into natural moisturizing compounds by various proteases, including caspase 14. A cornified cell envelope is formed on the inner surface of the corneocyte plasma membrane by transglutaminase-catalysed cross-linking of involucrin and loricrin. Ceramides form a lipid envelope by covalently binding to the cornified cell envelope, and extracellular lamellar lipids play an important role in permeability barrier function. Corneodesmosomes are the main adhesive structures in the SC and are degraded by certain serine proteases, such as kallikreins, during desquamation.

Clinical relevance – The roles of the different SC components, including the structural proteins in corneocytes, extracellular lipids and some proteins associated with lipid metabolism, have been investigated in genetically engineered mice and in naturally occurring hereditary skin diseases, such as ichthyosis, ichthyosis syndrome and atopic dermatitis in humans, cattle and dogs.

Introduction

The skin, which covers the entire body surface in mammals, is an anatomical and physiological barrier between the environment and the organism. The stratum corneum (SC) provides a barrier function for the skin. It is the outermost region of the epidermis and is composed of 'bricks' (i.e. flattened, protein-enriched corneocytes) and 'mortar' (i.e. intercellular lipid-enriched layers).[1] As a result of this 'bricks and mortar' structure, the SC in the mammalian skin can be considered as a 'rampart', which encloses 'citizens' (i.e. water and solutes) essential for physiological homeostasis and protects the 'castle' (i.e. the host) from physical, chemical and biological 'assaults'.

Within corneocytes are tight bundles of keratin intermediate filaments aggregated with filaggrin (FLG) monomers to provide a flattened shape and mechanical strength to the cells.[2–5] The cornified cell envelope is formed on the inner surface of the corneocyte plasma membrane and provides structural and mechanical integrity to the cells.[6,7] Covalent binding of the lipid envelope to the cornified cell envelope proteins provides a scaffold for extracellular lipid lamellae (ELL), which are crucial for maintaining permeability barrier function.[8,9] Various enzymes and plasma membrane proteins associated with the metabolism, uptake and secretion of lipids are also crucial in organizing intact ELL. Moreover, corneodesmosomes mediate cell–cell adhesion between corneocytes.[10–12] Degradation of corneodesmosome proteins in the uppermost SC is a key step in desquamation.[10,11]

The roles of the SC components in cutaneous barrier function have been studied in genetically engineered mice and in naturally occurring hereditary skin diseases in humans and animals. The aim of this review is to discuss recent progress in understanding the biological functions of the key SC components via the use of genetically engineered mouse models and to discuss the pathophysiology of spontaneous hereditary skin diseases related to genetic mutations or the altered expression of SC components in humans, cattle and dogs (summarized in Table 1).

Accepted 22 June 2012
Sources of Funding: This study was self-funded.
Conflict of Interest: No conflicts of interest have been declared.

Stratum corneum components crucial for barrier function

Structural proteins

Intermediate filament proteins.
Keratins (encoded by *KRT* genes) are fibrous structural proteins synthesized by epithelial cells, including keratinocytes. Keratin monomers assemble into web-like bundles

Table 1. Stratum corneum proteins and cutaneous abnormalities related to genetic alterations in mammals

Stratum corneum proteins			Cutaneous abnormalities in mammals		
Molecules	Genes	Functions	Mouse	Human	Other species
Intermediate filament cytoskeleton/filaggrin-related proteins					
Keratin 1	*KRT1*	Structural protein of IF	Death before weaning age in homozygous mutant mice; severe blistering; skin erosions and hyperkeratosis in heterozygous mutant mice	Epidermolytic ichthyosis	Not reported
Keratin 10	*KRT10*	Structural protein of IF	Death after birth in homozygous mutant mice; acanthosis and hyperkeratosis in heterozygous mutant mice	Epidermolytic ichthyosis	Mild recessive epidermolytic hyperkeratosis in Norfolk terrier
Keratin 2e	*KRT2*	Structural protein of IF	Scaly skin on tail, ears and feet	Superficial epidermolytic ichthyosis	Not reported
Filaggrin	*FLG*	Aggregation of IF in cornified cells	Increased desquamation; production of allergen-specific IgE by epicutaneous sensitization; contact dermatitis	Ichthyosis vulgaris; atopic dermatitis; contact dermatitis; alopecia areata	Canine atopic dermatitis?
Caspase-14	*CASP14*	Degradation of filaggrin monomers to natural moisturizing factors	Shiny and lichenified skin with increased TEWL	Not reported	Not reported
Cornified cell envelope-related proteins					
Involucrin	*IVL*	Structural protein of CCE	No histopathological changes	Not reported	Not reported
Loricrin	*LOR*	Structural protein of CCE	Increased susceptibility to mechanical stress	Loricrin keratoderma	Not reported
Transglutaminase-1	*TGM1*	Cross-linking of CCE proteins	Defective SC; early neonatal death owing to excessive water loss	Lamellar ichthyosis; congenital ichthyosiform erythroderma	Recessive lamellar ichthyosis in Jack Russell terrier
Cathepsin D	*CTSB*	Processing of transglutaminase-1 precursor protein	Reduced expression of involucrin, loricrin and filaggrin	Not reported	Not reported
Desquamation-related proteins					
Kallikrein-related peptidase 7 (KLK7)	*KLK7*	Proteolysis of corneodesmosome proteins	Not determined	Atopic dermatitis	Not reported
Lympho-epithelial Kazal-type-related inhibitor (LEKTI)	*SPINK5*	Inhibits KLKs etc.	Neonatal lethality, exfoliative erythroderma and severe dehydration with detached SC in homozygous mutant mice	Netherton syndrome	Not reported

Table 1. (*Continued*)

Stratum corneum proteins			Cutaneous abnormalities in mammals		
Molecules	Genes	Functions	Mouse	Human	Other species
Extracellular lipid-related proteins					
ATP-binding cassette subfamily A member 12 (ABCA12)	*ABCA12*	Lipid transporter responsible for cholesterol efflux from epidermal keratinocytes	Neonatal lethality with defective skin development in homozygous mutant mice	Harlequin ichthyosis; lamellar ichthyosis	Ichthyosis fetalis in cattle
Lipoxygenase 3	*ALOXE3*	Lipid metabolism of lamellar granule contents and/or intercellular lipid layers in the epidermis?	Not determined	Lamellar ichthyosis; congenital ichthyosiform erythroderma	Not reported
12R-Lipoxygenase	*ALOXE12B*	Releasing protein-bound ω-hydroxyceramides	Neonatal lethality with decreased protein-bound ω-hydroxyceramides and increased TEWL	Lamellar ichthyosis; congenital ichthyosiform erythroderma	Not reported
β-Glucocerebrosidase	*GBA*	Hydrolysis of glucosylceramides into free and protein-bound ceramides	Increased TEWL and incompetent ELL with decreased ceramides in Gaucher mice	Type II Gaucher disease	Not reported
Fatty acid transport protein 4 (FATP4)	*FATP4*	Uptake of exogenous fatty acids into cells	Neonatal lethality with disturbed cutaneous permeability barrier function	Ichthyosis prematurity syndrome	Not reported
Steroid sulphatase	*STS*	Degrading cholesterol sulphate to cholesterols for lipid barrier and desquamation	Cutaneous abnormalities have not been reported	Recessive X-linked ichthyosis	Not reported
Abhydrolase domain containing 5 (ABHD5)	*ABHD5*	Metabolism of triglycerides	Cutaneous abnormalities have not been reported	Chanarin–Dorfman syndrome	Not reported
Sphingosine-1-phosphate lyase (SGPL1)	*SGPL1*	Inactivation of sphingosin-1-phosphate	Cutaneous abnormalities have not been reported	Atopic dermatitis (upregulated gene transcription level)	Canine atopic dermatitis (upregulated gene transcription level)
Phospholipase domain-containing protein 1 (PNPLA1)	*PNPLA1*	Synthesis or remodelling of glycerophospholipids	Not determined	Autosomal recessive congenital ichthyosis	Autosomal recessive congenital ichthyosis in golden retriever
Cytochrome P450, family 4, subfamily F polypeptide 22 (CYP4F22)	*FLJ39501*	Role in 12R-lipoxygenase pathway?	Not determined	Lamellar ichthyosis	Not reported
Nuclear interaction partner of ALK-like domain containing 4 (NIPAL4)	*NIPAL4*	Membrane receptor for trioxilins A3 and B3?	Not determined	Lamellar ichthyosis; congenital ichthyosiform erythroderma	Not reported

Abbreviations: CCE, cornified cell envelope; ELL, extracellular lipid lamellae; IF, intermediate filament; SC, stratum corneum; TEWL, transepidermal water loss.

to form intermediate filaments, which are cytoskeletal components that terminate at desmosomes to form a cytoplasmic network. In the mammalian epidermis, type I (acidic) keratins and type II (neutral–basic) keratins form heterodimers via disulphide bonds. Specific keratins are found more prominently in various layers of the epidermis. For example, keratin 5 (K5) and keratin 14 (K14) form heterodimers in basal keratinocytes, whereas keratin 1 (K1) and keratin 10 (K10) form heterodimers in keratinocytes in suprabasal layers; keratin 2 (K2) is expressed in the stratum granulosum (SG).[13]

The functional importance of K1, K2 and K10 to cutaneous barrier function has been studied in mice by genetic engineering of keratin genes (*Krt*). Mice heterozygous for a mutation in the *Krt1* gene or transgenic mice expressing a truncated human *KRT1* gene exhibit suprabasalar blistering and skin erosions immediately after birth and develop marked scaling with increasing age.[14,15] In addition, mice homozygous for a mutation in the *Krt1* gene exhibit severe blistering and widespread desquamation at birth, and die due to severe dehydration.[14,15] Likewise, mice heterozygous for mutations in the *Krt10* gene or heterozygous transgenic mice generated by introduction of a *Krt10* mutation develop hyperkeratosis with age.[16–18] Mice homozygous for the gene knockout or transgene exhibit very fragile skin with severe suprabasalar blistering and erosions, and die shortly after birth.[16–18] In addition, a point mutation in the *Krt2* gene (T500P) in mice with dark skin (*Dsk2*) causes scaling on the tail, feet and ears owing to impaired intermediate filament assembly, in both homozygous and heterozygous mice, even though abnormalities in cutaneous barrier function in relation to the *Krt2* mutation have not been documented in the literature.[19]

These findings imply that keratins are crucial for the structural integrity of epidermal keratinocytes, and targeted ablation of some *Krt* genes causes fragility of the epidermis and/or a scaly phenotype.

Filaggrin and related proteins.
Profilaggrin, the precursor protein of FLG, is the major constituent of keratohyalin granules in the SG.[2,4,5] Profilaggrin (encoded by the *FLG* gene) is an insoluble, large, highly phosphorylated, histidine-rich protein, which contains tandemly arranged FLG repeats (10–12 repeats in humans) that are flanked on either side by two partial FLG repeats and N- and C-terminal domains.[4,5] The N- and C-terminal domains in profilaggrin are thought to be important in processing of profilaggrin to FLG monomers during epidermal differentiation.[4,20,21]

In humans, each FLG repeat consists of 324 amino acids and shows significant amino acid homology.[22–24] Meanwhile, two types of FLG repeats are distributed randomly in the mouse profilaggrin precursor protein.[25–27] The precursor protein itself has no keratinocyte-binding activity.[4] During the differentiation of keratinocytes, keratohyalin granules degranulate in response to increased Ca^{2+} levels, and profilaggrin is dephosphorylated and proteolysed into FLG monomers at the border between the SG and SC.[2–5] Filaggrin monomers specifically aggregate the keratin intermediate filament cytoskeleton into tight bundles (Figure 1a), thereby collapsing the cells into a flattened shape.[2–5] In the upper SC, FLG monomers undergo subsequent degradation into hygroscopic peptides (e.g. pyrrolidone carboxylic acid and urocanic acid), which are natural moisturizing factors (NMFs), by a variety of proteases, including caspase 14.[4,28,29]

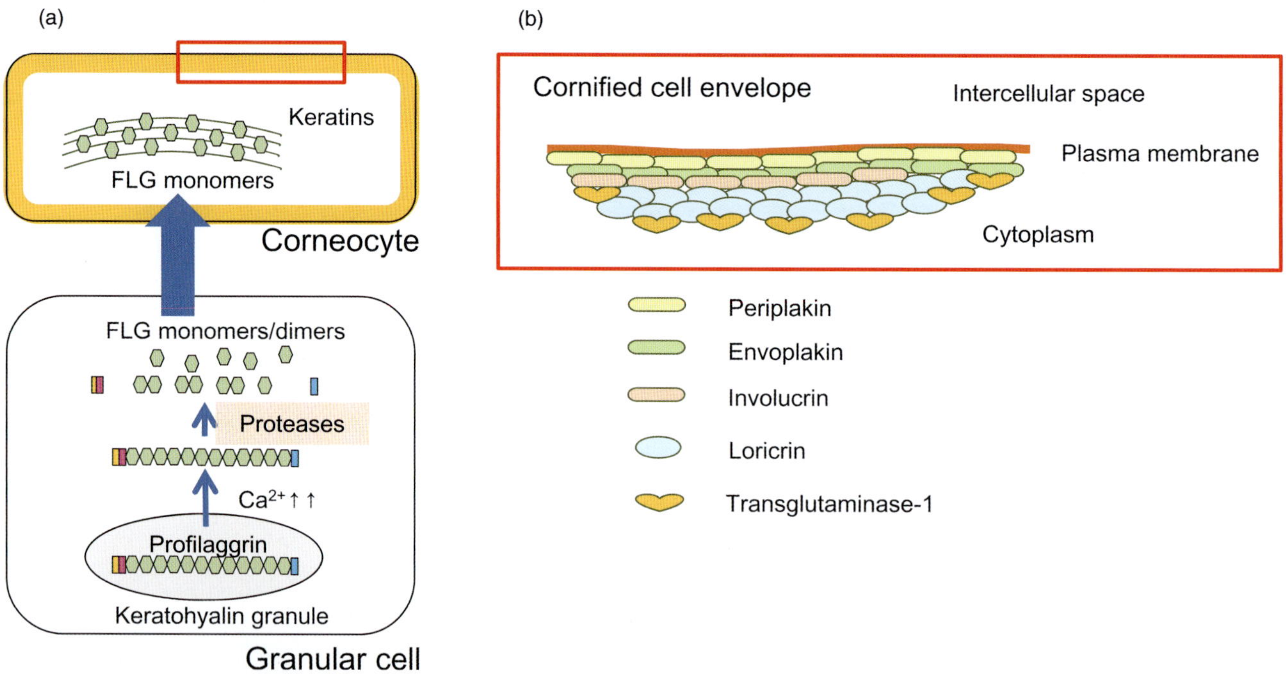

Figure 1. The key structural components of a corneocyte to form a solid 'brick'. (a) In corneocytes, filaggrin (FLG) monomers aggregate with keratin intermediate filaments and form tight bundles in the cytoplasm of corneocytes. Filaggrin monomers are the degradation product of profilaggrin, which contains tandemly arranged FLG repeats flanked on either side by two partial FLG repeats and N- and C-terminal domains. During the differentiation of keratinocytes, keratohyalin granules degranulate in response to increased Ca^{2+} levels, and profilaggrin is solubilized into FLG monomers by various proteases at the border between the stratum granulosum and the stratum corneum. (b) The cornified cell envelope located on the inner surface of the plasma membrane is formed by several proteins, including involucrin, loricrin, envoplakin and periplakin, which are cross-linked by transglutaminase-1.

The role of FLG in cutaneous barrier function has been studied by the use of two lines of mutant mice. Flaky tail mice, which have the two spontaneous genetic mutations *ft* and *ma*, have been reported to develop spontaneous atopic dermatitis (AD)-like disease.[30] Recently, it was found that a 1 bp deletion (5303delA) in the murine *Flg* gene is associated with the *ft* genotype in flaky tail mice.[27] Moreover, topical application of ovalbumin or *Dermatophagoides pteronyssinus* to *ft/ft* mice causes percutaneous allergen sensitization, with allergen-specific IgE production, increased transepidermal water loss (TEWL) and enhanced AD-like phenotyes.[27,31] The association of the *ma* mutation with the AD-like dermatitis phenotype, however, has not yet been demonstrated. Recently generated filaggrin gene knockout mice ($Flg^{-/-}$) exhibit dry skin and increased desquamation under mechanical stress.[32] Furthermore, $Flg^{-/-}$ mice exhibit enhanced penetration of foreign materials into the SC, leading to hapten-induced contact hypersensitivity and allergen-specific humoral immune responses.[32] In these mice, SC hydration and TEWL are normal, despite the fact that the NMF level is decreased in the SC of $Flg^{-/-}$ mice.[32]

Caspase 14, which belongs to a family of cysteine-dependent aspartate-directed proteases, is known to degrade profilaggrin and FLG monomers directly into NMF. Caspase-14-deficient mice show shiny and lichenified phenotypes, with decreased skin hydration and increased TEWL.[28,29]

In summary, FLG appears to be responsible for hampering a foreign invasion (e.g. penetration of allergens) through the SC rather than performing a water-holding function. In flaky tail mice and $Flg^{-/-}$ mice, data suggest that allergens passing through the SC may be captured by the dendrites of Langerhans cells that penetrate tight junctions located immediately beneath the SC, as previously demonstrated by three-dimensional visualization of mouse epidermis.[33] However, the water-holding capacity of FLG-degraded NMF products is debatable and needs to be evaluated further.

Cornified cell envelope proteins.
The cornified cell envelope is a 15-nm-thick layer of proteins (in humans) located on the inner surface of the keratinocyte plasma membrane. The cornified cell envelope is formed by the assembly of several precursor proteins, including involucrin, loricrin, envoplakin, periplakin and small proline-rich proteins (Figure 1b). Transglutaminases in the epidermis are thought to be responsible for the assembly of the precursor proteins that form the cornified cell envelope.[7,13,34,35] Among the three subtypes of transglutaminases, transglutaminase-1 is known to be a membrane-located transglutaminase in the epidermis.[36,37] Transglutaminase-1 is synthesized in the epidermis as an inactivated precursor protein, which is later processed by cathepsin D for activation.[38]

Transglutaminase-1-deficient mice exhibit a defective SC that causes neonatal death owing to increased TEWL. Additionally, cathepsin D-deficient mice exhibit reduced transglutaminase-1 activity and reduced expression of the cornified cell envelope proteins.[38] In contrast, loricrin-deficient mice exhibit transient congenital erythroderma, with a shiny, translucent skin at birth and increased susceptibility to mechanical stress.[39] However, the neonatal mutant mice do not exhibit increased TEWL, and lose the skin phenotypes at 4– 5 days after birth.[39] This phenotypic change may be associated with increased expression of other cornified cell envelope components. Targeted ablation of the murine involucrin gene alone does not cause any histopathological changes in the epidermis which shows an ultrastructurally normal cornified cell envelope.[40] However, triple knockout of involucrin, envoplakin and periplakin in mice leads to the development of phenotypes characterized by postnatal hyperkeratosis, defects in the assembled cornified cell envelope and increased susceptibility to mechanical stress.[41] Conversely, hyperkeratosis is not evident in the epidermis of involucrin, envoplakin or periplakin single knockout mice.[41]

Thus, evidence obtained through the use of genetically engineered mice suggests that the assembly of cornified cell envelope proteins is crucial for the normal desquamation process and the structural and mechanical integrity of corneocytes in the epidermis, even though targeted ablation of single protein genes did not cause lethal or lifelong cutaneous abnormalities.

Functional proteins in the stratum corneum

Desquamation-related proteins.
Corneodesmosomes are the main adhesive structure in the SC (Figure 2).[10–12] On the cytoplasmic side of corneodesmosomes, desmosomal plaque proteins are incorporated into the cornified cell envelope and separated from tonofilaments attached to the intermediate filament cytoskeleton.[6,42] The extracellular part of corneodesmosomes is comprised of desmosomal cadherins, such as desmoglein (Dsg)1 and desmocollin (Dsc)1, as well as corneodesmosin, a unique extracellular component of corneodesmosomes.[11,43–46] During desquamation, the

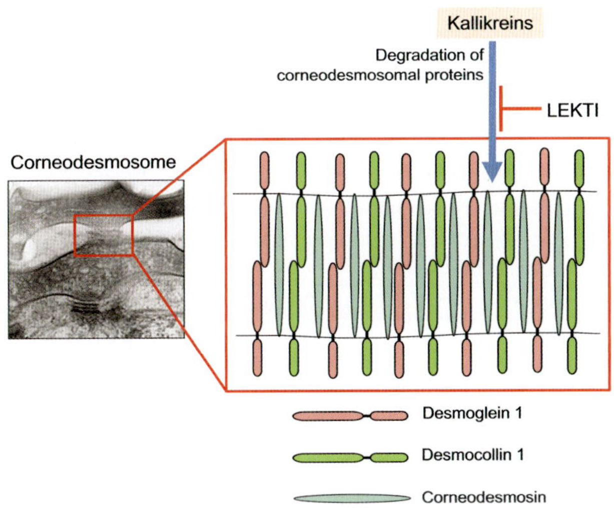

Figure 2. Corneodesmosomes mediate adhesion of corneocyte 'bricks'. The extracellular components of corneodesmosomes include two desmosomal cadherins, desmoglein 1 and desmocollin 1, as well as corneodesmosin. The extracellular components of corneocytes are degraded by kallikreins, which leads to desquamation. The enzymatic activity of kallikreins is inhibited by lymphoepithelial Kazal-type 6 serine protease inhibitor (LEKTI), which is crucial for maintaining the normal desquamation process.

extracellular components of corneodesmosomes are degraded by kallikreins (KLKs) and cathepsins.[47–49]

The KLKs are a family of 15 trypsin- or chymotrypsin-like serine proteases (KLK1–KLK15).[50–53] In human skin, at least eight KLKs, including KLK5 and KLK7, are expressed and secreted into the extracellular space between the SG and SC.[54] Kallikrein 5 degrades all extracellular components of corneodesmosomes, while KLK7 degrades only Dsc1 and corneodesmosin but not Dsg1.[42,53] The enzymatic activities of KLK5 and KLK7 are known to be inhibited by lymphoepithelial Kazal-type 6 serine protease inhibitor (LEKTI), which is encoded by the *SPINK5* gene (Figure 2).[55,56] The LEKTI is synthesized in the SG and released by lamellar granules into the extracellular space.[57]

The generation of *Spink5* gene knockout mice has provided insight into the detailed biological functions of LEKTI and KLKs in the skin. *Spink5*$^{-/-}$ newborn mice have very fragile skin, with severe erosions, and die within a few hours of birth.[58] A deficiency of LEKTI in the epidermis causes hyperactivity of KLK5 and KLK7, as well as desmosomal separation at the SG–SC interface.[58] In addition, *Spink5*$^{-/-}$ embryo skin grafted onto nude mice exhibits parakeratotic hyperkeratosis and desmosomal cleavage resembling human Netherton syndrome.[58,59] It is therefore suggested that regulation of the enzymatic activity of KLKs by LEKTI is crucial for maintaining the normal desquamation process and thus cutaneous barrier formation.

Extracellular lipids and related proteins.
In the upper stratum spinosum (SS) and SG, lamellar granules, which originate from a part of the Golgi apparatus, contain precursors of intercellular lipids in the SC, such as phospholipids, glucosylceramides, sphingomyelin and cholesterol.[7,60,61] During the differentiation of keratinocytes, lamellar granules move to the apex of granular cells, fuse with the plasma membrane and secrete their contents into the extracellular space at the SG–SC border by exocytosis.[34] Two epidermal lipoxygenases, lipoxygenase 3 and 12R-lipoxygenase, are presumed to be associated with lipid metabolism of the lamellar granule contents and/or extracellular lipid layers in the epidermis.[35] Targeted ablation of the murine 12R-lipoxygenase gene results in neonatal death, with progressive dehydration, increased TEWL and decreased protein-bound ω-hydroxyceramides.[62,63]

Secreted lipids are subsequently processed and arranged into ELL in the intercellular space of the SC (Figure 3a).[64] Some lipid classes are covalently bound to cornified cell envelope proteins, such as involucrin, envoplakin and periplakin, and form a lipid envelope that acts as a scaffold for the ELL.[7,65] Ceramides (CERs), cholesterol and long-chain free-fatty acids are the three major lipid constituents in the SC and critical ingredients to form the 'mortar' of the epidermal 'rampart'.[64,66]

Ceramides are a class of lipid molecules consisting of sphingoid bases that are amide linked to fatty acids. It is generally accepted that CERs are the main constituents of the SC and play important roles in maintaining permeability barrier function.[67,68] In the suprabasal layer, CERs newly synthesized by the *de novo* pathway are immediately converted to glucosylceramides and sphingomyelins. The glucosylceramides and sphingomyelins are then incorporated into lamellar granules and secreted into the interface of the SG and SC, where they are converted back to CERs by β-glucocerebrosidase and amide sphingomyelinase (Figure 3b).[69–73] Deficiency of β-glucocerebrosidase in type 2 Gaucher mice results in increased TEWL, increased glucosylceramides, decreased SC CERs and incompetent structure of ELL.[72,74] The ATP-binding cassette subfamily A member 12 (ABCA12) is a lipid transporter that plays a role, at least in part, in the incorporation of glucosylceramides into lamellar granules (Figure 3b).[75] Mice homozygous for the *Abca12* null allele exhibit neonatal lethality, with skin fissures and severe weight loss that are probably due to increased TEWL.[76]

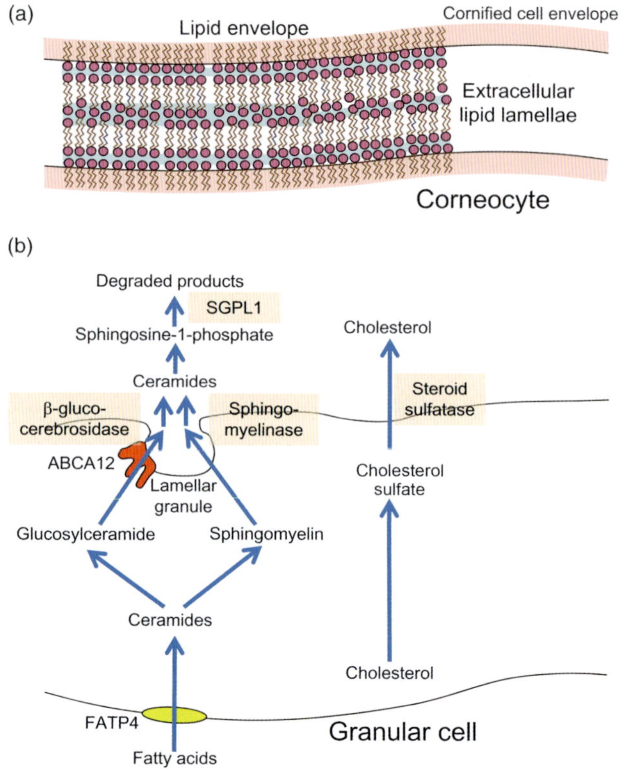

Figure 3. Lipids in the intercellular spaces are arranged into extracellular lipid lamellae and compose 'mortar' in the stratum corneum. (a) Lipids secreted into intercellular spaces during cornification are subsequently processed and arranged into extracellular lipid lamellae in the intercellular space of the stratum corneum. Some lipid classes are covalently bound to cornified cell envelope proteins and form a lipid envelope that acts as a scaffold for the extracellular lipid lamellae. (b) In granular cells, fatty acids are incorporated into the cytoplasm through fatty acid transport protein 4 (FATP4) and converted to ceramides. Ceramides are subsequently converted to glucosylceramides and sphingomyelins. The two precursor lipids are then packed into lamellar granules. The ATP-binding cassette subfamily A member 12 (ABCA12) is a membrane-transporter protein that, at least in part, plays a role in the incorporation of glucosylceramide into lamellar granules. When lamellar granules secrete their contents into the extracellular space, precursor lipids are catalysed by β-glucocerebrosidase and sphingomyelinase and are converted back to ceramides. Ceramides are degraded into shingosine-1-phosphate and irreversibly inactivated by sphingosine-1-phosphate lyase (SGPL1). Cholesterol in the cytoplasm is catalysed into cholesterol sulphate and further converted back to cholesterol by steroid sulphatase in the extracellular space.

In the epidermis of *Abca12*$^{-/-}$ mice, there was remarkable hyperkeratosis, lipid droplets in the SG suggestive of lipid congestion in lamellar granules, and sparse SC CERs.[76]

Free extractable CERs in the human SC were formerly divided into eight fractions corresponding to 10 classes.[77,78] However, recent studies using liquid chromatography–mass spectrometry revealed that free extractable CERs in human and canine SC could be divided into 11 groups according to their sphingoid and fatty acid structures, as follows: CER[EOH] (combination of ω-hydroxy fatty acids and 6-hydroxylsphingosines), CER[EOP] (combination of ω-hydroxy fatty acids and phytosphingosines), CER[EOS] (combination of ω-hydroxy fatty acids and sphingosines), CER[AH] (combination of α-hydroxy fatty acids and 6-hydroxyl sphingosines), CER[AP] (combination of α-hydroxy fatty acids and phytosphingosines), CER[AS] (combination of α-hydroxy fatty acids and sphingosines), CER[ADS] (combination of α-hydroxy fatty acids and dihydrosphingosines), CER[NH] (combination of nonhydroxy fatty acids and 6-hydroxyl sphingosines), CER[NP] (combination of nonhydroxy fatty acids and phytosphingosines), CER[NS] (combinations of nonhydroxy fatty acids and sphingosines) and CER[NDS] (combination of nonhydroxy fatty acids and dihydrosphingosines; Figure 4).[79,80] Among the 11 classes of human SC CERs, seven CER classes, including esterified ω-hydroxyceramides with very long carbon chains (CER[EOS], CER[EOP] and CER[EOH]), are expressed exclusively in the SC.[79,80] It is well recognized that the esterified ω-hydroxyceramides play important roles in epidermal barrier function owing to their extremely long fatty acid chains, although their composition ratios are relatively low among all free extractable SC CERs.[79–83] Moreover, nonesterified ω-hydroxyceramides (CER[OS], CER[OP] and CER[OH]), which are degraded products of esterified ω-hydroxyceramides, covalently bind to the cornified cell envelope and form a lipid envelope.[84] In human SC, CER[OS] and CER[OH] are two major protein-bound CERs.[85] In contrast, CER[OS] and CER[OP] are two major protein-bound CERs in canine SC.[86] Ceramides are cleaved to generate sphingosine, which is then phosphorylated to sphingosine-1-phosphate (S1P) by sphingosine kinase. Sphingosine-1-phosphate is irreversibly inactivated by a S1P lyase (SGPL1; Figure 3b).[87,88]

The epidermis also contains free fatty acids, as well as fatty acids bound to triglycerides, phospholipids, glycosylceramides and CERs.[34] Fatty acid transport protein 4 (FATP4) is known to be a lipid transporter that plays a crucial role in the uptake of fatty acids into keratinocytes (Figure 3b).[61] Mice with spontaneous mutations in, or targeted disruption of, the gene encoding FATP4 exhibited disturbed epidermal barrier function and neonatal lethality.[89,90]

Cholesterol, the third major lipid class in the SC, is synthesized in keratinocytes, and at least a part of the cholesterol is metabolized into cholesterol sulphate. During cornification, steroid sulphatase is secreted into the intercellular spaces of the SC, where it degrades cholesterol sulphate into cholesterol (Figure 3b), which is incorporated into the ELL.[34,61]

In summary, interactions between heterogeneous lipid classes and metabolic pathways are important for providing structural and functional integrity to the ELL and their scaffold structure lipid envelopes. Genetic engineering of some protein genes associated with lipid transfer/metabolism has led to an understanding of not only the biological function of the proteins but also the importance of lipid constituents (e.g. mortal) to permeability barrier function (e.g. to curb the population drain from the castle).

Cutaneous manifestations associated with the alteration of SC components in humans and other mammalian species

Ichthyosis and ichthyosis syndrome in humans

Ichthyosis is a clinically and aetiologically heterogeneous group of hereditary cornification disorders. Ichthyosis in

Fatty acid \ Sphingoid	6-hydroxy sphingosine [H]	Phytosphingosine [P]	Sphingosine [S]	Dihydrosphingosine [D]
Esterified ω-hydroxy fatty acid [EO]	CER[EOH]	CER[EOP]	CER[EOS]	CER[EODS] (Not detected in SC)
α-hydroxy fatty acid [A]	CER[AH]	CER[AP]	CER[AS]	CER[ADS]
Nonhydroxy fatty acid [N]	CER[NH]	CER[NP]	CER[NS]	CER[NDS]

Figure 4. Ceramide (CER) classes recognized in human and canine stratum corneum (SC). Human and canine CERs can be divided into 11 groups according to their sphingoid and fatty acid structures. Ceramide classes recognized exclusively in the SC are surrounded by a red rectangle. CER[ADS], which is recognized exclusively in the SC and hairs in humans, is surrounded by a green rectangle. CER[EODS] has not been detected in mammalian SC.

humans is classified into six major distinct clinical subtypes: harlequin ichthyosis (HI), congenital ichthyosiform erythroderma (CIE) and lamellar ichthyosis (LI), epidermolytic ichthyosis (EI; formerly called bullous congenital ichthyosiform erythroderma), recessive X-linked ichthyosis (RXLI) and ichthyosis vulgaris (IV).[35]

Harlequin ichthyosis is the most devastating, often fatal, autosomal recessive congenital ichthyosis (ARCI) in humans. Affected newborns exhibit cracks in the skin, ectropion (turning outwards of the lower eylids), eclabium (turning outwards of a lip) and flattened ears. Ultrastructurally, human HI is characterized by abnormal lamellar granules in the SG and the absence of the ELL in the SC. In 2005, truncation or deletion mutations in the *ABCA12* gene were first reported to underlie human HI.[91] These findings indicate that defects in the key lipid transporter, ABCA12, in lamellar granules cause malformation of the ELL and disrupt cutaneous barrier function in human HI.

Congenital ichthyosiform erythroderma and LI in humans are other forms of ARCI that share similar clinical features, but the scales in LI patients are rougher and larger than those in CIE patients. Affected babies are born in a collodion membrane, which is a shiny extra layer of the skin. After the membrane is shed, the skin becomes erythematous, with extensive hyperkeratotic scales. The molecular pathogenesis of human CIE and LI varies among cases. Mutations in a gene encoding transglutaminase-1, a cornified cell envelope-associated protein, have been reported since the mid-1990s in humans with LI and CIE.[92–95] Moreover, a combination of missense mutations in the *ABCA12* gene has been reported to underlie human LI.[96] Mutations in the genes encoding lipoxygenase 3 and 12R-lipoxygenase,[97] as well as nuclear interaction partner of ALK-like domain containing 4 (NIPAL4),[98] have also been reported to underlie certain cases of human CIE and LI. Furthermore, mutations in *FLJ39501*, which encodes cytochrome P450, family 4, subfamily F polypeptide 22 (CYP4F22), were identified as causative genetic defects in human LI.[99] The exact physiological roles of NIPAL4 and CYP4F22 in the SC have not been fully elucidated.

Epidermolytic ichthyosis in humans is caused by mutations in either *KRT1* or *KRT10*.[100–102] Affected patients exhibit widespread blisters and erosions, with a histopathology of keratinocyte vacuolation in the upper epidermis from birth. The blisters subsequently cease, and generalized hyperkeratotic scales become prominent. Ultrastructurally, irregular, clumped intermediate filaments are seen in the keratinocytes in the upper SS and SG. Epidermolytic ichthyosis in humans usually exhibits an autosomal dominant inheritance.

Genetic defects in the steroid sulphatase gene[103,104] and *KRT2*[105,106] have been identified to underlie human RXLI and superficial EI (formerly called ichthyosis bullosa of Siemens), respectively. Also, the homozygous and compound heterozygous mutations R501X and 2282del4 in *FLG* have been identified to cause human IV.[107] In addition, mutation in the gene encoding FATP4 has been reported to underlie human ichthyosis prematurity syndrome.[108] Mutations in *SPINK5*[109] and *ABHD5*[110] have been reported to underlie human Netherton syndrome and Chanarin–Dorfman syndrome, respectively. These two diseases are classified into the disease group 'ichthyosis syndrome', in which cornification disorders are accompanied by internal organ failure.

Ichthyosis in other mammals

Hereditary keratinization disorders comparable to HI, LI and EI in humans have also been reported in veterinary research publications.

Ichthyosis fetalis has been reported in Chianina cattle as an autosomal recessive skin disorder. Affected calves show deep skin fissures, ectropion and eclabium reminiscent of human HI.[111] Genome-wide association studies and sequence analysis identified a homozygous missense mutation in A5804G that resulted in a H1935R substitution in the *ABCA12* gene in three affected cattle.[112] Comparison of the genetic evidence with the severe clinical phenotype suggests that the histidine 1935 residue in *ABCA12* has key structural or functional importance.

An autosomal recessive LI associated with a LINE-1 insertion in the transglutaminase-1 gene has been reported in the Jack Russell terrier dog.[113] Very recently, a novel homozygous insertion–deletion mutation in the gene encoding phospholipase domain-containing protein 1 (PNLPA1), which is expressed in the upper epidermis and synthesises or remodels glycerophospholipids that play an important role in epidermal lipid barrier function, has been identified in 120 golden retrievers affected by a form of LI resembling human ARCI.[114] This discovery led to the identification of novel mutations in *PNLPA1* in six human individuals affected by ARCI.[114] Moreover, a homozygous mutation in the consensus donor splice site of intron 5 in *KRT10* has been identified in seven Norfolk terrier dogs affected by mild recessive EI.[115]

Hereditary keratinization disorders compatible with other forms of ichthyosis or ichthyosis syndrome have not been reported in the veterinary literature.

Human AD

Atopic dermatitis is a genetically associated, chronically relapsing and pruritic skin disease that is commonly recognized in humans and dogs. It is believed that multiple factors, such as immunological abnormalities, environmental factors and impaired cutaneous barrier functions, are involved in the onset and/or aggravation of AD.

In human AD, lower levels of CERs in the SC are believed to be associated with a change in the organization of ELL, acceleration of TEWL and reduced water capacitance, leading to atopic dry skin.[116] In addition, the profiles of the SC CER classes are altered in humans with AD, and a significant negative correlation has been found between the TEWL value and the quantities of total CERs and some CER classes, such as CER[NP], CER[EOS] and CER[EOP].[117–119] Moreover, it has been reported that the quantities of protein-bound ω-hydroxyceramides are decreased both in lesional and in clinically nonlesional skin of humans with AD.[120]

Possible mechanisms that underlie decreased SC CERs have been proposed in the literature. Jensen *et al.*[121] reported that the activity of epidermal acid sphingomyelinase was decreased in lesional and clinically nonlesional skin in human AD, correlating with reduced SC

CER content and disturbed barrier function. In addition, Imokawa and his group proposed that novel sphingomyelin and glucosylceramide deacylases, which hydrolyse sphingomyelin and glucosylceramide into degraded products, compete with sphingomyelinase and β-glucocerebrosidase and lead to SC CERs deficiency in human AD.[122–124] This increased enzymatic activity is recognized specifically in AD but not in contact dermatitis. Moreover, it has been reported that the transcription level of the *SGPL1* gene encoding S1P lyase, which hydrolyses the CER degradation product S1P, is increased in human AD.[125]

Human AD is known to develop frequently in patients with IV, probably owing to disrupted cutaneous barrier function. In 2006, an association of loss-of-function mutations (R501X and 2282del4) in *FLG*, which were initially identified in human IV,[107] in human AD and/or asthma cohorts, was first reported.[126] To date, the association of more than 40 *FLG* mutations with AD has been reported, and approximately 25–50% of AD patients possess *FLG* mutations.[3,35] Most of the human patients with AD have heterozygous mutations in *FLG*.[3]

A mutation in the gene encoding KLK7 has been reported in human patients with AD.[127] In addition, increased protein expression and protease activity of KLKs in human AD have also been reported.[128,129]

Canine AD

Decreased CER contents in the SC of dogs with AD have also been reported in the veterinary literature. Electron microscopic analysis revealed that the continuity and thickness of the ELL were significantly reduced in clinically nonlesional SC of dogs with spontaneous AD and an experimental model of canine AD sensitized with house dust mites.[130–132] Previously, we reported that the proportion of free extractable CERs, but not that of cholesterol or free fatty acids, in the SC was negatively correlated with TEWL in dogs with AD.[133]

Reiter *et al.*[134] reported that the proportions of free extractable CER1 (CER[EOS]) and CER9 (CER[EOP]) were lower in clinically nonlesional skin of dogs with AD than in skin from breed- and age-matched healthy dogs. We recently reported that the quantities of total free extractable CERs and their CER[EOS], CER[EOP] and CER[NP] subclasses, as well as mixtures of CER[NDS/NS] and CER[AS/NH], were significantly lower in clinically nonlesional skin of dogs with AD than in breed- and age-matched healthy dogs.[80] In that study, the greatest differences between CER content in atopic dogs and control animals were in the quantities of CER[EOP] (3.2-fold), a mixture of CER[AS/NH] (2.3-fold) and CER[-EOS] (2.2-fold), whereas the differences in other CER classes were <1.6-fold.[80]

Popa *et al.*[135] recently reported that the amounts of protein-bound CER[OS] and CER[OP], which are degradation products of free extractable CER[EOS] and CER[-EOP], respectively, were decreased in clinically nonlesional skin of dogs with AD compared with healthy dogs. Furthermore, recent studies indicated that dogs with AD have lower amounts of S1P in the skin and plasma, and increased transcription of the *SGPL1* gene.[88,136]

These findings indicate that free and protein-bound CERs, particularly the ω-hydroxyceramides believed to be crucial for maintaining permeability barrier function, are decreased in the SC of dogs with AD. In addition, the above findings suggest the importance of S1P lyase in the pathophysiology of canine AD.

The association of FLG with canine AD has also been investigated. Wood *et al.*[137] reported that a single nucleotide polymorphism within *FLG* is associated with AD in Labrador retrievers in the UK. The association of *FLG* with canine AD has not been reported in other breeds.[137–139] Changes in the immunostaining pattern of FLG and its C-terminus in dogs with AD have been reported;[140,141] however, mutations in *FLG* have not yet been identified in canine AD. Moreover, changes in KLKs have not been reported in the veterinary literature.

Other diseases in humans

Loss-of-function mutations in *FLG* may be associated with contact dermatitis[142–144] and alopecia areata[145] in humans.

Gaucher disease is the most common type of lysosomal storage disease in humans and is associated with a genetic deficiency of β-glucocerebrosidase. It has been reported that a subset of infants with type II Gaucher disease exhibit congenital ichthyosis and neonatal death.[146]

A disease entity of loricrin keratoderma, in which 1 bp insertions in *LOC* cause aberrant loricrin synthesis, has been proposed in human medicine. Histopathologically, affected patients exhibit marked hyperkeratosis and hypergranulosis. Nuclear accumulation of loricrin was confirmed by immunohistochemistry and immunoelectron microscopy.[147] These disease entities have not been reported in the veterinary literature.

Implications and future perspectives for biological and clinical research

Investigations using genetically engineered mouse models and spontaneous skin diseases in humans and other mammals have shed light on the biological properties of SC-related proteins and lipids, which are crucial in forming the impregnable epidermal 'rampart' to protect the mammalian 'castle'. In particular, genetic mutations in hereditary ichthyosis and ichthyosis syndrome in humans, as well as their mouse models, have provided greater understanding of the roles of targeted proteins in the maintenance of cutaneous barrier function. In contrast, there is limited evidence to explain the gene mutations in naturally occurring ichthyosis in other mammalian species. Future studies, including genome-wide analysis, will lead to the discovery of genetic mutations that underlie hereditary keratinization disorders with unknown aetiology in domestic and companion animals. This approach will accelerate the development of perinatal diagnosis and gene therapies for hereditary diseases, and prevent the breeding of animals with unaffected carriers.

Atopic dermatitis is heterogeneous owing to genetic, environmental and immunological factors. Although mutations in *FLG* are clearly associated with the pathogenesis of human AD, the mutation does not fully describe the pathogenesis of AD, because approximately half of the humans with AD do not possess *FLG* mutations. In addition, it has not been fully elucidated whether CER deficiency is the primary factor that causes AD or whether it is secondary to AD. It has been reported that bacterial ceramidases cause reduction of SC CERs; thus, CERs are not always reduced as a result of congenital abnormalities.[148] Moreover, it has not been fully elucidated whether the reduction of CERs in human and canine AD accelerates the percutaneous entry of allergens through the SC (outside-to-inside barrier dysfunction), even though the reduction is associated with increased water permeability (inside-to-outside barrier dysfunction). Future studies are expected to determine whether reduction of CERs is recognized from early life and permits percutaneous allergen entry in AD. Moreover, future genome-wide analysis to identify undiscovered mutations in genes crucial for structural integrity or lipid metabolism in the SC of humans or animals with AD will be expected.

References

1. Elias PM. Epidermal lipids, barrier function, and desquamation. *J Invest Dermatol* 1983; 80: 44s–49s.
2. Steinert PM, Cantieri JS, Teller DC *et al.* Characterization of a class of cationic proteins that specifically interact with intermediate filaments. *Proc Natl Acad Sci USA* 1981; 78: 4097–4101.
3. Kawasaki H, Kubo A, Sasaki T *et al.* Loss-of-function mutations within the filaggrin gene and atopic dermatitis. *Curr Probl Dermatol* 2011; 41: 35–46.
4. Sandilands A, Sutherland C, Irvine AD *et al.* Filaggrin in the frontline: role in skin barrier function and disease. *J Cell Sci* 2009; 122: 1285–1294.
5. Dale BA, Resing KA, Lonsdale-Eccles JD. Filaggrin: a keratin filament associated protein. *Ann N Y Acad Sci* 1985; 455: 330–342.
6. Nemes Z, Steinert PM. Bricks and mortar of the epidermal barrier. *Exp Mol Med* 1999; 31: 5–19.
7. Candi E, Schmidt R, Melino G. The cornified envelope: a model of cell death in the skin. *Nat Rev Mol Cell Biol* 2005; 6: 328–340.
8. Swartzendruber DC, Wertz PW, Madison KC *et al.* Evidence that the corneocyte has a chemically bound lipid envelope. *J Invest Dermatol* 1987; 88: 709–713.
9. Swartzendruber DC, Wertz PW, Kitko DJ *et al.* Molecular models of the intercellular lipid lamellae in mammalian stratum corneum. *J Invest Dermatol* 1989; 92: 251–257.
10. Chapman SJ, Walsh A. Desmosomes, corneosomes and desquamation. An ultrastructural study of adult pig epidermis. *Arch Dermatol Res* 1990; 282: 304–310.
11. Serre G, Mils V, Haftek M *et al.* Identification of late differentiation antigens of human cornified epithelia, expressed in re-organized desmosomes and bound to cross-linked envelope. *J Invest Dermatol* 1991; 97: 1061–1072.
12. Skerrow CJ, Clelland DG, Skerrow D. Changes to desmosomal antigens and lectin-binding sites during differentiation in normal human epidermis: a quantitative ultrastructural study. *J Cell Sci* 1989; 92: 667–677.
13. Shimizu H. Structure and Function of the Skin. In: *Shimizu's Textbook of Dermatology*. 1st edition. Tokyo: Nakayama Shoten, 2007; 1–26.
14. McGowan KA, Aradhya S, Fuchs H *et al.* A mouse keratin 1 mutation causes dark skin and epidermolytic hyperkeratosis. *J Invest Dermatol* 2006; 126: 1013–1016.
15. Bickenbach JR, Longley MA, Bundman DS *et al.* A transgenic mouse model that recapitulates the clinical features of both neonatal and adult forms of the skin disease epidermolytic hyperkeratosis. *Differentiation* 1996; 61: 129–139.
16. Reichelt J, Bauer C, Porter R *et al.* Out of balance: consequences of a partial keratin 10 knockout. *J Cell Sci* 1997; 110: 2175–2186.
17. Arin MJ, Longley MA, Wang XJ *et al.* Focal activation of a mutant allele defines the role of stem cells in mosaic skin disorders. *J Cell Biol* 2001; 152: 645–649.
18. Porter RM, Leitgeb S, Melton DW *et al.* Gene targeting at the mouse cytokeratin 10 locus: severe skin fragility and changes of cytokeratin expression in the epidermis. *J Cell Biol* 1996; 132: 925–936.
19. Fitch KR, McGowan KA, van Raamsdonk CD *et al.* Genetics of dark skin in mice. *Genes Dev* 2003; 17: 214–228.
20. Nemoto-Hasebe I, Akiyama M, Nomura T *et al.* *FLG* mutation p.Lys4021X in the C-terminal imperfect filaggrin repeat in Japanese patients with atopic eczema. *Br J Dermatol* 2009; 161: 1387–1390.
21. Sandilands A, Terron-Kwiatkowski A, Hull PR *et al.* Comprehensive analysis of the gene encoding filaggrin uncovers prevalent and rare mutations in ichthyosis vulgaris and atopic eczema. *Nat Genet* 2007; 39: 650–654.
22. Gan SQ, McBride OW, Idler WW *et al.* Organization, structure, and polymorphisms of the human profilaggrin gene. *Biochemistry* 1990; 29: 9432–9440.
23. McKinley-Grant LJ, Idler WW, Bernstein IA *et al.* Characterization of a cDNA clone encoding human filaggrin and localization of the gene to chromosome region 1q21. *Proc Natl Acad Sci USA* 1989; 86: 4848–4852.
24. Presland RB, Haydock PV, Fleckman P *et al.* Characterization of the human epidermal profilaggrin gene. Genomic organization and identification of an S-100-like calcium binding domain at the amino terminus. *J Biol Chem* 1992; 267: 23772–23781.
25. Rothnagel JA, Steinert PM. The structure of the gene for mouse filaggrin and a comparison of the repeating units. *J Biol Chem* 1990; 265: 1862–1865.
26. Zhang D, Karunaratne S, Kessler M *et al.* Characterization of mouse profilaggrin: evidence for nuclear engulfment and translocation of the profilaggrin B-domain during epidermal differentiation. *J Invest Dermatol* 2002; 119: 905–912.
27. Fallon PG, Sasaki T, Sandilands A *et al.* A homozygous frameshift mutation in the mouse *Flg* gene facilitates enhanced percutaneous allergen priming. *Nat Genet* 2009; 41: 602–608.
28. Hoste E, Kemperman P, Devos M *et al.* Caspase-14 is required for filaggrin degradation to natural moisturizing factors in the skin. *J Invest Dermatol* 2011; 131: 2233–2241.
29. Denecker G, Hoste E, Gilbert B *et al.* Caspase-14 protects against epidermal UVB photodamage and water loss. *Nat Cell Biol* 2007; 9: 666–674.
30. Presland RB, Boggess D, Lewis SP *et al.* Loss of normal profilaggrin and filaggrin in flaky tail (*ft/ft*) mice: an animal model for the filaggrin-deficient skin disease ichthyosis vulgaris. *J Invest Dermatol* 2000; 115: 1072–1081.
31. Moniaga CS, Egawa G, Kawasaki H *et al.* Flaky tail mouse denotes human atopic dermatitis in the steady state and by topical application with *Dermatophagoides pteronyssinus* extract. *Am J Pathol* 2010; 176: 2385–2393.
32. Kawasaki H, Nagao K, Kubo A *et al.* Altered stratum corneum barrier and enhanced percutaneous immune responses in filaggrin-null mice. *J Allergy Clin Immunol* 2012; 129: 1538–1546.
33. Kubo A, Nagao K, Yokouchi M *et al.* External antigen uptake by Langerhans cells with reorganization of epidermal tight junction barriers. *J Exp Med* 2009; 206: 2937–2946.
34. Proksch E, Brandner JM, Jensen JM. The skin: an indispensable barrier. *Exp Dermatol* 2008; 17: 1063–1072.
35. Akiyama M. Updated molecular genetics and pathogenesis of ichthiyoses. *Nagoya J Med Sci* 2011; 73: 79–90.
36. Kim IG, McBride OW, Wang M *et al.* Structure and organization of the human transglutaminase 1 gene. *J Biol Chem* 1992; 267: 7710–7717.

37. Yamanishi K, Inazawa J, Liew FM *et al.* Structure of the gene for human transglutaminase 1. *J Biol Chem* 1992; 267: 17858–17863.
38. Egberts F, Heinrich M, Jensen JM *et al.* Cathepsin D is involved in the regulation of transglutaminase 1 and epidermal differentiation. *J Cell Sci* 2004; 117: 2295–2307.
39. Koch PJ, de Viragh PA, Scharer E *et al.* Lessons from loricrin-deficient mice: compensatory mechanisms maintaining skin barrier function in the absence of a major cornified envelope protein. *J Cell Biol* 2000; 151: 389–400.
40. Djian P, Easley K, Green H. Targeted ablation of the murine involucrin gene. *J Cell Biol* 2000; 151: 381–388.
41. Sevilla LM, Nachat R, Groot KR *et al.* Mice deficient in involucrin, envoplakin, and periplakin have a defective epidermal barrier. *J Cell Biol* 2007; 179: 1599–1612.
42. Ishida-Yamamoto A, Kishibe M. Involvement of corneodesmosome degradation and lamellar granule transportation in the desquamation process. *Med Mol Morphol* 2011; 44: 1–6.
43. Suzuki Y, Koyama J, Moro O *et al.* The role of two endogenous proteases of the stratum corneum in degradation of desmoglein-1 and their reduced activity in the skin of ichthyotic patients. *Br J Dermatol* 1996; 134: 460–464.
44. Simon M, Montezin M, Guerrin M *et al.* Characterization and purification of human corneodesmosin, an epidermal basic glycoprotein associated with corneocyte-specific modified desmosomes. *J Biol Chem* 1997; 272: 31770–31776.
45. Caubet C, Jonca N, Brattsand M *et al.* Degradation of corneodesmosome proteins by two serine proteases of the kallikrein family, SCTE/KLK5/hK5 and SCCE/KLK7/hK7. *J Invest Dermatol* 2004; 122: 1235–1244.
46. Descargues P, Deraison C, Prost C *et al.* Corneodesmosomal cadherins are preferential targets of stratum corneum trypsin- and chymotrypsin-like hyperactivity in Netherton syndrome. *J Invest Dermatol* 2006; 126: 1622–1632.
47. Simon M, Jonca N, Guerrin M *et al.* Refined characterization of corneodesmosin proteolysis during terminal differentiation of human epidermis and its relationship to desquamation. *J Biol Chem* 2001; 276: 20292–20299.
48. Bernard D, Méhul B, Thomas-Collignon A *et al.* Analysis of proteins with caseinolytic activity in a human stratum corneum extract revealed a yet unidentified cysteine protease and identified the so-called "stratum corneum thiol protease" as cathepsin L2. *J Invest Dermatol* 2003; 120: 592–600.
49. Igarashi S, Takizawa T, Takizawa T *et al.* Cathepsin D, but not cathepsin E, degrades desmosomes during epidermal desquamation. *Br J Dermatol* 2004; 151: 355–361.
50. Brattsand M, Stefansson K, Lundh C *et al.* A proteolytic cascade of kallikreins in the stratum corneum. *J Invest Dermatol* 2005; 124: 198–203.
51. Lundwall A, Brattsand M. Kallikrein-related peptidases. *Cell Mol Life Sci* 2008; 65: 2019–2038.
52. Sotiropoulou G, Pampalakis G, Diamandis EP. Functional roles of human kallikrein-related peptidases. *J Biol Chem* 2009; 284: 32989–32994.
53. Borgono CA, Michael IP, Komatsu N *et al.* A potential role for multiple tissue kallikrein serine proteases in epidermal desquamation. *J Biol Chem* 2007; 282: 3640–3652.
54. Komatsu N, Tsai B, Sidiropoulos M *et al.* Quantification of eight tissue kallikreins in the stratum corneum and sweat. *J Invest Dermatol* 2006; 126: 925–929.
55. Magert HJ, Standker L, Kreutzmann P *et al.* LEKTI, a novel 15-domain type of human serine proteinase inhibitor. *J Biol Chem* 1999; 274: 21499–21502.
56. Deraison C, Bonnart C, Lopez F *et al.* LEKTI fragments specifically inhibit KLK5, KLK7, and KLK14 and control desquamation through a pH-dependent interaction. *Mol Biol Cell* 2007; 18: 3607–3619.
57. Ishida-Yamamoto A, Deraison C, Bonnart C *et al.* LEKTI is localized in lamellar granules, separated from KLK5 and KLK7, and is secreted in the extracellular spaces of the superficial stratum granulosum. *J Invest Dermatol* 2005; 124: 360–366.
58. Descargues P, Deraison C, Bonnart C *et al.* *Spink5*-deficient mice mimic Netherton syndrome through degradation of desmoglein 1 by epidermal protease hyperactivity. *Nat Genet* 2005; 37: 56–65.
59. Briot A, Deraison C, Lacroix M *et al.* Kallikrein 5 induces atopic dermatitis-like lesions through PAR2-mediated thymic stromal lymphopoietin expression in Netherton syndrome. *J Exp Med* 2009; 206: 1135–1147.
60. Downing DT, Stewart ME, Wertz PW *et al.* Skin lipids: an update. *J Invest Dermatol* 1987; 88: 2s–6s.
61. Feingold KR. Lipid metabolism in the epidermis. *Dermatoendocrinology* 2011; 3: 52.
62. Epp N, Fürstenberger G, Müller K *et al.* 12R-lipoxygenase deficiency disrupts epidermal barrier function. *J Cell Biol* 2007; 177: 173–182.
63. Moran JL, Qiu H, Turbe-Doan A *et al.* A mouse mutation in the 12R-lipoxygenase, *Alox12b*, disrupts formation of the epidermal permeability barrier. *J Invest Dermatol* 2007; 127: 1893–1897.
64. Bouwstra JA, Ponec M. The skin barrier in healthy and diseased state. *Biochim Biophys Acta* 2006; 1758: 2080–2095.
65. Marekov LN, Steinert PM. Ceramides are bound to structural proteins of the human foreskin epidermal cornified cell envelope. *J Biol Chem* 1998; 273: 17763–17770.
66. Jungersted JM, Hellgren LI, Jemec GB *et al.* Lipids and skin barrier function – a clinical perspective. *Contact Dermatitis* 2008; 58: 255–262.
67. Holleran WM, Man MQ, Gao WN *et al.* Sphingolipids are required for mammalian epidermal barrier function. Inhibition of sphingolipid synthesis delays barrier recovery after acute perturbation. *J Clin Invest* 1991; 88: 1338–1345.
68. Coderch L, López O, de la Maza A *et al.* Ceramides and skin function. *Am J Clin Dermatol* 2003; 4: 107–129.
69. Mizutani Y, Mitsutake S, Tsuji K *et al.* Ceramide biosynthesis in keratinocyte and its role in skin function. *Biochimie* 2009; 91: 784–790.
70. Uchida Y, Hara M, Nishio H *et al.* Epidermal sphingomyelins are precursors for selected stratum corneum ceramides. *J Lipid Res* 2000; 41: 2071–2082.
71. Holleran WM, Takagi Y, Menon GK *et al.* Processing of epidermal glucosylceramides is required for optimal mammalian cutaneous permeability barrier function. *J Clin Invest* 1993; 91: 1656–1664.
72. Holleran WM, Ginns EI, Menon GK *et al.* Consequences of β-glucocerebrosidase deficiency in epidermis. Ultrastructure and permeability barrier alterations in Gaucher disease. *J Clin Invest* 1994; 93: 1756–1764.
73. Hamanaka S, Hara M, Nishio H *et al.* Human epidermal glucosylceramides are major precursors of stratum corneum ceramides. *J Invest Dermatol* 2002; 119: 416–423.
74. Doering T, Proia RL, Sandhoff K. Accumulation of protein-bound epidermal glucosylceramides in β-glucocerebrosidase deficient type 2 Gaucher mice. *FEBS Lett* 1999; 447: 167–170.
75. Mitsutake S, Suzuki C, Akiyama M *et al.* ABCA12 dysfunction causes a disorder in glucosylceramide accumulation during keratinocyte differentiation. *J Dermatol Sci* 2010; 60: 128–129.
76. Yanagi T, Akiyama M, Nishihara H *et al.* Harlequin ichthyosis model mouse reveals alveolar collapse and severe fetal skin barrier defects. *Hum Mol Genet* 2008; 17: 3075–3083.
77. Farwanah H, Wohlrab J, Neubert RH *et al.* Profiling of human stratum corneum ceramides by means of normal phase LC/APCI-MS. *Anal Bioanal Chem* 2005; 383: 632–637.
78. Ponec M, Weerheim A, Lankhorst P *et al.* New acylceramide in native and reconstructed epidermis. *J Invest Dermatol* 2003; 120: 581–588.
79. Masukawa Y, Narita H, Sato H *et al.* Comprehensive quantification of ceramide species in human stratum corneum. *J Lipid Res* 2009; 50: 1708–1719.
80. Yoon JS, Nishifuji K, Sasaki A *et al.* Alteration of stratum corneum ceramide profiles in spontaneous canine model of atopic dermatitis. *Exp Dermatol* 2011; 20: 732–736.

81. Uchida Y, Holleran WM. Omega-*O*-acylceramide, a lipid essential for mammalian survival. *J Dermatol Sci* 2008; 51: 77–87.
82. Bouwstra JA, Gooris GS, Dubbelaar FE *et al.* Role of ceramide 1 in the molecular organization of the stratum corneum lipids. *J Lipid Res* 1998; 39: 186–196.
83. de Jager M, Gooris G, Ponec M *et al.* Acylceramide head group architecture affects lipid organization in synthetic ceramide mixtures. *J Invest Dermatol* 2004; 123: 911–916.
84. Behne M, Uchida Y, Seki T *et al.* Omega-hydroxyceramides are required for corneocyte lipid envelope (CLE) formation and normal epidermal permeability barrier function. *J Invest Dermatol* 2000; 114: 185–192.
85. Farwanah H, Pierstorff B, Schmelzer CE *et al.* Separation and mass spectrometric characterization of covalently bound skin ceramides using LC/APCI-MS and Nano-ESI-MS/MS. *J Chromatogr B Analyt Technol Biomed Life Sci* 2007; 852: 562–570.
86. Popa I, Thuy LH, Colsch B *et al.* Analysis of free and protein-bound ceramides by tape stripping of stratum corneum from dogs. *Arch Dermatol Res* 2010; 302: 639–644.
87. Herzinger T, Kleuser B, Schäfer-Korting M *et al.* Sphingosine-1-phosphate signaling and the skin. *Am J Clin Dermatol* 2007; 8: 329–336.
88. Baumer W, Rossbach K, Mischke R *et al.* Decreased concentration and enhanced metabolism of sphingosine-1-phosphate in lesional skin of dogs with atopic dermatitis: disturbed sphingosine-1-phosphate homeostasis in atopic dermatitis. *J Invest Dermatol* 2011; 131: 266–268.
89. Moulson CL, Martin DR, Lugus JJ *et al.* Cloning of wrinkle-free, a previously uncharacterized mouse mutation, reveals crucial roles for fatty acid transport protein 4 in skin and hair development. *Proc Natl Acad Sci USA* 2003; 100: 5274–5279.
90. Herrmann T, van der Hoeven F, Grone HJ *et al.* Mice with targeted disruption of the fatty acid transport protein 4 (Fatp 4, Slc27a4) gene show features of lethal restrictive dermopathy. *J Cell Biol* 2003; 161: 1105–1115.
91. Akiyama M, Sugiyama-Nakagiri Y, Sakai K *et al.* Mutations in lipid transporter ABCA12 in harlequin ichthyosis and functional recovery by corrective gene transfer. *J Clin Invest* 2005; 115: 1777–1784.
92. Russell LJ, DiGiovanna JJ, Rogers GR *et al.* Mutations in the gene for transglutaminase 1 in autosomal recessive lamellar ichthyosis. *Nat Genet* 1995; 9: 279–283.
93. Parmentier L, Blanchet-Bardon C, Nguyen S *et al.* Autosomal recessive lamellar ichthyosis: identification of a new mutation in transglutaminase 1 and evidence for genetic heterogeneity. *Hum Mol Genet* 1995; 4: 1391–1395.
94. Laiho E, Ignatius J, Mikkola H *et al.* Transglutaminase 1 mutations in autosomal recessive congenital ichthyosis: private and recurrent mutations in an isolated population. *Am J Hum Genet* 1997; 61: 529–538.
95. Akiyama M, Takizawa Y, Kokaji T *et al.* Novel mutations of TGM1 in a child with congenital ichthyosiform erythroderma. *Br J Dermatol* 2001; 144: 401–407.
96. Lefevre C, Audebert S, Jobard F *et al.* Mutations in the transporter ABCA12 are associated with lamellar ichthyosis type 2. *Hum Mol Genet* 2003; 12: 2369–2378.
97. Jobard F, Lefèvre C, Karaduman A *et al.* Lipoxygenase-3 (*ALOXE3*) and 12(*R*)-lipoxygenase (*ALOX12B*) are mutated in non-bullous congenital ichthyosiform erythroderma (NCIE) linked to chromosome 17p13.1. *Hum Mol Genet* 2002; 11: 107–113.
98. Lefèvre C, Bouadjar B, Karaduman A *et al.* Mutations in *ichthyin* a new gene on chromosome 5q33 in a new form of autosomal recessive congenital ichthyosis. *Hum Mol Genet* 2004; 13: 2473–2482.
99. Lefèvre C, Bouadjar B, Ferrand V *et al.* Mutations in a new cytochrome P450 gene in lamellar ichthyosis type 3. *Hum Mol Genet* 2006; 15: 767–776.
100. Cheng J, Syder AJ, Yu QC *et al.* The genetic basis of epidermolytic hyperkeratosis: a disorder of differentiation-specific epidermal keratin genes. *Cell* 1992; 70: 811–819.
101. Rothnagel JA, Dominey AM, Dempsey LD *et al.* Mutations in the rod domains of keratins 1 and 10 in epidermolytic hyperkeratosis. *Science* 1992; 257: 1128–1130.
102. Chipev CC, Korge BP, Markova N *et al.* A leucine → proline mutation in the H1 subdomain of keratin 1 causes epidermolytic hyperkeratosis. *Cell* 1992; 70: 821–828.
103. Koppe G, Marinković-Ilsen A, Rijken Y *et al.* X-linked icthyosis. A sulphatase deficiency. *Arch Dis Child* 1978; 53: 803–806.
104. Webster D, France JT, Shapiro LJ *et al.* X-linked ichthyosis due to steroid-sulphatase deficiency. *Lancet* 1978; 1(8055): 70–72.
105. Arin MJ, Longley MA, Epstein EH Jr *et al.* A novel mutation in the 1A domain of keratin 2e in ichthyosis bullosa of Siemens. *J Invest Dermatol* 1999; 112: 380–382.
106. Suga Y, Arin MJ, Scott G *et al.* Hot spot mutations in keratin 2e suggest a correlation between genotype and phenotype in patients with ichthyosis bullosa of Siemens. *Exp Dermatol* 2000; 9: 11–15.
107. Smith FJ, Irvine AD, Terron-Kwiatkowski A *et al.* Loss-of-function mutations in the gene encoding filaggrin cause ichthyosis vulgaris. *Nat Genet* 2006; 38: 337–342.
108. Klar J, Schweiger M, Zimmerman R *et al.* Mutations in the fatty acid transport protein 4 gene cause the ichthyosis prematurity syndrome. *Am J Hum Genet* 2009; 85: 248–253.
109. Chavanas S, Bodemer C, Rochat A *et al.* Mutations in *SPINK5*, encoding a serine protease inhibitor, cause Netherton syndrome. *Nat Genet* 2000; 25: 141–142.
110. Badeloe S, van Geel M, Nagtzaam I *et al.* Chanarin–Dorfman syndrome caused by a novel splice site mutation in *ABHD5*. *Br J Dermatol* 2008; 158: 1378–1380.
111. Molteni L, Dardano S, Parma P *et al.* Ichthyosis in Chianina cattle. *Vet Rec* 2006; 158: 412–414.
112. Charlier C, Coppieters W, Rollin F *et al.* Highly effective SNP-based association mapping and management of recessive defects in livestock. *Nat Genet* 2008; 40: 449–454.
113. Credille KM, Minor JS, Barnhart KF *et al.* Transglutaminase 1-deficient recessive lamellar ichthyosis associated with a LINE-1 insertion in Jack Russell terrier dogs. *Br J Dermatol* 2009; 161: 265–272.
114. Grall A, Guaguère E, Planchais S *et al.* *PNPLA1* mutations cause autosomal recessive congenital ichthyosis in golden retriever dogs and humans. *Nat Genet* 2012; 44: 140–147.
115. Credille KM, Barnhart KF, Minor JS *et al.* Mild recessive epidermolytic hyperkeratosis associated with a novel keratin 10 donor splice-site mutation in a family of Norfolk terrier dogs. *Br J Dermatol* 2005; 153: 51–58.
116. Janssens M, van Smeden J, Gooris GS *et al.* Lamellar lipid organization and ceramide composition in the stratum corneum of patients with atopic eczema. *J Invest Dermatol* 2011; 131: 2136–2138.
117. Imokawa G, Abe A, Jin K *et al.* Decreased level of ceramides in stratum corneum of atopic dermatitis: an etiologic factor in atopic dry skin? *J Invest Dermatol* 1991; 96: 523–526.
118. Di Nardo A, Wertz P, Giannetti A *et al.* Ceramide and cholesterol composition of the skin of patients with atopic dermatitis. *Acta Derm Venereol* 1998; 78: 27–30.
119. Ishikawa J, Narita H, Kondo N *et al.* Changes in the ceramide profile of atopic dermatitis patients. *J Invest Dermatol* 2010; 130: 2511–2514.
120. Macheleidt O, Kaiser HW, Sandhoff K. Deficiency of epidermal protein-bound ω-hydroxyceramides in atopic dermatitis. *J Invest Dermatol* 2002; 119: 166–173.
121. Jensen JM, Fölster-Holst R, Baranowsky A *et al.* Impaired sphingomyelinase activity and epidermal differentiation in atopic dermatitis. *J Invest Dermatol* 2004; 122: 1423–1431.
122. Hara J, Higuchi K, Okamoto R *et al.* High-expression of sphingomyelin deacylase is an important determinant of ceramide deficiency leading to barrier disruption in atopic dermatitis. *J Invest Dermatol* 2000; 115: 406–413.

123. Imokawa G. A possible mechanism underlying the ceramide deficiency in atopic dermatitis: expression of a deacylase enzyme that cleaves the *N*-acyl linkage of sphingomyelin and glucosylceramide. *J Dermatol Sci* 2009; 55: 1–9.
124. Murata Y, Ogata J, Higaki Y *et al.* Abnormal expression of sphingomyelin acylase in atopic dermatitis: an etiologic factor for ceramide deficiency? *J Invest Dermatol* 1996; 106: 1242–1249.
125. Seo EY, Park GT, Lee KM *et al.* Identification of the target genes of atopic dermatitis by real-time PCR. *J Invest Dermatol* 2006; 126: 1187–1189.
126. Palmer CN, Irvine AD, Terron-Kwiatkowski A *et al.* Common loss-of-function variants of the epidermal barrier protein filaggrin are a major predisposing factor for atopic dermatitis. *Nat Genet* 2006; 38: 441–446.
127. Vasilopoulos Y, Cork MJ, Murphy R *et al.* Genetic association between an AACC insertion in the 3′UTR of the stratum corneum chymotryptic enzyme gene and atopic dermatitis. *J Invest Dermatol* 2004; 123: 62–66.
128. Komatsu N, Saijoh K, Kuk C *et al.* Human tissue kallikrein expression in the stratum corneum and serum of atopic dermatitis patients. *Exp Dermatol* 2007; 16: 513–519.
129. Voegeli R, Rawlings AV, Breternitz M *et al.* Increased stratum corneum serine protease activity in acute eczematous atopic skin. *Br J Dermatol* 2009; 161: 70–77.
130. Inman AO, Olivry T, Dunston SM *et al.* Electron microscopic observations of stratum corneum intercellular lipids in normal and atopic dogs. *Vet Pathol* 2001; 38: 720–723.
131. Piekutowska A, Pin D, Rème CA *et al.* Effects of a topically applied preparation of epidermal lipids on the stratum corneum barrier of atopic dogs. *J Comp Pathol* 2008; 138: 197–203.
132. Marsella R, Samuelson D, Doerr K. Transmission electron microscopy studies in an experimental model of canine atopic dermatitis. *Vet Dermatol* 2010; 21: 81–88.
133. Shimada K, Yoon JS, Yoshihara T *et al.* Increased transepidermal water loss and decreased ceramide content in lesional and non-lesional skin of dogs with atopic dermatitis. *Vet Dermatol* 2009; 20: 541–546.
134. Reiter LV, Torres SM, Wertz PW. Characterization and quantification of ceramides in the nonlesional skin of canine patients with atopic dermatitis compared with controls. *Vet Dermatol* 2009; 20: 260–266.
135. Popa I, Remoue N, Hoang LT *et al.* Atopic dermatitis in dogs is associated with a high heterogeneity in the distribution of protein-bound lipids within the stratum corneum. *Arch Dermatol Res* 2011; 303: 433–440.
136. Wood SH, Clements DN, Ollier WE *et al.* Gene expression in canine atopic dermatitis and correlation with clinical severity scores. *J Dermatol Sci* 2009; 55: 27–33.
137. Wood SH, Ollier WE, Nuttall T *et al.* Despite identifying some shared gene associations with human atopic dermatitis the use of multiple dog breeds from various locations limits detection of gene associations in canine atopic dermatitis. *Vet Immunol Immunopathol* 2010; 138: 193–197.
138. Barros Roque J, O'Leary CA, Kyaw-Tanner M *et al.* Haplotype sharing excludes canine orthologous *Filaggrin* locus in atopy in West Highland White Terriers. *Anim Genet* 2009; 40: 793–794.
139. Salzmann CA, Olivry TJ, Nielsen DM *et al.* Genome-wide linkage study of atopic dermatitis in West Highland White Terriers. *BMC Genet* 2011; 12: 37.
140. Marsella R, Samuelson D, Harrington L. Immunohistochemical evaluation of filaggrin polyclonal antibody in atopic and normal beagles. *Vet Dermatol* 2009; 20: 547–554.
141. Chervet L, Galichet A, McLean WH *et al.* Missing C-terminal filaggrin expression, NFkappaB activation and hyperproliferation identify the dog as a putative model to study epidermal dysfunction in atopic dermatitis. *Exp Dermatol* 2010; 19: e343–e346.
142. Carlsen BC, Johansen JD, Menne T *et al.* Filaggrin null mutations and association with contact allergy and allergic contact dermatitis: results from a tertiary dermatology clinic. *Contact Dermatitis* 2010; 63: 89–95.
143. Thyssen JP, Johansen JD, Linneberg A *et al.* The association between null mutations in the filaggrin gene and contact sensitization to nickel and other chemicals in the general population. *Br J Dermatol* 2010; 162: 1278–1285.
144. Novak N, Baurecht H, Schafer T *et al.* Loss-of-function mutations in the filaggrin gene and allergic contact sensitization to nickel. *J Invest Dermatol* 2008; 128: 1430–1435.
145. Betz RC, Pforr J, Flaquer A *et al.* Loss-of-function mutations in the filaggrin gene and alopecia areata: strong risk factor for a severe course of disease in patients comorbid for atopic disease. *J Invest Dermatol* 2007; 127: 2539–2543.
146. Finn LS, Zhang M, Chen SH *et al.* Severe type II Gaucher disease with ichthyosis, arthrogryposis and neuronal apoptosis: molecular and pathological analyses. *Am J Med Genet* 2000; 91: 222–226.
147. Ishida Yamamoto A. Loricrin keratoderma: a novel disease entity characterized by nuclear accumulation of mutant loricrin. *J Dermatol Sci* 2003; 31: 3–8.
148. Ohnishi Y, Okino N, Ito M *et al.* Ceramidase activity in bacterial skin flora as a possible cause of ceramide deficiency in atopic dermatitis. *Clin Diagn Lab Immunol* 1999; 6: 101–104.

To cite this article, please use DOI: 10.1111/j.1365-3164.2012.01073.x

3.2

Fixing the skin barrier: past, present and future – man and dog compared

Rosanna Marsella

Department of Small Animal Clinical Sciences, College of Veterinary Medicine, 2015 SW 16th Avenue, University of Florida, Gainesville, FL 32610, USA

Correspondence: Rosanna Marsella, Department of Small Animal Clinical Sciences, College of Veterinary Medicine, 2015 SW 16th Avenue, University of Florida, Gainesville, FL 32610, USA. E-mail: marsella@ufl.edu

Skin barrier dysfunction exists in both human and canine atopic dermatitis, leading to increased water loss and potentially facilitating allergen penetration and sensitization. Both lipid (e.g. ceramides) and protein (e.g. filaggrin) abnormalities have been described. Some are genetically inherited (e.g. filaggrin mutations are one of the major risk factors in humans) and some are secondary and linked to inflammation.

In humans, numerous studies have shown efficacy of emollients and moisturizers in barrier restoration, and this approach has been for years the mainstay of therapy. Recently, this strategy has shown promise as a preventative function.

In veterinary medicine, evidence regarding skin barrier impairment is rapidly building. Decreased ceramides and filaggrin (in some subsets of dogs) have been described. Altered metabolism of ceramides has also been proposed. Despite these preliminary data and the availability of products marketed to improve the skin barrier, evidence regarding the clinical benefit of skin repair intervention is still limited. Preliminary studies have demonstrated that topical application of fatty acids and ceramides and systemic administration of fatty acids improve lipid deficiencies in the skin of dogs with atopic dermatitis, but limited clinical evidence exists.

Disease remission in humans is paralleled by an improved skin barrier, both with calcineurin inhibitors and glucocorticoids. In veterinary medicine, a preliminary study on ciclosporin and prednisone failed to detect significant improvement of water loss, while successful immunotherapy correlated with an improved skin barrier. Controlled, large studies are needed to address the question of which skin repair approach is clinically most effective and whether this can be used as a preventative strategy.

What is known in human medicine

The importance of addressing skin dryness in humans with atopic dermatitis (AD) has been known for decades. A direct relationship exists between skin dryness and disease severity in AD patients.[1] Both moisturizers and emollients have been shown to improve the skin barrier and clinical signs.[2] Skin barrier creams increase the time between flare-ups and reduce relapses by about one-third compared with no treatment.[3] Skin care has also a preventative function. Early implementation of emollient therapy (petrolatum based) decreases the frequency of development of AD in high-risk children to 15%, compared with 30–50% when no skin care is done.[4] Despite the fact that skin barrier repair has been practised for a long time, the debate on the best ingredient to use is ongoing.

Accepted 11 May 2012

Sources of Funding: The author has received funds for research from Sogeval and Virbac.

Conflict of Interest: The author has received funds for research from Sogeval and Virbac.

Emollients, moisturizers and products based on lipids/ceramides: which one is the best?

The terms moisturizers and emollients are frequently used interchangeably, although moisturizers typically contain water as the main ingredient mixed with humectants to hydrate the stratum corneum, while emollients classically contain some form of lipid. Water itself can contribute to dryness and worsen the skin barrier, because prolonged contact with water can disrupt the stratum corneum and water rapidly evaporates after application.[5] Watery lotions can worsen the skin barrier and predispose to development of AD.[6] Therefore, ointments or thick creams rather than watery lotions are preferred in humans with AD.

Ingredients used in skin repair include combinations of petrolatum, vegetable oils, glycerin and urea.[7] Petrolatum has an immediate barrier-repairing effect[8] and is used in many over-the-counter products (e.g. Vaseline®, Hangzhou Jinque Home Product Co. Ltd, Xiaoshan, Hangzhou, China; Aquaphor®, Beiersdorf Inc., Wilton, CT, USA; and Cetaphil®, Galderma Laboratories L.P., Fort Worth, TX, USA). Paraffin oil and vegetable oils penetrate into the upper layers of the stratum corneum, and this is paralleled by a decrease in transepidermal water loss (TEWL), with the most effective occlusion seen with petrolatum.[9]

Large differences exist between products, and efficacy depends on the type of product and frequency of application. The choice and composition of the moisturizer are crucial in the long term. A study investigating the impact of long-term treatment with moisturizers on skin barrier function in healthy skin demonstrated that the effect is determined by the composition of the moisturizer.[10] Moisturizers have the ability to affect epidermal mRNA expression of genes for involucrin, transglutaminase 1 and kallikrein 5 and 7, either improving or worsening skin barrier function.[11]

Urea, a common moisturizing agent, is an endogenous metabolite that enhances stratum corneum hydration and has antimicrobial activity.[12] Topical application reduces dryness[13] and decreases TEWL.[14] Urea is not merely a passive metabolite, but a small-molecule regulator of epidermal structure and function by enhancing the expression of antimicrobial peptides, a property beneficial in patients with AD.[15]

In recent years, several no-steroidal barrier creams have been approved for AD treatment. EpiCeram® (PuraCap™; Pharmaceutical LCC, South Plainfield, NJ, USA) contains a combination of ceramides, cholesterol and fatty acids and was approved by the Federal Drug Administration (USA) in 2006.[16] Its efficacy was documented in a case series[17] and in a trial in patients with moderate-to-severe AD.[18] Remission of disease as established by the investigator under the global assessment was achieved by 58% of subjects after 3 weeks. Pruritus decreased markedly from baseline to week 3, regardless of severity at baseline. The efficacy of EpiCeram® was comparable to that observed with fluticasone propionate cream.[19] EpiCeram® reduced clinical disease severity and pruritus and improved sleep habits after both 14 and 28 days of therapy. Although the fluticasone group showed greater improvement at 14 days, improvement with EpiCeram® did not differ significantly from fluticasone by 28 days.

Atopiclair® (Galderma S.A., Lausanne, Switzerland) contains a combination of plant extracts, including glycyrrhetinic acid and *Vitis vinifera*. Atopiclair® is effective in the treatment of AD and has antipruritic properties in patients with mild-to-moderate AD.[20] Glycyrrhetinic acid, abundant in liquorice, can inhibit pruritus elicited by protease-activated receptor-2 agonists.[21] Humans with AD have higher levels of protease-activated receptor-2,[22] and this leads to increased permeability, barrier dysfunction, itching and inflammation.[23] Besides being antipruritic, glycyrrhetinic acid has antibacterial and antifungal properties that are beneficial in patients with AD.[24]

A recent study stirred debate because it showed a lack of significant difference in the clinical efficacy between a glycyrrhetinic acid-containing barrier repair cream (Atopiclair®), a ceramide-dominant barrier repair cream (EpiCeram®) and an over-the-counter petroleum-based skin protectant moisturizer (Aquaphor Healing Ointment®) applied three times daily for 3 weeks in children with mild-to-moderate AD.[25] These results clearly demonstrated that there are multiple valid approaches to skin repair.

Topical glucocorticoids and calcineurin inhibitors

As inflammation worsens the skin barrier, it is reasonable to propose that control of inflammation improves skin barrier function. Indeed, both topical calcineurin inhibitors and topical glucocorticoids (e.g. betamethasone) improve TEWL.[26] While both treatments decreased TEWL, electron microscopy of the skin after 3 weeks showed that only pimecrolimus-treated patients had an ordered stratum corneum with regular lamellar body extrusion, while the betamethasone-treated skin had inconsistent extracellular by-layers and only partly filled lamellar bodies. These results are consistent with the cutaneous atrophy observed clinically with betamethasone use, indicating that pimecrolimus is more appropriate for long-term therapy in terms of preservation of skin barrier. Pimecrolimus can also beneficially modulate expression of several genes involved directly in the skin barrier.[27] Tacrolimus, on the contrary, was reported to have negative effects on the skin barrier, including permeability and antimicrobial functions.[28] These effects were mediated by decreasing epidermal lipid synthesis, lamellar body secretion and expression of antimicrobial peptides.

What is known in dogs

Skin barrier dysfunction exists in AD[29,30] and may increase the risk of allergic sensitization.[31] Decreased ceramides[32,33] and abnormal stratum corneum ultrastructure have been described.[34,35] An increase in free and protein-bound glycosylceramides suggests an abnormality in metabolism of ceramides.[36] A significant decrease and altered metabolism of sphingosine-1-phosphate are described in lesional atopic skin compared with healthy skin.[37] All these studies emphasize the relevance of exploring skin barrier repair in veterinary medicine.

In dogs, the skin barrier is often assessed by TEWL, although the reliability of this methodology is not good.[38] A relationship between deficiency of ceramides and an increase in TEWL has been described,[39] while a relationship between disease severity and skin barrier dysfunction measured by TEWL has yet to be proved in dogs.[40] Thus, while it is reasonable to speculate that restoration of lipid deficiency should improve skin barrier function, it is still largely unknown whether skin barrier repair would directly translate into an improvement of clinical signs.

Lipid/ceramide-rich products

Topical application of ceramides, free fatty acids and cholesterol (Allerderm spot-on®; Virbac Animal Health, Fort Worth, TX, USA) improves the ultrastructure of the stratum corneum and increases the number of lipid lamellae.[41] Three weeks of topical application led to an increase in ceramide content and decrease in glucosylceramides. Normalization of protein-bound lipid content was also observed.[42] While these two studies showed a positive effect on lipid composition, demonstration of clinical benefit is still limited. An open study in dogs with chronic AD showed clinical improvement with twice-weekly application for 12 weeks, with a significant improvement of erythema noticeable after 6 weeks.[43] Although these results are promising, the impact of this study is limited by the small number of patients and the lack of a control group. A yet unpublished double-blinded, placebo-controlled study, applying the same emulsion three times weekly for 4 weeks, reported a significant decrease of clinical signs when compared with the control group, although the results on TEWL were mixed.[44] The lack of significant improvement in TEWL may be an indication of poor reliability of TEWL measurements rather than lack of skin barrier amelioration in light of the ultrastructural studies, although the ultrastructural studies did not evaluate the correlation between ultrastructure and TEWL measurements.[41]

An open study using a spot-on (once weekly) and a spray (once daily) containing essential oils and unsaturated fatty acids (Dermoscent Essential®; Laboratoire de Dermo-Cosmetique Animale, Castres, France) for 8 weeks[45] showed a significant decrease of clinical scores and pruritus in both groups, with no difference between groups. No improvement on TEWL was found. Oral administration of essential fatty acids [omega-6 (linoleic acid 350 mg/mL and γ-linolenic acid 45 mg/mL) and omega-3 (eicosapentaenoic acid 25 mg/mL and docosahexaenoic acid 28 mg/mL), mixed 5:1 (v/v); Megaderm®/EFA-Z® (Virbac S.A., Carros, France)] for 2 months also improved the ultrastructure and increased the lipid content in the skin of atopic dogs.[46] This feature was observed with both free and protein-bound lipids. No evaluation of the correlation with clinical improvement was reported.

Evidence to support the topical application of phytosphingosine is lacking at this time. A blinded, randomized controlled trial in atopic dogs using a phytosphingosine-containing shampoo (Douxocalm®; Sogeval Laboratories Inc., Irving, TX, USA) or a phytosphingosine-containing shampoo plus spray with similar ingredients or a control shampoo containing antiseptics, fatty acids and complex sugars (Allermyl®; Virbac Animal Health)[47] showed clinical improvement in all groups. No significant difference was found between groups. As all the interventions were theoretically able to affect the skin barrier, it is unknown whether using phytosphingosine provides extra benefit compared with any emollient or simple bathing. No assessment of skin barrier function was done in this study.

Barrier creams and other strategies

'Barrier cream' or skin protectants provide an exogenous barrier to water loss.[48,49] Dimethicone is an over-the-counter skin protectant.[50] Although this could be an effective and inexpensive strategy, a recent double-blinded, placebo-controlled study using dimethicone for 4 weeks in dogs with AD failed to demonstrate an improvement in clinical signs and TEWL.[51]

Ultrapure soft water, which is water in which calcium and magnesium ions have been replaced by sodium ions, has beneficial effects on the skin barrier compared with tap water.[52] In a randomized, controlled, cross-over study, shampoo treatment with ultrapure soft water significantly decreased pruritus and dermatitis scores, whereas shampoo treatment with tap water did not.[52]

Glucocorticoids, calcineurin inhibitors and allergen-specific immunotherapy

A preliminary study evaluating anti-inflammatory doses of oral prednisolone versus ciclosporin in dogs with AD failed to report a significant effect of time or group for TEWL after 4 weeks.[53] Clinical signs improved in both groups, but TEWL was not correlated with clinical improvement. On the contrary, successful allergen-specific immunotherapy was correlated with decreased TEWL when compared with atopic dogs that did not respond to allergen-specific immunotherapy.[54]

Concluding remarks

Skin barrier repair is a promising yet still incompletely explored approach to the management of canine AD. This approach could prove to be very beneficial when initiated early on in life and could possibly alter the course and minimize development of allergic sensitization. However, this approach needs to be evaluated carefully, because the choice of the wrong ingredients could have negative long-term effects and ultimately worsen an already impaired skin barrier. Thus, large controlled studies are still needed to identify the best treatment and the long-term effects on skin barrier function.

References

1. Aalto-Korte K. Improvement of skin barrier function during treatment of atopic dermatitis. *J Am Acad Dermatol* 1995; 33: 969–972.
2. Lodén M. Role of topical emollients and moisturizers in the treatment of dry skin barrier disorders. *Am J Clin Dermatol* 2003; 4: 771–788.
3. Wirén K, Nohlgård C, Nyberg F *et al.* Treatment with a barrier-strengthening moisturizing cream delays relapse of atopic dermatitis: a prospective and randomized controlled clinical trial. *J Eur Acad Dermatol Venereol* 2009; 23: 1267–1272.
4. Simpson EL, Berry TM, Brown PA *et al.* A pilot study of emollient therapy for the primary prevention of atopic dermatitis. *J Am Acad Dermatol* 2010; 63: 587–593.
5. Tsai TF, Maibach HI. How irritant is water? An overview. *Contact Dermatitis* 1999; 41: 311–314.
6. Rendell ME, Baig-Lewis SF, Berry TM *et al.* Do early skin care practices alter the risk of atopic dermatitis? A case-control study. *Pediatr Dermatol* 2011; 28: 593–595.
7. Simpson EL. Atopic dermatitis: a review of topical treatment options. *Curr Med Res Opin* 2010; 26: 633–640.
8. Matsumoto T, Yuasa H, Kai R *et al.* Skin capacitance in normal and atopic infants, and effects of moisturizers on atopic skin. *J Dermatol* 2007; 34: 447–450.
9. Patzelt A, Lademann J, Richter H *et al. In vivo* investigations on the penetration of various oils and their influence on the skin barrier. *Skin Res Technol* 2012; 18: 364–369.
10. Buraczewska I, Berne B, Lindberg M *et al.* Changes in skin barrier function following long-term treatment with moisturizers, a randomized controlled trial. *Br J Dermatol* 2007; 156: 492–498.
11. Buraczewska I, Berne B, Lindberg M *et al.* Long-term treatment with moisturizers affects the mRNA levels of genes involved in keratinocyte differentiation and desquamation. *Arch Dermatol Res* 2009; 301: 175–181.
12. Puschmann M, Gogoll K. Improvement of skin moisture and skin texture with urea therapy. *Hautarzt* 1989; 40(Suppl 9): 67–70.
13. Amichai B, Grunwald MH. A randomized, double-blind, placebo-controlled study to evaluate the efficacy in AD of liquid soap containing 12% ammonium lactate + 20% urea. *Clin Exp Dermatol* 2009; 34: e602–e604.
14. Lodén M, Andersson AC, Lindberg M. Improvement in skin barrier function in patients with atopic dermatitis after treatment with a moisturizing cream (Canoderm). *Br J Dermatol* 1999; 140: 264–267.

15. Grether-Beck S, Felsner I, Brenden H *et al.* Urea uptake enhances barrier function and antimicrobial defense in humans by regulating epidermal gene expression. *J Invest Dermatol* 2012; 132: 1561–1572.
16. Madaan A. Epiceram for the treatment of atopic dermatitis. *Drugs Today (Barc)* 2008; 44: 751–755.
17. Bikowski J. Case studies assessing a new skin barrier repair cream (epiceram) for the treatment of atopic dermatitis. *Drugs Dermatol* 2009; 8: 1037–1041.
18. Kircik LH, Del Rosso JQ. Nonsteroidal treatment of atopic dermatitis in pediatric patients with a ceramide-dominant topical emulsion formulated with an optimized ratio of physiological lipids. *J Clin Aesthet Dermatol* 2011; 4: 25–31.
19. Sugarman JL, Parish LC. Efficacy of a lipid-based barrier repair formulation in moderate-to-severe pediatric atopic dermatitis. *J Drugs Dermatol* 2009; 8: 1106–1111.
20. Veraldi S, De Micheli P, Schianchi R *et al.* Treatment of pruritus in mild-to-moderate atopic dermatitis with a topical non-steroidal agent. *J Drugs Dermatol* 2009; 8: 537–539.
21. Akasaka Y, Yoshida T, Tsukahara M *et al.* Glycyrrhetinic acid prevents cutaneous scratching behavior in mice elicited by substance P or PAR-2 agonist. *Eur J Pharmacol* 2011; 670: 175–179.
22. Lee SE, Jeong SK, Lee SH. Protease and protease-activated receptor-2 signaling in the pathogenesis of atopic dermatitis. *Yonsei Med J* 2010; 51: 808–822.
23. Steinhoff M, Neisius U, Ikoma A *et al.* Proteinase-activated receptor-2 mediates itch: a novel pathway for pruritus in human skin. *J Neurosci* 2003; 23: 6176–6680.
24. Asl MN, Hosseinzadeh H. Review of pharmacological effects of *Glycyrrhiza* sp. and its bioactive compounds. *Phytother Res* 2008; 22: 709–724.
25. Miller DW, Koch SB, Yentzer BA *et al.* An over-the-counter moisturizer is as clinically effective as, and more cost-effective than, prescription barrier creams in the treatment of children with mild-to-moderate atopic dermatitis: a randomized, controlled trial. *J Drugs Dermatol* 2011; 10: 531–537.
26. Jensen JM, Pfeiffer S, Witt M *et al.* Different effects of pimecrolimus and betamethasone on the skin barrier in patients with atopic dermatitis. *J Allergy Clin Immunol* 2009; 123: 1124–1133.
27. Grzanka A, Zebracka-Gala J, Rachowska R *et al.* The effect of pimecrolimus on expression of genes associated with skin barrier dysfunction in atopic dermatitis skin lesions. *Exp Dermatol* 2012; 21: 184–188.
28. Kim M, Jung M, Hong SP *et al.* Topical calcineurin inhibitors compromise stratum corneum integrity, epidermal permeability and antimicrobial barrier function. *Exp Dermatol* 2010; 19: 501–510.
29. Marsella R, Olivry T, Carlotti DN *et al.* Current evidence of skin barrier dysfunction in human and canine atopic dermatitis. *Vet Dermatol* 2011; 22: 239–248.
30. Olivry T. Is the skin barrier abnormal in dogs with atopic dermatitis? *Vet Immunol Immunopathol* 2011; 144: 11–16.
31. Olivry T, Wofford J, Paps JS *et al.* Stratum corneum removal facilitates experimental sensitization to mite allergens in atopic dogs. *Vet Dermatol* 2011; 22: 188–196.
32. Yoon JS, Nishifuji K, Sasaki A *et al.* Alteration of stratum corneum ceramide profiles in spontaneous canine model of atopic dermatitis. *Exp Dermatol* 2011; 20: 732–736.
33. Reiter LV, Torres SM, Wertz PW. Characterization and quantification of ceramides in the nonlesional skin of canine patients with atopic dermatitis compared with controls. *Vet Dermatol* 2009; 20: 260–266.
34. Inman AO, Olivry T, Dunston SM *et al.* Electron microscopic observations of stratum corneum intercellular lipids in normal and atopic dogs. *Vet Pathol* 2001; 38: 720–723.
35. Marsella R, Samuelson D, Doerr K. Transmission electron microscopy studies in an experimental model of canine atopic dermatitis. *Vet Dermatol* 2010; 21: 81–88.
36. Popa I, Remoue N, Hoang LT *et al.* Atopic dermatitis in dogs is associated with a high heterogeneity in the distribution of protein-bound lipids within the stratum corneum. *Arch Dermatol Res* 2011; 303: 433–440.
37. Bäumer W, Rossbach K, Mischke R *et al.* Decreased concentration and enhanced metabolism of sphingosine-1-phosphate in lesional skin of dogs with atopic dermatitis: disturbed sphingosine-1-phosphate homeostasis in atopic dermatitis. *J Invest Dermatol* 2011; 131: 266–268.
38. Lau-Gillard PJ, Hill PB, Chesney CJ *et al.* Evaluation of a handheld evaporimeter (VapoMeter) for the measurement of transepidermal water loss in healthy dogs. *Vet Dermatol* 2010; 21: 136–145.
39. Shimada K, Yoon JS, Yoshihara T *et al.* Increased transepidermal water loss and decreased ceramide content in lesional and nonlesional skin of dogs with atopic dermatitis. *Vet Dermatol* 2009; 20: 541–546.
40. Marsella R. Are transepidermal water loss and clinical signs correlated in canine atopic dermatitis: a compilation of studies. *Vet Dermatol* 2012; 23: 238–e49.
41. Piekutowska A, Pin D, Rème CA *et al.* Effects of a topically applied preparation of epidermal lipids on the stratum corneum barrier of atopic dogs. *J Comp Pathol* 2008; 138: 197–203.
42. Popa I, Remoue N, Osta B *et al.* The lipid alterations in the stratum corneum of dogs with atopic dermatitis are alleviated by topical application of a sphingolipid-containing emulsion. *Clin Exp Dermatol* 2012; 37: 665–671.
43. Fujimura M, Nakatsuji Y, Fujiwara S *et al.* Spot-on skin lipid complex as an adjunct therapy in dogs with atopic dermatitis: an open pilot study. *Vet Med Int* 2011; 2011: 281846.
44. Marsella R, Genovese D, Gilmer L *et al.* Investigations on the effects of a topical ceramide and free fatty acid solution (Allerderm Spot on®) on clinical signs and skin barrier function in dogs with atopic dermatitis: a double blinded, randomized, controlled study. *Vet Dermatol* 2012; 23: (Suppl 1): (abstract).
45. Tretter S, Mueller RS. The influence of topical unsaturated fatty acids and essential oils on normal and atopic dogs. *J Am Anim Hosp Assoc* 2011; 47: 236–240.
46. Popa I, Pin D, Remoué N *et al.* Analysis of epidermal lipids in normal and atopic dogs, before and after administration of an oral omega-6/omega-3 fatty acid feed supplement. A pilot study. *Vet Res Commun* 2011; 35: 501–509.
47. Bourdeau P, Bruet V, Gremillet C. Evaluation of phytosphingosine-containing shampoo and microemulsion spray in the clinical control of allergic dermatoses in dogs: preliminary results of a multicentre study. *Vet Dermatol* 2007; 18: 177–178.
48. Mao-Qiang M, Brown BE, Wu-Pong S *et al.* Exogenous nonphysiologic vs physiologic lipids: divergent mechanisms for correction of permeability barrier dysfunction. *Arch Dermatol* 1995; 131: 809–816.
49. Ghadially R, Halkier-Sorensen L, Elias PM. Effects of petrolatum on stratum corneum structure and function. *J Am Acad Dermatol* 1992; 26: 387–396.
50. Federal Register. Skin protectant drug products for over-the-counter human use. 1983: Part 347: 48: 6832.
51. Pellicoro C, Marsella R, Ahrens K. Evaluation of the clinical and skin barrier effects of topical therapy with dimethicone in dogs with naturally occurring atopic dermatitis. *Vet Dermatol* 2011; 22: 291.
52. Ohmori K, Tanaka A, Makita Y *et al.* Pilot evaluation of the efficacy of shampoo treatment with ultrapure soft water for canine pruritus. *Vet Dermatol* 2010; 21: 477–483.
53. Feldt D, Marsella R, Ahrens K. A prospective, blinded, controlled pilot study to evaluate the effects of cyclosporine (Atopica) on skin barrier function in canine atopic dermatitis by measurement of trans-epidermal water loss. Accepted abstract at World congress.
54. Cornegliani L, Vercelli A, Sala E *et al.* Transepidermal water loss in healthy and atopic dogs, treated and untreated: a comparative preliminary study. *Vet Dermatol* 2012; 23: 41–44.

To cite this article, please use DOI: 10.1111/j.1365-3164.2013.12019.x

3.3

Autosomal recessive ichthyosis in golden retriever dogs: distribution and frequency of the *PNPLA1* mutant allele in different populations

Eric Guaguere*, Anne Thomas†, Anais Grall‡, Emmanuelle Bourrat§, Laetitia Lagoutte‡, Frederique Degorce-Rubiales¶, Christophe Hitte‡, Emmanuel Bensignor, Jacques Fontaine††, Didier Pin§§, Guillaume Queney† and Catherine Andre‡**

*Clinique Vétérinaire Saint Bernard, Lomme, France
†Antagene, Animal Genetics Laboratory, La Tour de Salvagny, France
‡Centre National de la Recherche Scientifique, University of Rennes, Rennes, France
§Hôpital St Louis, Paris, France
¶Laboratoire d'Anatomie Pathologique Vétérinaire du Sud-Ouest, Toulouse, France
**Clinique Vétérinaire de la Boulais, Cesson-Sévigné, France
††Clinique Vétérinaire, Bruxelles, Belgium
§§VetAgroSup Ecole Vétérinaire de Lyon, Lyon, France

Correspondence: Catherine Andre, Institut de Génétique et Développement de Rennes, UMR6290-CNRS/Université de Rennes 1, 2, Avenue du Professeur Léon Bernard, 35043 Rennes, Cedex, France. E-mail: catherine.andre@univ-rennes1.fr

Background – Ichthyoses are genodermatoses that mainly occur in dogs and humans. To date four genes have been identified in dogs; all are also involved in homologous human ichthyoses. A new autosomal recessive ichthyosis gene, *PNPLA1*, was recently identified in the golden retriever breed.

Objective – The aim of this study was to report the allele frequency and penetrance of the *PNPLA1* gene mutation causing ichthyosis in golden retriever dogs from Europe, Australia and the USA.

Animals – Blood or cheek swab samples were collected from 1600 healthy or affected golden retriever dogs.

Methods – Golden retriever dogs were tested for the *PNPLA1* mutation using a commercially available genetic test.

Results The results showed that in the French population of golden retrievers the mutation is almost fully penetrant. Moreover, the *PNPLA1* mutation has a high frequency in France and is generally more frequent in European dogs compared to dogs in the USA and Australia, occurring in approximately 30% of homozygous affected dogs and 40% of heterozygous (carrier) dogs. Interestingly, the first estimates showed that the mutation frequency is lower in the USA and Australia.

Conclusion and clinical importance – A commercially available genetic test for the *PNPLA1* mutation can be used to identify affected, homozygous healthy and carrier dogs, and helps with the diagnosis of mild ichthyosis cases. Moreover, it assists breeders to rationally decrease the frequency of the disease in golden retriever dogs.

Introduction

Ichthyoses encompass a heterogeneous group of genodermatoses characterized by abnormal desquamation over the entire body due to defects of terminal keratinocyte differentiation and desquamation.[1–3] This disease occurs in people and in animals (dogs, horses, cattle). Breed-associated ichthyoses have been identified in the Norfolk terrier (*KRT10* gene[4]), Jack Russell terrier (*TGM1* gene[5]) and cavalier King Charles spaniel (*FAM83H* gene[6]). Lamellar ichthyosis has been reported in the golden retriever breed,[7–10] and the genetic cause has been recently identified.[1] Affected golden retriever dogs have a homozygous insertion-deletion in the *PNPLA1* gene that leads to a premature stop codon and a 74 amino-acid

This study was not published in the special issue of the *Veterinary Dermatology* journal (VDE 2013; 24:1).

Sources of Funding: This study was mainly supported by the CNRS and the University of Rennes 1, France, and by the European Commission LUPA project on canine genetics (FP7-LUPA, GA-201370).

Conflicts of Interest: The Centre National de la Recherche Scientifique (CNRS) and Université Rennes 1 have applied for an international patent (André *et al.*, PCT/EP2010/067569) covering the use of the canine *PNPLA1* mutation for the genetic screening of ichthyosis in golden retriever dogs. The Antagene laboratory has the international licence for providing the ichthyosis DNA test in golden retriever dogs.

shortened PNPLA1 protein. This protein belongs to a family of enzymes regulating lipid metabolism.[11] The consequence of this mutation in the homozygous state is an impairment of the cutaneous-barrier lipid metabolism that affects normal differentiation of keratinocytes and ultimately leads to a dysfunction of epidermal desquamation.

The goal of this study was to determine the frequency and penetrance of the *PNPLA1* mutation in geographically distinct golden retriever populations using a recent commercially available genetic test.

Materials and methods

Institutional approval

This study was approved by the Centre National de la Recherche Scientifique (CNRS) ethical board approval, France (35-238-13), and samples were voluntarily provided by private dog owners and breeders.

Samples

Blood and cheek swabs were obtained by veterinarians from affected and unaffected dogs.

Genetic testing

Dogs were tested for the *PNPLA1* mutation using a commercially available test based on a fluorescent dye end-point polymerase chain reaction (PCR) method, from Antagene (Animal Genetics Laboratory, La Tour de Salvagny, France; http://www.antagene.com). The presence or absence of the mutation was previously validated in 320 golden retriever dogs (120 affected, 200 unaffected), 180 healthy dogs belonging to other retriever breeds and 300 dogs from 25 other breeds.[1]

Dogs

To estimate the mutation frequency two groups of dogs were tested. Group one consisted of golden retriever dogs of unknown clinical status that were randomly selected from different kennels and different regions of each country. This was to obtain data representative of the general population, so-called 'research data'. Genetic testing was conducted at the Centre National de la Recherche Scientifique, University of Rennes. The second group consisted of dogs tested by the commercial laboratory providing the diagnostic test following requests from veterinarians or owners for confirmation of the diagnosis or for screening purposes, so-called 'commercial data'. A total of 1600 golden retriever DNA samples from France, Switzerland,[12] the USA and Australia were tested for the *PNPLA1* mutation. For the dogs whose clinical status was assessed, a correlation of the phenotype/genotype was performed to determine penetrance.

Diagnosis of ichthyosis

All dogs diagnosed with the disease had been examined by a veterinarian or veterinary dermatologist. The diagnosis was based on clinical and histopathological findings. Dermatological clinical signs included a mild to moderate or severe generalized scaling with initially small to large white scales becoming progressively black, and a hyperpigmented and rough ventral glabrous skin similar to sandpaper. Histopathological features were characterized by moderate to severe laminated or compact orthokeratotic hyperkeratosis and isolated vacuolated keratinocytes regularly visible in the stratum granulosum. In all cases, other possible causes for the skin lesions were ruled out.

Data analysis

Data analysis was descriptive. Based on the results of the genetic tests, percentages of homozygous normal, homozygous mutated or heterozygous dogs were calculated for both 'research' and 'commercial' data. The percentage of the mutated allele was also calculated in a given population.

Results

The French population of golden retrievers was analysed by using data obtained from the genetic test of 180 randomly selected dogs ('research data') and 600 nonrandomly selected dogs tested at the request of veterinarians or owners ('commercial data'). Dogs randomly selected for testing had a frequency of the *PNPLA1* mutation of 48.5% compared to 63.5% for the ones nonrandomly selected. In Switzerland, the frequency of the mutation in the randomly selected population was 56% and in the nonrandomly selected population it was 64.5%. In the USA and Australia, 500 and 115 dogs, respectively, were nonrandomly selected for testing. The results indicated that even though dogs from these geographical regions were not randomly selected as in the French and Swiss dog populations, the frequency of the mutated allele was only 38.5% and 31.5%, respectively. This result indicates that the proportion of affected golden retrievers with the *PNPLA1* mutated allele is lower in the USA and Australia than in France or Switzerland (Table 1).

With the clinical and genetic knowledge gained to date, of more than 500 dogs carrying the mutation in the homozygous state, less than 1% (four dogs) were asymptomatic suggesting that this mutation is almost fully penetrant.

Table 1. Numbers of dogs tested with the ichthyosis genetic test and frequencies of the ichthyosis causal *PNPLA1* mutated allele in golden retrievers from different geographical areas

Dog source	Number of dogs tested	Homozygous normal (% of dogs)	Heterozygous (% of dogs)	Homozygous mutated (% of dogs)	Frequency of the *PNPLA1* mutated allele (%)*
France – research data	180	30	43	27	48.5
France – commercial data	600	17	39	44	63.5
Switzerland – research data	179	20	48	32	56
Switzerland – commercial data	26	4	63	33	64.5
USA – commercial data	500	37	49	14	38.5
Australia – commercial data	115	48	41	11	31.5
Total dogs tested	1600				

Research data: data from randomly selected dogs; commercial data: data from dogs tested at the request of veterinarians or owners (i.e. nonrandomly selected).

*Calculated as: 1 × number of dogs heterozygous for the mutated gene + 2 × number of dogs homozygous for the mutated gene/2 × number of dogs tested × 100.

Discussion

The identification of the *PNPLA1* mutated gene provides veterinarians and breeders with a diagnostic and screening test for ichthyosis. Prior to the development of this test, it was not possible to detect carrier and asymptomatic cases. Breeding programmes can now test their sires and dams before breeding, with the goal of progressively diminishing the incidence of this disease in golden retriever dogs. It is the authors' recommendation that carrier dogs are not systematically removed from the population if they have other desirable traits, but instead are bred to homozygous normal dogs. Testing the sire and dam will detect the homozygous normal dogs and the rare asymptomatic dog.

The frequency of the mutation in the population of golden retrievers from the countries investigated was generally high, with 31.5% in Australia, 38.5% in the USA, 48.5% in France and 56% in Switzerland (Table 1). The data from this study clearly indicate significant numbers of affected and carrier dogs worldwide and a difference for the disease allele frequency between the USA and Australia compared to Europe. However, it is important to mention that samples from the USA and Australia originated from dogs suspected of the disease (i.e. not randomly selected), which likely increased the frequency of the mutated gene in these populations.

The penetrance of the *PNPLA1* mutated allele is almost 100%; all affected dogs harbour the mutation in the homozygous state making the use of the genetic test easier and directly useful for the breeding selection since a simple autosomal scheme is expected (i.e. homozygous dogs for the mutated allele will develop the disease and will transmit the mutated allele to 100% of their offspring; homozygous dogs for the normal allele will not develop the disease and will transmit a normal allele to 100% of their offspring, and heterozygous dogs will not develop the disease but will transmit the mutated allele to 50% of their offspring). However, not all 'unaffected' dogs will be homozygous normal, since the authors have identified four of 500 dogs that were homozygous for the mutation while showing no clinical signs of ichthyosis. This discrepancy indicates the need to perform thorough and frequent clinical examinations as well as genetic tests to detect such rare cases. However, it is important to remember that asymptomatic dogs harbouring a homozygous *PNPLA1* mutation will transmit the mutation to all offspring and caution should be taken with such dogs especially if they are champions.

Acknowledgements

We thank the French veterinarians, especially T. Bord, X. Langon, A. Muller, P. Prelaud and M.D. Vaillant, for providing us with clinical data and samples, as well as dog owners and breeders who provided samples and genealogical data. We also thank P. Bellaud (histopathology platform H^2P^2, IFR140 Biogenouest, Rennes, France) for histology stainings, and P. Quignon (Institut de Génétique et Développement de Rennes, France) for careful readings and helpful discussions.

References

1. Grall A, Guaguère E, Planchais S, et al. PNPLA1 mutations cause autosomal recessive congenital ichthyosis in golden retriever dogs and humans. *Nat Genet* 2012; 44: 140–147.
2. Fischer J. Autosomal recessive congenital ichthyosis. *J Invest Dermatol* 2009; 129: 1319–1321.
3. Oji V, Tadini G, Akiyama M, et al. Revised nomenclature and classification of inherited ichthyoses: results of the First Ichthyosis Consensus Conference in Soreze 2009. *J Am Acad Dermatol* 2010; 63: 607–641.
4. Credille KM, Barnhart KF, Minor JS, et al. Mild recessive epidermolytic hyperkeratosis associated with a novel keratin 10 donor splice-site mutation in a family of Norfolk terrier dogs. *Br J Dermatol* 2005; 153: 51–58.
5. Credille KM, Minor JS, Barnhart KF, et al. Transglutaminase 1-deficient recessive lamellar ichthyosis associated with a LINE-1 insertion in Jack Russell terrier dogs. *Br J Dermatol* 2009; 161: 265–272.
6. Forman OP, Penderis J, Hartley C, et al. Parallel mapping and simultaneous sequencing reveals deletions in BCAN and FAM83H associated with discrete inherited disorders in a domestic dog breed. *PLoS Genet* 2012; 8: 1–9.
7. Guaguere E, Bensignor E, Muller A, et al. Epidemiological, clinical, histopathological and ultrastructural aspects of ichthyosis in golden retrievers: a report of 50 cases. *Vet Dermatol* 2007; 18: 382–383.
8. Cadiergues MC, Patel A, Shearer DH, et al. Cornification defect in the golden retriever: clinical, histopathological, ultrastructural and genetic characterisation. *Vet Dermatol* 2008; 19: 120–129.
9. Mauldin EA, Credille KM, Dunstan RW, et al. The clinical and morphologic features of nonepidermolytic ichthyosis in the golden retriever. *Vet Pathol* 2008; 45: 174–180.
10. Guaguere E, Bensignor E, Küry S, et al. Clinical, histopathological and genetic data of ichthyosis in the golden retriever: a prospective study. *J Small Anim Pract* 2009; 50: 227–235.
11. Baulande S, Langlois C. Proteins sharing PNPLA domain, a new family of enzymes regulating lipid metabolism. *Med Sci (Paris)* 2010; 26: 177–184.
12. Owczarek-Lipska M, Thomas A, André C, et al. Frequency of gene defects in selected European retriever populations. *Schweiz Arch Tierheilkd* 2011; 9: 418–420.

To cite this article, please use DOI: 10.1111/j.1365-3164.2012.01097.x

3.4

Epidermal structure created by canine hair follicle keratinocytes enriched with bulge cells in a three-dimensional skin equivalent model *in vitro*: implications for regenerative therapy of canine epidermis

Tetsuro Kobayashi*[1], Kaoru Enomoto†[1], Yu Hsuan Wang†, Ji Seon Yoon†, Ryoko Okamura‡, Kaori Ide†, Manabu Ohyama*, Toshio Nishiyama‡, Toshiroh Iwasaki† and Koji Nishifuji†

*Department of Dermatology, Keio University School of Medicine, 35 Shinanomachi, Shinjuku, Tokyo, Japan
†Department of Veterinary Medicine and ‡Scleroprotein and Leather Research Institute, Faculty of Agriculture, Tokyo University of Agriculture and Technology, 3-5-8 Saiwai-cho, Fuchu, Tokyo, Japan

Correspondence: Koji Nishifuji, Department of Veterinary Medicine, Faculty of Agriculture, Tokyo University of Agriculture and Technology, 3-5-8 Saiwai-cho, Fuchu, Tokyo 183-8509, Japan. E-mail: kojimail@cc.tuat.ac.jp

Background – Keratinocytes in the hair follicle bulge region have a high proliferative capacity, with characteristics of epithelial stem cells. This cell population might thus be an ideal source for generating the interfollicular epidermis in a canine skin equivalent.

Hypothesis/Objectives – This study was designed to determine the ability of canine hair follicle bulge cell-enriched keratinocytes to construct canine living skin equivalents with interfollicular epidermis *in vitro*.

Animals – Four healthy beagle dogs from a research colony.

Methods – Bulge cell-enriched keratinocytes showing keratin 15 immunoreactivity were isolated from canine hair follicles and cultured on dermal equivalent containing canine fibroblasts. Skin equivalents were subjected to histological, immunohistochemical, western blot and RT-PCR analyses after 10–14 days of culture at the air–liquid interface.

Results – The keratinocyte sheets showed an interfollicular epidermal structure comprising four to five living cell layers covered with a horny layer. Immunoreactivities for keratin 14 and desmoglein 3 were detected in the basal and immediate suprabasilar layers of the epidermis, while keratin 10 and desmoglein 1 occurred in more superficial layers. Claudin 1 immunoreactivity was seen in the suprabasalar layer of the constructed epidermis, and filaggrin monomers and loricrin were detected in the uppermost layer. Basal keratinocytes in the skin equivalent demonstrated immunoreactivity to antibodies against basement membrane zone molecules.

Conclusions and clinical importance – A bulge stem cell-enriched population from canine hair follicles formed interfollicular epidermis within 2 weeks *in vitro*, and thus represents a promising model for regenerative therapy of canine skin.

Introduction

The skin is the outermost surface of the animal's body and plays a crucial role in providing a mechanical and biological barrier against microbial organisms, chemical components and ultraviolet light. The skin also protects the body from dehydration and maintains the physiological environment inside the body. Large skin defects caused by extensive wounding, trauma, burns, chronic ulcers or surgical procedures involved in removing large tumours are major concerns in veterinary medicine.

Wound healing is a complex process that includes inflammation, angiogenesis, re-epithelialization and remodeling of the extracellular matrix processes.[1,2] Re-epithelialization is a crucial step in wound healing, and the development of a new therapeutic approach to accelerate re-epithelialization is a key goal for successful wound management.[3] It is notable that hair-covered areas recover sooner than hairless areas following skin injury, as re-epithelialization spreads from the hair follicle infundibulum.[4,5] This suggests that hair follicle keratinocytes may contribute to re-epithelialization of the interfollicular epidermis.

Accepted 4 July 2012
[1]T.K. and K.E. contributed equally to this work.
Sources of Funding: M.O., T.I. and K.N. received funding from the Ministry of Education, Culture, Sports, Science and Technology of Japan.
Conflict of Interest: No conflicts of interest have been declared.

The hair follicle bulge region constitutes the outermost layer of the outer root sheath and the attachment site of the arrector pili muscle. In addition, it was recently reported to harbour epithelial stem cells in mice.[6–8] This cell population has been shown to contribute to the regeneration of the interfollicular epidermis after wounding.[9] These findings suggest that hair follicle stem cells may represent a promising target for the development of new treatment approaches for skin wounds. The bulge region in canine hair follicles contains keratin 15 (K15)-positive keratinocytes with characteristics of epithelial stem cells.[10,11] These K15-positive cells have a greater proliferative capacity than interfollicular epidermal keratinocytes *in vitro*, and a better ability to reconstitute pilosebaceous units and interfollicular epidermis *in vivo*.[11] Canine hair follicle bulge cells may therefore represent a more effective cell source for the regeneration of skin wounds than canine interfollicular epidermal keratinocytes.

Three-dimensional (3D) skin equivalents have been developed as *ex vivo* dermatological research materials[12] and as new therapeutic materials for wound treatment.[13,14] Keratinocytes in these 3D skin equivalents can recapitulate *in vivo* epithelial cell differentiation *in vitro* and generate stratum corneum and the dermoepidermal junction.[12] These 3D skin equivalents are considered to possess similar physiological properties to normal skin. The goal of the present study was to investigate the potential of canine hair follicle bulge cells to construct interfollicular epidermis in skin equivalents and assess the ability of the cell population to differentiate into intact interfollicular epidermis *in vitro*.

Materials and methods

Skin samples

Three healthy beagle dogs (3–4 years old) were used in this study. Keratinocytes and fibroblasts were isolated from skin samples obtained from the dorsolateral skin (20 mm × 20 mm) after sedation with medetomidine hydrochloride (20–80 μg/kg; Domitor; Pfizer Japan, Tokyo, Japan) and local anaesthesia with lidocaine hydrochloride (Xylocaine; AstraZeneca Japan, Osaka, Japan). For immunohistochemical staining of normal canine skin, samples were obtained from the nose and footpads of a healthy beagle dog using a skin biopsy punch after euthansia for reasons unrelated to this study, and were embedded in optimal cutting temperature (OCT) compound (Sakura Finetek, Tokyo, Japan) or fixed with 10% neutral buffered formalin for paraffin embedding. All experimental procedures were officially approved by the Animal Research Committee and were carried out in accordance with the ethical guidelines of Tokyo University of Agriculture and Technology.

Isolation and culture of bulge cell-enriched keratinocytes

Canine bulge cell-enriched keratinocytes, which were positive for the bulge stem-cell marker K15, were isolated from hair follicles as previously described.[10,11] Skin samples were cut vertically into small pieces. The middle parts of the fragments, containing the isthmus and suprabulbar parts of the hair follicles, including the bulge region,[10] were carefully microdissected and incubated with 1500 U/mL of dispase II (Godo Syusei, Tokyo, Japan) overnight at 4°C. Hair follicle epithelia were separated manually from the adjacent dermis and incubated with 0.05% trypsin EDTA for 15–20 min at 37°C to isolate single hair follicle keratinocytes. Isolated cells were filtered using a 100 μm cell strainer (Becton Dickson, Franklin Lakes, NJ, USA) and counted.

Isolated keratinocytes were cultured in William's medium (Invitrogen, Carlsbad, CA, USA) supplemented with 10% NuSerum IV (Becton Dickson), 5 ng/mL epidermal growth factor (Sigma-Aldrich, St Louis, MO, USA) and 10^{-10} mol/L cholera toxin (List Biological Laboratories, Campbell, CA, USA) on type 1 collagen-coated dishes (Iwaki, Chiba, Japan) at 37°C in a humidified atmosphere of air supplemented with 5% CO_2 as previously reported.[10,11] Culture medium was changed every 3–4 days. Cultured keratinocytes at passages two to three were stored in liquid nitrogen until use.

Isolation and culture of canine dermal fibroblasts

Canine dermal pieces comprising 2 mm cubes were placed on culture dishes and incubated with Dulbecco's modified Eagle's medium (DMEM; Invitrogen) containing 10% fetal bovine serum (FBS) at 37°C in a humidified atmosphere of air supplemented with 5% CO_2. Outgrowth of fibroblasts from the dermal pieces was observed within 2 weeks. Canine dermal fibroblasts at passages two to four were used in the following experiments.

Establishment of canine skin equivalent using bulge cell-enriched keratinocytes

Canine fibroblasts (1 × 10^5 cells/mL) were suspended in FBS. Collagen gel solution was made, containing a mixture of bovine collagen type I (Cellmatrix; Nitta Gelatin Inc., Osaka, Japan), 5x-concentrated DMEM (Cellmatrix), 10x-concentrated Ham's F-12 medium (Cellmatrix) and fibroblast-containing FBS at a ratio of 7:1:1:1. The collagen gel solution was placed on silicon sheets in six-well culture plates, and incubated at 37°C in a humidified atmosphere of air supplemented with 5% CO_2 for 1 h until the solution gelled to form a dermal equivalent. The dermal equivalent was then detached from the silicon sheet and cultured for a further 2–3 days.

The canine dermal equivalent was placed on stainless-steel mesh (0.29 mm mesh) to avoid further shrinkage of the gel. A polycarbonate ring was placed on the dermal equivalent, and 4 × 10^5 keratinocytes were added into the ring. Fresh culture medium [DMEM containing 10% FBS, 10^{-10} mol/L cholera toxin (List Biological Laboratories), 10 ng/mL epidermal growth factor (Sigma-Aldrich), 0.4 μg/mL hydrocortisone (Sigma-Aldrich), 5 μg/mL transferrin (Sigma-Aldrich), 10^{-8} mol/L retinoic acid (Sigma-Aldrich), 2 nmol/L 3,3′-5 tri-iodothyronine (Sigma-Aldrich), 5 μg/mL insulin (Sigma-Aldrich), 100 U/mL penicillin, 100 μg/mL streptomycin and 0.25 μg/mL amphotericin (CellnTEC, Bern, Switzerland)] was applied outside the ring. The ring was removed after 1–2 days, and 2 mL of fresh culture medium was added into the dish to start the cell culture at the air–liquid interface. Cells were incubated at 37°C, in a humidified atmosphere of air supplemented with 5% CO_2, and the culture medium was changed every 3 days, with the addition of 10 μmol/L matrix metalloproteinase III inhibitor (Merck Millipore, Billerica, MA, USA) and 1.5 μmol/L aprotinin (Roche Diagnostics, Almere, The Netherlands) 8 days after initiation of the culture.

Skin equivalents were harvested and embedded in the OCT compound or fixed with 10% neutral buffered formalin for paraffin embedding for further histological, immunofluorescence and western blot analyses.

Immunofluorescence staining

Frozen sections were prepared for staining of keratin 10 (K10), keratin 14 (K14), loricrin, claudin 1, α6 integrin, type XVII collagen, Bullous pemphigoid antigen 1 (BP230/BPAG1) and laminins by fixing with acetone at −20°C for 10 min or with methanol:acetone (1:1 v/v) at room temperature, and incubating with primary antibodies overnight at 4°C. For staining of desmoglein 1 (Dsg1) and desmoglein 3 (Dsg3), nonfixed frozen sections were incubated with primary antibodies recognizing canine Dsg1 and Dsg3 for 1 h at room temperature. Filaggrin monomers were stained in paraffin-embedded sections. The primary antibodies used are listed in Table 1. Cross-reactivities of anti-K10, anti-claudin 1 and anti-laminin antibodies against canine antigens have been described by the manufacturers. Immunoreactivities of human pemphigus foliaceus sera and AK15 anti-Dsg3 monoclonal antibody to canine Dsg1 and Dsg3, respec-

Table 1. Antibodies

Protein	Antibody	Clone	Source (catalogue number)
Keratin 14	Mouse anti-keratin 14 MAb	LL002	Abcam, Cambridge, UK (#ab7800)
Keratin 10	Mouse anti-keratin 10 MAb	RKSE60	Progen, Heidelberg, Germany (#10501)
Filaggrin	Rabbit anti-filaggrin PAb		Kanda S *et al.*,[29]
Loricrin	Rabbit anti-loricrin PAb		Abcam (#ab24722)
Desmoglein 1	Human pemphigus foliaceus sera		Masayuki Amagai, Keio University School of Medicine, Tokyo, Japan
Desmoglein 3	Mouse anti-Dsg3 MAb	AK15	Masayuki Amagai
Claudin 1	Rabbit anti-claudin 1 PAb		Abcam (#ab15098)
α6 Integrin	Rat anti-α6 integrin MAb	GoH3	American Research Products, Waltham, MA, USA (#03-10709)
Type XVII collagen	Mouse anti-type XVII collagen MAb	1A8c	Katsushi Owaribe, Nagoya University, Nagoya, Japan
BP230/BPAG1	Mouse anti-BP230/BPAG1 MAb	279	Katsushi Owaribe
Laminins	Rabbit anti-laminin PAb		Abcam (#ab11575)
Desmoglein 1 and 3	Mouse anti-Dsg 1 & 3 MAb	32-2B	David Garrod, University of Manchester, Manchester, UK

Abbreviations: MAb, monoclonal antibody; PAb, polyclonal antibody.

tively, were determined by immunoprecipitation using baculovirus-expressed recombinant canine Dsg1[15] and Dsg3 (K. Nishifuji, unpublished observation). The amino acid sequence of the loricrin peptide used as an immunogen to generate the anti-loricrin antibody in this study was mostly conserved according to the predicted amino acid sequence of canine loricrin (93%; Genbank accession no. XP 864440.2). Sections were subsequently incubated with fluorescence-conjugated secondary antibodies and Hoechst 33258 (Invitrogen) for 1 h at room temperature. All sections were subjected to microscopic analysis with a fluorescence microscope (TE2000-U; Nikon, Tokyo, Japan).

Western blot analysis

Total cell lysates from the skin equivalent were applied to SDS–PAGE and blotted to polyvinylidene fluoride membranes. The bands corresponding to K14, filaggrin monomers, claudin 1 and Dsgs were visualized using the antibodies listed in Table 1.

RT-PCR analysis

Total RNA was purified from the canine skin equivalents using a RNeasy Mini Kit (Qiagen, Hilden, Germany) and used to synthesize complementary DNA using a PrimeScript RT reagent kit (Takara Bio, Shiga, Japan) according to the manufacturer's protocol. The PCR was conducted using the AmpliTaq Gold 360 Master Mix (Applied Biosystems, Foster City, CA, USA). Reactions were performed using the following cycling conditions: 30 cycles of 30 s at 95°C, 30 s at 60°C and 60 s at 72°C. The primer sets used are shown in Table 2.

Table 2. Primer sequences for RT-PCR

Gene	Primer sequences
Type XVII collagen	Forward: 5′-AAGGAGCCAAACACGAGAGA-3′ Reverse: 5′-GGACTCACACTTGCTGATCG-3′
β4 Integrin	Forward: 5′-TGGACAACCTCAAGCAGATG-3′ Reverse: 5′-CAGGCCTCATGTCTGTCTGA-3′
Laminin α3	Forward: 5′-AGTTGAGGTTCACCGGTTTG-3′ Reverse: 5′-GGGTGACTTGCAGGCTATGT-3′
Laminin β3	Forward: 5′-GATTGACCAAGCCTGAGACC-3′ Reverse: 5′-CCCGAAGATGAAACCACATT-3′
Laminin γ2	Forward: 5′-GAAACCCAGCAGCTCTTACG-3′ Reverse: 5′-AAAAGTGGCATTGCCCATAC-3′
Keratin 10	Forward: 5′-TTGAGACGCACTGTTCAAGG-3′ Reverse: 5′-ACGCAGTAGCGACCTTCTGT-3′
Keratin 14	Forward: 5′-GAGATGCGTGACCAGTACGA-3′ Reverse: 5′-GCAATTCGCTATTAGAGACCAC-3′
Keratin 1	Forward: 5′-CAACCAGAGCCTTCTCCAAC-3′ Reverse: 5′-TCCGAGTGGAGGTGTCTACC-3′
Keratin 5	Forward: 5′-GACGCTGCCTACATGAACAA-3′ Reverse: 5′-TCATACTGGGCCTTGACCTC-3′

Results

Canine bulge cell-enriched hair follicle keratinocytes undergo normal differentiation of interfollicular epidermal keratinocytes in a skin equivalent

Canine bulge-enriched keratinocytes were seeded onto canine dermal equivalents and cultured at the air–liquid interface. Reconstituted skin equivalents were harvested on days 7–14 and subjected to histological analysis. Keratinocytes in skin equivalents became stratified into three or four layers covered with a cornified layer on days 10–14, as shown by haematoxylin and eosin staining (Figure 1). Basophilic cytoplasmic granules resembling keratohyalin granules were observed in the superficial layer of the reconstituted epithelium.

The differentiation pattern of keratinocytes in the canine skin equivalents was evaluated by immunofluorescence analysis of keratinocyte differentiation markers. Immunoreactivity for K14, an intermediate filament preferentially expressed in basal keratinocytes of normal epidermis, was recognized in the basal and immediate suprabasal layers in the canine skin equivalent (Figure 2), and immunoreactivity for K10, which is expressed in differentiated keratinocytes in normal epidermis, was recognized in the more superficial layers of the constituted epidermis (Figure 2).

Profilaggrin is an essential component of keratohyalin granules in the stratum granulosum and is processed to filaggrin monomers during cornification. Immunoreactivity for filaggrin monomers was recognized as a cytoplasmic granular pattern in the superficial living cell layer in the canine skin equivalent (Figure 2), while lori-

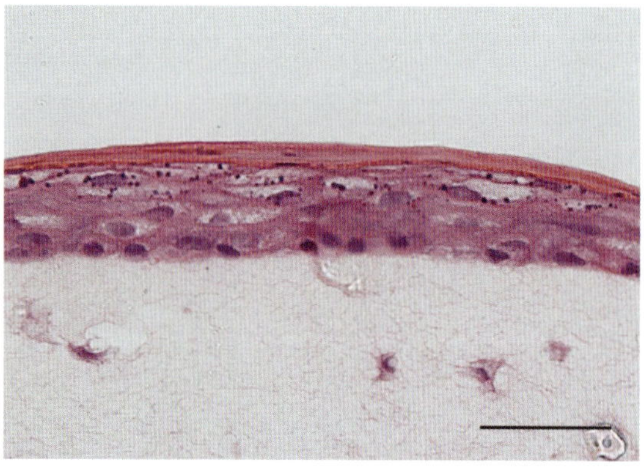

Figure 1. Histological findings for canine skin equivalent. Canine bulge cell-enriched keratinocytes were placed on a canine dermal equivalent and cultured for 14 days. The keratinocytes formed three to four layers of stratified epidermis. Cytoplasmic granules resembling keratohyalin granules were visible immediately beneath the stratum corneum. Mayer's haematoxylin and eosin stain. Scale bar represents 50 μm.

crin, which is produced in the stratum granulosum and forms the cornified cell envelope in the stratum corneum, was recognized in the uppermost, anucleated cell layer (Figure 2). The immunostaining pattern for filaggrin monomers and loricrin was similar to that seen in normal canine nasal planum and footpad.

Epidermis in canine skin equivalents expresses cell adhesion and tight junction molecules

The Dsg, desmosomal cell–cell adhesion molecules, are expressed on the surface of epidermal keratinocytes in a differentiation-specific manner. Desmoglein 1 immunoreactivity was recognized in the suprabasal layer of the epithelium in the canine skin equivalents, whereas Dsg3 immunoreactivity was detected in the basal and immediate suprabasal layers of the epidermis. These staining patterns were similar to those in canine nasal planum and footpad (Figure 3). Immunoreactivity for claudin 1, which is a major transmembrane constituent of tight junctions, was recognized preferentially in the suprabasal layer of the epidermis in both canine skin equivalents and canine nasal planum (Figure 3).

Canine skin equivalent derived from hair follicle bulge-enriched cells expresses epidermal basement membrane zone (BMZ) molecules

Immunofluorescence analysis was also performed to determine whether the canine skin equivalent derived from hair follicle bulge-enriched cells expressed key components of the BMZ. Immunoreactivities for hemidesmosomal proteins, α6 integrin, type XVII collagen and BP230, were detected in the BMZ in normal canine skin and in basal keratinocytes in the canine skin equivalents (Figure 4). Immunoreactivity for laminins, which are major proteins of the lamina densa, was also recognized in basal cells in the skin equivalents.

Western blot and RT-PCR analyses to confirm protein expression

Western blot analysis revealed bands corresponding to K14, filaggrin monomers, Dsg1, Dsg3 and claudin 1 in canine skin equivalent lysate (Figure 5).

The RT-PCR analysis revealed transcription of genes encoding for K10, K14, K1, K5, type XVII collagen, β4 integrin and laminin α3, β3 and γ2 in the canine skin equivalents (Figure 6).

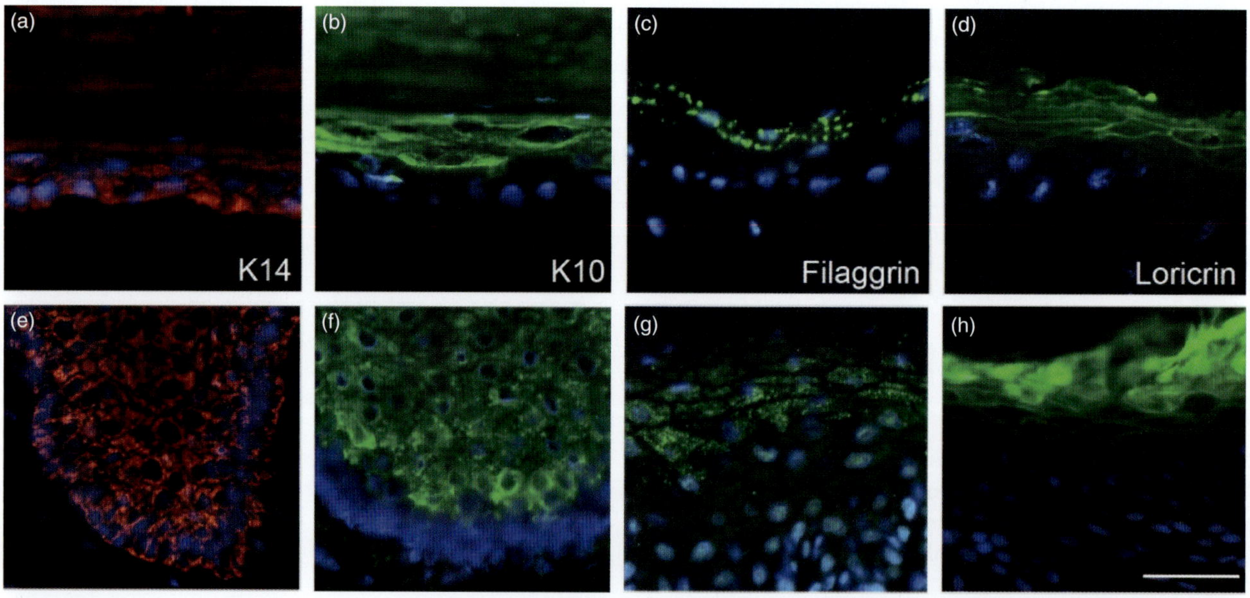

Figure 2. Immunofluorescence analysis to assess the expression patterns of epidermal components in canine skin equivalents. Cytoplasmic keratin 14 (K14) immunoreactivity was recognized in the basal and immediate suprabasal layers (a), whereas keratin 10 (K10) immunoreactivity was recognized in the upper layers of the skin equivalent (b). Immunoreactivity for filaggrin monomers was recognized in the superficial layer of keratinocytes, as a cytoplasmic granular pattern (c). Loricrin immunoreactivity was recognized in the plasma membranes of anucleated cells in the superficial epidermis (d). Immunoreactivities for K14 (e), K10 (f), filaggrin monomers (g) and loricrin (h) in the nasal planum of a normal dog. Scale bar represents 50 μm.

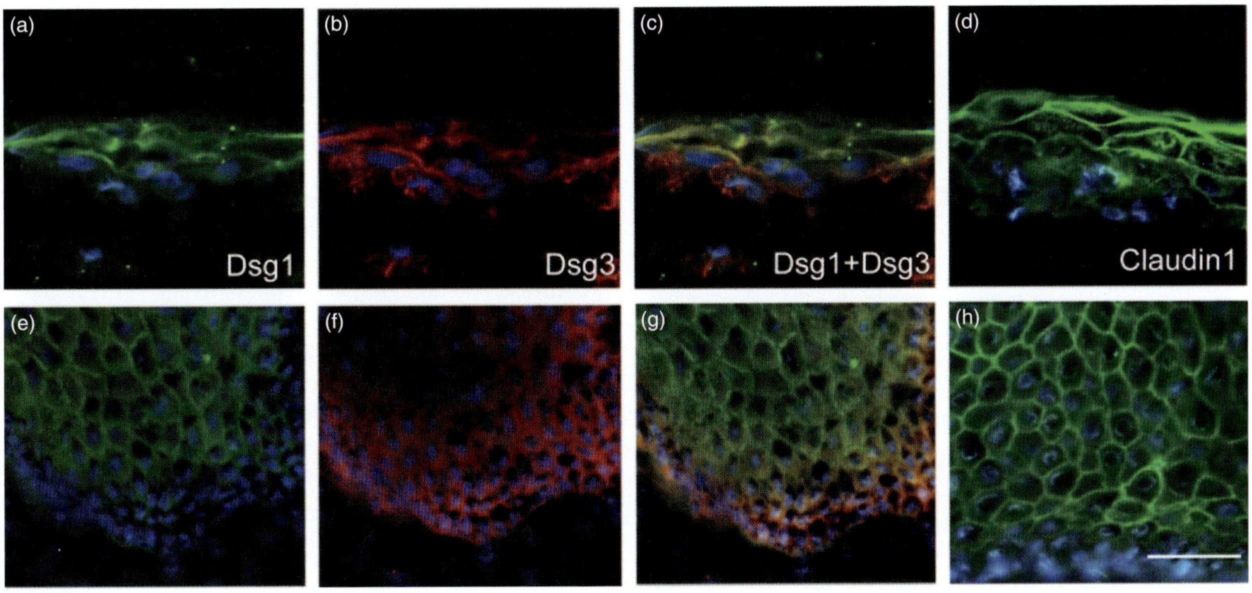

Figure 3. Immunofluorescence analysis to assess the expression of cell adhesion and tight junction molecules in canine skin equivalents. Desmoglein 1 (Dsg1) immunoreactivity was recognized on keratinocyte surfaces in the middle to superficial epidermal layers (a), whereas desmoglein 3 (Dsg3) immunoreactivity was recognized in the lower part of the epidermis (b). (c) Merged figure showing Dsg1 and Dsg3. (d) Claudin 1 immunoreactivity was recognized in whole layers of epidermis, except for the basal layer. Immunoreactivities for Dsg1 (e), Dsg3 (f), merged Dsg1 and Dsg3 (g) and claudin 1 (h) in the nasal planum of a normal dog. Scale bar represents 50 μm.

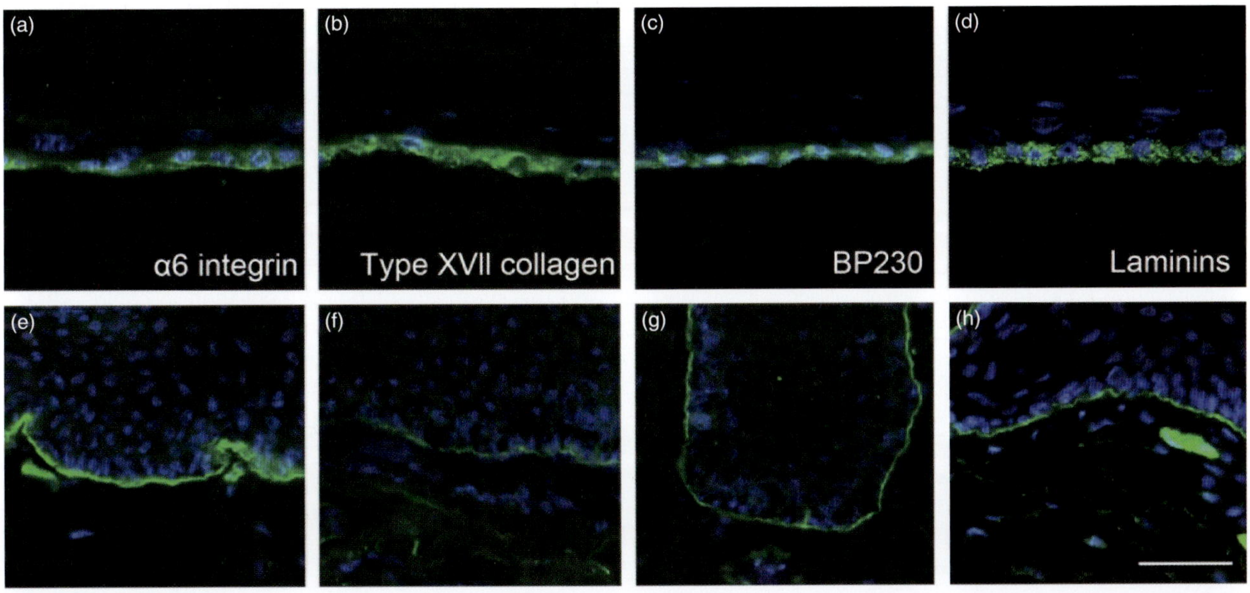

Figure 4. Immunofluorescence analysis to assess the expression of basement membrane zone molecules in canine skin equivalent. Immunoreactivities of antibodies against α6 integrin (a), type XVII collagen (b), BP230 (c) and laminins (d) were recognized in the basal keratinocytes. Immunoreactivities of antibodies against α6 integrin (e), type XVII collagen (f), BP230 (g) and laminins (h) in the nasal planum of a normal dog. Scale bar represents 50 μm.

Discussion

Human skin equivalents are available commercially and have demonstrated successful results in the repair of skin defects.[14,16] In addition, canine 3D skin equivalents derived from keratinocytes isolated from haired skin, which may contain both follicular and interfollicular keratinocytes, have been reported in the literature.[17,18] However, these previous methods may not be suitable for harvesting proliferated keratinocytes in an efficient manner. Contamination of the differentiated keratinocyte population in the spinous and granular layers may result in unstable proliferation and incomplete formation of epidermal structures in the skin equivalent. It is therefore necessary to develop a method of harvesting keratinocytes with high proliferative capacity. The bulge region in canine hair follicles was previously reported to harbour specialized keratinocytes that express some hair follicle stem cell markers, as seen in mice and humans, and which possess a greater proliferative capacity than interfollicular epidermal keratinocytes.[10,11] Bulge stem cell-enriched keratinocytes might thus represent a suitable cell source for constructing a canine 3D skin equivalent. We used hair fol-

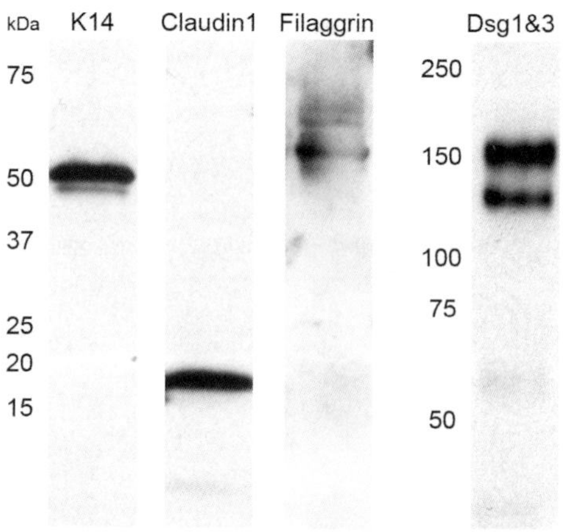

Figure 5. Western blot analysis of epidermal proteins expressed in canine skin equivalent. Protein bands corresponding to K14 (56 kDa), claudin 1 (19 kDa), filaggrin monomers (59 kDa), Dsg1 (160 kDa) and Dsg3 (130 kDa) were expressed in lysates of canine skin equivalents.

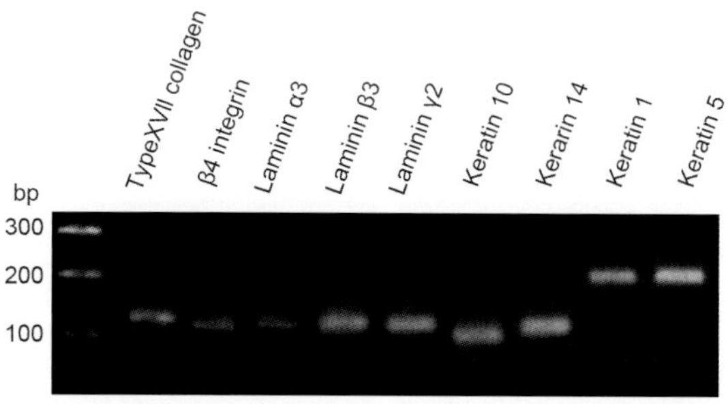

Figure 6. RT-PCR analysis to determine mRNA expression of the epidermal basement membrane zone proteins in canine skin equivalent. Complementary DNA for type XVII collagen, β4 integrin, laminins α3, β3 and γ2, and K10, K14, K1 and K5 were amplified by RT-PCR using mRNA extracted from the skin equivalent as a template. Bands in the left lane indicate molecular weight standards.

licle bulge cells to establish a novel canine skin equivalent. Canine bulge cell-enriched keratinocytes formed stratified epithelia covered with a horny layer within 2 weeks, and the expression patterns of some keratinocyte differentiation markers, including keratins, filaggrin, loricrin and Dsgs, were similar to those in canine nasal planum. Conversely, immunoreactivities for canine bulge cell markers, which were positive when the cells were harvested, become negative in the skin equivalents (data not shown). These findings imply that the hair follicle bulge cells undergo normal differentiation and cornification processes of the interfollicular epidermis in the skin equivalent. Others have reported that murine bulge cells formed interfollicular epidermis and contribute to wound healing in full-thickness skin defects.[9] Thus, although the efficiencies of bulge cell-enriched keratinocytes and interfollicular epidermal keratinocytes to form a canine skin equivalent have not been compared directly, the results of the present study suggest that canine hair follicle bulge cells could be a promising cell source for promoting re-epithelialization of skin defects *in vivo*. Further investigations are needed to compare the efficiencies of bulge cell-enriched keratinocytes and interfollicular epidermal keratinocytes for the construction of 3D skin equivalents.

Although autologous skin grafts have been used to promote re-epithelialization in skin defects in humans and dogs,[19,20] this technique is limited in terms of the size of the skin grafts. To overcome this limitation, autografts of epidermal cell sheets using cultured keratinocytes have been tested in human patients suffering from chronic ulcers.[14,16] However, the epidermal cell sheets are usually thin and fragile, and lack the epidermal BMZ components that stabilize the grafts. In contrast, immunoreactivity for laminins, which provide connections between transmembrane molecules via hemidesmosomes with anchoring fibrils, was, in the present study, recognized in the basal keratinocytes of the skin equivalents derived from bulge cell-enriched keratinocytes. In addition, immunoreactivities of antibodies against α6 integrin, type XVII collagen and BP230 were detected in basal keratinocytes, even though cross-reactivities between these antibodies and the corresponding canine BMZ molecules have not yet been confirmed. The RT-PCR analysis revealed transcription of genes encoding for β4 integrin and laminins α3, β3 and γ2 in the canine skin equivalents, suggesting the expression of some key components of hemidesmosomes and lamina densa. In contrast, the expression of type VII collagen, which forms anchoring fibrils immediately beneath the BMZ, was not observed in the skin equivalents (data not shown). Previous studies reported that compartmentalization of type VII collagen in the BMZ in human skin equivalents required culture for more than 3 weeks;[21] keratinocytes were cultured on dermal equivalents for 2 weeks or less in the present study, and this short culture period might thus explain the lack of type VII collagen immunoreactivity in these canine skin equivalents. It is also possible that bovine collagen I may exert a negative effect on the synthesis of type VII collagen in canine keratinocytes or fibroblasts. Further optimization of the culture conditions, including a longer cultivation period and the use of allogenic materials, is expected to produce complete anchoring fibrils in the canine skin equivalents.

The results of the present study also indicated that the skin equivalents produced from canine bulge cell-derived keratinocytes formed a stratum corneum, and immunoreactivities for filaggrin and loricrin, which are major constituents of the stratum corneum, were recognized in the uppermost layer of keratinocytes. Moreover, immunoreactivity for claudin 1, a major transmembrane tight junction molecule, was also recognized in the canine skin equivalent. Taken together, these canine skin equivalents were shown to possess a normal stratum corneum and tight junction proteins, which are crucial for maintaining cutaneous barrier function.[22,23]

Although these canine skin equivalents open up the possibility of skin regenerative medicine in veterinary fields, several issues remain regarding their future clinical application. First, dermal equivalents contain bovine materials as scaffolding for canine fibroblast growth; this heterogeneous material may cause immunogenic reactions in recipient dogs and raises potential concerns about infectious diseases derived from bovine proteins.[14] New approaches for generating dermal equivalents, including the use of other scaffolding materials or a self-assembly approach by fibroblasts with no exogenous scaffolding elements, must therefore be assessed.[12] Second, it took 2 weeks to generate the complete skin equivalent in the present study, which is too long for the management of acute wounds. Cryopreserved allogenic cultured skin grafts have offered the possibility of initial treatment;[24,25] even though they are ultimately rejected, the allogenic graft can accelerate the wound-healing process, probably by inducing some important growth factors.[26] The lack of pilosebaceous units in the cultured skin equivalent is another problematic issue. However, a previous study reported that canine bulge cell-enriched keratinocytes grafted with mouse dermal cells in nude mice resulted in reconstitution of hair follicles, as well as sebaceous glands,[11] indicating that canine bulge cells have the capacity to reconstitute pilosebaceous units *in vivo*. In contrast, no previous studies have reported the reconstitution of pilosebaceous units either *in vitro* or *ex vivo*. The lack of several important factors, such as hair-inducing mesenchymal cells (dermal papilla cells), a scaffolding structure for hair follicle formation and a dermal vascular network, may be responsible for the lack of reconstitution of pilosebaceous units in skin equivalents.[27] It would be interesting to determine whether the addition of dermal papillae cells into the dermal equivalents could help to reconstitute pilosebaceous units in the skin equivalents. Further studies are needed to evaluate the long-term stability and the risk of carcinogenesis of canine skin equivalents *in vivo* prior to clinical application.

In conclusion, canine skin equivalents derived from bulge cell-enriched keratinocytes represent a promising option for wound-healing treatment. In addition, the highly efficient transduction of genetically engineered genes into target cells is crucial for successful gene therapy,[28] and bulge cells, which have the characteristics of stem cells, might thus be ideal cell targets for gene therapy of hereditary skin disorders. Efficient canine skin equivalents represent an important development in regenerative medicine of canine skin.

Acknowledgements

The authors are grateful to Masayuki Amagai for human pemphigus foleaceus serum and AK15 anti-Dsg3 monoclonal antibody, David Garrod for 32-2B anti-Dsgs monoclonal antibody and Katsushi Owaribe for monoclonal antibodies against type XVII collagen and BP230.

References

1. Gurtner GC, Werner S, Barrandon Y *et al.* Wound repair and regeneration. *Nature* 2008; 453: 314–321.
2. Lau K, Paus R, Tiede S *et al.* Exploring the role of stem cells in cutaneous wound healing. *Exp Dermatol* 2009; 18: 921–933.
3. Coulombe PA. Wound epithelialization: accelerating the pace of discovery. *J Invest Dermatol* 2003; 121: 219–230.
4. Brown JB, McDowell F. Epithelial healing and the transplantation of skin. *Ann Surg* 1942; 115: 1166–1181.
5. Langton AK, Herrick SE, Headon DJ. An extended epidermal response heals cutaneous wounds in the absence of a hair follicle stem cell contribution. *J Invest Dermatol* 2008; 128: 1311–1318.
6. Cotsarelis G, Sun TT, Lavker RM. Label-retaining cells reside in the bulge area of pilosebaceous unit: implications for follicular stem cells, hair cycle, and skin carcinogenesis. *Cell* 1990; 61: 1329–1337.
7. Cotsarelis G. Epithelial stem cells: a folliculocentric view. *J Invest Dermatol* 2006; 126: 1459–1468.
8. Blanpain C, Fuchs E. Epidermal homeostasis: a balancing act of stem cells in the skin. *Nat Rev Mol Cell Biol* 2009; 10: 207–217.
9. Ito M, Liu Y, Yang Z *et al.* Stem cells in the hair follicle bulge contribute to wound repair but not to homeostasis of the epidermis. *Nat Med* 2005; 11: 1351–1354.
10. Kobayashi T, Shimizu A, Nishifuji K *et al.* Canine hair-follicle keratinocytes enriched with bulge cells have the highly proliferative characteristic of stem cells. *Vet Dermatol* 2009; 20: 338–346.
11. Kobayashi T, Iwasaki T, Amagai M *et al.* Canine follicle stem cell candidates reside in the bulge and share characteristic features with human bulge cells. *J Invest Dermatol* 2010; 130: 1988–1995.
12. Auxenfans C, Fradette J, Lequeux C *et al.* Evolution of three dimensional skin equivalent models reconstructed *in vitro* by tissue engineering. *Eur J Dermatol* 2009; 19: 107–113.
13. Cooper ML, Spielvogel RL. Artificial skin for wound healing. *Clin Dermatol* 1994; 12: 183–191.
14. Hunziker T, Limat A. Cultured keratinocyte grafts. *Curr Probl Dermatol* 1999; 27: 57–64.
15. Nishifuji K, Amagai M, Nishikawa T *et al.* Production of recombinant extracellular domains of canine desmoglein 1 (Dsg1) by baculovirus expression. *Vet Immunol Immunopathol* 2003; 15: 177–182.
16. Clark RA, Ghosh K, Tonnesen MG. Tissue engineering for cutaneous wounds. *J Invest Dermatol* 2007; 127: 1018–1029.
17. Barnhart KF, Credille KM, Ambrus A *et al.* Preservation of phenotype in an organotypic cell culture model of a recessive keratinization defect of Norfolk terrier dogs. *Exp Dermatol* 2005; 14: 481–490.
18. Serra M, Brazis P, Puigdemont A *et al.* Development and characterization of a canine skin equivalent. *Exp Dermatol* 2007; 16: 135–142.
19. Adams DC, Ramsey ML. Grafts in dermatologic surgery: review and update on full- and split-thickness skin grafts, free cartilage grafts, and composite grafts. *Dermatol Surg* 2005; 31: 1055–1067.
20. Fowler D. Distal limb and paw injuries. *Vet Clin North Am Small Anim Pract* 2006; 36: 819–845.
21. Woodley DT, Krueger GG, Jorgensen CM *et al.* Normal and gene-corrected dystrophic epidermolysis bullosa fibroblasts alone can produce type VII collagen at the basement membrane zone. *J Invest Dermatol* 2003; 121: 1021–1028.
22. Elias PM. Stratum corneum defensive functions: an integrated view. *J Invest Dermatol* 2005; 125: 183–200.
23. Niessen CM. Tight junctions/adherens junctions: basic structure and function. *J Invest Dermatol* 2007; 127: 2525–2532.
24. De Luca M, Albanese E, Cancedda R *et al.* Treatment of leg ulcers with cryopreserved allogeneic cultured epithelium. A multicenter study. *Arch Dermatol* 1992; 128: 633–638.
25. Teepe RG, Koebrugge EJ, Ponec M *et al.* Fresh versus cryopreserved cultured allografts for the treatment of chronic skin ulcers. *Br J Dermatol* 1990; 122: 81–89.
26. Myers S, Navsaria H, Sanders R *et al.* Transplantation of keratinocytes in the treatment of wounds. *Am J Surg* 1995; 170: 75–83.
27. Stenn KS, Cotsarelis G. Bioengineering the hair follicle: fringe benefits of stem cell technology. *Curr Opin Biotechnol* 2005; 16: 493–497.
28. Gache Y, Pin D, Gagnoux-Palacios L *et al.* Correction of dog dystrophic epidermolysis bullosa by transplantation of genetically modified epidermal autografts. *J Invest Dermatol* 2011; 131: 2069–2078.
29. Kanda S, Sasaki T, Shiohama A *et al.* Characterization of canine filaggrin: gene structure and protein expression in dog skin. *Vet Dermatol* 2013; 24: 25–e7.

To cite this article, please use DOI: 10.1111/j.1365-3164.2012.01102.x

3.5

Skin lipid profiling in normal and seborrhoeic shih tzu dogs

Ji-Seon Yoon, Koji Nishifuji, Sinpei Ishioroshi, Kaori Ide and Toshiroh Iwasaki

Department of Veterinary Medicine, Faculty of Agriculture, Tokyo University of Agriculture and Technology, 3-5-8 Saiwai-cho, Fuchu, Tokyo 183-8509, Japan

Correspondence: Toshiroh Iwasaki, Tokyo University of Agriculture and Technology, 3-5-8 Saiwai-cho, Fuchu, Tokyo 183-8509, Japan. E-mail: bpag2180@cc.tuat.ac.jp

Background – Seborrhoea is a clinical condition resulting in excessive lipid and/or scale on the skin and is a common and important skin disease of dogs. However, there is little information on the skin surface lipid composition of dogs with seborrhoea.

Hypothesis/Objectives – To compare skin surface lipid profiles in normal and seborrhoeic shih tzu dogs.

Methods – Fourteen client-owned dogs (seven seborrhoeic and seven normal) were investigated. Lipids in sebaceous glands (SGs) were extracted from homogenized tissues of SG hyperplasia. Surface lipid was collected by tape stripping [stratum corneum (SC)-enriched fraction] and acetone-wetted cotton swab (acetone-extracted fraction). Lipids in SGs, SC-enriched fractions and acetone-extracted fractions were evaluated by high-performance thin-layer chromatography.

Results – Lipids in SGs mainly consisted of cholesterol esters, wax esters and triglycerides, whereas lipids in the SC-enriched fraction mainly consisted of ceramides. The acetone-extracted fraction contained a mixture of lipid classes recognized in SG- and SC-enriched fractions. In seborrhoeic dogs, concentrations of wax esters and triglycerides in the acetone-extracted fraction were significantly higher than in control dogs ($P = 0.0285$). Amounts of total ceramides (in micrograms) per milligram of SC were not significantly different between the two groups ($P = 0.5204$). Interestingly, two unknown ceramide fractions, which accounted for 20% of the total ceramides, were recognized exclusively in seborrhoeic dogs.

Conclusions and clinical importance – These results provide evidence that the skin surface lipid profiles are altered in shih tzu dogs with seborrhoea.

Introduction

In mammals, the sebaceous glands (SGs) and the keratinocytes produce a protective lipid layer that covers the skin. Studies in humans have shown that the lipid composition of SGs differs from that of keratinocytes.[1–3] For example, human sebum is primarily comprised of low-polar lipids, such as esters, triglycerides (TGs), diglyceride and squalene, fatty acids and cholesterol (CHOL).[1] Meanwhile, human keratinocytes in the stratum granulosum produce ceramides (CERs), CHOL and free fatty acids (FFAs), which comprise the extracellular lipid layers in the stratum corneum (SC) crucial for maintaining the barrier function of the skin.[2,3]

Seborrhoea is a clinical condition characterized as excessive greasiness and increased scale formation on the skin. This is an important and common skin disease of dogs and it can be secondary to inflammation or be a primary skin disease. In dogs, primary seborrhoea is an inherited disorder of abnormal cornification. Commonly affected dog breeds include the American cocker spaniel, English springer spaniel, West Highland white terrier and Basset hound.[4,5] Secondary seborrhoea can result from a wide range of causes, such as ectoparasites, bacterial pyoderma, *Malassezia* overgrowth, atopic dermatitis, endocrinopathies or nutritional imbalances.[4,6] Although primary and secondary seborrhoea are common, very little is known about the composition of skin lipid in this skin disease.

The shih tzu dog breed commonly exhibits seborrhoea, often in association with underlying triggers, such as *Malassezia* dermatitis or atopic dermatitis.[6] The goal of this study was to compare the skin surface lipids of normal and seborrhoeic shih tzu dogs. This information may provide a better understanding of lipid profiles in seborrhoea in dogs.

Accepted 10 July 2012

Present address: Ji-Seon Yoon, Department of Dermatology, College of Medicine, Seoul National University, 28 Yongon-dong, Chongno-gu, Seoul, 110-744, South Korea.

Sources of Funding: This study was partly funded by the Kao Corporation, who covered some research expenses.

Conflict of Interest: No conflicts of interest have been declared.

Material and methods

All dogs were privately owned, and owners gave their written informed consent. All experimental procedures were approved by the Animal Research Committee and were carried out in accordance with the ethical guidelines of Tokyo University of Agriculture and Technology.

Dogs

The normal group of dogs (n = 7) consisted of shih tzu dogs without evidence of skin disease, specifically seborrhoea or *Malassezia* overgrowth (Table 1). The affected group of dogs (n = 7) consisted of dogs with clinical signs compatible with seborrhoea. The age and gender of the dogs in both groups were matched. Skin cytology revealed *Malassezia* overgrowth (>10 per high-power field) for all dogs on initial presentation. To minimize the contaminating SC surface lipids with lipids from yeast, all dogs were treated with an antimicrobial shampoo (Malaseb™; Dermcare-Vet Pty Ltd, Springwood, Queensland, Australia) and/or oral itraconazole (5 mg/kg, once daily, Itorizole®; Janssen Pharmaceutical KK, Tokyo, Japan) until the number of Malassezia organisms found on skin cytology were less than two per high-power field (at least 4 weeks). Complete blood counts, serum chemistries, abdominal ultrasound imaging and computer tomography were suggestive of an unilateral adrenal gland tumour in one dog. Three dogs were considered to have atopy, because these dogs had elevated serum allergen-specific IgE. No cause for the *Malassezia* overgrowth was found in the remaining four seborrhoeic dogs.

For this study, skin surface lipids and the SC were collected from the seven shih tzu dogs whose clinical conditions were compatible with seborrhoea and the seven normal dogs.

Sebaceous gland tissue

Tissue for SG isolation was collected from two dogs (a 12-year-old male and an 11-year-old spayed female) with SG hyperplasia via skin biopsy procedure using local anaesthesia. Intact hyperplastic SGs were used to maximize collection of pure SG lipids. Skin biopsy specimens were also collected for histological examination; tissue was fixed in 10% neutral buffered formalin and processed routinely.

Lipid extractions

Sebaceous glands.

Lipids were extracted from the SG tissue using a modification of the method reported by Bligh and Dyer.[7,8] Briefly, the epithelium was first separated from the SG by incubation with 1500 U/mL dispase II (Godo Syusei, Tokyo, Japan) for 1 h at 37°C. The remaining SG tissue was then homogenized and suspended in a mixture of chloroform, methanol and water (1:2:0.8, by volume) at room temperature for 30 min. Next, chloroform and water were added to the homogenized mixture to change the volume ratio of chloroform, methanol and water to a 1:1:1 mixture. After centrifugation, the lipid-containing supernatant was collected and transferred to new glass test tubes.

Skin surface.

Two methods were used to collect skin surface lipids. In the first, skin surface lipids were collected by vigorously rubbing an area of inguinal skin (2 cm × 4 cm) five times using an approximately 2 cm × 4 cm × 0.5 cm piece of acetone-wetted cotton. This method enabled collection of a mixture of SGs and free extractable SC lipids. The cotton material was then placed into glass tubes, sealed and preserved at −20°C until analysed. For lipid extraction, the cotton swabs were dissolved in 10 mL of a chloroform and methanol mixture (2:1, by volume) at room temperature, and the solvent containing a lipid extract was transferred to a new glass test tube.

In the second procedure, using previously described methods,[9] lipids from the SC-enriched fractions were collected via tape stripping. Briefly, after removing sebum by scrubbing a 2 cm × 4 cm area of inguinal skin with acetone using cotton swabs, five consecutive tape strippings were performed. In a previously published study, 10 consecutive tape strips removed almost all layers of the SC in dogs.[10] Tape strips were then immersed in *n*-hexane (Sigma-Aldrich, St Louis, MO, USA) and sonicated to collect the SC extracts. The SC components extracted from the tape strips were filtered through a 0.45 μm DURAPORE-membrane filter (HVHP type; Millipore, Billerica, MA, USA). The SC extracts were weighed, placed in glass test tubes and dissolved in 5 mL of chloroform and methanol (2:1, by volume) at room temperature and shaken for 30 min for lipid extraction. After centrifugation at 1000***g*** for 5 min, the supernatant containing the lipid extracts was transferred to a new glass test tube. Lipid extracts from SG hyperplasia, acetone-containing cotton swabs and tape stripping were dried using a nitrogen stream at 38°C, reconstituted in 50 μL of chloroform and methanol (2:1, by volume), and used for analysis. To avoid technical variance between investigators, all lipid extraction procedures were performed by the same investigator (J.-S.Y.).

High-performance thin-layer chromatography (HPTLC)

Lipid analysis was performed using HPTLC. Briefly, 5 μL reconstituted lipid extract was applied to HPTLC plates (Merck, Darmstadt, Germany). The lipid bands of different polarity were developed using hexane followed by a solvent mixture of chloroform, methanol and acetic acid (190:9:1, by volume). In addition, for the quantitative analysis of ceramide classes, the bands of size-fractionated CER classes were developed by three separate applications of a mixture of chloroform, methanol and acetic acid (190:9:1, by volume). Nonpolar lipid mixtures, bovine-derived CER[NS] (combination of nonhydroxy fatty acids and 6-hydroxyl sphingosines) and CER[AS] (combination of α-hydroxy fatty acids and 6-hydroxyl sphingosines; Matreya, Pleasant Gap, PA, USA) were used as standards to determine the polarity and quantity of each HPTLC band. For colour development, the plates were sprayed with 10% $CuSO_4$ (Wako Pure Chemical Industries, Ltd, Osaka, Japan) and 8% H_3PO_4 (Wako Pure Chemical Industries, Ltd) aqueous solution and then heated at 180°C for 7 min. The HPTLC fractions were scanned and subjected to a density plot analysis using Bio1D-ver.12.11 software (Vilber Lourmat, Marne-la-Vallée, France). The quantity of each CER fraction per milligram of the SC was determined by comparing the density plots with those of serially diluted (0.1, 0.3, 0.6 and 1 μg/μL) CER standards in chloroform and methanol (2:1, by volume).[9]

Normal-phase liquid chromatography connected to electrospray ionization-mass spectrometry (NPLC-ESI-MS)

In order to analyse CERs, NPLC-ESI-MS was conducted as previously described.[9] Briefly, lipids extracted from SC were redissolved in 10 mL of chloroform and methanol (99.5:0.5, by volume) and applied to Sep-Pak Vac RC Silica cartridges (Waters, Milford, MA, USA). In this method, flow-through fractions contain low-polar lipids (e.g. CHOL), while high-polar lipids (e.g. CERs) appear in the eluate that is extracted from the cartridge using chloroform and methanol (95:5, by

Table 1. Signalment of shih tzu dogs at the time of examination

	Control		Seborrhoea	
Dog no.	Sex	Age	Sex	Age
1	M	7 years 2 months	M	6 years 6 months
2	F	10 years 4 months	F	10 years
3	F	4 years 6 months	FS	5 years
4	F	10 years 2 months	F	9 years 8 months
5	F	9 years	F	9 years
6	M	11 years 6 months	MN	11 years 7 months
7	F	9 years	FS	8 years 4 months

Abbreviations: F, female; FS, female spayed; M, male; MN, male neutered.

volume). The fractions containing CERs were dried using a nitrogen stream and submitted to Yukiguni Aguri Co. (Gunma, Japan) for NPLC-ESI-MS using a LTQ-Orbitrap mass spectrometry system operating in electrospray ionization mode (Thermo Fisher Scientific, Waltham, MA, USA). Parameters for scan measurement of the electrospray ionization using unit mass resolution mode were determined at the following settings: polarity, negative; temperature of nitrogen gas, 300°C; flow of heated dry nitrogen gas, 8.0 L/min; nebulized gas pressure, 137.9 kPa.; capillary voltage, 3500 V; fragmenter voltage, 150 V; and scan range, 250–1500 atomic mass unit.

Statistical analyses

Student's unpaired t-test (StatView® 5.0; SAS Institute Inc., Cary, NC, USA) was used to compare the relative amounts of lipid fractions, quantities of total CERs, and each CER class per milligram of SC between seborrhoeic dogs and control dogs. A P-value of <0.05 was considered to be statistically significant.

Results

Profiling of skin lipids

Initially, the major lipid components in the SG and surface lipids (i.e. SC-enriched and acetone-extracted fractions) in shih tzu dogs without seborrhoea were determined. Lipids extracted from tissues of SG hyperplasia, SC-enriched fractions and acetone-extracted fractions were subjected to HPTLC analysis. If the polarity of the fractions in canine samples were almost identical to those of the lipid standards, including cholesterol esters (CEs), TGs, CHOL, FFAs and CERs, the fractions were assigned to canine CEs, TGs, CHOLs, FFAs and CERs corresponding to the standard (Figure 1a). A dense band recognized between CEs and TGs was assigned to wax esters (WEs) according to a previous report.[11] It was found that lipids extracted from SGs consisted of mainly CEs (18.3%), WEs (19.2%) and TGs (45.2%), as well as small proportions of CHOL (8.5%) and FFAs (5.3%; Figure 1b). In contrast, lipids in the SC-enriched fraction mainly consisted of CERs (65.6%) and small proportions of CHOL (7.7%) and FFAs (11.6%; Figure 1b). Lipids in the acetone-extracted fraction consisted of a mixture of SG- and SC-derived lipids (Figure 1b).

Comparison of skin surface lipid profiles (acetone-extracted fractions) in dogs with seborrhoea and healthy dogs

Next, we determined whether the skin surface lipid profile was altered in shih tzu dogs with seborrhoea. Histological examination of skin biopsy samples from the two dogs with seborrhoea revealed parakeratotic hyperkeratosis, epidermal acanthosis, spongiosis and lymphocytic exocytosis, no yeast organisms were recognized in the tissue samples (Figure 2). Relative amounts of CEs, WEs, TGs, CHOLs, FFAs and total CERs in acetone-extracted fractions obtained from shih tzu dogs with seborrhoea were analysed based on the results of densitometry analysis, and compared with those in control dogs (Figure 3a). Findings revealed that the relative amounts of WEs and TGs in dogs with seborrhoea were significantly higher than in control dogs ($P < 0.05$; Figure 3b). In contrast, relative amounts of FFAs and total CERs were significantly lower in dogs with seborrhoea than in control dogs ($P < 0.05$; Figure 3b).

Comparison of the SC CER profiles in dogs with seborrhoea and control dogs

The next investigation was to determine whether the quantities of the SC CER classes were altered in dogs with seborrhoea compared with normal dogs. Eight fractions of the SC CERs, which were assigned to corresponding CER

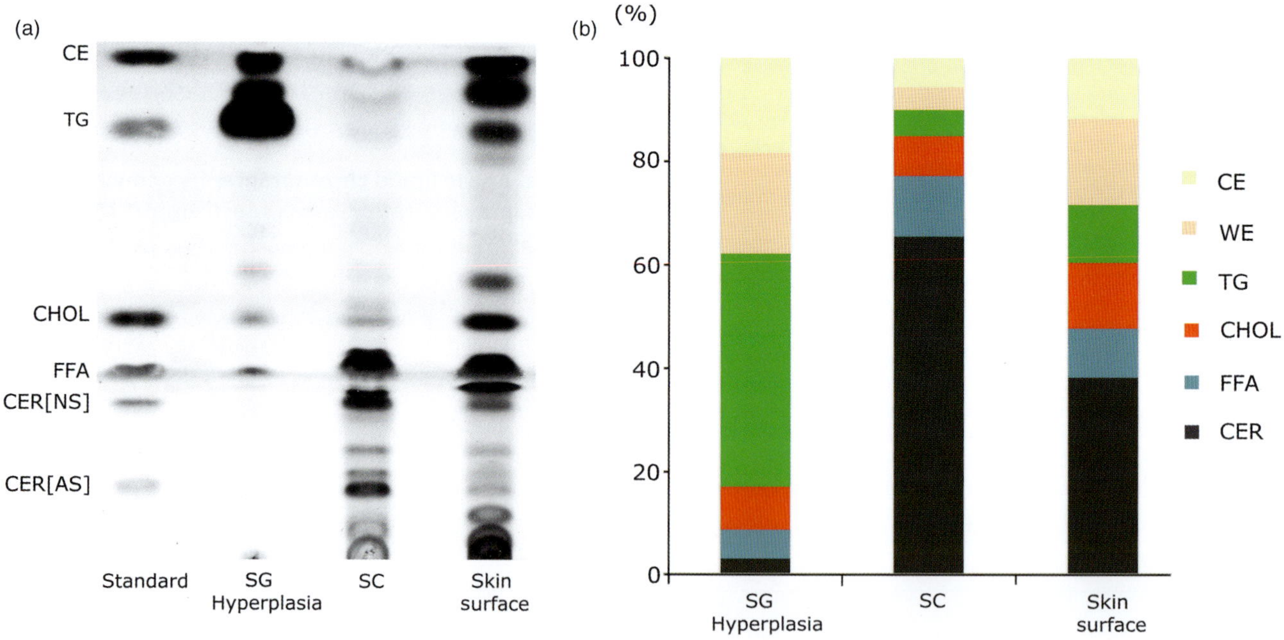

Figure 1. High-performance thin-layer chromatography (HPTLC) analysis of lipids extracted from sebaceous gland (SG) hyperplasia, stratum corneum (SC) and the skin surface in shih tzu dogs without seborrhoea. (a) Representative data from HPTLC analysis of lipids in SG hyperplasia (SG-enriched fraction), SC (SC-enriched tape stripped fraction) and skin surface (acetone-extracted fraction). (b) Composition ratio of lipids in SG hyperplasia, SC and skin surface. Abbreviations: CE, cholesterol ester; CER, ceramide; CER[AS], combination of α-hydroxy fatty acid and sphingosine; CER[NS], combination of nonhydroxy fatty acid and sphingosine; CHOL, cholesterol; FFA, free fatty acid; TG, triglyceride; WE, wax ester.

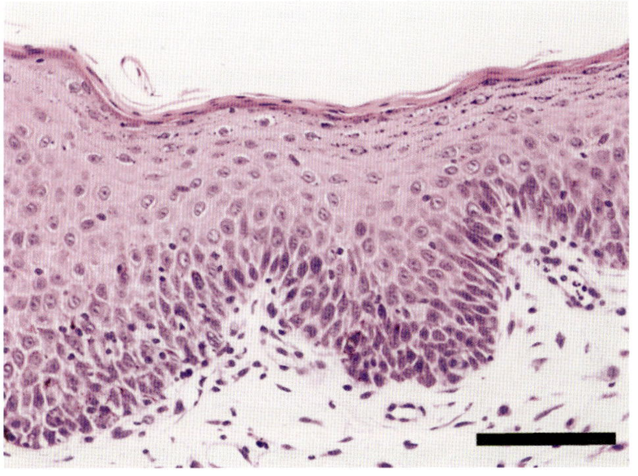

Figure 2. Histopathological findings from a shih tzu with seborrhoea (dog no. 6). The epidermis showed parakeratotic hyperkeratosis, epidermal acanthosis, spongiosis and lymphocytic exocytosis. Scale bar indicates 100 mm. Mayer's haematoxylin and eosin stain.

classes according to a previous report,[7] were recognized in dogs with seborrhoea and in the age- and sex-matched control dogs (Figure 4a). Quantities of total CERs per milligram of SC in control dogs (14.9 ± 2.3 μg) were not significantly different from those in seborrhoeic dogs (14.0 ± 2.4 μg, $P = 0.5204$; (Figure 4b). Quantities of CER[EOS] (1.1 ± 0.3 μg), CER[EOP] (0.7 ± 0.3 μg), CER[EOH] (1.1 ± 0.3 μg) and a mixture of CER[AS] and CER[NH] (1.7 ± 0.3 μg) per milligram of SC were significantly lower in the SC of seborrhoeic dogs than control dogs (CER[EOS], 1.6 ± 0.4 μg; CER[EOP], 1.1 ± 0.3 μg; CER[EOH], 1.7 ± 0.3 μg; and a mixture of CER[AS] and CER[NH], 3.2 ± 0.8 μg; Figure 4b). Interestingly, two unknown SC CER fractions, whose polarities did not correspond to any of the SC CER classes recognized in healthy dogs, appeared exclusively in the seven dogs with seborrhoea (Figure 4a,b). Density plot analysis revealed that quantities of the unknown fractions accounted for approximately 20% of total SC CERs in the shih tzu dogs with seborrhoea (unknown 1, 0.9 ± 0.2 μg; and unknown 2, 1.8 ± 0.5 μg; both expressed per milligram of SC).

Furthermore, lipids in the SC-enriched fractions collected from dogs with seborrhoea and control dogs were subjected to NPLC-ESI-MS, which enables one to distinguish CERs with different carbon chains based upon retention time and mass/charge ratio. The total carbon chain numbers of SC CERs in dogs with seborrhoea and control dogs are shown in Table 2. In dogs with seborrhoea, CER[NDS], CER[NS], CER[AS], CER[NH] and CER[AP] contained subspecies with short carbon chains (<40 total carbons), which did not appear in the SC of control dogs.

Discussion

The present study revealed the detailed composition of lipids in SG, SC-enriched and acetone-extracted fractions in normal and seborrhoeic shih tzu dogs. Based on our findings, low-polar lipids, such as CEs, WEs and TGs, appear to be the main lipid constituents in SGs of shih tzu dogs. These findings are comparable with the lipid composition in human sebum.[1,12,13] In this study, we could not demonstrate the presence of squalene in canine sebum, even though squalene has been reported as a lipid constituent of human sebum.[12,13]

Our study also revealed that the profiles of SG lipids and SC CERs were altered in seborrhoeic shih tzu dogs. The relative amounts of WEs and TGs in the total skin surface lipids were increased, while that of total CERs appeared to be decreased in shih tzu dogs with seborrhoea. However, the quantities of total SC CERs per milligram of SC in shih

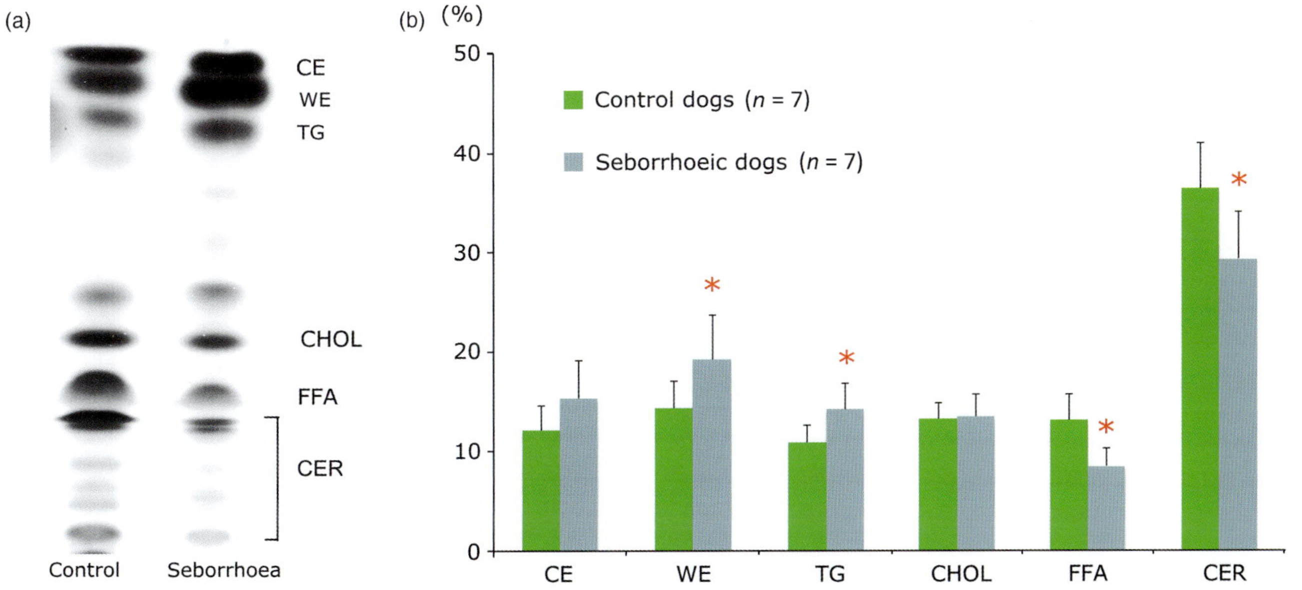

Figure 3. Skin surface lipid profile (acetone-extracted fractions) in shih tzu dogs with seborrhoea and control dogs. (a) Representative data of HPTLC analysis of lipids in the skin surface in control dogs and in dogs with seborrhoea. Abbreviations: CE, cholesterol esters; CER, ceramides; CHOL, cholesterol; FFA, free fatty acids; TG, triglycerides; and WE, wax esters. (b) Relative amounts of skin surface lipids in control animals ($n = 7$) and shih tzu dogs with seborrhoea ($n = 7$). Note that the relative amounts of WEs and TGs are significantly increased, whereas those of FFAs and total CERs are significantly decreased, in dogs with seborrhoea compared with those in the control dogs (*$P < 0.05$, Student's unpaired t-test).

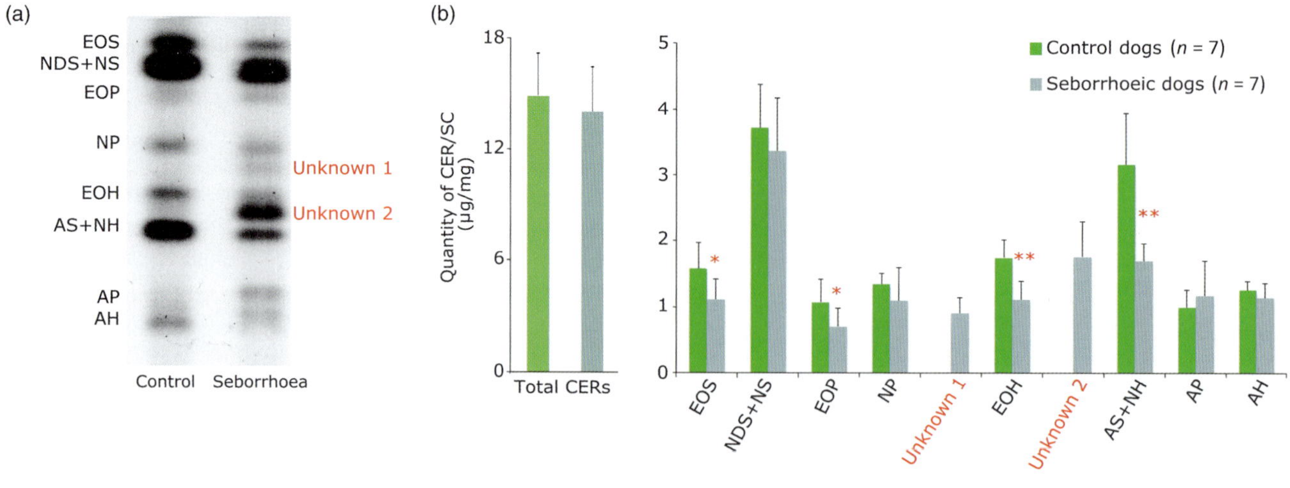

Figure 4. Skin surface ceramide (CER) profiles in shih tzu dogs with seborrhoea and control dogs. (a) Representative data of HPTLC analysis of free extractable CER fractions in shih tzu dogs with seborrhoea and control dogs. Two aberrant fractions (unknown 1 and unknown 2) are recognized exclusively in dogs with seborrhoea. (b) Comparison of quantities of total CERs and CER fractions in control dogs and seborrhoeic dogs. Quantities of total CERs are not significantly different between the two groups. Quantities of CER[EOS], CER[EOP], CER[EOH] and a mixture of CER[AS] and CER[NH] were significantly lower in dogs with seborrhoea than those in control dogs ($*P < 0.05$, $**P < 0.01$, Student's unpaired *t*-test). Two unknown fractions are recognized exclusively in seborrhoeic dogs. Abbreviations: CER[EOS], combination of ω-hydroxy fatty acids and sphingosines; CER[EOP], combination of ω-hydroxy fatty acids and phytosphingosines; CER[EOH], combination of ω-hydroxy fatty acids and 6-hydroxylsphingosines; CER[AS], combination of α-hydroxy fatty acids and sphingosines; CER[NH], combination of nonhydroxy fatty acids and 6-hydroxyl sphingosines.

tzu dogs with seborrhoea were comparable to those in control dogs. These findings imply that secretion of SG contents increased in the skin surface of shih tzu dogs with seborrhoea, while the quantity of total SC CERs was not altered. Our findings also indicate that quantities of some CER classes, including CER[EOS], CER[EOP], CER[EOH] and a mixture of CER[AS] and CER[NH], were significantly lower in shih tzu dogs with seborrhoea than normal dogs. The ceramides CER[EOS], CER[EOP] and CER[EOH] are known as esterified ω-hydroxy CERs, which are formed by an amide bond of linoleic acid with ω-hydroxy fatty acids.[14,15] As the esterified ω-hydroxy CERs are thought to be essential for formation of multilamellar structures in the extracellular spaces of the SC,[16–18] it is conceivable that the structure and continuity of the extracellular lamellar structure is altered in shih tzu dogs with seborrhoea. It is also possible that these changes may be the cause of aberrant barrier function of the SC, which leads to secondary bacterial infections in seborrhoeic dogs. Future studies using electron microscopy will help to elucidate ultrastructural changes in the extracellular lipid lamellae in seborrhoeic dogs.

Our study also identified two unknown CER fractions, whose polarities were not equivalent to those of any CER fraction in healthy dogs. The polarities of the two unknown CER fractions were also not comparable to those of CER fractions in dogs with atopic dermatitis previously reported,[9] indicating that these two unknown fractions are characteristic of seborrhoea not shared with atopic dermatitis. In addition, NPLC-ESI-MS analysis in this study revealed that some CER classes in seborrhoeic SC contained subspecies with short carbon chains, which did not appear in control SC samples. Ceramides with different carbon chains might have different polarity and can be fractionated as aberrant bands by HPTLC.[19] The exact CER classes fractionated as unknown bands are unconfirmed in the present study. However, comparison of the results of HPTLC with those of NPLC-ESI-MS leads one to speculate that unknown fraction 2 may be CER[AS] with short carbon chains. We recently found that the two

Table 2. Total number of carbons and degree of unsaturation (number of double bonds) of ceramide classes detected in the stratum corneum of shih tzu dogs

Ceramide classe	Control	Seborrhoea
CER[NDS]	41, 42, 44, 47, 48, 52	36, 38, 40, 41, 42, 44
CER[NS]	40, 41, 42, 43, 44 45, 46, 47, 48, 49, 50, 51, 55	33, 34, 35, 36, 37, 38, 39, 40, 41, 42, 43, 44, 45, 46, 47, 48, 50, 55
CER[NP]	32, 33, 34, 35, 36, 38, 40, 42, 43, 44, 45, 46	34, 36, 37, 38, 39, 40, 41, 42, 43, 44, 45, 46
CER[ADS]	32, 33, 34, 35, 36, 38, 40	32, 33, 34, 38
CER[AS]	38, 39, 41, 42	33, 34, 35, 36, 37, 38, 39, 40, 41, 42, 43, 44, 45, 46, 47, 48
CER[NH]	36, 38, 39, 40, 41, 42, 43, 44, 45, 46, 47, 48, 49, 50	31, 32, 34, 36, 37, 38, 39, 40, 41, 42, 43, 44, 45, 46, 48, 50
CER[AP]	41, 42, 43, 45, 47	33, 34, 36, 38, 40, 42, 44, 47
CER[AH]	41, 42, 43, 44, 45, 46, 48, 49	42, 44, 46, 48
CER[EOS]	64:2, 66:2, 68:2	64:2, 66:2, 68:2
CER[EOP]	66:2	66:2
CER[EOH]	68:2,70:2	68:2,70:2

Abbreviations: CER, ceramide; CER[ADS], combination of α-hydroxy fatty acids and dihydrosphingosines; CER[AH], combination of α-hydroxy fatty acids and 6-hydroxyl sphingosines; CER[AP], combination of α-hydroxy fatty acids and phytosphingosines; CER[AS], combination of α-hydroxy fatty acids and sphingosines; CER[EOH], combination of ω-hydroxy fatty acids and 6-hydroxylsphingosines; CER[EOP], combination of ω-hydroxy fatty acids and phytosphingosines; CER[EOS], combination of ω-hydroxy fatty acids and sphingosines; CER[NDS], combination of nonhydroxy fatty acids and dihydrosphingosines; CER[NH], combination of nonhydroxy fatty acids and 6-hydroxyl sphingosines; CER[NP], combination of nonhydroxy fatty acids and phytosphingosines; and CER[NS], combination of nonhydroxy fatty acids and sphingosines.

unknown CER fractions with identical polarities were also synthesized in cultured canine keratinocytes, in which the SC was not formed (J. S. Yoon, unpublished observations 2012). It is generally known that parakeratosis, in which keratinocytes are improperly cornified and contain nuclei in their cytoplasm, is commonly recognized in seborrhoea.[4] Although histopathological analysis was performed only in two seborrhoeic dogs in the present study, these findings imply that unknown CER fractions might be associated with incomplete keratinization of the epidermal keratinocytes in dogs with seborrhoea.

In conclusion, our findings indicate that the greasy and scaly skin condition in shih tzu dogs with seborrhoea appears to be associated with an alteration of the lipid profile of SGs and the SC. In addition, it is suggested that the alteration of the SC CER profile might affect the composition of the extracellular lipid lamellae and lipid envelope in seborrhoeic shih tzu dogs. Future studies are needed to investigate the effect of changes in the CER profile to cutaneous barrier function in seborrhoeic dogs.

Acknowledgements

The authors are grateful to Yukiguni Agri Co. for carrying out the chromatography and spectrophotometry analysis (NPLC-ESI-MS).

References

1. Pappas A. Epidermal surface lipids. *Dermatoendocrinol* 2009; 1: 72–76.
2. Holleran WM, Takagi Y, Uchida Y. Epidermal sphingolipids: metabolism, function, and roles in skin disorders. *FEBS Lett* 2006; 580: 5456–5466.
3. Proksch E, Fölster-Holst R, Jensen JM. Skin barrier function, epidermal proliferation and differentiation in eczema. *J Dermatol Sci* 2006; 43: 159–169.
4. Scott DW, Miller WH, Griffin CE. Keratinization defects. In: *Muller and Kirk's Small Animal Dermatology*. 6th edition. Philadelphia, PA: Saunders Co., 2000; 1030–1036.
5. Kwochka KW, Rademakers AM. Cell proliferation kinetics of epidermis, hair follicles, and sebaceous glands of cocker spaniels with idiopathic seborrhea. *Am J Vet Res* 1989; 50: 1918–1922.
6. Mauldin EA, Scott DW, Miller WH *et al. Malassezia* dermatitis in the dog: a retrospective histopathological and immunopathological study of 86 cases (1990–95). *Vet Dermatol* 1997; 8: 191–202.
7. Bligh EG, Dyer WJ. A rapid method of total lipid extraction and purification. *Can J Biochem Physiol* 1959; 37: 911–917.
8. Uchida Y, Hara M, Nishio H *et al.* Epidermal sphingomyelins are precursors for selected stratum corneum ceramides. *J Lipid Res* 2000; 41: 2071–2082.
9. Yoon JS, Nishifuji K, Sasaki A *et al.* Alteration of stratum corneum ceramide profiles in spontaneous canine model of atopic dermatitis. *Exp Dermatol* 2011; 20: 732–736.
10. Shimada K, Yoshihara T, Yamamoto M *et al.* Transepidermal water loss reflects skin barrier function of dog. *J Vet Med Sci* 2008; 70: 841–843.
11. De Luca C, Valacchi G. Surface lipids as multifunctional mediators of skin responses to environmental stimuli. *Mediators Inflamm* 2010; 2010: 321–494.
12. Rissmann R, Groenink HW, Weerheim AM *et al.* New insights into ultrastructure, lipid composition and organization of vernix caseosa. *J Invest Dermatol* 2006; 126: 1823–1833.
13. Nikkari T. Comparative chemistry of sebum. *J Invest Dermatol* 1974; 62: 257–267.
14. Masukawa Y, Narita H, Shimizu E *et al.* Characterization of overall ceramide species in human stratum corneum. *J Lipid Res* 2008; 49: 1466–1476.
15. Sandhoff R. Very long chain sphingolipids: tissue expression, function and synthesis. *FEBS Lett* 2010; 584: 1907–1913.
16. Bouwstra JA, Gooris GS, Dubbelaar FE *et al.* Role of ceramide 1 in the molecular organization of the stratum corneum lipids. *J Lipid Res* 1998; 39: 186–196.
17. Kessner D, Brezesinski G, Funari SS *et al.* Impact of the long chain ω-acylceramides on the stratum corneum lipid nanostructure. Part 1: thermotropic phase behaviour of CER[EOS] and CER[EOP] studied using X-ray powder diffraction and FT-Raman spectroscopy. *Chem Phys Lipids* 2010; 163: 42–50.
18. Li W, Sandhoff R, Kono M *et al.* Depletion of ceramides with very long chain fatty acids causes defective skin permeability barrier function, and neonatal lethality in ELOVL4 deficient mice. *Int J Biol Sci* 2007; 3: 120–128.
19. Ponec M, Weerheim A, Lankhorst P *et al.* New acylceramide in native and reconstructed epidermis. *J Invest Dermatol* 2003; 120: 581–588.

Part 4

Therapy

To cite this article, please use DOI: 10.1111/vde.12000

4.1

Stem cell therapy in veterinary dermatology

Robert J. Harman

Vet-Stem, Inc., 12860 Danielson Court, Poway, CA 82064, USA

Correspondence: Robert J. Harman, Vet-Stem, Inc., 12860 Danielson Court, Poway, CA 82064, USA. E-mail: bharman@vet-stem.com

Background – Adult stem cells come from many sources and have the capacity to differentiate into many cell types, including those of the skin. The most commonly studied stem cells are those termed mesenchymal stem cells (MSCs), which are easily isolated from bone marrow and adipose tissue. Mesenchymal stem cells are known to produce a wide array of cytokines that modulate the regeneration process. The ease of collection, propagation and use of these MSCs in therapy of traumatic, ischaemic and immune-mediated skin conditions is emerging.

Approach and evidence – In traumatic and ischaemic skin damage, MSCs are used in tissue-engineered skin and by direct injection into damaged tissue. For immune-mediated diseases, systemic administration of stem cells can modulate the immune system. The earliest clinical work has been with autologous stem cell sources, such as adipose tissue and bone marrow. In immune-mediated diseases, the MSCs are used to downregulate production of inflammatory cytokines and to block T-cell activation. Cells are generally given intravenously. Multiple sclerosis, rheumatoid arthritis and lupus have been successfully treated in human clinical trials. Mesenchymal stem cells can also stimulate resident local cells, such as keratinocytes and progenitor cells, to proliferate, migrate and repair skin injury and disease.

Looking ahead – The discovery of the MSC in adipose tissue has spawned a global effort to utilize these cells in therapy of a wide range of diseases of the skin. Reconstructive surgery, scar blocking and resolution and skin regeneration have all been shown to be possible in human and animal studies.

Introduction

Stem cell therapy is not a new discipline. The first stem cell transplants were performed in the 1950s using bone marrow to reconstitute the marrow of chemotherapy patients.[1] These stem cells were primarily haematopoietic and were used to replace the damaged or dead marrow stem cells so that the patient could replenish the white and red cell lineages. In the 1980s, a new subpopulation of marrow cells was discovered and named the mesenchymal stem cells (MSCs), in the belief that this cell type was from the mesenchyme and could be induced to differentiate into a mesenchymal tissue cell type, such as bone or cartilage.[2] In the ensuing decades, stem/progenitor cells have been identified in nearly every tissue of the body. In 1998, James Thompson at the University of Wisconsin was the first researcher to isolate and propagate human embryonic stem cells (ESCs) and ushered in the era of 'stem cell medicine'. Although thought to be the most pleuripotent stem cell, the ESC has not yet proved to be a clinically useful cell type, owing to major risks of tumourigenesis and immune rejection.[3] On the contrary, the adult MSC has been shown to be nontumourigenic and nonimmunogenic. The clinical interest in MSCs has focused on their ability to modulate the immune system, to stimulate tissue regeneration and to differentiate into all three germ layer lineages. *In vitro* models, preclinical animal models and early clinical translation provide evidence that stem cells can prove to be safe and efficacious in the therapy of dermatological conditions in human and veterinary medicine. This review chronicles the progression of basic and clinical research in support of the clinical use of the MSC.

Accepted 19 July 2012

Sources of Funding: This study was self-funded.

Conflict of Interest: The author is an employee and shareholder of Vet-Stem, Inc., which is in the commercial business of veterinary stem cell therapy.

Sources and types of stem cells

What are stem cells? In traditional textbooks, it was taught that stem cells were the origin of all major tissue types and that once cells became partly or totally differentiated into a cell type they were now terminal cells and could not dedifferentiate. It is now known that cells are very 'plastic' and can transform more than originally thought.[4] As usual, the situation is much more intricate and complicated than the initial studies indicated. Table 1 summarizes the characteristics of several classes of stem cells. There are two major types of stem cells, the ESCs and adult stem cells (ASCs). Embryonic stem cells come from the inner cell mass of an early embryo. Once removed, they can be grown *in vitro* and are generally immortal in cell culture. They can be induced *in vitro* to form a very large number of cell/tissue types; however, their nature is to form a whole organism. In research, they are already a very powerful tool in the discovery of mechanisms of healing, disease pathogenesis and organ formation. However, to the clinician, they still have two very critical flaws that block their use in the clinic, as

Table 1. A summary of stem cell types and general characteristics

Characteristics	Adult stem cell*	Embryonic stem cell	Induced pluripotent stem cell
Sources	Fat, bone marrow, cord blood or other tissues	Inner cell mass of an early embryo	Adult stem cell genetically modified to act like embryonic stem cell
Form teratomas	No	Yes	Yes
Rejected as foreign tissue	No	Yes	Yes
Self-renewal	Yes	Yes	Yes
Differentiation capacity	Yes	Yes	Yes
Immortal cell lines	No	Yes	Yes

*A specific type of adult stem cell, the mesenchymal stem cell, is found in mesenchymal tissues, such as bone marrow and adipose tissue.

follows: (i) they form teratomas when implanted into a patient; and (ii) they are a foreign genotype and can potentially be rejected by the recipient's immune system.[3] In addition, there is a major controversy about the use of embryos to harvest these cells.

Adult stem cells are different from ESCs. They are found in almost every tissue of every human and animal and are used by the body to make repairs in everyday life. Some of these stem cells, particularly MSCs, have the ability to produce large amounts of growth factors and can differentiate into many body tissues. They do not form teratomas when injected into patients unless they have been damaged in the laboratory and, if they are from the same patient (autologous), they will not be rejected as foreign. Neonatal stem cells from the placenta, umbilical cord, amnion, etc. are generally considered to be ASCs, because they behave in the manner described above. Induced pleuripotent stem cells are adult cells that have been genetically reprogrammed to revert to a more undifferentiated state. Like ESCs, they can form teratomas and they have also recently been reported to be immunogenic, even if the source of adult cells is from the same patient.[5]

What are the sources of adult stem cells? They are found in nearly every tissue, including bone marrow, fat, skin, nerve tissue, muscle and many others. If the source is from a different species than the recipient (e.g. pig valves for people) they are called xenogeneic. If they are from the same species but a different individual (e.g. kidney for transplant) they are called allogeneic. If the donor is the recipient then they are termed autologous. The only tissue with adequate concentrations of ASCs for direct (uncultured) use is the adipose depot. All other sources need to be expanded *ex vivo* in order to have a therapeutic dosage available to treat a patient.

An interesting canine stem cell source was recently identified in the hair follicle bulge.[6] Human bulge stem cells have been previously identified, but this is the first verification that there are canine bulge stem cells that share many characteristics with the human bulge cells. This bulge region is found as a subtle swelling of the outer root sheath in both the canine and human hair follicle, near the insertion point of the arrector pili muscle.[6] The stem cells were found using labelling techniques at this site during anagen phase, but also in the secondary germ at the bottom of the follicle during telogen, leading to the hypothesis that these are the cells responsible for regeneration of the dermal component of hair follicles during cycling.[6] Further discussion of the canine bulge stem cell will be covered in the section on alopecia below.

Identification and characterization of the mesenchymal stem cell

Although there is no single 'marker' or identifying characteristic that clearly identifies the MSC, there are a combination of characteristics that are generally accepted to be representative of this cell type. The International Society of Cell Therapy has published their guidelines on the characterization of the MSC.[7] The proposed primary characteristics are as follows: (i) the MSC must be plastic adherent when maintained in standard culture conditions; (ii) the MSC must express cell surface markers CD105, CD73 and CD90; lack expression of CD45, CD34, CD14 or CD11b, CD79a or CD19, and HLA-DR surface molecules; and (iii) the MSC must be capable of differentiating into osteoblasts, adipocytes and chondroblasts *in vitro*. Although stem cell scientists continue to develop more stringent criteria, these basic criteria are generally accepted as the baseline for declaring a cell type as a MSC.

Figure 1 demonstrates the third primary characteristic of the MSC, namely differentiation. These four photomicrographs show adipogenic, chondrogenic, neurogenic and osteogenic differentiation of adipose-derived stem cells (ADSCs).[8]

Additionally, researchers use gene arrays to evaluate whether the cell type in question is able to express the genes thought to be related to the abilities of stem cells. Common genes expressed in progenitor cells include nerve growth factor receptor, basic fibroblast growth factor 2, frizzled homolog 9 and activated leukocyte cell adhesion molecule. In a recent publication, the authors used these genes in a dolphin skin regeneration clinical study to verify that the cells of interest expressed these genes.[8] The International Society of Cell Therapy has not adopted any gene array criteria for MSCs at this time.

Mechanisms of action of the mesenchymal stem cell

In contrast to drug or growth factor therapy, stem cell therapy does not rely upon a single target receptor or a single pathway for its action. In stem cell therapy, the ASCs are delivered either directly to the area of trauma or disease (e.g. wounds, tendonitis or osteoarthritis) or are

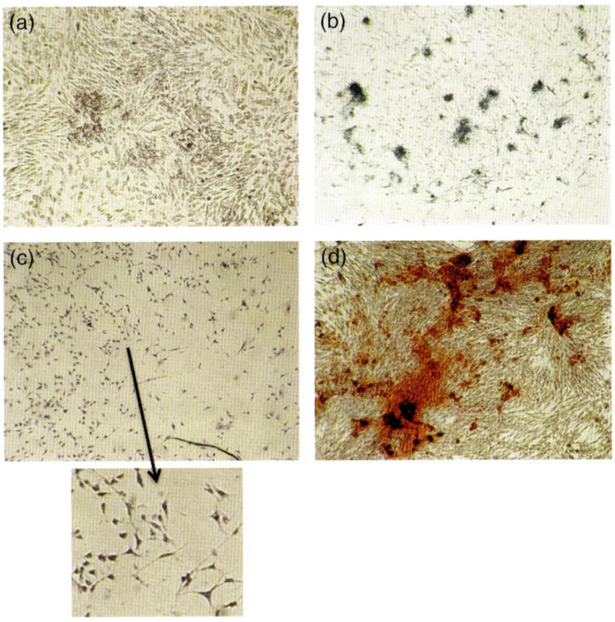

Figure 1. Photomicrographs of positive differentiation assays for the following adipose-derived stem cells: adipogenic (a); chondrogenic (b); neurogenic (c); and osteogenic (d). The inset photomicrograph below (c) is a higher magnification view of the neurogenic differentiation slide showing the typical neuronal phenotype. This study used standardized induction media known to induce each specific phenotype, and immunostaining was not employed (reprinted with permission from Stem Cells and Development (Vol 21(16)), published by Mary Ann Liebert, Inc., New Rochelle, NY).[8]

delivered systemically (e.g. liver disease, renal disease or immune-mediated disease). Both delivery methods take advantage of the ability of stem cells to differentiate into many tissue types and their ability to 'communicate' with the cells of their local environment through paracrine modalities to create the optimal environment for natural healing.[4]

While therapeutically successful, the detailed molecular mechanisms of stem cell-related healing are complex and remain under investigation. Repair occurs through a complex variety of demonstrated stem cell functions, including the following: (i) trophic support;[4,9,10] (ii) -anti-inflammatory and immunomodulatory functions;[11,12] (iii) revascularization;[13] (iv) anti-apoptotic activity;[13] (v) differentiating capacity;[14] and (vi) homing.[15] Although the mechanisms remain under investigation, clinical efficacy is documented in preclinical human and animal trials.[16] The public have long used aspirin to decrease fever and control pain, beginning in the late 1800s, but the mechanisms of action were not discovered until 1971 when British pharmacologist John Robert Vane discovered the suppression of prostaglandins and received the Nobel Prize in 1981.[17]

Stem cell therapy delivers a population of cells able to communicate with other cells in their local environment. Until recently, differentiation was thought to be the primary function of stem cells. However, the functions of regenerative cells are now known to be much more diverse, including immune modulation[18] and secretion of cell signalling factors and cytokines that influence both local and remote cell populations.[4] These cellular functions are implicated in a highly integrated and complex network. Cellular therapy should be viewed as a complex, yet balanced, approach to a therapeutic goal where the cells take their signals from the microenvironment of the injured tissue. Unlike traditional medicine, in which one drug targets one or a few receptors, a single stem cell therapy can be applied in a wide variety of injuries and diseases.

Trophic support

Multiple studies demonstrate that ASCs secrete bioactive levels of cytokines and growth factors that support angiogenesis, tissue remodelling, differentiation and anti-apoptotic events.[10,13] Adipose and bone marrow stem cells secrete a number of angiogenesis-related cytokines, such as vascular endothelial growth factor, hepatocyte growth factor, basic fibroblast growth factor, granulocyte–macrophage colony-stimulating factor and transforming growth factor-β.[10,13]

Anti-inflammatory/immunomodulatory functions

In general, *in vitro* studies demonstrate that bone marrow stem cells (BMSCs) and ADSCs limit inflammatory responses and promote anti-inflammatory pathways. When present in an inflammatory environment, BMSCs may alter the cytokine secretion profile of dendritic cell subsets and T-cell subsets, causing a shift from a pro-inflammatory environment to an anti-inflammatory or tolerant environment.[12] Bone marrow stem cells and ADSCs do not express MHC class II antigens or costimulatory molecules and they suppress T-cell proliferation.[19] Adult stem cells suppress mixed lymphocyte reactions and inhibit T-cell proliferation induced by a third cell type or by mitogenic factors.[20] Both types of stem cells are able to control lethal graft-versus-host disease that occurs in mice after haploidentical haematopoietic transplantation.[18,20]

Revascularization

The stromal vascular fraction extracted from adipose tissue contains ADSCs and endothelial progenitor cells that promote angiogenesis and neovascularization by the secretion of cytokines, such as hepatocyte growth factor, vascular endothelial growth factor, placental growth factor, transforming growth factor, fibroblast growth factor and angiopoietin.[21] In an *in vivo* model of hindlimb ischaemia, intravenous injection of ADSCs was associated with an increase in blood flow and vascular density and incorporation of the cells in the leg vasculature.[22]

Anti-apoptosis

Apoptosis is defined as a programmed cell death or 'cell suicide', an event that is genetically controlled. In normal conditions, apoptosis determines the lifespan and coordinated removal of cells. When acutely injured tissue is denied critical blood flow, ischaemia will result. Adipose-derived stem cells significantly reduced endothelial cell apoptosis during ischaemic events in animal studies.[13] Rehman *et al.*[13] demonstrated that ADSCs express factors that support cell survival and avoid apoptosis.

Differentiating capacity

Studies using stem cells from a variety of sources demonstrate a diverse plasticity, including differentiation into adipogenic, osteogenic, chondrogenic, myogenic, cardiomyogenic, endothelial, hepatogenic, neurogenic, epithelial and haematopoietic lineages.[4] These data are supported by *in vivo* experiments and functional studies that demonstrated the regenerative capacity of stem cells to repair damaged or diseased tissue via transplant engraftment and differentiation.[23] Nixon *et al.*[24] demonstrated statistically significant improvement in histological repair of a collagenase-induced injury in the superficial digital flexor tendon in horses treated with autologous regenerative cells harvested from fat.

Homing

Homing (chemotaxis) is an event by which a cell migrates from one area of the body to a distant site, where it may be needed for a given physiological event. Homing is an important function of adult stem cells and one mechanism by which intravenous or parenteral administration of MSCs permits a therapeutic cell to target a specific diseased area effectively. A cerebral arterial occlusion model of stroke demonstrated that labelled BMSCs administered intravenously 24 h and 7 days postinjury migrated to the area of injury, dramatically reducing the stroke infarct size.[25] Mesenchymal stem cells homed to the lung in response to injury and reduced inflammation and collagen deposition in a mouse model of pulmonary fibrosis.[26]

The mechanism of how stem cells home to injured tissues and migrate across endothelium is not fully understood. It is likely that injured tissues express specific receptors for chemokines and ligands to facilitate trafficking, adhesion and infiltration of stem cells, as is the case with recruitment of leukocytes to sites of inflammation. Chemokines and adhesion molecules play a significant role in the trafficking of leukocytes, and BMSCs have been shown to express some of these molecules.[15]

Engineered skin

The discipline of tissue engineering attempts to use scaffolding and cells to create a tissue construct, grown *ex-vivo*. In the case of skin, the construct can be epidermis, dermis or some combination, to create a transplantable tissue. This engineered tissue can be used in place of autografts or noncellular scaffolding to repair damaged skin, such as in trauma, burns or ischaemic tissue. The largest barrier to the successful transplantation of engineered skin is vascularization. An epidermal graft must be nourished by the passive diffusion of nutrients from dermal capillaries. Early studies by Boyce[27] demonstrated that engineered grafts required 10–15 days before dermal capillaries could effectively form. This length of time is not compatible with graft survival. Adipose-derived stem cells co-cultured with human fibroblasts can create a vascularized skin construct.[28] This type of construct shows the use of the revascularization capability of stem cells in a combination engineered graft.

Although there are no commercially available canine, equine or feline tissue-engineered products, the human market gives evidence that such grafts are possible, practical and commercially successful (Dermagraft; Advanced Biohealing, Westport, CT, USA, recently purchased by Shire Pharmaceuticals). Dermagraft provides neonatal tissue-derived fibroblasts cultured on a degradable matrix.

Mesenchymal stem cell therapy of chronic nonhealing wounds

Healing of wounds requires the coordination of cell migration, cellular proliferation and differentiation and the assembly of scaffolding (extracellular matrix). Additionally, angiogenesis is required to create the vascular supply route. Typically, a granulation bed forms, and re-epithelialization occurs. In chronic wounds, a dysregulation occurs, resulting in a wound that does not heal by the normal course. As described in the preceding subsections, stem cells have the ability to home to areas of inflammation, interact with the local microenvironment, attract other progenitor cells, differentiate into various tissues types and produce a wide variety of cytokines and growth factors that could influence healing in a chronic wound. Human ADSCs can influence the migration and proliferation of human dermal fibroblasts and, in rodent models, can reduce the time for wound closure.[29]

A number of rodent models have shown that MSCs applied intravenously,[30] topically[31] and subcutaneously[32] can improve wound healing. Human clinical studies have demonstrated the healing of chronic fistulas in patients with Crohn's disease, both by local delivery and by the intravenous route.[33] Reports on the clinical application of BMSCs in human wound therapies have demonstrated that grafted MSCs facilitate skin regeneration, both in acute and in chronic wounds.[34–36] Falanga *et al.*[35] used autologous bone marrow MSCs delivered in a fibrin spray to accelerate healing in human cutaneous wounds.

In a recent study, standardized skin wounds in the dolphin (*Turchiops truncates*) were treated with cultured ADSCs in a blinded, placebo-controlled clinical study.[8] Wound tissue biopsy samples were evaluated by a blinded, independent histopathologist, with analysis of cell proliferation (number of mitoses) and healing rate on days 1, 5 and 15 after treatment. Wounds in dolphins treated with autologous ADSCs showed improved healing compared with the saline placebo-treated dolphins (Figure 2).[8]

Mesenchymal stem cell therapy of immune-mediated skin diseases

MSC populations have the ability to modulate the immune system as described in the mechanisms of action section above. In particular, they have the ability to suppress T-cell alloreactivity. In patients with transplant rejection graft-versus-host disease, MSCs have shown the ability to suppress the activated T cells and to prevent activation of the T cells. This phenomenon has been used to prolong skin graft survival[37] and in the treatment of severe graft-versus-host disease.[38]

Atopic dermatitis is a complicated disease. Atopy is defined as the heritable predisposition of the production of IgE to otherwise ordinary environmental substances, such as pollens, moulds and house dust mites.[39] There is

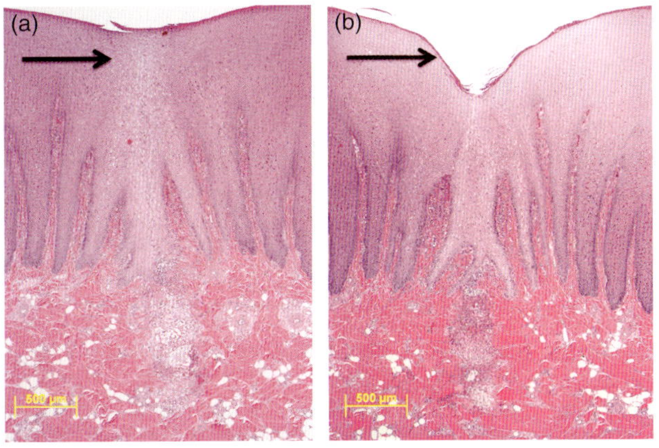

Figure 2. Dolphin skin wound biopsy samples obtained on day 15 after intralesional treatment with adipose-derived cultured autologous stem cells (a) and phosphate-buffered saline (b). There was improved healing in the stem cell-treated group. The arrows show the site of the original wound and illustrate the superior filling in the treated versus control lesion. Images courtesy of Vet-Stem, Inc., Poway, CA, USA.

evidence to support transcutaneous presentation of allergen both to initiate and to perpetuate atopic inflammation and pruritus.[40] When present in an inflammatory environment, data demonstrate that MSCs may alter the cytokine secretion profile of dendritic cell subsets and T-cell subsets, causing a shift from a pro-inflammatory environment to an anti-inflammatory or tolerant environment.[12] Mesenchymal stem cells do not express MHC class II antigens or costimulatory molecules and they suppress T-cell proliferation.[20] Adipose-derived stem cells suppress mixed lymphocyte reactions and inhibit T-cell proliferation induced by a third cell type or by mitogenic factors.[20] Additionally, BMSCs and ADSCs suppress T-cell activation.[41]

Most recently, Riordan *et al.*[42] reported on ADSC therapy of multiple sclerosis patients and reviewed the literature on the cells from the vascular stromal fraction and their function in modulation of inflammation and autoimmunity. Kang *et al.*[43] replicated much of this proof of immunomodulation of the stem cell using canine ADSCs, showing that the dog has a similar MSC to other reported species. Taken together, these data support the idea that ASCs could provide the immunoregulation necessary to control atopic dermatitis in dogs. The only published data on canine stem cell therapy are from a small pilot study using a small adipose biopsy and cell culture.[44] This study used autologous stem cells and the intravenous route, with no statistical improvement in clinical signs of atopic dermatitis. On the contrary, Liang *et al.*,[45] in a human clinical study, showed improvement in the cutaneous clinical redundant signs of refractory lupus when treated with allogeneic MSCs.

Mesenchymal stem cell therapy of scar tissue

The MSC has been shown to produce hepatocyte growth factor, a basic fibroblast growth factor that can inhibit scar tissue formation.[46] In human plastic surgery, it is reported that ADSCs, or even the stromal vascular fraction processed from lipoaspirate, have the ability to block or remodel scar tissue when used alone or in conjunction with a fat graft.[47] In models of liver disease in rodents, MSC infusion can modulate metalloproteinase activity and reduce deposition of collagen, reducing the fibrosis seen with histopathology.[48] Lung fibrosis can also be blocked by MSC infusion in the bleomycin model of pulmonary fibrosis and the mechanisms appear to include blockade of interleukin-1 and tumour necrosis factor-α.[26]

Mesenchymal stem cell therapy in alopecia

There is a cyclical regeneration of hair follicles during the life of an animal that is believed to be modulated by stem cells.[49] Kobayashi *et al.*[6] reported the similarity of the canine and human bulge cells and was able to show multipotency of these cells in the reconstitution of pilosebaceous glands. Immunohistochemistry of the bulge region in canine skin samples demonstrated a population of CD34 glycoprotein-positive cells.[50] This marker is most commonly found on the surface of haematopoietic stem cells. The best approach for therapy of alopecia has been debated. Options include using cytokines to stimulate these resident multipotent cells, injection of cultured bulge cells and injection of a MSC preparation that might stimulate activity of these resident progenitors.

The large size of the market for therapy for human male pattern baldness has spawned a number of biotechnology companies that are employing these various approaches to treatment. Dermal papilla cells are thought to be a major regulator of the keratinocytes and hair growth.[51] At least one company (Intercytex, Manchester, UK) has entered human clinical testing with autologous cultured dermal papilla cells and fibroblasts, based upon preclinical data showing that this approach can stimulate new hair growth. Replicel Life Science (Vancouver, BC, Canada) has taken a similar approach but uses autologous dermal sheath cup cells and has also entered human clinical testing. Bone marrow stem cells and umbilical cord stem cells have been employed *in vitro* and in an athymic nude mouse model to create dermal papilla-like structures and hair follicles.[52] The general concepts of paracrine anti-inflammatory and mitotic effects of ASCs already discussed could be employed in strategies to heal and stimulate the damaged bulge and related cells in patients with alopecia. Furthermore, autoimmune damage to the hair follicle region might be treated using the ability of stem cells to reduce T-cell activation and cause activated T cells to become apoptotic.[20,43]

Bulge stem cell markers in oncology

In a letter to the editor of *Veterinary Dermatology*, Grandi *et al.* [53] noted that use of immunohistochemical markers found on bulge stem cells might help to elucidate the histogenesis of certain tumours. In particular, ceratokeratin (CK15), CD34 and nestin have been reported in the veterinary literature.[6,50,54,55] An example of a study of human tumours found CD15-positive cells in trichoepitheliomas and certain basal cell carcinomas, while squamous cell carcinomas were negative.[56] Further investigation of these markers and others markers found on bulge stem cells needs to be performed on veterinary tumours. In contrast to the suggestive literature on bulge stem cells above, the MSC literature has not reported tumour formation in association with MSC clinical therapy.[57]

US Food and Drug Administration (FDA) regulation of stem cell therapy in veterinary medicine

In the USA, the FDA Centre for Veterinary Medicine regulates all veterinary drugs. Stem cell products are considered to be drugs and are regulated as such by the FDA.[58] Service businesses are being allowed to operate under regulatory discretion at the present time, but any products, such as allogeneic cells, must be approved under the New Animal Drug Approval (NADA process) according to Lynne Oliver of the FDA, Centre for Veterinary Medicine.[59]

Future perspectives of stem cell therapy in veterinary dermatology

It is clear from the substantial amount of research, both past and ongoing, that there will be translation of basic research into clinical protocols in the coming years. Current clinical practices in human dermatology will be likely to find their way into veterinary medicine, as have many other clinical practices. The prospect of MSC use in therapy of veterinary dermatological conditions is promising and we await appropriate clinical studies to provide guidance for clinical use. The veterinary species will continue to provide sound data that can be used to further the approval process for translation into the human clinics. 'One Medicine' is truly a partnership between human and veterinary medicine, with the goal of improvement of the health of human and veterinary patients.

References

1. Thomas ED, Lochte LH Jr, Lu WC *et al.* Intravenous infusion of bone marrow in patients receiving radiation and chemotherapy. *New Engl J Med* 1957; 157: 491–496.
2. Caplan A. Mesenchymal stem cells. *J Orthop Res* 1991; 9: 641–650.
3. Gruen L, Grabel L. Scientific and ethical roadblocks to human embryonic stem cell therapy. *Stem Cells* 2006; 24: 2162–2169.
4. Caplan A. Mesenchymal stem cells as trophic mediators. *J Cell Biochem* 2006; 98: 1076–1084.
5. Zhao T, Zhang Z, Rong Z *et al.* Immunogenecity of induced pluripotent stem cells. *Nature* 2011; 474: 212–215.
6. Kobayashi T, Iwasaki T, Amagai M *et al.* Canine follicle stem cell candidates reside in the bulge and share characteristic features with human bulge cells. *J Invest Dermatol* 2010; 130: 1988–1995.
7. Dominici M, Le Blanc K, Mueller I *et al.* Minimal criteria for defining multipotent mesenchymal stromal cells. The International Society for Cellular Therapy position statement. *Cytotherapy* 2006; 8: 315–317.
8. Johnson SP, Catania JM, Harman RJ, *et al.* Adipose-derived stem cell collection and characterization in bottlenose dophins (*Tursiops truncates*). *Stem Cells Dev* 2012; 21: 2949–2957.
9. Kras K, Hausman D, Martin R. Tumor necrosis factor-alpha stimulates cell proliferation in adipose tissue-derived stromal-vascular cell culture: promotion of adipose tissue expansion by paracrine growth factors. *Obes Res* 2000; 8: 186–193.
10. Kilroy G, Foster S, Wu X *et al.* Cytokine profile of human adipose-derived stem cells: expression of angiogenic, hematopoietic, and pro-inflammatory factors. *J Cell Physiol* 2007; 212: 702–709.
11. Togel F, Hu Z, Weiss K *et al.* Administered mesenchymal stem cells protect against ischemic acute renal failure through differentiation-independent mechanisms. *Am J Physiol Renal Physiol* 2005; 289: F31–F42.
12. Aggarwal S, Pittenger M. Human mesenchymal stem cells modulate allogeneic immune cell responses. *Blood* 2005; 105: 1815–1822.
13. Rehman J, Traktuev D, Li J *et al.* Secretion of angiogenic and antiapoptotic factors by human adipose stromal cells. *Circulation* 2004; 109: 1292–1298.
14. Kolf C, Cho E, Tuan R. Mesenchymal stromal cells. Biology of adult mesenchymal stem cells: regulation of niche, self-renewal and differentiation. *Arthritis Res Ther* 2007; 9: 204.
15. Francois S, Bensidhoum M, Mouiseddine M *et al.* Local irradiation not only induces homing of human mesenchymal stem cells at exposed sites but promotes their widespread engraftment to multiple organs: a study of their quantitative distribution after irradiation damage. *Stem Cells* 2006; 24: 1020–1029.
16. Black L, Gaynor J, Gahring D *et al.* Effect of adipose-derived mesenchymal stem and regenerative cells on lameness in dogs with chronic osteoarthritis of the coxofemoral joints: a randomized, double-blinded, multicenter controlled trial. *Vet Ther* 2007; 8: 272–284.
17. Jefferys D. *Aspirin: The Remarkable Story of a Wonder Drug.* New York: Bloomsbury Publishing USA, 2005.
18. Yañez R, Lamana M, García-Castro J *et al.* Adipose tissue-derived mesenchymal stem cells have *in vivo* immunosuppressive properties applicable for the control of the graft-versus-host disease. *Stem Cells* 2006; 24: 2582–2591.
19. McIntosh K, Zvonic S, Garrett S *et al.* The immunogenecity of human adipose-derived cells: temporal changes *in vitro*. *Stem Cells* 2006; 24: 1246–1253.
20. Parker A, Katz A. Adipose-derived stem cells for the regeneration of damaged tissues. *Expert Opin Biol Ther* 2006; 6: 567–578.
21. Nakagami H, Morishita R, Maeda K *et al.* Adipose tissue-derived stromal cells as a novel option for regenerative cell therapy. *J Atheroscler Thromb* 2006; 13: 77–81.
22. Miranville A, Heeschen C, Sengenes C *et al.* Improvement of postnatal neovascularization by human adipose tissue-derived stem cells. *Circulation* 2004; 110: 249–355.
23. Awad HA, Butler DL, Boivin GP *et al.* Autologous mesenchymal stem cell-mediated repair of tendon. *Tissue Eng* 1999; 5: 267–277.
24. Nixon A, Dahlgren L, Haupt L *et al.* Adipose-derived pluripotent stem cells for tendon repair. *Am J Vet Res* 2008; 69: 928–937.
25. Chen J, Li Y, Wang L. Therapeutic benefit of intravenous administration of bone marrow stromal cells after cerebral ischemia in rats. *Stroke* 2001; 32: 1005–1011.
26. Ortiz L, DeTreil M, Fattman C *et al.* Interleukin 1 receptor antagonist mediates the anti-inflammatory and antifibrotic effect of mesenchymal stem cells during lung injury. *Proc Natl Acad Sci USA* 2007; 104: 11002–11007.
27. Boyce S. Cultured skin substitutes: a review. *Tissue Eng* 1996; 2: 255–266.
28. Auxenfans C, Lequeux C, Perrusel E *et al.* Adipose-derived stem cells (ASCs) as a source of endothelial cells in the reconstruction of endothelialized skin equivalents. *J Tissue Eng Regen Med* 2012; 6: 512–518.
29. Kim W, Park B, Sung J. Wound healing effect of adipose-derived stem cells: a critical role of secretory factors on human dermal fibroblasts. *J Dermatol Sci* 2007; 48: 15–24.
30. Sasaki M, Abe R, Fujita Y. Mesenchymal stem cells are recruited into wounded skin and contribute to wound repair by transdifferentiation into multiple skin cell type. *J Immunol* 2008; 180: 2581–2587.
31. Javazon E, Keswani S, Badillo A *et al.* Enhanced epithelial gap closure and increased angiogenesis in wounds of diabetic mice

treated with adult murine bone marrow stromal progenitor cells. *Wound Repair Regen* 2007; 15: 350–359.

32. Chen L, Tredget E, Liu C *et al.* Analysis of allogenicity of mesenchymal stem cells in engraftment and wound healing in mice. *PLoS One* 2009; 4: e7119.
33. García-Olmo D, Herreros D, De-La-Quintana P *et al.* Adipose-derived stem cells in Crohn's rectovaginal fistula. *Case Report Med* 2010; 2010: 961758.
34. Badiavas E, Abedi M, Butmarc J *et al.* Participation of bone marrow derived cells in cutaneous wound healing. *J Cell Physiol* 2003; 196: 245–250.
35. Falanga V, Iwamoto S, Chartier M *et al.* Autologous bone marrow-derived cultured mesenchymal stem cells delivered in a fibrin spray accelerate healing in murine and human cutaneous wounds. *Tissue Eng* 2007; 13: 1299–1312.
36. Yoshikawa T, Mitsuno H, Nonaka I *et al.* Wound therapy by marrow mesenchymal cell transplantation. *Plast Reconstr Surg* 2008; 121: 860–877.
37. Bartholomew A, Sturgeon C, Siatskas M *et al.* Mesenchymal stem cells suppress lymphocyte proliferation *in vitro* and prolong skin graft survival *in vivo*. *Exp Hematol* 2002; 30: 42–48.
38. Le Blanc K, Rasmusson I, Sundberg B *et al.* Treatment of severe acute graft-versus-host disease with third party haploidentical mesenchymal stem cells. *Lancet* 2004; 363: 1439–1441.
39. Olivry T, DeBoer DJ, Favrot C *et al.* Treatment of canine atopic dermatitis: 2010 clinical practice guidelines form the International Task Force on Canine Atopic Dermatitis. *Vet Dermatol* 2010; 21:233–248.
40. Olivry T. The ACVD task force on canine atopic dermatitis (IX): the controversy surrounding the route of allergen challenge in canine atopic dermatitis. *Vet Immunol Immunopathol* 2001; 81: 219–225.
41. Rasmusson I. Immune modulation by mesenchymal stem cells. *Exp Cell Res* 2006; 312: 2169–2179.
42. Riordan N, Ichim T, Min W *et al.* Non-expanded adipose stromal vascular fraction cell therapy for multiple sclerosis. *J Transl Med* 2009; 7: 29.
43. Kang J, Kang K, Koo H *et al.* Soluble factors-mediated immunomodulatory effects of canine adipose tisssue-derived mesenchymal stem cells. *Stem Cells Dev* 2008; 17: 681–694.
44. Hall M, Rosencrantz W, Griffin C *et al.* Evaluation of the potential use of adipose-derived mesenchymal stromal cells in the treatment of canine atopic dermatitis: a pilot study. *Vet Ther* 2010; 11: E1–E4.
45. Liang J, Zhang H, Hua B *et al.* Allogeneic mesenchymal stem cells transplantation in refractory systemic lupus erythematosus: a pilot study. *Ann Rheum Dis* 2010; 69: 1423–1429.
46. Caplan A. The MSC: an injury drugstore. *Cell Stem Cell* 2011; 9: 11–15.
47. Jeong J. Adipose stem cells and skin repair. *Curr Stem Cell Res Ther* 2010; 5: 137–140.
48. Banas A, Teratani T, Yamamoto Y *et al.* IFATS Series: *In vivo* therapeutic potential of human adipose tissue mesenchymal stem cells (AT-MSCs) after transplantation into mice with liver injury. *Stem Cells* 2008; 26: 2705–2712.
49. Fuchs E, Merrill B, Jamora C *et al.* At the roots of a never-ending cycle. *Dev Cell* 2001; 1: 13–25.
50. Pascucci L, Mercati F, Gargiulo AM *et al.* CD34 glycoprotein identifies putative stem cells located in the isthmic region of canine hair follicles. *Vet Dermatol* 2006; 17: 244–251.
51. Al-Refu K. Stem cells and alopecia: a review of pathogenesis. *Br J Dermatol* 2012; 167: 479–484.
52. Yoo BY, Shin YH, Yoon HH *et al.* Application of mesenchymal stem cells derived from bone marrow and umbilical cord in human hair multiplication. *J Dermatol Sci* 2010; 60: 74–83.
53. Grandi F, Firmo B, Colodel MM *et al.* The importance of follicular stem cells in veterinary medicine in the context of skin tumours. *Vet Dermatol* 2011; 23: 81–83.
54. Kobayashi T, Shimizu A, Nishifuji K *et al.* Canine hair-follicle keratinocytes enriched for bulge cells have the highly proliferative characteristic of stem cells. *Vet Dermatol* 2009; 20: 338–346.
55. Mercati F, Pascucci L, Gargiulo AM *et al.* Immunohistochemical evaluation of intermediate filament nestin in dog hair follicles. *Histol Histopathol* 2008; 23: 1035–1041.
56. Jin DM, Lyle S, Elenitsas R *et al.* Cytokeratin 15 expression in trichoepitheliomas and a subset of basal cell carcinomas suggests they originate from hair follicle stem cells. *J Cutan Pathol* 1999; 26: 113–118.
57. Klopp A, Gupta A, Spaeth E *et al.* Dissecting a discrepancy in the literature: do mesenchymal stem cells support or suppress tumor growth? *Stem Cells* 2011; 29: 11–19.
58. Norbert K. The regulation of veterinary regenerative medicine and the potential impact of such regulation on clinicians and firms commercializing these treatments. *Vet Clin North Am Equine Pract* 2011; 27: 383–391.
59. Oliver L. FDA: The new animal drug approval process, in *Proceedings*. Second Ann Conf North Am Vet Regen Med 2011.

To cite this article, please use DOI: 10.1111/j.1365-3164.2012.01088.x

4.2

A systematic review of randomized controlled trials for prevention or treatment of atopic dermatitis in dogs: 2008–2011 update

Thierry Olivry and Petra Bizikova

Department of Clinical Sciences and Center for Comparative Medicine and Translational Research, College of Veterinary Medicine, North Carolina State University, Raleigh, NC, USA

Correspondence: Thierry Olivry, Department of Clinical Sciences, North Carolina State University, College of Veterinary Medicine, 1060 William Moore Drive, Raleigh, NC 27607, USA. E-mail: tolivry@ncsu.edu

Background – The management of atopic dermatitis (AD) in dogs relies mainly on the use of interventions to reduce pruritus and skin lesions.

Objectives – To provide a critical analysis of recent clinical trials reporting the efficacy and safety of interventions for canine AD.

Methods – Systematic review of randomized controlled trials (RCTs) published, presented or completed between 2008 and 2011, which enrolled dogs with AD. The search was done using electronic databases, reviewing published meeting abstracts and sending queries to professional email lists. Trials reporting the efficacy of interventions aimed at treating, preventing or reducing glucocorticoid usage in atopic dogs were selected.

Results – Twenty-one RCTs were included. We found further moderate-quality evidence of efficacy and safety of oral glucocorticoids and ciclosporin for treatment of canine AD. There was additional moderate-quality evidence of the efficacy of a topical glucocorticoid spray containing hydrocortisone aceponate. Low-quality evidence was found for the efficacy and safety of injectable recombinant interferons, a budesonide leave-on conditioner, a ciclosporin topical nano-emulsion and oral fexofenadine. There is low-quality evidence of efficacy of oral masitinib, with a need for monitoring for protein-losing nephropathy. Finally, we uncovered low-quality evidence of efficacy of a commercial diet as a glucocorticoid-sparing intervention and of a glucocorticoid spray as a flare-delaying measure. Very low-quality evidence was found for the efficacy of other interventions.

Conclusions and clinical importance – Topical or oral glucocorticoids and oral ciclosporin remain the interventions with highest evidence for efficacy and relative safety for treatment of canine AD.

Introduction

Atopic dermatitis (AD) is a common allergic skin disease of dogs that is currently defined as a genetically predisposed inflammatory and pruritic skin disease, with characteristic clinical features and an association with IgE antibodies most commonly directed against environmental allergens.[1] This disease has recently been shown to have a strong impact on the quality of life of both affected dogs and their owners[2,3] and, as such, it is probably one of the most important chronic skin diseases of dogs.

Recent international practice guidelines have highlighted the need for a multifaceted line of attack for the management of canine AD.[4] Approaches to consider currently include the avoidance of flare factors, an increase in skin and coat hygiene and care, the control of skin infections and the use of pharmacotherapy to alleviate skin lesions and manifestations of pruritus.[4] To reduce signs immediately during acute flares of AD, topical and/or oral glucocorticoids are suggested.[4] For long-term pharmacological treatment of chronic or recurrent signs of canine AD, oral and/or topical glucocorticoids, topical tacrolimus, oral ciclosporin and injectable interferons are currently recommended.[4] Finally, additional strategies are also used to prevent the recurrence of clinical signs.[4]

The recommendations for specific drugs included in the 2010 guidelines derived principally from two systematic reviews of interventions to treat dogs with AD. The first review, published in 2003,[5] analysed results of clinical trials testing pharmacological interventions, whether the trials were randomized or not; it did not discuss studies evaluating the efficacy of essential fatty acid (EFA) formulations or allergen-specific immunotherapy, and it was limited to clinical trials published in peer-reviewed jour-

Accepted 12 June 2012

Sources of Funding: This study was self-funded.

Conflict of Interest: From 2008 to 2011, Thierry Olivry participated in North Carolina State University-approved consulting activities (C) for or has received a lecturing honorarium (LH) or obtained research funding (RF) from the following companies whose products are discussed herein: AB-Science (France; C), Novartis Animal Health (Switzerland; C, LH and RF) and Virbac (France; C and RF). Petra Bizikova has received research funding from Virbac (France) via North Carolina State University.

nals.[5] In 2010, an international collaboration published a second systematic review using the more stringent methodology and the support of the Cochrane Skin Group.[6] That study was limited to randomized controlled trials (RCTs), and there were no restrictions on publication type and status, languages or types of interventions.[6] In that review, database searches were done in 2005 for trials from 1980 to 2004, and RCTs published in 2005, 2006 and 2007 were included in a prospective fashion. In all, 49 RCTs were scrutinized.[6]

Objectives

To determine the efficacy of interventions to treat or prevent skin lesions and/or pruritic manifestations of canine AD, we carried out a systematic review of recent RCTs that had enrolled atopic dogs of any age and disease severity. These trials had to be completed, presented or published between 2008 and 2011. This paper serves, therefore, as an update of the previous systematic review.[6] This article is written according to the reporting standards for systematic reviews and meta-analyses set up by the latest 2009 Preferred Reporting Items for Systematic Reviews and Meta-Analyses (PRISMA) statement.[7]

Methods

Protocol and registration

With minor changes in outcome measures and study selection criteria, the protocol for this systematic review was nearly identical to that of a recent publication.[6] Owing to the lack of availability of online repositories accepting the advanced publication of veterinary systematic review protocols, it could not be published before this review was conducted.

Eligibility criteria

Types of studies.
In this systematic review, we included solely RCTs of interventions aimed at treating or preventing AD in dogs. As our latest systematic review focused on trials published or presented from the early 1980s until the end of 2007,[6] we limited our present analysis to trials published, presented or completed between 2008 and 2011, both years included. There were no language or publication status restrictions. Finally, we excluded studies that had been presented at meetings before 2007, and which had already been discussed in our 2010 review.[6]

Types of participants.
As done previously,[6] dogs had to be diagnosed with AD based on (as minimal criteria) the presence of characteristic clinical signs and the exclusion of pruritic dermatoses of similar appearance.[8,9] The fulfilment of published diagnostic criteria such as those of Willemse[10], Prélaud *et al.*[11] or Favrot *et al.*[12] was considered acceptable if non-AD pruritic diseases had also been excluded according to current standards. If the RCT had enrolled dogs with different diagnoses (e.g. AD and other diseases or pruritic dogs without further diagnostic characterization), the study was excluded. We also eliminated four trials that enrolled laboratory dogs with experimentally induced atopic skin lesions.

Types of interventions.
Randomized controlled trials had to report either the treatment or prevention of manifestations of pruritus and/or skin lesions of canine AD. There was no restriction on the route or type of intervention. Comparators could either consist of a relevant placebo or an active medication, be it a different dose of the same drug or an intervention already recommended for treatment of canine AD.[4]

As done in our preceding systematic review,[6] RCTs were categorized at 'short-term' if they lasted 8 weeks or less and 'long-term' if their duration extended beyond 8 weeks. We also separated studies aimed at preventing flares of canine AD from those designed to relieve existing signs (i.e. treatment *sensu stricto*).

Types of outcome measures.
As in our recent review,[6] included studies had to report an assessment of the extent and/or intensity of pruritus and/or skin lesions after a preventive or therapeutic intervention. Trials solely reporting the safety of an intervention were not reviewed further.

Primary outcome measures were similar to those used recently, while secondary outcome measures were expanded from previous ones.[6] Primary outcome measures consisted of the proportion of dogs with a good-to-excellent improvement at study end using a categorical global assessment scale assessed by either investigators (primary outcome 1a) or dog owners (primary outcome 1b).

As secondary outcome measures, we determined the percentage of dogs with complete – or near complete – remission of signs, as estimated by a reduction of 90% or more from baseline investigator-graded lesional (secondary outcome 1a) or owner-rated pruritus scores (secondary outcome 1b). We also extracted from the RCTs the percentage of dogs with a 50% or greater reduction from baseline of investigator-graded lesional (secondary outcome 2a) or owner-rated pruritus scores (secondary outcome 2b). In the absence of universally accepted validated severity scales for evaluating skin and pruritus in dogs with AD, the outcome measures listed above were determined from values assessed with any scoring scheme used by the study authors, but only if there were more than 10 possible grades of severity in the scales utilized.

Furthermore, whenever RCTs employed validated scales, such as the Canine Atopic Dermatitis Extent and Severity Index version 3 (CADESI-03)[13,14] and Hill's Pruritus Visual Analog Scale (PVAS),[15,16] for which thresholds for normal dogs have been established, we added four other secondary outcome measures. For these RCTs, we calculated the percentage of dogs that, at trial's end, had CADESI-03 values in the range of those of normal dogs (0–15; secondary outcome 3a) or of dogs with mild AD (16–59; secondary outcome 4a). Likewise, we determined the percentage of dogs with a PVAS in the range of that of normal dogs (0–1.9; secondary outcome 3b) or dogs with mild pruritus (i.e. the value anchored by the third lowermost descriptor, 2–3.5; secondary outcome 4b). We also calculated these outcome measures for other scales if there were clearly indicated benchmarks for the absence of signs (or normal dog status) and/or for mild AD.

Finally, for glucocorticoid-sparing effect trials and prevention studies, we used different outcome measures that appeared to be more clinically relevant for these unique study designs. These *ad hoc* outcome measures were the glucocorticoid dosage at study end and the time to relapse, respectively.

Whenever possible and to provide a better comparison of the efficacy between different interventions tested in placebo-controlled RCTs, we calculated numbers needed to treat (NNT) based on each of the available outcome measures. However, to limit the lack of relevance of NNTs because of a high random chance placebo effect in RCTs with small group sizes,[17] NNTs were calculated only for large trials with more than 50 dogs per group.

Each NNT was calculated as follows.[18]

1 The average benefit increase (ABI) of the intervention over placebo equals the percentage of dogs with positive outcome in the active intervention-treated group (i.e. the experimental event rate) minus the percentage of dogs with positive outcome in the placebo-treated group (i.e. the control event rate)
2 The NNT, which is the inverse (i.e. reciprocal) of the ABI, equals one divided by the ABI.
3 The NNT was rounded up to the next integer.

As an example, in the context of this review, an NNT of '*n*' could be interpreted as follows: a veterinarian would have to treat '*n*' dogs with AD with the active intervention to obtain one additional positive outcome over treatment with placebo. The lower the NNT, the stronger the treatment effect over placebo.

Finally, in this review, we extracted and reviewed adverse events following each nonplacebo intervention.

Information sources

Studies were identified by searching three databases (Medline via PubMed, Thomson Reuters' Web of Science and CAB Abstract via EBSCO Host) for the period between 1 January 2008 and 31 December 2011. Searches were done once on 2 January 2012.

Additionally, we searched online published abstracts from the three leading veterinary dermatology international congresses: the World Congress of Veterinary Dermatology (WCVD, 2008), the annual joint congresses of the European Society of Veterinary Dermatology (ESVD) and European College of Veterinary Dermatology (ECVD) of 2009, 2010 and 2011, as well as those of the North American Veterinary Dermatology Forum (NAVDF) held annually between 2008 and 2011.

To identify RCTs that had not yet been published or presented, we sent an email twice (18 December 2011 and 3 January 2012) to the three main veterinary dermatology lists (Vetderm, DipECVD and Dipderm) requesting colleagues to provide information on recently completed studies. Finally, we contacted, by email, representatives of three companies known to the authors to have completed relevant RCTs.

Search

The same search was done with the three electronic databases, with the goal of having a simple yet very sensitive strategy that yielded a maximum of species- and disease-specific citations. The terms employed were as follows: (dog or dogs or canine) and (atopic and dermatitis). We added a date limit from 1 January 2008 to 31 December 2012, but there were no language or publication type restrictions. The search was done by one author (T.O.) and verified by the co-author (P.B.).

Study selection

As done for our 2010 Cochrane-style systematic review,[6] the titles of all electronic citations and meeting abstracts were first scanned for identification of clinical trials. Then, abstracts and/or article full texts were assessed to determine whether or not the study was an RCT, if it had enrolled solely dogs with AD, and if it had reported efficacy outcome measures. Furthermore, meeting abstracts and electronic article citations were matched for the identification of duplicate studies. The trial selection was not blinded, but it was done independently by the two authors; disagreements were resolved by consensus. Reasons for exclusion were recorded.

Data collection process

One of the authors first assessed study characteristics and extracted outcome measures, while the other assessed the risks of bias; then they reversed roles and verified each other's extracted data. Discrepancies were identified and resolved by consensus.

When information was insufficient to assess outcome measures from the published or presented data, study authors were contacted by email. In the event of a lack of reply within 2 weeks, a second request was sent. When authors further declined to provide the requested information or original data, the mention 'not provided upon request' was added to the tables or the study was excluded from review, depending upon the amount of information available for analysis. The extracted data were entered in tables similar to those of the 2010 review.[6]

Data items

The following parameters were extracted from each article and/or from information obtained from the authors: objective of the study (treatment or prevention of AD); study design (parallel or crossover); duration of the trial; type of duration (short or long term); characteristics of study participants (number of dogs, their age range, type of AD etc.); type of intervention (treatment or prevention, including dose, duration and frequency); type of outcome measure; and funding source.

Risk of bias in individual studies

To determine the validity of eligible RCTs, the adequacy of several parameters known to affect bias was assessed as done previously.[5,6] The following parameters were rated as 'none', 'adequate', 'unclear' or 'inadequate': (i) method of generation of randomization sequences; (ii) method of concealment of allocation to treatment groups; (iii) masking of intervention for observers (e.g. clinicians) and participants (e.g. dog owners); (iv) inclusion of cases lost to follow-up in intention-to-treat (ITT) analyses; and (v) degree of certainty that the participants were affected with AD, as judged by the author's description.

The parameters 'comparison of groups at baseline' and 'assessment of compliance' were also added to the appraisal of study design.

Three of the parameters above (randomization method, masking and ITT) were used for an overall evaluation of study quality. When these parameters had been rated as 'adequate or performed', the RCT was graded as 'high quality'; when they were all rated as 'inadequate or unclear', the study was graded as 'poor'; and when only one or two of three parameters was assessed as 'inadequate or unclear', the RCT was graded as being of 'intermediate' quality.

Planned methods of analysis

As no two studies appeared to test similar interventions and/or used sufficiently similar designs, pooling of data for meta-analysis was not attempted. As a result, between-RCT variability (i.e. heterogeneity or inconsistencies) was not calculated. Nevertheless, whenever available, we compared dichotomous primary outcome measures between interventions using the Mantel–Haenszel (M-H) test; results are presented as risk ratios (RRs) with 95% confidence intervals (CIs) in the figures. These analyses were done using RevMan 5.0 analysis software (The Nordic Cochrane Centre, Copenhagen, Denmark).

Risk of bias across studies

In the absence of availability of published clinical trial protocols before the final results were eventually reported, the authors could not compare whether the outcome measures published matched those planned at study onset. However, the outcome measures reported in the study methods were matched to those of the results section. We also assessed whether the reported outcome measures were consistent with those employed in recent RCTs enrolling dogs with AD and if they appeared clinically relevant.

Additional analyses

Owing to the heterogeneity of interventions and study designs, sensitivity, subgroup and meta-regression analyses were not conducted.

Results

Study selection

The search of Medline, Web of Science and CAB Abstract databases yielded a total of 672 citations, while 406 congress abstracts were available after examination of their online publication (Figure 1). Five replies were received from queries sent to the three veterinary dermatology lists. Among all citations, there were 48 clinical trials with atopic dogs, of which 18 were excluded because of lack of fulfilment of inclusion criteria. We subsequently eliminated seven RCTs that had been presented at congresses and later published as full papers (Figure 1). Owing to insufficient data available for full review and

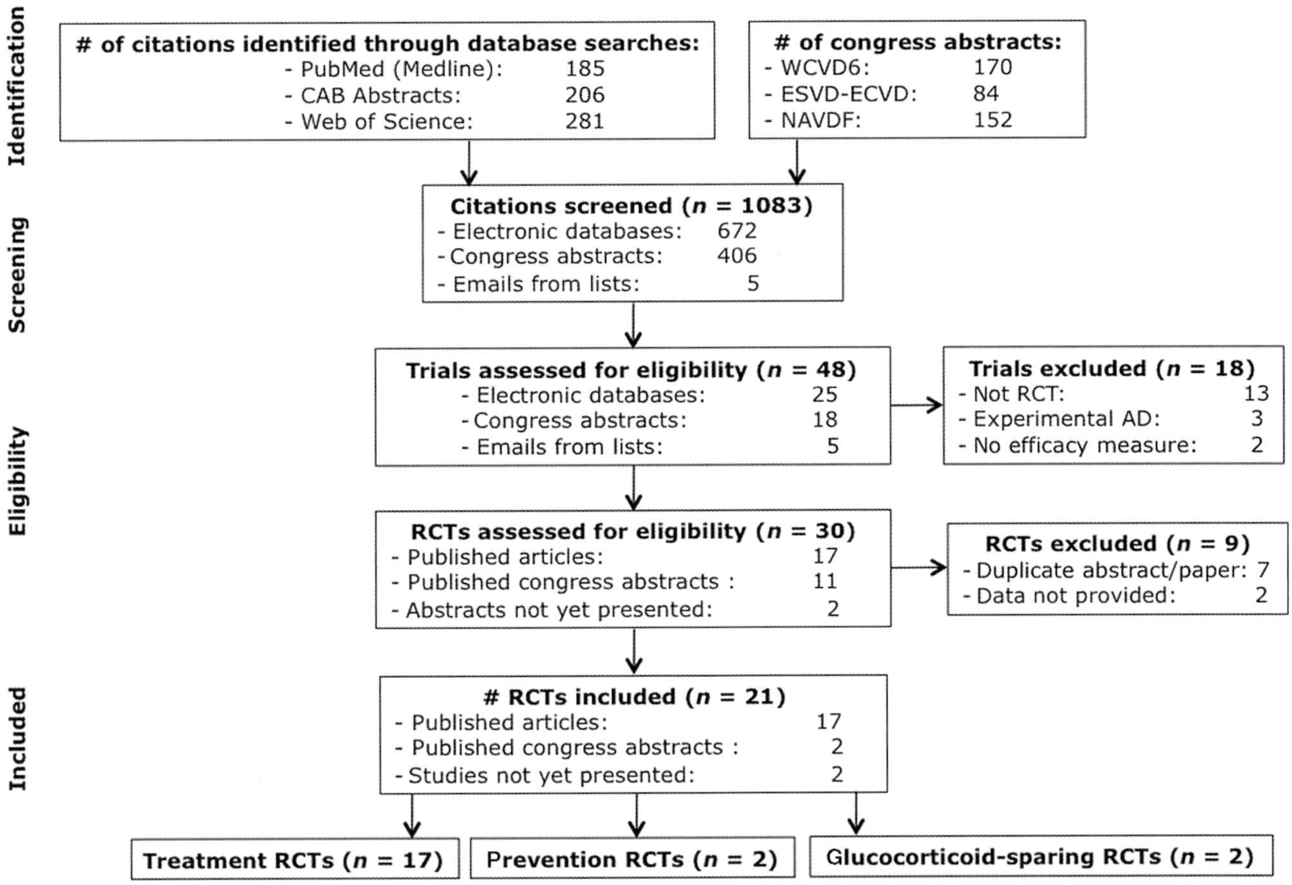

Figure 1. Flow diagram of study selection. Abbreviations: AD, atopic dermatitis; and RCTs, randomized controlled trials.

analysis, we also removed one published and one presented RCT.[19,20] The remaining 21 RCTs are reviewed herein.

Study characteristics

Details of study methodology, participants, interventions and funding sources can be found in Table 1.

Publication status.

All but one study included in this review were RCTs reported in English; one was in Italian. At the time of writing, 16 trials had been published in full in peer-reviewed journals, three were published only as abstracts,[21–23] one was accepted for publication at the time of selection[24] and one had neither been published nor presented, but study details were provided for our review in response to an email request to the vetderm list (A. Puigdemont, personal communication 2012).

Methods.

Of 21 RCTs, there were 17 that used a parallel design of two groups or more, while the remaining four were cross-over trials (Table 1). Fourteen studies had interventions that were shorter than 8 weeks, hence were categorized as 'short term'; the other seven lasted from 2 to 9 months (i.e. 'long-term' studies). While the abstract from one relapse prevention study did not specify the duration of the trial,[24] it clearly lasted more than 2 months.

Participants.

The number of subjects varied among RCTs (average, 42; median, 30; range, 10–316; Table 1). The lowest number of dogs in a treatment group was five (T-cell receptor peptide group[22]) and the highest was 202 (masitinib group[25]). Only six of 21 RCTs (29%) performed or reported a power analysis to justify subject numbers in each treatment group.[25–30] All but one trial enrolled dogs with nonseasonal AD, while the last looked at the effect of an intervention to prevent recurrence of signs in dogs with predefined seasonal AD.[31]

Several studies added further limitations to their enrolment criteria. One trial of allergen-specific immunotherapy (ASIT) selected only dogs with demonstrable hypersensitivity to *Dermatophagoides farinae* house dust mites.[32] One RCT selected only dogs with pedal lesions,[21] another selected dogs with at least mild signs,[30] while four studies enrolled dogs with moderate to severe AD (A. Puigdemont, personal communication 2012).[25–27] Finally, two trials needed dogs to have signs for a minimal duration before selection (6 months[33] and 1 year[22]).

Interventions.

All but four studies tested the efficacy – and safety – of various types of topical, oral or injectable interventions for treatment of canine AD (Table 1). Two trials investigated the effect of dietary interventions for their potential reducing effect on concurrently given oral glucocorticoids.[23,27] Finally, two RCTs examined the outcome of

Table 1. Characteristics of included studies

First author (year)	Methods (duration, month)	Participants	Interventions	Prevention or treatment?	Short or long term?	Outcomes	Funding	Comments
Bensignor (2008)[36]	Crossover, 2 × 1 month	20 dogs with nonseasonal nonfood-induced AD	Commercial or home-made fish and potato diet	Treatment	Short-term	Change in lesion and pruritus scores	Procter and Gamble Pet Care	—
Glos (2008)[34]	Parallel, 2 months	50 dogs with nonseasonal AD	Four different commercial diets	Treatment	Short-term	Change in lesion and pruritus scores, coat quality and stool characteristics	Procter and Gamble Pet Care	—
Bryden (2008)[21]	Crossover, 2 × 0.5 month	10 dogs with nonseasonal AD and pedal lesions	Hydrocortisone aceponate spray or placebo	Treatment	Short-term	Change in lesion and pruritus scores, IGA, OGA	Virbac	Only affected feet treated
Willemse (2009)[32]	Parallel, 9 months	38 dogs with *D. farinae* sensitive AD	*D. farinae* restricted subcutaneous immunotherapy or placebo	Treatment	Long-term	Change in lesion and pruritus scores	Artu Biologicals	Dogs also had hypersensitivities other than *D. farinae*
Nuttall (2009)[26]	Parallel, 1 month	29 dogs with nonseasonal AD and CADESI-03 > 50	Hydrocortisone aceponate spray or placebo	Treatment	Short-term	Change in lesion and pruritus scores, OGA	Virbac	Part 1 RCT data only
Horvath-Ungerboeck (2009)[38]	Crossover, 2 × 1 month	30 dogs with nonseasonal AD	Tepoxalin or placebo	Treatment	Short-term	Change in lesion and pruritus scores	Intervet/ Schering-Plough Animal Health	—
Carlotti (2009)[35]	Parallel, 6 months	31 dogs with AD	Recombinant feline interferon-ω or ciclosporin	Treatment	Long-term	Change in lesion and pruritus scores	Virbac	—
Plevnik (2009)[37]	Parallel, 1.5 months	30 dogs with AD	Methylprednisolone or fexofenadine	Treatment	Short-term	Change in lesion and pruritus scores	Government of Republic of Slovenia	—
Noli (2009)[31]	Parallel, 6 months	14 dogs with seasonal AD recurrent for at least 2 years	Blackcurrant seed oil or placebo	Prevention	Long-term	Change in lesion and pruritus scores	NBF Lanes	—
Yasukawa (2010)[40]	Parallel, 2 months	31 dogs with AD	Two different dosages of recombinant canine interferon-γ	Treatment	Short-term	Change in lesion and pruritus scores	Toray Industries	—

Table 1. (*Continued*)

First author (year)	Methods (duration, month)	Participants	Interventions	Prevention or treatment?	Short or long term?	Outcomes	Funding	Comments
Schmidt (2010)[27]	Parallel, 2 months	22 dogs with nonseasonal moderate/ severe AD	Methylprednisolone + Phytopica herbal preparation or placebo	Treatment (steroid-sparing effect)	Short-term	Change in lesion and pruritus scores, OGA, methylprednisolone dosage	Intervet/ Schering-Plough Animal Health	—
Singh (2010)[33]	Parallel, 2 months	30 dogs with AD >0.5 year duration	Pentoxifylline, EFA or placebo	Treatment	Short-term	Change in lesion and pruritus scores	Unclear	—
Ahlstrom (2010)[28]	Crossover, 2 × 3 weeks	29 dogs with AD	Budesonide conditioner or placebo	Treatment	Short term	Change in lesion and pruritus scores, QoL	Dermcare-Vet	—
Kovalik (2011)[39]	Parallel, 1.5 months	20 dogs with AD	Generic ciclosporin or prednisone	Treatment	Short-term	Change in lesion and pruritus scores	Teva Pharmaceuticals	—
Mueller (2011)[29]	Parallel, 3 months	21 dogs with AD	*Trichuris vulpis* eggs or placebo	Treatment	Long-term	Change in lesion and pruritus scores	Canine Research Society	—
Sanchez (2011)[23]	Parallel, 2 months	22 dogs with nonseasonal nonfood-associated AD	Prednisone and fatty acid-rich or commercial diets	Treatment (steroid-sparing effect)	Short-term	Change in lesion and pruritus scores, prednisone dosage	Affinity Petcare	—
Gingerich (2011)[22]	Parallel, 1.5 months	11 dogs with nonseasonal AD >1 year duration	TCR-Vß8.1 or placebo	Treatment	Short-term	Change in lesion and pruritus scores	Immulan BioTherapeutics	—
Nuttall (2012)[30]	Parallel, 3 months	48 dogs with at least mild nonseasonal AD	Hydrocortisone aceponate spray or ciclosporin	Treatment	Long-term	Change in lesion and pruritus scores, OGA	Virbac	—
Cadot (2011)[25]	Parallel, 3 months	316 dogs with nonseasonal AD and CADESI-02 > 25	Masitinib or placebo	Treatment	Long-term	Change in lesion and pruritus scores, IGA, OGA	AB-Science	306 dogs analysed (modified ITT)

Table 1. *(Continued)*

First author (year)	Methods (duration, month)	Participants	Interventions	Prevention or treatment?	Short or long term?	Outcomes	Funding	Comments
Lourenço (2012)[24]	Parallel, variable	41 dogs with AD	Hydrocortisone aceponate spray or placebo	Prevention	Long-term	Time to relapse necessitating treatment	Virbac	—
Puigdemont (2012) Unpublished	Parallel, 1.5 months	32 dogs with moderate or severe nonseasonal AD	Topical ciclosporin or placebo	Treatment	Short-term	Change in lesion and pruritus scores	Advancell	—

Abbreviations: AD, atopic dermatitis; EFA, essential fatty acids; IGA, Investigator Global Assessment; ITT, intention to treat; OGA, Owner Global Assessment; QoL, quality of life.

interventions aimed at preventing the recurrence of flares of AD (i.e. prevention studies).[24,31]

Outcome measures.
As indicated in Table 1 and per selection criteria, all studies reported one or more outcome measures of efficacy. In general, these included the evolution, over the duration of the tested intervention(s), of pruritus and/or skin lesions scores (Table 1). To these were added, in five RCTs (Table 1), owner- and/or investigator-assessed global assessment ratings.[21,25–27,30] In one study, the evaluation of quality of life (QoL) was also added.[28] The two studies on glucocorticoid-sparing effect logically included the evaluation of the reduction in the dosage of oral glucocorticoids.[23,27] Finally, one of the two prevention studies used 'time to relapse necessitating treatment' as a logical and relevant outcome measure for that particular design.[24]

Of the RCTs that tested the evolution of skin lesions over time, the validated third version of the CADESI score was used in 10 studies,[21–24,26,27,29,30,34,35] while five trials employed the second version of this scale, which had limited validation.[25,31,33,36,37] Four trials employed unvalidated scales modified from the first, second or third versions of the CADESI – the so called 'modified CADESI' or 'mCADESI' – having changed the type of lesions, the body sites and/or the severity rating used (A. Puigdemont, personal communication 2012).[28,38,39] One trial employed a scale derived from the 'six area six signs AD' (SASSAD) used in human patients with AD even though this scale had not been validated beforehand for canine AD.[32] Finally, one study used a simple but not validated six-point categorical scale.[40]

Of 20 RCTs that tested the efficacy of interventions on pruritus, 16 used the evolution of scores obtained on a visual analog scale (VAS), which varied between 5 and 20 cm; only three[22,29,30] used the PVAS developed and validated by Hill and colleagues,[15] even though it was first published in 2007 before some of these RCTs were designed. Finally, three trials used other *ad hoc* unvalidated pruritus scales.[35,38,40]

Funding.
One trial was funded by a grant from the government of the Republic of Slovenia,[37] while all others were funded by pharmaceutical companies.

Risk of bias in individual studies
Details on each study's randomization method, intervention masking, loss to follow-up, diagnosis certainty, baseline group comparison, compliance assessment and overall quality rating can be found in Table 2.

In summary, out of 21 RCTs, only one had an overall quality rated as 'poor',[33] seven were given an 'intermediate' rating,[31,35–40] and the remaining 13 had the highest quality mark (Table 2). The most common reason for not attributing this 'high-quality' rating was a lack of performance of ITT analyses.[33,35,36,38]

Results of individual studies

As in our recent systematic review,[6] individual trials will be discussed below in groups testing similar interven-

Table 2. Assessment of study design

First author (year)	Generation of randomization sequence	Allocation concealment	Intervention masking	Loss to follow-up	Diagnosis certainty	Groups comparable at baseline	Assessment of compliance	Quality
Bensignor (2008) [36]	Adequate (coin toss)	Adequate	Investigator only	ITT not performed	Adequate	Yes	Not assessed	Intermediate
Glos (2008) [34]	Adequate (randomization table)	Adequate	Adequate	ITT performed	Adequate	Yes	Not assessed	High
Bryden (2008) [21]	Adequate (computer)	Adequate	Adequate	ITT on all data provided by author	Adequate	Yes	Not assessed	High
Willemse (2009) [32]	Adequate (computer)	Adequate	Adequate	ITT performed	Adequate	Yes	Adequate	High
Nuttall (2009) [26]	Adequate (computer)	Adequate	Adequate	ITT performed	Adequate	Yes	Adequate	High
Horvath-Ungerboeck (2009) [38]	Adequate (block)	Adequate	Adequate	ITT not performed	Adequate	Yes	Not assessed	Intermediate
Carlotti (2009) [35]	Adequate (computer)	Adequate	Adequate	ITT not performed	Adequate	Yes	Adequate	Intermediate
Plevnik (2009) [37]	Inadequate	Inadequate	Inadequate	ITT on all data provided by author	Adequate	Yes	Not assessed	Intermediate
Noli (2009)[31]	Inadequate	Inadequate	Adequate	ITT on all data provided by author	Adequate	Yes	Not assessed	Intermediate
Yasukawa (2010) [40]	Adequate (table)	Adequate	Not performed	ITT performed	Adequate	Higher pruritus in 5000 units group at baseline	Not provided upon request	Intermediate
Schmidt (2010) [27]	Adequate (computer)	Adequate	Adequate	ITT performed	Adequate	Yes	Adequate	High
Singh (2010) [33]	Inadequate	Inadequate	Not performed	ITT not performed	Adequate	Yes	Not assessed	Poor
Ahlstrom (2010) [28]	Adequate (coin toss)	Adequate	Adequate	ITT performed	Adequate	Carry over of budesonide effect if given before placebo	Adequate	High
Kovalik (2011) [39]	Inadequate	Adequate	Investigator only	ITT performed	Adequate	Yes	Unclear	Intermediate
Mueller (2011) [29]	Adequate (randomization table)	Adequate	Adequate	ITT performed	Adequate	Yes	Adequate	High
Sanchez (2011) [23]	Adequate (table)	Adequate	Adequate	ITT performed	Adequate	Yes	Not assessed	High
Gingerich (2011) [22]	Adequate (block)	Adequate	Adequate	ITT on all data provided by author	Adequate	Yes	Adequate	High
Nuttall (2012) [30]	Adequate (computer)	Adequate	Investigator only	ITT performed	Adequate	Yes	Adequate	High
Cadot (2011) [25]	Adequate (computer)	Adequate	Adequate	Modified ITT performed	Adequate	Yes	Adequate	High
Lourenço (2012) [24]	Adequate	Adequate	Adequate	ITT performed	Adequate	Yes	Adequate	High
Puigdemont (2012) Unpublished	Adequate (computer)	Adequate	Adequate	ITT performed	Adequate	Yes	Adequate	High

Abbreviation: ITT, intention to treat.

tions within three larger subheadings: (i) treatment; (ii) glucocorticoid sparing; and (iii) prevention RCTs. Details on study design and quality assessment can be found in Tables 1 and 2, respectively.

Interventions for treatment of clinical signs

Glucocorticoids.

Two RCTs used an oral glucocorticoid as control for another intervention,[37,39] while four tested the efficacy of a topical glucocorticoid (Table 3).[21,26,28,30]

One study reported the efficacy of methylprednisolone (Medrol; Pharmacia, Luxemburg, Luxemburg),[37] while the second used prednisone (Encorton; Polfa Pharmaceuticals, Lublin, Poland).[39] In both studies, drug dosages and protocols corresponded to those employed and recommended in recent practice guidelines.[4] In these two small trials, the frequencies of dogs that achieved positive outcomes (Table 3) are in the range of those found after similar interventions (reviewed by Olivry *et al.*[6]). The results suggest treatment efficacy even though the glucocorticoids were not compared with placebo but were used as positive comparators for another intervention. Adverse effects reported in the publications were those expected for oral glucocorticoids.[37,39]

Three RCTs reported efficacy data for the same novel diester glucocorticoid spray that contains 0.0584% hydrocortisone aceponate (Cortavance; Virbac, Carros, France),[21,26,30] while one tested the effectiveness of a novel glucocorticoid leave-on conditioner containing 0.025% budesonide (Barazone; Dermcare-Vet, Springwood, Queensland, Australia; Table 3).[28] Three studies were placebo controlled,[21,26,28] while one used ciclosporin as the active control.[30] One trial focused on pedal pruritus and skin lesions;[21] two had a crossover design.[21,28]

In two studies, the hydrocortisone aceponate spray appeared to be more effective than placebo for nearly all outcome measures (Table 3 and Figures 2 and 3).[21,26] The magnitude of the effect was dampened by the small size of each treatment group, this being shown by the very large confidence interval bracketing the relative risk (Figures 2 and 3). In the largest trial, the outcome measures of efficacy were comparable between the glucocorticoid spray and ciclosporin.[30] The safety of this diester glucocorticoid spray was found to be acceptable, with the lack of report of relevant adverse drug events.[21,26,30] Remarkably, skin thinning was not reported with this formulation, even after 3 months of usage at frequencies varying from once daily to twice weekly.[30]

A once-weekly application of the 0.025% budesonide leave-on conditioner appeared more effective than placebo for the achievement of outcome measures of partial (≥50%) but not complete (≥90%) reduction of pruritus and skin lesions (Table 3). In this crossover study, there was a carry-over effect of budesonide on skin lesions when it had been applied before placebo. Quality of life was reported to be significantly higher with the glucocorticoid conditioner than after placebo application.[28] This conditioner was discussed as having a good-to-excellent tolerance, and there were no differences between placebo and actively treated dogs for scores of polydipsia, polyphagia and skin thinning.

Ciclosporin.

Oral ciclosporin (Atopica; Novartis Animal Health, Basel, Switzerland) was used in two RCTs as an active comparator for two other interventions (Table 3).[30,35] In another trial, a generic microemulsified formulation of ciclosporin (Equoral; Teva Pharmaceuticals, Warsaw, Poland) was tested against prednisone (see glucocorticoid section above for details on the prednisone arm),[39] and a fourth RCT evaluated the efficacy of a novel topical 2.25% nano-emulsion of ciclosporin (Cyclostopic-Vet; Advancell, Barcelona, Spain) versus placebo (A. Puigdemont, personal communication 2012). In trials were ciclosporin was used as a positive comparator,[30,35] secondary outcome measures were found to be in the range of those reported in the previous systematic review that had analysed data from six RCTs (Table 3).[6] Positive outcome measures obtained using the generic formulation of ciclosporin were also similar to those reported previously for the brand approved for the treatment of canine AD.[6] This generic formulation also appeared to be of an efficacy equivalent to that of oral prednisone.[39] In these three studies, adverse effects of ciclosporin were mainly the expected occurrences of mild, usually self-limiting vomiting, loose stools and diarrhoea.

Positive outcome measures were more frequently achieved after the twice-daily application of the novel topical ciclosporin nano-emulsion for 6 weeks than after that of placebo (Table 3). Adverse events were not seen.

Interferons.

There were two intermediate-quality-graded small RCTs testing the efficacy of recombinant interferons for the treatment of canine AD (Table 3).

In one study,[35] dogs were treated with either injections of recombinant feline interferon-ω (Virbagen Omega; Virbac, Carros, France), a type I interferon, plus capsules of placebo, or they received oral ciclosporin capsules (Atopica; Novartis Animal Health, Basel, Switzerland) and placebo injections. Positive secondary outcome measures were seen more often after treatment with oral ciclosporin than with injectable feline interferon-ω (Table 3), but the improvement between groups was of the same order of magnitude. Relevant adverse events were not seen except for one dog that repeatedly exhibited increased pruritus 3 days after interferon injections.

In the second RCT, dogs received injections of one of two different dosages of recombinant canine interferon-γ (KT-100; Toray Industries, Tokyo, Japan) in a nonblinded fashion.[40] For evaluation of skin lesions, we reviewed only data for the parameter 'erythema', because the other two lesions ('excoriations' and 'alopecia') were secondary to pruritus, which was evaluated separately. The reduction of erythema and pruritus was greater with the higher dosage of canine interferon-γ (5000 units/kg/injection; Table 3), even though the pruritus scores had been significantly higher in that group at baseline. Safety appeared excellent, except for one dog from the high dosage group that exhibited immediate allergic signs shortly after an injection.

Diets.

Two studies looked at the benefit of using commercial diets for treatment of canine AD.[34,36]

Table 3. Randomized controlled trials evaluating interventions for treatment effect

First author (year)	Intervention	Primary outcome measure (NNT)		Secondary outcome measure (NNT)								Comments
		1a	1b	1a	1b	2a	2b	3a	3b	4a	4b	
		Percentage of dogs with good-to -excellent response (clinician)	Percentage of dogs with good-to -excellent response (owner)	Percentage of dogs in complete remission (>90% reduction lesions)	Percentage of dogs in complete remission (>90% reduction pruritus)	Percentage of dogs in partial remission (>50% reduction lesions)	Percentage of dogs in partial remission (>50% reduction pruritus)	Percentage of dogs with lesions in the range of normal dogs	Percentage of dogs with pruritus in the range of normal dogs	Percentage of dogs with lesions in the range of dogs with mild AD	Percentage of dogs with pruritus in the range of dogs with mild AD	
Bensignor (2008)[36]	Commercial or home-made fish and potato diet	n.a.	n.a.	Commercial, 0/16 (0%). Home-made, 0/16 (0%)	Commercial, 0/16 (0%). Home-made, 0/16 (0%)	Commercial, 0/16 (0%). Home-made, 0/16 (0%)	Commercial, 2/16 (1%). Home-made, 1/16 (1%)	n.a.	n.a.	n.a.	n.a.	Reported reduction in average pruritus and skin lesions scores while on commercial but not home-made diet
Glos (2008)[34]	Diet A, Hill's canine d/d salmon & rice. Diet B, Eukanuba FP fish and potato. Diet C, Royal Canin Hypoallergenic DR21. Diet D, Pedigree Complete Maxi chicken and rice	n.a.	n.a.	A, 1/14 (7%). B, 2/12 (17%). C, 2/12 (17%). D, 1/12 (8%)	A, 1/14 (7%). B, 1/12 (8%). C, 1/12 (8%). D, 0/12 (0%).	A, 7/14 (50%). B, 9/12 (75%). C, 5/12 (42%). D, 6/12 (50%).	A, 5/14 (36%). B, 6/12 (50%). C, 2/12 (17%). D, 4/12 (33%)	A, 4/14 (29%). B, 10/12 (83%). C, 3/12 (25%). D, 7/12 (59%)	n.a.	A, 6/14 (43%). B, 1/12 (8%). C, 9/12 (75%). D, 5/12 (42%)	n.a.	Eight dogs also treated with prednisolone, 1 with ciclosporin; coat became more lustrous with diet A; outcome measures provided by authors
Bryden (2008)[21]	HCA once daily for 7 days then every other day for 7 days or placebo topically	HCA, 3/10 (30%). Placebo, 0/10 (0%)	HCA, 3/10 (30%). Placebo, 0/10 (0%)	n.a.	n.a.	n.a.	n.a.	HCA, 3/10 (30%). Placebo, 1/10 (10%) (erythema)	HCA, 1/10 (10%). Placebo, 1/10 (10%)	HCA, 5/10 (50%). Placebo, 1/10 (10%) (erythema)	HCA, 7/10 (70%). Placebo, 1/10 (10%)	Outcome measures calculated from raw data provided by authors
Willemse (2009)[32]	*D. farinae* specific subcutaneous immunotherapy (standard protocol)	n.a.	n.a.	n.a.	n.a.	n.a.	n.a.	n.a.	n.a.	n.a.	n.a.	No significant differences in pruritus and lesion scores between immunotherapy and placebo groups

Table 3. *(Continued)*

First author (year)	Intervention	Primary outcome measure (NNT) 1a: Percentage of dogs with good-to -excellent response (clinician)	Primary 1b: Percentage of dogs with good-to -excellent response (owner)	Secondary outcome measure (NNT) 1a: Percentage of dogs in complete remission (>90% reduction lesions)	1b: Percentage of dogs in complete remission (>90% reduction pruritus)	2a: Percentage of dogs in partial remission (>50% reduction lesions)	2b: Percentage of dogs in partial remission (>50% reduction pruritus)	3a: Percentage of dogs with lesions in the range of normal dogs	3b: Percentage of dogs with pruritus in the range of normal dogs	4a: Percentage of dogs with lesions in the range of dogs with mild AD	4b: Percentage of dogs with pruritus in the range of dogs with mild AD	Comments
Nuttall (2009)[26]	HCA once daily or placebo topically	n.a.	HCA, 6/15 (40%). Placebo, 2/13 (15%)	HCA, 1/15 (7%). Placebo, 0/13 (0%)	HCA, 4/15 (27%). Placebo, 0/13 (0%)	HCA, 11/15 (73%). Placebo, 3/13 (23%)	HCA, 7/15 (47%). Placebo, 1/13 (8%)	HCA, 4/15 (27%). Placebo, 0/13 (0%)	n.a.	HCA, 7/15 (47%). Placebo, 5/13 (39%)	n.a.	Primary outcome 1b: grades 4 and 5 combined; other outcome measures provided by authors
Horvath-Ungerboeck (2009)[38]	Tepoxalin 10 mg/kg once daily or placebo p.o.	n.a.	n.a.	Tepoxalin, 1/28 (4%). Placebo, 2/25 (8%)	n.a.	Tepoxalin, 7/28 (25%). Placebo, 4/25 (16%)	Tepoxalin, 10/28 (36%). Placebo, 4/25 (16%)	n.a.	Tepoxalin, 4/28 (14%). Placebo, 1/25 (4%)	n.a.	Tepoxalin, 11/28 (39%). Placebo, 5/25 (20%)	Normal dog: EPS = 0; mild AD: EPS = 1
Carlotti (2009)[35]	Recombinant feline interferon-ω 1–4 million units/injection s.c. or ciclosporin 50–200 mg/day p.o.	n.a.	n.a.	Interferon, 3/18 (17%). Ciclosporin, 4/8 (50%)	Interferon, 3/18 (17%). Ciclosporin, 2/8 (25%)	Interferon, 9/18 (50%). Ciclosporin, 4/8 (50%)	Interferon, 7/18 (39%). Ciclosporin, 5/8 (63%)	Interferon, 4/18 (22%). Ciclosporin, 2/8 (25%)	n.a.	Interferon, 4/18 (22%). Ciclosporin, 2/8 (25%)	n.a.	—
Plevnik (2009)[37]	MP 0.5 mg/kg once daily for 5 days, then every other day. FEX 18 mg/kg once daily. Both p.o.	n.a.	n.a.	MP, 0/15 (0%). FEX, 3/15 (20%)	MP, 5/15 (33%). FEX, 4/15 (27%)	MP, 12/15 (80%). FEX, 14/15 (93%)	MP, 10/15 (67%). FEX, 12/15 (80%)	n.a.	n.a.	n.a.	n.a.	Outcome measures calculated from raw data provided by authors
Yasukawa (2010)[40]	Recombinant canine interferon-γ 2000 or 5000 units/kg three times weekly for 4 weeks, then once weekly for 4 weeks s.c.	n.a.	n.a.	n.a.	n.a.	2000 units, 4/11 (36%). 5000 units, 9/14 (64%)	2000 units, 5/11 (46%). 5000 units, 11/14 (79%)	n.a.	n.a.	n.a.	n.a.	8 week per protocol data extracted from table; erythema and pruritus parameters only

Table 3. (*Continued*)

First author (year)	Intervention	Primary outcome measure (NNT) 1a: Percentage of dogs with good-to -excellent response (clinician)	1b: Percentage of dogs with good-to -excellent response (owner)	Secondary outcome measure (NNT) 1a: Percentage of dogs in complete remission (>90% reduction lesions)	1b: Percentage of dogs in complete remission (>90% reduction pruritus)	2a: Percentage of dogs in partial remission (>50% reduction lesions)	2b: Percentage of dogs in partial remission (>50% reduction pruritus)	3a: Percentage of dogs with lesions in the range of normal dogs	3b: Percentage of dogs with pruritus in the range of normal dogs	4a: Percentage of dogs with lesions in the range of dogs with mild AD	4b: Percentage of dogs with pruritus in the range of dogs with mild AD	Comments
Singh (2010)[33]	PTX 20 mg/kg three times daily, PTX + EFA mix or placebo, all p.o.	n.a.	n.a.	n.a.	n.a.	n.a.	n.a.	PTX, 3/11 (27%). PTX + EFA, 5/12 (42%). Placebo, 0/4 (0%)	n.a.	n.a.	Data shown are dogs with 100% remission of both CADESI-02 and pruritus VAS; author reported no longer having access to study data	
Ahlstrom (2010)[28]	Budesonide 0.025% conditioner once weekly or placebo topically	n.a.	n.a.	Budesonide, 3/29 (10%). Placebo, 0/29 (0%)	Budesonide, 6/29 (21%). Placebo, 5/29 (17%)	Budesonide, 20/29 (69%). Placebo, 5/29 (17%)	Budesonide, 19/29 (66%). Placebo, 9/29 (31%)	n.a.	n.a.	n.a.	n.a.	Higher quality -of-life values after budesonide; ITT data sets
Kovalik (2011)[39]	Ciclosporin 5 mg/kg once daily or prednisone 1 mg/kg once daily for 7 days then every other day, both p.o.	n.a.	n.a.	Ciclosporin, 7/13 (54%). Prednisone, 2/7 (29%)	Ciclosporin, 4/13 (31%). Prednisone, 0/7 (0%)	Ciclosporin, 11/13 (85%). Prednisone, 6/7 (86%)	Ciclosporin, 10/13 (77%). Prednisone, 6/7 (86%)	n.a.	n.a.	n.a.	n.a.	—
Mueller (2011)[29]	*Trichuris vulpis* 2500 embryonated eggs or placebo p.o.	n.a.	n.a.	*Trichuris*, 0/11 (0%). Placebo, 0/10 (0%)	*Trichuris*, 0/11 (0%). Placebo, 1/10 (10%)	*Trichuris*, 4/11 (36%). Placebo, 1/10 (10%)	*Trichuris*, 3/11 (27%). Placebo, 0/10 (0%)	*Trichuris*, 7/11 (64%). Placebo, 6/10 (60%)	*Trichuris*, 2/11 (18%). Placebo, 2/10 (20%)	*Trichuris*, 2/11 (18%). Placebo, 2/10 (20%)	*Trichuris*, 3/11 (27%). Placebo, 2/10 (20%)	Outcome measures provided by the authors
Gingerich (2011)[22]	TCR-Vß8.1 100 mg injected twice or placebo s.c.	n.a.	n.a.	TCR, 0/5 (0%). Placebo, 0/6 (0%)	TCR, 1/5 (20%). Placebo, 0/6 (0%)	TCR, 4/5 (80%). Placebo, 1/6 (17%)	TCR, 4/5 (80%). Placebo, 1/6 (17%)	TCR, 2/5 (40%). Placebo, 3/6 (50%)	TCR, 3/5 (60%). Placebo, 2/6 (33%)	TCR, 2/5 (40%). Placebo, 1/6 (17%)	TCR, 1/5 (20%). Placebo, 1/6 (17%)	Two dogs treated with placebo had normal CADESI-03 at baseline and at study end

Table 3. (*Continued*)

		Primary outcome measure (NNT)		Secondary outcome measure (NNT)								
		1a	1b	1a	1b	2a	2b	3a	3b	4a	4b	
First author (year)	Intervention	Percentage of dogs with good-to -excellent response (clinician)	Percentage of dogs with good-to -excellent response (owner)	Percentage of dogs in complete remission (>90% reduction lesions)	Percentage of dogs in complete remission (>90% reduction pruritus)	Percentage of dogs in partial remission (>50% reduction lesions)	Percentage of dogs in partial remission (>50% reduction pruritus)	Percentage of dogs with lesions in the range of normal dogs	Percentage of dogs with pruritus in the range of normal dogs	Percentage of dogs with lesions in the range of dogs with mild AD	Percentage of dogs with pruritus in the range of dogs with mild AD	Comments
Nuttall (2012)[30]	HCA once daily topically or ciclosporin 5 mg/kg once daily p.o.; frequencies decreased to every other day or twice weekly if effective	n.a.	HCA, 19/24 (79%). Ciclosporin 10/21 (48%)	HCA, 9/24 (38%). Ciclosporin, 8/21 (38%)	HCA, 5/24 (21%). Ciclosporin, 5/21 (24%)	HCA, 18/24 (75%). Ciclosporin, 18/21 (86%)	HCA, 16/24 (67%). Ciclosporin, 12/21 (57%)	HCA, 8/24 (33%). Ciclosporin, 9/21 (43%)	HCA, 10/24 (42%). Ciclosporin, 7/21 (33%)	HCA, 5/24 (21%). Ciclosporin, 2/21 (10%)	HCA, 0/24 (0%). Ciclosporin, 1/21 (5%)	Outcome measures provided by authors, ITT with last value carried forward
Cadot (2011)[25]	Masitinib 12.5 mg/kg or placebo once daily p.o.	Masitinib, 90/202 (45%). Placebo, 26/104 (25%) (NNT, 6)	Masitinib, 80/202 (40%). Placebo, 31/104 (30%) (NNT, 11)	n.p.	n.p.	Masitinib, 86/202 (43%). Placebo, 27/104 (26%) (NNT, 6)	n.p.	n.a.	n.a.	n.a.	n.a.	All outcome measures from modified ITT with missing data as failure
Puigdemont (2012) Unpublished	Ciclosporin 2.25% nano-emulsion twice daily or placebo topically	n.a.	n.a.	Ciclosporin, 5/17 (29%). Placebo, 1/15 (7%)	Ciclosporin, 2/17 (12%). Placebo, 1/15 (7%)	Ciclosporin, 11/17 (65%). Placebo, 4/15 (27%)	Ciclosporin, 10/17 (59%). Placebo, 5/15 (33%)	n.a.	n.a.	n.a.	n.a.	Outcome measures provided by authors; ITT with last value carried forward

Abbreviations: AD, atopic dermatitis; EFA, essential fatty acids; EPS, Edinburgh Pruritus Score; FEX, fexofenadine; HCA, hydrocortisone aceponate; ITT, intention to treat; MP, methylprednisolone; n.a., not available or not assessable; NNT, number needed to treat; n.p., not provided by authors upon request; p.o., *per os*; PTX, pentoxifylline; s.c, subcutaneousy; TCR, T-cell receptor; VAS, visual analog scale

Study	Interventions 1/2	Intervention 1 Events	Intervention 1 Total	Intervention 2 Events	Intervention 2 Total	Risk ratio M-H, Random, 95% CI
Bryden 2008[21]	HCA / placebo	3	10	0	10	7.00 [0.41, 120.16]
Cadot 2011[25]	Masitinib / placebo	90	202	26	104	1.78 [1.24, 2.57]

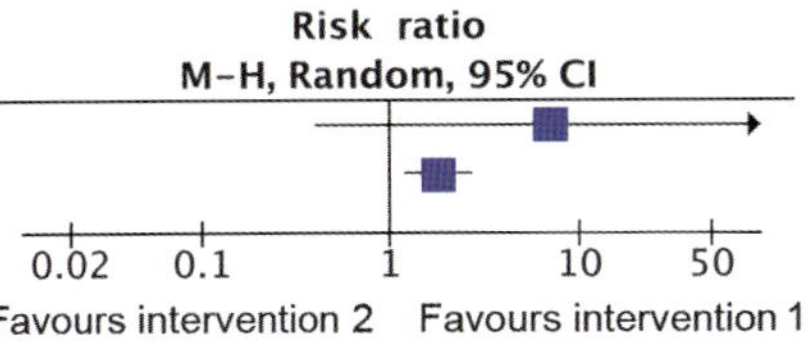

Figure 2. Forest plot of the primary outcome measure 1a: clinician global assessment of efficacy. In this figure, the event rate represents the number of dogs for which clinicians reported a good-to-excellent response at trials' end. In these plots, the vertical line ('1') represents the 'no effect' line. The horizontal bar spanning the blue squares highlights the confidence interval of the risk ratio (i.e. treatment effect). In this graph, the size of the blue square was not made proportional to the size of the study. Interventions 1 and 2 are the ones listed in the second column. Abbreviations: CI, confidence interval; HCA, hydrocortisone aceponate; and M-H, Mantel–Haenszel test.

In the first RCT, which had a crossover design without washout, dogs with nonfood-induced AD were given either a home-made fish and potato diet or a commercially available diet with similar ingredients (Eukanuba FP dry; Iams, Procter & Gamble Pet Care, Schwalbach, Germany). The main difference between these two interventions was the lack of supplementation with EFA, minerals and vitamins in the home-made diet. The study authors reported that skin lesion and pruritus scores decreased more often after the commercial than the home-made diet, but there were no difference in rates of achievement of secondary outcome measures between the two interventions (Table 3). Adverse events were not discussed in this paper.

The second RCT compared the effect of three diets marketed for allergic dogs with that of a widely used commercial diet.[34] Dogs were randomized to be fed Hill's prescription diet Canine d/d Salmon & Rice (Hill's Pet Nutrition, Hamburg, Germany), Eukanuba Dermatosis FP (Procter & Gamble Pet Care, Schwalbach, Germany) Royal Canin Hypoallergenic DR21 (Royal Canin, Köln, Germany) or the Pedigree Complete Maxi Chicken & Rice (Masterfoods, Verden, Germany) control diet (Table 3). Of importance is that enrolled dogs had not all been subjected to a dietary restriction–provocation test beforehand, and this could have affected treatment benefit if any dog had eaten a diet containing ingredients to which it was hypersensitive. In all, positive secondary outcome measures were reached in a highly variable percentage of dogs being fed the test or control diets, and these outcome measures were also inconsistently achieved within each diet group (Table 3). Clinically relevant and constant differences in benefit from any of the 'allergic' diets over the control diet were not found.

Miscellaneous.
Seven trials evaluated the efficacy of a variety of interventions to treat dogs with AD. The tested interventions included *D. farinae* restricted immunotherapy in dogs hypersensitive to this plus other allergens,[32] the cyclooxygenase-1, cyclooxygenase-2 and 5-lipoxygenase inhibitor tepoxalin (Zubrin; Intervet/Schering-Plough Animal Health, Boxmeer, The Netherlands),[38] the type 1 histamine receptor inverse agonist (antihistamine) fexofenadine (Telfast; Sanofi-Aventis, Ljubljana, Slovenia),[37] the phosphodiesterase inhibitor pentoxifylline with or without EFA (brands not specified),[33] embryonated eggs of *Trichuris vulpis*,[29] synthetic T-cell receptor V-β peptides,[22] and the tyrosine kinase inhibitor masitinib (Masivet or Kinavet; AB-Science, Paris, France).[25] Outcome measures are reported in Table 3. Except for fexofenadine and masitinib, whose results are discussed below, the evaluation of our standardized measures of efficacy did not suggest any clinical benefit of these interventions. In general, this lack of efficacy was due to an inconsistency between positive outcome measures,[22,29,38] too low an effect compared with placebo,[29,32,38] a lack of available data to assess[33] and/or to a very small subject number per group, resulting in a study that was probably underpowered.[22,29,33]

One small RCT of intermediate quality suggested, for all outcome measures, a consistent benefit of the antihistamine fexofenadine (Telfast; Sanofi-Aventis), with an efficacy that was of the same magnitude as that of oral methylprednisolone (Medrol; Pharmacia, Luxemburg, Luxemburg).[37] Unfortunately, there was no report of a power analysis done beforehand to justify such a small number of dogs in this noninferiority trial; this study was probably underpowered. Clinically relevant adverse effects of fexofenadine were not noted.

Study	Interventions 1/2	Intervention 1 Events	Intervention 1 Total	Intervention 2 Events	Intervention 2 Total	Risk ratio M-H, Random, 95% CI
Bryden 2008[21]	HCA / placebo	3	10	0	10	7.00 [0.41, 120.16]
Cadot 2011[25]	Masitinib / placebo	80	202	31	104	1.33 [0.95, 1.87]
Nuttall 2009[26]	HCA / placebo	6	15	2	13	2.60 [0.63, 10.73]
Nuttall 2012[30]	HCA / ciclosporine	19	24	10	21	1.66 [1.02, 2.72]

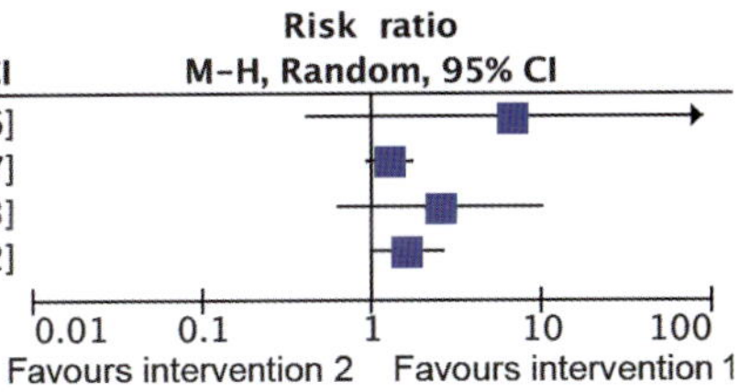

Figure 3. Forest plot of the primary outcome measure 1b: owner global assessment of efficacy. In this figure, the event rate represents the number of dogs for which owners reported a good-to-excellent response at trials' end. In these plots, the vertical line ('1') represents the 'no effect' line. The horizontal bar spanning the blue squares highlights the confidence interval of the risk ratio (i.e. treatment effect). In this graph, the size of the blue square was not made proportional to the size of the study. Interventions 1 and 2 are the ones listed in the second column. Abbreviations: CI, confidence interval; HCA, hydrocortisone aceponate; M-H, Mantel–Haenszel test.

The largest RCT reviewed herein is a 3 month high-quality study that tested the efficacy of masitinib (Masivet or Kinavet; AB-Science, Paris, France) versus placebo in 316 dogs with nonseasonal AD, of whom 306 were retained for modified intention-to-treat analyses (202 masitinib and 104 placebo).[25] In Table 3, we calculated outcome measures using the set of 'missing data as failure'. Data for calculation of our standardized outcome measures were not provided upon request. Overall, the published outcome measures were satisfied more often after oral administration of masitinib than after placebo, and the confidence interval of the effect suggests a modest treatment benefit (Table 3 and Figures 2 and 3). The calculation of NNTs, which was done only for this large trial, is also consistent with a small treatment effect (i.e. between six and 11 dogs would have to be treated to gain one additional positive outcome over placebo). This modest efficacy over the control intervention was most likely due to an unusually large benefit seen in the placebo group, which was probably caused by the allowance of microbial infection control in this trial, as well as the enrolment of dogs with no pruritus or mild pruritus at baseline in both groups (see online supplemental information in the study by Cadot *et al.*[25]). The intake of masitinib led to a higher proportion of severe and nonfatal adverse events compared with placebo. In dogs receiving masitinib, a severe protein-losing nephropathy developed in two (1%), proteinuria in 12 (6%) and hypoalbuminaemia in five of 206 dogs (2%). If detected early, this urinary protein loss was reversible.

Interventions for glucocorticoid dose reduction.
Our search identified two small high-quality RCTs aimed at testing an intervention that, given along with oral glucocorticoids, was hoped to result in a decrease in glucocorticoid dosage (Table 4).[23,27]

In the first trial,[27] dogs received daily oral methylprednisolone with a plant-derived extract (Phytopica; Intervet Schering-Plough Animal Health, Milton Keynes, UK) or placebo dry granules. Once daily, the owners were instructed to decrease the dose of methylprednisolone based on the dog's pruritus levels assessed using a VAS. While there was a similar change in global efficacy rating and lesional and pruritus scores in both groups (Table 4), the decrease in methylprednisolone dose was significantly higher in dogs given Phytopica rather than placebo.[27] Furthermore, after 2 months, twice as many dogs (80%) given the herbal supplement had had a 50% reduction in their dose of methylprednisolone compared with that taken at baseline (Table 4).[27] Five of 21 dogs (24%) did not complete this trial, mainly because of adverse effects. These consisted principally of polyuria–polydipsia, which was seen equally in both groups, and soft stools mostly after Phytopica. To the best of our knowledge, this herbal supplement is no longer available commercially.

The second study employed a design similar to the one above.[23] Dogs with nonseasonal nonfood-induced AD were given prednisone along with a novel EFA-rich diet (Advance Veterinary Diets Atopic Care; Affinity Petcare, Sant Cugat del Vallès, Spain) or a control commercial dog food (Brekkies Excel Complet; Affinity Petcare, Sant Cugat del Vallès, Spain) for 2 months, and the dose of the glucocorticoid was then reduced according to a predetermined protocol. Altogether, the EFA-rich test diet appeared to lead to a greater reduction in skin lesion and pruritus scores compared with the control diet. Moreover, at study end, eight of 11 dogs (73%) eating the control diet were still receiving prednisone, while none of the dogs given the EFA-rich test diet was given this medication (Table 4). Adverse effects of the diets were not discussed in either study abstract or poster transmitted by the authors.

Interventions for prevention of flares.
There are two studies that investigated if an intervention could prevent relapses of signs of canine AD (Table 5).[24,31] The first RCT was a small intermediate-quality study enrolling dogs with recurrent seasonal AD.[31] One to 2 months before the expected seasonal exacerbation, dogs were given a supplementation of either blackcurrant seed oil (Vegetable Seedoil Product, Paesi Bassi) or a non-oil placebo (brands not specified). Using the parameters set out in Table 5, recurrences were found to have occurred at comparable rates in dogs treated with blackcurrant seed oil or placebo. Adverse effects were not discussed in the paper.

The second trial was a high-quality RCT that employed a novel design.[24] Dogs with AD were treated once daily, until remission of signs, with the 0.0584% hydrocortisone aceponate spray already discussed in the preceding section discussing glucocorticoids (Cortavance; Virbac, Carros, France). Once their disease was controlled, dogs were randomized to have previously lesional areas sprayed once daily for two consecutive days each week with either the active glucocorticoid or a placebo. The time to relapse needing treatment was found to be significantly longer after treatment with the glucocorticoid compared with the placebo spray (Table 5). Adverse drug events were not observed with this glucocorticoid proactive intermittent regimen.

Syntheses of results

In this updated systematic review, because study designs, interventions and outcome measures varied vastly, we focused on individual study description rather than pooling of results in meta-analyses. The summary of available evidence can be found in the first section of the Discussion below.

Risk of bias across study

As protocols were not made available publically beforehand, *post hoc* modifications of outcome measures at the time of publication/presentation could not be verified. In all trials, outcome measures were matched to those reported in the Results section. In only one study was one data set defined in the Methods ('imputation of missing values according to the last observation carried forward') neither reported in the results section of that study nor further discussed.[25] In general, the outcome measures reported in the studies were consistent with those used in a recent systematic review.[6] Additional outcome measures were added whenever relevant to the study design (e.g. the dosage of glucocorticoid at trial's end in

Table 4. Randomized controlled trials evaluating interventions for glucocorticoid-sparing effect

		Primary outcome measure (NNT)		Secondary outcome measure (NNT)								
		1a	1b	1a	1b	2a	2b	3a	3b	4a	4b	
First author (year)	Intervention	Percentage of dogs with good-to-excellent response (clinician)	Percentage of dogs with good-to-excellent response (owner)	Percentage of dogs in complete remission (≥90% reduction lesions)	Percentage of dogs in complete remission (≥90% reduction pruritus)	Percentage of dogs in partial remission (≥50% reduction lesions)	Percentage of dogs in partial remission (≥50% reduction pruritus)	Percentage of dogs with lesions in the range of normal dogs	Percentage of dogs with pruritus in the range of normal dogs	Percentage of dogs with lesions in the range of dogs with mild AD	Percentage of dogs with pruritus in the range of dogs with mild AD	Comments
Schmidt (2010)[27]	Methylprednisolone 0.4 mg/kg once daily + Phytopica 200 mg/kg once daily or placebo, all p.o.	n.a.	Phytopica, 8/10 (80%). Placebo, 8/11 (73%)	Phytopica, 0/10 (0%). Placebo, 1/11 (9%)	Phytopica, 4/10 (40%). Placebo, 1/11 (9%)	Phytopica, 10/10 (100%). Placebo, 9/11 (82%)	Phytopica, 9/10 (90%). Placebo, 7/11 (64%)	Phytopica, 0/10 (0%). Placebo, 0/11 (0%)	n.a.	Phytopica, 10/10 (100%). Placebo, 9/11 (82%)	n.a.	Dogs with 50% reduction of methylprednisolone dosage at day 56: Phytopica, 8/10 (80%); placebo, 4/11 (36%)
Sanchez (2011)[23]	Prednisone 0.5 mg/kg once daily p.o. then decreased plus EFA-rich (Atopic Care) test or control (Brekkies Excel Complet) diets	n.a.	n.a.	Test diet, 6/11 (55%). Control diet, 1/11 (9%)	Test diet, 8/11 (73%). Control diet, 0/11 (0%)	Test diet, 11/11 (100%). Control diet, 6/11 (55%)	Test diet, 11/11 (100%). Control diet, 8/11 (73%)	Test diet, 7/11 (64%). Control diet, 2/11 (18%)	n.a.	Test diet, 4/11 (36%). Control diet, 6/11 (55%)	n.a.	Dogs on prednisone at study end: test diet, 0/11 (0%); control diet, 8/11 (73%); outcome measures provided by authors

Abbreviations: EFA, essential fatty acids; n.a., not available or not assessable; NNT, number needed to treat; p.o., *per os*.

Table 5. Randomized controlled trials (RCTs) evaluating interventions for prevention effect

First author (year)	Intervention	Primary outcome measure (NNT)		Secondary outcome measure (NNT)								Comments
		Percentage of dogs with good-to-excellent response (clinician)	Percentage of dogs with good-to-excellent response (owner)	Percentage of dogs in complete remission (≥90% reduction lesions)	Percentage of dogs in complete remission (≥90% reduction pruritus)	Percentage of dogs in partial remission (≥50% reduction lesions)	Percentage of dogs in partial remission (≥50% reduction pruritus)	Percentage of dogs with lesions in the range of normal dogs	Percentage of dogs with pruritus in the range of normal dogs	Percentage of dogs with lesions in the range of dogs with mild AD	Percentage of dogs with pruritus in the range of dogs with mild AD	
		1a	1b	1a	1b	2a	2b	3a	3b	4a	4b	
Noli (2009)[31]	BSO 100 mg/kg once daily or placebo p.o.	n.a.	n.a.	n.a.	n.a.	n.a.	n.a.	No recurrence (lesions): BSO, 4/7 (57%); placebo, 3/7 (43%)	No recurrence (pruritus): BSO, 3/7 (43%); placebo, 2/7 (29%)	n.a.	n.a.	No recurrence parameters: <10 (CADESI-02) or <2 (VAS)
Lourenço (2012)[24]	HCA for two consecutive days per week or placebo topically	n.a.	n.a.	n.a.	n.a.	n.a.	n.a.	n.a.	n.a.	n.a.	n.a.	Mean (range) number of days to relapse needing treatment: HCA, 115 (31–260); placebo, 33 (15–61)

Abbreviations: AD, atopic dermatitis; BSO, blackcurrant seed oil; HCA, hydrocortisone aceponate; n.a., not available or not assessable; p.o., *per os*; VAS, visual analog scale.

studies testing a steroid-sparing effect,[23,27] or the 'time to relapse needing treatment' in a flare prevention study[24]). For the first time among previous RCTs with atopic dogs, authors evaluated a 'quality-of-life' outcome measure, albeit using an unvalidated scale.[28] Whenever not reported in study abstracts or papers, authors were contacted to obtain needed outcome measures and/or raw data to allow their calculation. Authors complied with this request in 18 of 21 studies (86%). Of the three studies with missing data, two were eventually excluded because of insufficient information available for appropriate evaluation;[19,20] missing outcome measures were replaced by 'not provided upon request' for the last study.[25]

Discussion

Summary of evidence

In the following paragraphs of this section, the quality of evidence was defined according to that proposed in the recent GRADE consensus (Box 1).[41] Specific recommendations for usage will be made in the Conclusion of this review.

Herein, we found further moderate-quality evidence of efficacy of oral glucocorticoids and microemulsified ciclosporin (Atopica; Novartis Animal Health) at dosages comparable to those used in trials already included in an earlier systematic review.[6] There is new low-quality evidence, based on a single small trial,[39] that a generic microemulsified ciclosporin (Equoral; Teva Pharmaceuticals) has an efficacy in the range of that of the brand approved for use in canine AD (Atopica; Novartis Animal Health). Surprisingly, in spite of the large size of this molecule, there is low-quality evidence that a nano-emulsion containing 2.25% of ciclosporin (Cyclostopic-Vet; Advancell) might be effective topically (A. Puigdemont, personal communication 2012).

Based on one RCT each, there is low-quality evidence of the efficacy and safety of injectable recombinant feline interferon-ω (Virbagen Omega; Virbac),[35] injectable recombinant canine interferon-γ (KT-100; Toray Industries)[40] and oral fexofenadine (Telfast; Sanofi-Aventis)[37] to treat canine AD. Likewise, there is low-quality evidence of the efficacy of oral masitinib (Masivet or Kinavet; AB-Science) for management of this disease, but there is a need for close monitoring for rare but potentially fatal protein-losing nephropathy after using this drug.[25]

There is only very low-quality evidence of the possible modest clinical effectiveness of synthetic T-cell receptor V-β peptides, this reduced evidence grade stemming principally from a very small number of subjects per treatment group.[22]

The clinical benefit of the other interventions [tepoxalin (Zubrin; Intervet/Schering-Plough Animal Health),[38] *Trichuris* eggs,[29] single mite allergen immunotherapy[32] and pentoxifylline with or without EFA][33] was not readily apparent in single trials only providing very low-quality evidence. The same conclusion was reached for the benefit of blackcurrant seed oil to prevent the recurrence of signs of seasonal canine AD.[31]

Finally, a new EFA-rich diet (Atopic Care; Affinity Petcare) seems promising as a glucocorticoid-sparing dietary intervention (low-quality evidence).[23] Another interven-

Box 1. Quality of evidence and definitions according to the Grading of Recommendations Assessment, Development and Evaluation (GRADE) system (reproduced with permission of BMJ Publishing Group Ltd).[41]

High quality	Further research is very unlikely to change our confidence in the estimate of effect
Moderate quality	Further research is likely to have an important impact on our confidence in the estimate of effect and may change the estimate
Low quality	Further research is very likely to have an important impact on our confidence in the estimate of effect and is likely to change the estimate
Very low quality	Any estimate of effect is very uncertain

tion that would successfully permit the lowering of the dosage of required glucocorticoids, Phytopica (Intervet-Schering Plough Animal Health),[27] might no longer be available commercially.

Limitations

In comparison with our two previous publications on interventions for canine AD, this review has fewer limitations.[5,6] Our sensitive search method and lack of restriction of publication status and languages reduced publication bias. The finding that all RCTs now enrolled only dogs with better-defined AD is likely to permit a better extrapolation of study results to the wider population of dogs with AD. The award of a 'high-quality' study design rating for 13 of 21 RCTs (62%) is a marked improvement over older RCTs, given that only 12 of 49 (24%) had received this grade in the previous review.[6] This higher quality of trials is intrinsically associated with a reduction of selection, detection and attrition biases.[6] Importantly, the main reason for not obtaining the highest design quality rating was the lack of performance of ITT analyses. Future publications of RCTs should address this insufficiency and report either ITT alone (with included dogs having received at least one dose of the tested interventions and missing values reported as 'last observed carried forward'). Alternatively, authors could report both ITT and 'per protocol' data sets, the latter including only dogs that finished the trial without deviation.

The main limitation of RCTs included herein is that many had very low numbers of subjects per group (15 or less). Moreover, power analyses to determine an appropriate subject number beforehand were performed in fewer than 30% of the trials. Without a power calculation, the selection of the number patients is arbitrary, and low numbers would likely render trials unable to determine anything but a marked treatment effect. It is likely that, in this systematic review, most studies were underpowered; small but real treatment effects were thus likely missed.

Given that there is currently no avenue and no requirement for investigators to publish their study protocol before a RCT is started, there is no possibility for reviewers to verify changes made in outcome measures and/or subgroup analyses after randomization codes are unblinded and results analysed statistically. This limitation might allow some authors to selectively choose more favourable outcome measures thereby potentially making low-potency interventions appear more effective and in a better light than they really are.

A second limitation of trials reviewed herein is the common usage of unvalidated novel or modified published severity scales. Furthermore, reported outcome measures varied greatly, and this made their extraction and standardization difficult. In this systematic review, and to allow the comparison with studies included in the preceding systematic review, we used a set of primary and secondary outcome measures similar to that reported previously.[6] Traditionally, one has mainly evaluated the efficacy of an intervention for canine AD by determining the proportion of dogs achieving a '≥50% reduction' in skin lesion and pruritus severity during the trial. The satisfaction of such a lesion reduction benchmark appears to be associated with a good-to-excellent evaluation of treatment response by dog owners.[42] However, the validity of this reduction threshold for determining a satisfactory antipruritic effect has been questioned recently.[16] As a result of this observation, and as suggested before,[16] we added herein two new outcome measures. These consist of the evaluation of the proportion of dogs that, at trial's end, have skin lesion and pruritus scores in the range of those of normal dogs or of dogs with mild AD. Those outcome measures could be an additional clinically relevant assessment of effective interventions.

Conclusions

Implications for practice

Adding the evidence summarized in this work to that discussed in the two preceding systematic reviews of treatments for canine AD permits the following updated recommendations.[5,6]

Multiple high-quality RCTs have now shown the consistent efficacy, with minor and predictable adverse effects, of the oral glucocorticoids prednisone, prednisolone and methylprednisolone, with a starting dosage of approximately 0.5 mg/kg once to twice daily to be tapered as needed. Several high-quality RCTs have also confirmed the efficacy of topical glucocorticoid formulations, with the strongest evidence existing for the novel 0.0584% hydrocortisone aceponate spray (Cortavance; Virbac). The potency of topical glucocorticoids is likely to vary between formulations and brands; skin thinning with prolonged daily usage is the major safety risk. Intermittent application of these topical formulations appears to prevent this problem, and it might delay the recurrence of flares if applied proactively (i.e. applied even if lesions are no longer seen) to previously affected areas.

Overall, multiple high-quality RCTs have established the efficacy and safety, apart from minor reversible adverse effects, of oral microemulsified ciclosporin given at a starting dosage of 5 mg/kg once daily and tapered after treatment effect is seen. The benefit appears comparable to, but slower to appear than, that of oral glucocorticoids.

In all, a small number of intermediate-quality RCTs has documented the efficacy of recombinant interferons for treatment of canine AD, but protocols for optimal benefit and safety are still unknown. The most favourable regimen (i.e. type of interferon, dosage and frequency of injections) and its cost–benefit have not yet been determined.

The previous evidence of allergen-specific immunotherapy was not strengthened by the RCT reviewed herein,[32] because the protocol of this recent study employed a mite allergen-restricted formulation in dogs hypersensitive to this and other allergens. Such a strategy had not been employed before.

Implications for research

In light of the results of the studies discussed in the present review, additional high-quality RCTs are needed to confirm the efficacy and safety of oral masitinib (Masivet or Kinavet; AB-Science), oral generic or brand-named pentoxifylline at high dosages (i.e. >60 mg/kg/day), oral generic or brand-named fexofenadine, the injectable recombinant interferons (KT-100; Toray Industries; and Virbagen Omega; Virbac), the topical ciclosporin nanoemulsion (Cyclostopic-Vet; Advancell), the budesonide leave-on conditioner (Barazone; Dermcare-Vet) and T-cell receptor peptides. Likewise, the glucocorticoid-sparing effect of the new EFA-rich diet (Atopic Care; Affinity-Petcare) and the preventive effectiveness of topical glucocorticoids (i.e. proactive therapy) must be verified. A parallel study comparing generic and brand-named microemulsified (modified) ciclosporin is warranted.

Additional RCTs to test the efficacy and safety of oral microemulsified ciclosporin and glucocorticoids for the treatment of canine AD are unlikely to provide additional benefit unless these explore new treatment regimens (i.e. different dosages or frequencies of administration) or their efficacy in different subsets of patients (e.g. dogs with mild or severe AD, or those with severe pruritus but few lesions). Ciclosporin and oral glucocorticoids are, nevertheless, the active drugs to which other new interventions should be compared in future trials. As only ciclosporin, but not oral glucocorticoids, has been tested against placebo in previous RCTs, it should be the medication preferred as active comparator for noninferiority trials.[43]

There is a need to conduct high-quality RCTs to assess the efficacy of other commonly used interventions for the treatment of canine AD. For example, trials comparing the effectiveness and safety of different protocols of immunotherapy should be performed (e.g. subcutaneous versus sublingual routes, standard versus rush frequencies, specific versus 'regional nonspecific' formulations). The effectiveness of the plethora of commercially available topical formulations containing oatmeal, antihistamines, topical anaesthetics and lipids deserves more scrutiny and stricter testing. Importantly, the impact of using oral and/or topical antimicrobials (antibacterial or antifungal) has never been assessed as sole or concomitant therapy in dogs with AD.

Further studies aimed at preventing relapses of AD when signs are in remission are also needed. Determining whether additional diets or supplements possess a glucocorticoid-sparing effect would be of great help to patients. Interventions limited to subjects whose signs did not respond to glucocorticoids or ciclosporin would be important, but this research would be likely to benefit only few patients. Finally, studying the cost of all interventions compared with their benefit, safety and improvement in the quality of life of the patients would be likely to influence the care of dogs with AD.

To decrease the risk of perception of a positive treatment effect in placebo control groups, enrolled subjects must have, at baseline, at least mild AD skin lesions and pruritus; dogs with pruritus in normal ranges should not be included. To lower the risk of high placebo effect, further study designs should limit the number of hygiene and anti-infective interventions that could result in improvement of clinical signs. If the duration of the study (i.e. if it lasts 3 months or more) justifies the need for an active control of infections, then a noninferiority trial with a proven effective intervention – preferably oral ciclosporin, because it has been tested against placebo – might be better indicated.[43] Such a trial would be likely to require a higher number of subjects, especially if small noninferiority margins are used.[43]

To enable a better comparison of efficacy among RCTs, and to permit the regrouping of these RCTs in meta-analyses, it is critical that outcome measures be standardized. Investigators are encouraged to use only validated severity scales, such as the third version of the CADESI[13] and Hill's PVAS.[15,16] Furthermore, these two scales are currently the only ones for which AD severity thresholds have been determined.[14,15] Importantly, these scales must be used without a single modification, because *ad hoc* 'modified CADESI' are not validated scales, and the use of this specific denomination implies a scale tested for reliability and validity. Finally, unvalidated scales might not be precise enough to detect a small treatment effect, or they might not be reproducible enough to permit the detection of a lack of treatment efficacy.

In follow-up to the discussion in the 'Limitations' section above, we propose to set up primary outcome measures for future RCTs to be both investigator and owner global assessments of treatment efficacy (IGA-E/OGA-E). Clinically relevant benchmarks would be the frequency of dogs with AD having a subjective good-to-excellent global response to tested interventions. As pruritus and acute skin lesions (i.e. erythema) are not always evolving in parallel in dogs with AD,[44] the separate evaluation of skin lesions and pruritus during treatment should serve as secondary outcome measures. We recommend first an assessment of the proportion of dogs with complete or near complete response to treatment [that is, one associated with a reduction ≥90% of the initial CADESI ($CADESI_{90}$) or PVAS ($PVAS_{90}$) values]. One could also add an evaluation of partial treatment responses (i.e. ≥50% reduction from baseline of severity scale values; $CADESI_{50}$ and $PVAS_{50}$). We also encourage further determination and reporting of the proportion of dogs which, at study end, have normal CADESI-03 (i.e.$CADESI_{norm}$ of 0–15) or PVAS values (i.e. $PVAS_{norm}$ of 0–1.9), as well as those that reach benchmarks of only mild AD (i.e. $CADESI_{mild}$, 16–59; and $PVAS_{mild}$, 2–3.5). These benchmarks can only be calculated with these two unmodified and validated severity scales.[13,15] The assessment of pre- and post-treatment quality-of-life scores using previously reported scales could also be of value to pet owners.[2,3,45,46]

For trials testing the glucocorticoid-sparing effect of interventions, the proportion of dogs without glucocorticoids at study end, as well as the final dosage of glucocorticoids, appears to be relevant outcome measures.[23,27] Finally, for studies evaluating interventions aimed at preventing flares of canine AD, determining the 'time to relapse' seems to be an easily understood outcome measure, as long as such relapse is clearly defined, for example, when pruritus in the preceding day increases to above a 'grade 2' of Hill's PVAS.

Concluding statement

This systematic review confirmed the previously shown benefit of oral and topical glucocorticoids and oral microemulsified ciclosporin for treatment of canine AD. Masitinib appears to have a promising effect, but further studies are needed to confirm its efficacy and safety. Protocols for using injectable interferons must be optimized. Likewise, the use of nutritional interventions for glucocorticoid-sparing effect must be studied further. Finally, other studies are needed to further document the effect of intermittent proactive applications of topical glucocorticoids to prevent flares of AD.

References

1. Halliwell R. Revised nomenclature for veterinary allergy. *Vet Immunol Immunopathol* 2006; 114: 2007–2008.
2. Linek M, Favrot C. Impact of canine atopic dermatitis on the health-related quality of life of affected dogs and quality of life of their owners. *Vet Dermatol* 2010; 21: 456–462.
3. Noli C, Minafo G, Galzerano M. Quality of life of dogs with skin diseases and their owners. Part 1: development and validation of a questionnaire. *Vet Dermatol* 2011; 22: 335–343.
4. Olivry T, DeBoer DJ, Favrot C *et al.* Treatment of canine atopic dermatitis: 2010 clinical practice guidelines from the international task force on canine atopic dermatitis. *Vet Dermatol* 2010; 21: 233–248.
5. Olivry T, Mueller RS, The International Task Force on Canine Atopic Dermatitis. Evidence-based veterinary dermatology: a systematic review of the pharmacotherapy of canine atopic dermatitis. *Vet Dermatol* 2003; 14: 121–146.
6. Olivry T, Foster AP, Mueller RS *et al.* Interventions for atopic dermatitis in dogs: a systematic review of randomized controlled trials. *Vet Dermatol* 2010; 21: 4–22.
7. Liberati A, Altman DG, Tetzlaff J *et al.* The PRISMA statement for reporting systematic reviews and meta-analyses of studies that evaluate health care interventions: explanation and elaboration. *PLoS Med* 2009; 6: e1000100.
8. DeBoer DJ, Hillier A. The ACVD Task Force on Canine Atopic Dermatitis (XV): fundamental concepts in clinical diagnosis. *Vet Immunol Immunopathol* 2001; 81: 271–276.
9. Griffin CE, DeBoer DJ. The ACVD Task Force on Canine Atopic Dermatitis (XIV): clinical manifestations of canine atopic dermatitis. *Vet Immunol Immunopathol* 2001; 81: 255–269.
10. Willemse T. Atopic skin disease: a review and a reconsideration of diagnostic criteria. *J Small Anim Pract* 1986; 27: 771–778.
11. Prélaud P, Guaguère E, Alhaidari Z *et al.* Réévaluation des critères de diagnostic de la dermite atopique [reevaluation of diagnostic criteria of atopic dermatitis]. *Rev Med Vet* 1998; 149: 1057–1064.
12. Favrot C, Steffan J, Seewald W *et al.* A prospective study on the clinical features of chronic canine atopic dermatitis and its diagnosis. *Vet Dermatol* 2010; 21: 23–30.
13. Olivry T, Marsella R, Iwasaki T *et al.* Validation of CADESI-03, a severity scale for clinical trials enrolling dogs with atopic dermatitis. *Vet Dermatol* 2007; 18: 79–96.
14. Olivry T, Mueller R, Nuttall T *et al.* Determination of CADESI-03 thresholds for increasing severity levels of canine atopic dermatitis. *Vet Dermatol* 2008; 19: 115–119.
15. Hill PB, Lau P, Rybnicek J. Development of an owner-assessed scale to measure the severity of pruritus in dogs. *Vet Dermatol* 2007; 18: 301–308.
16. Rybnicek J, Lau-Gillard PJ, Harvey R *et al.* Further validation of a pruritus severity scale for use in dogs. *Vet Dermatol* 2009; 20: 115–122.
17. Moore RA, Gavaghan D, Tramèr MR *et al.* Size is everything – large amounts of information are needed to overcome random effects in estimating direction and magnitude of treatment effects. *Pain* 1998; 78: 209–216.
18. McQuay HJ, Moore RA. Using numerical results from systematic reviews in clinical practice. *Ann Intern Med* 1997; 126: 712–720.
19. Marsella R, Messinger L, Zabel S *et al.* A randomized, double-blind, placebo-controlled study to evaluate the effect of EFF1001, an *Actinidia arguta* (hardy kiwi) preparation, on CADESI score and pruritus in dogs with mild to moderate atopic dermatitis. *Vet Dermatol* 2010; 21: 50–57.
20. Pellicoro M, Marsella R, Ahrens K. Evaluation of the clinical and skin repair effects of dimethicone topical therapy in dogs with naturally occurring atopic dermatitis. *Vet Dermatol* 2011; 22: 291 (abstract).
21. Bryden SL, Burrows AK, Rème C *et al.* Efficacy of a 0.0584% hydrocortisone aceponate spray (Cortavance) for the management of pedal pruritus in atopic dogs: a pilot study. *Vet Dermatol* 2008; 19: 40 (abstract).
22. Gingerich DA, Woods CR. T-cell receptor (TCR) peptides – an immunotherapeutic approach for canine atopic dermatitis. In: *American Academy of Veterinary Pharmacology and Therapeutics 17th Biannual Symposium.* 2011; 6. Available at: http://www.aavpt.org/17thBiennial.shtml. Accessed June 18, 2012.
23. Sanchez N, Villanueva S, Torre C *et al.* Efficacy of a specific diet in the management of canine atopic dermatitis: a randomized, blinded, controlled clinical study. *Vet Dermatol* 2011; 22: 472 (abstract).
24. Lourenço-Martins AM, São-Braz B, Schmidt V *et al.* Long-term maintenance therapy of canine atopic dermatitis with a 0.0584% hydrocortisone aceponate spray (Cortavance) used on two consecutive days each week. *Vet Dermatol* 2012; 23: (Suppl 1): 39 (abstract).
25. Cadot P, Hensel P, Bensignor E *et al.* Masitinib decreases signs of canine atopic dermatitis: a multicentre, randomized, double-blind, placebo-controlled phase 3 trial. *Vet Dermatol* 2011; 22: 554–564.
26. Nuttall T, Mueller R, Bensignor E *et al.* Efficacy of a 0.0584% hydrocortisone aceponate spray in the management of canine atopic dermatitis: a randomised, double blind, placebo-controlled trial. *Vet Dermatol* 2009; 20: 191–198.
27. Schmidt V, McEwan N, Volk A *et al.* The glucocorticoid sparing efficacy of Phytopica™ in the management of canine atopic dermatitis: a randomised, double blind, placebo controlled trial. *Vet Dermatol* 2010; 21: 91–104.
28. Ahlstrom LA, Mason KV, Mills PC. Barazone decreases skin lesions and pruritus and increases quality of life in dogs with atopic dermatitis: a randomized, blinded, placebo-controlled trial. *J Vet Pharmacol Ther* 2010; 33: 573–582.
29. Mueller RS, Specht L, Helmer M *et al.* The effect of nematode administration on canine atopic dermatitis. *Vet Parasitol* 2011; 181: 203–209.
30. Nuttall TJ, McEwan NA, Bensignor E *et al.* Comparable efficacy of a topical 0.0584% hydrocortisone aceponate spray and oral ciclosporin in treating canine atopic dermatitis. *Vet Dermatol* 2012; 23: 4–10,e1–e2.

31. Noli C, Galzerano M, Toma S. Efficacia della somministrazione di olio di semi di ribes nero nella prevenzione del prurito e dei segni clinici della dermatite atopica stagionale (efficacy of the administration of blackcurrant seed oil in the prevention of pruritus and clinical signs of seasonal atopic dermatitis). *Summa Anim Comp* 2009; 9: 21–27.
32. Willemse T, Bardagi M, Carlotti DN *et al.* *Dermatophagoides farinae*-specific immunotherapy in atopic dogs with hypersensitivity to multiple allergens: a randomised, double blind, placebo-controlled study. *Vet J* 2009; 180: 337–342.
33. Singh SK, Dimri U, Saxena SK *et al.* Therapeutic management of canine atopic dermatitis by combination of pentoxifylline and PUFAs. *J Vet Pharmacol Ther* 2010; 33: 495–498.
34. Glos K, Linek M, Loewenstein C *et al.* The efficacy of commercially available veterinary diets recommended for dogs with atopic dermatitis. *Vet Dermatol* 2008; 19: 280–287.
35. Carlotti DN, Boulet M, Ducret J *et al.* The use of recombinant omega interferon therapy in canine atopic dermatitis: a double-blind controlled study. *Vet Dermatol* 2009; 20: 405–411.
36. Bensignor E, Morgan DM, Nuttall T. Efficacy of an essential fatty acid-enriched diet in managing canine atopic dermatitis: a randomized, single-blinded, cross-over study. *Vet Dermatol* 2008; 19: 156–162.
37. Plevnik A, Kobal S, Domanjko-Petric A *et al.* The efficacy of antihistamine fexofenadine versus methylprednisolone in the treatment of atopic dermatitis in dogs. *Slovenian Vet Res - Slovenski Veterinarski Zbornik* 2009; 46: 5–11.
38. Horvath-Ungerboeck C, Thoday KL, Shaw DJ *et al.* Tepoxalin reduces pruritus and modified CADESI-01 scores in dogs with atopic dermatitis: a prospective, randomized, double-blinded, placebo-controlled, cross-over study. *Vet Dermatol* 2009; 20: 233–242.
39. Kovalik M, Taszkun I, Pomorski Z *et al.* Evaluation of a human generic formulation of ciclosporin in the treatment of canine atopic dermatitis with *in vitro* assessment of the functional capacity of phagocytic cells. *Vet Rec* 2011; 168: 537–542.
40. Yasukawa K, Saito S, Kubo T *et al.* Low-dose recombinant canine interferon-γ for treatment of canine atopic dermatitis: an open randomized comparative trial of two doses. *Vet Dermatol* 2010; 21: 42–49.
41. Guyatt GH, Oxman AD, Vist GE *et al.* GRADE: an emerging consensus on rating quality of evidence and strength of recommendations. *BMJ* 2008; 336: 924–926.
42. Steffan J, Parks C, Seewald W *et al.* Clinical trial evaluating the efficacy and safety of cyclosporine in dogs with atopic dermatitis. *J Am Vet Med Assoc* 2005; 226: 1855–1863.
43. D'Agostino RB Sr, Massaro JM, Sullivan LM. Non-inferiority trials: design concepts and issues – the encounters of academic consultants in statistics. *Stat Med* 2003; 22: 169–186.
44. Hill P, Rybnicek J, Lau-Gillard P. Correlation between pruritus score and grossly visible erythema in dogs. *Vet Dermatol* 2010; 21: 450–455.
45. Favrot C, Linek M, Mueller R *et al.* Development of a questionnaire to assess the impact of atopic dermatitis on health-related quality of life of affected dogs and their owners. *Vet Dermatol* 2010; 21: 63–69.
46. Noli C, Colombo S, Cornegliani L *et al.* Quality of life of dogs with skin disease and of their owners. Part 2: administration of a questionnaire in various skin diseases and correlation to efficacy of therapy. *Vet Dermatol* 2011; 22: 344–351.

To cite this article, please use DOI: 10.1111/j.1365-3164.2012.01064.x

4.3

The effect of ketoconazole on whole blood and skin ciclosporin concentrations in dogs

Laura L. Gray*, Andrew Hillier*, Lynette K. Cole* and Päivi J. Rajala-Schultz†

Departments of *Veterinary Clinical Sciences and †Veterinary Preventive Medicine, College of Veterinary Medicine, The Ohio State University, Columbus, OH 43210, USA

Correspondence: Laura L. Gray, Department of Veterinary Clinical Sciences, College of Veterinary Medicine, The Ohio State University, 601 Vernon L. Tharp Street, Columbus, OH 43210, USA. E-mail: gray.704@osu.edu

Background – Ciclosporin (CSA) is approved for the treatment of canine atopic dermatitis. Ciclosporin is metabolized by liver cytochrome P450 enzymes, a process inhibited by ketoconazole (KTZ).

Hypothesis/Objectives – The aims of this study were to determine skin and blood CSA concentrations when CSA was administered alone at 5.0 (Treatment 1) or 2.5 mg/kg (Treatment 2) and when CSA was administered at 2.5 mg/kg concurrently with KTZ at 5 (Treatment 3) or 2.5 mg/kg (Treatment 4). We hypothesized that skin and blood CSA concentrations in Treatment 1 would not differ from those obtained with T3 or T4.

Animals – In a randomized cross-over study, six healthy research dogs received each of the treatments (Treatment 1, 2, 3 and 4) once daily for 7 days.

Methods – After the first, fourth and seventh dose for each treatment, a peak and trough skin punch biopsy sample and whole blood sample were collected and analysed with high-performance liquid chromatography–tandem mass spectrometry. Data were analysed using a repeated measures approach with PROC MIXED in SAS. Pairwise comparisons were performed with least squares means and Tukey–Kramer adjustment for multiple comparisons.

Results – Mean blood CSA concentrations in Treatment 1 were not different from those in Treatment 2 or 4, but were less than in Treatment 3. Mean skin CSA concentrations in Treatment 1 were greater than in Treatment 2, not different from those in Treatment 4, and less than those in Treatment 3.

Conclusions and clinical importance – Administration of CSA and KTZ concurrently at 2.5 mg/kg each may be as effective as CSA alone at 5.0 mg/kg for treatment of canine atopic dermatitis.

Introduction

Ciclosporin (CSA) is an immune-modulating drug currently labelled in the USA as Atopica® (Novartis Animal Health, Greensboro, NC, USA) for use in the treatment of canine atopic dermatitis (CAD).[1] As a calcineurin inhibitor, the primary mechanism of action of CSA is prevention of transcriptional activation of genes responsible for interleukin-2 production, a necessary step for full activation of the T-helper cell pathway.[2,3] The absence of interleukin-2 synthesis prevents the activation and proliferation of T cells, in addition to the secondary synthesis of cytokines involved in CAD, such as interleukin-4, interleukin-5, interleukin-8 and interferon-γ.[2] A systematic review and meta-analysis of 10 controlled clinical trials, enrolling approximately 800 dogs, provided strong evidence for the efficacy of CSA in the treatment of CAD and concluded that the efficacy of CSA was comparable to that of oral corticosteroids.[4] The clinically effective dose of CSA for the treatment of CAD has been determined to be 5 mg/kg orally once daily.[5,6] Treatment with CSA is typically maintained lifelong (as with all treatments for CAD), and 40–50% of dogs have continued control of their disease with every other day dosing at 5 mg/kg after 4–8 weeks of induction daily dosing.[4]

The cost of therapeutic agents as well as potential adverse effects are important factors for consideration, particularly when coupled with the fact that CAD commonly manifests at a young age and requires lifelong treatment. Long-term administration of Atopica® on a daily or every other day basis, particularly in medium-sized to large dogs, can be cost prohibitive. The cost of Atopica® was listed as a reason for discontinuing treatment in 10% (five of 51) of dogs with CAD being treated for at least 6 months in a study of long-term use of CSA.[7] The authors are not aware of any published studies assessing the effect of drug cost on owners' initial choice of therapy for their dog with CAD.

As the cost of Atopica® may be a limiting factor for its use, methods to reduce the dose of CSA without loss of clinical efficacy have been evaluated. Ciclosporin is

Accepted 21 March 2012

Sources of Funding: The Ohio State University, College of Veterinary Medicine, Canine Intramural Grant.

Conflict of Interest: Andrew Hillier is a speaker and consultant for Novartis Animal Health. No conflicts of interest have been declared for the other authors.

primarily metabolized in the liver by cytochrome P450 enzymes 2B11 and 3A12/26.[8,9] Consequently, research thus far has focused on pharmacotherapeutic manipulation of this enzyme system by co-administration of drugs known to be P450-enzyme inhibitors. Recent studies indicate that neither metoclopramide nor cimetidine, both P450 inhibitors, have any effect on the pharmacokinetic profile of concurrently administered CSA.[10,11] Grapefruit juice and powdered whole grapefruit may variably affect the pharmacokinetic parameters of CSA in dogs.[11,12]

Ketoconazole (KTZ) is a potent inhibitor of numerous cytochrome P450 enzymes, including CYP 2B11 and 3A12/26.[8,9] Numerous *in vitro* and *in vivo* studies have demonstrated that co-administration of KTZ with CSA results in increased whole blood CSA concentrations in dogs.[13–18] The inhibitory effect of KTZ on CSA clearance from blood was determined to be dose dependent, with the critical KTZ dosage range identified as 2.5–10 mg/kg daily.[18] A study on normal research beagles investigating the dose of KTZ necessary to maintain whole blood CSA trough levels between 400 and 600 mg/mL showed that KTZ at 13.6 mg/kg daily enabled a 75% reduction of CSA dose, with estimated monetary savings of 57.8% at that time, and KTZ at 4.7mg/kg daily reduced CSA dose by 38% and thus reduced cost by 23.8%.[14] These results have been applied clinically in studies on the efficacy of combination KTZ and CSA for the treatment of canine perianal fistulas, with excellent short-term results and a significant decrease in the dose of CSA required for clinical efficacy. One study involving 12 dogs with perianal fistulas showed that doses of KTZ between 5 and 11 mg/kg daily allowed a 50–75% dose reduction of CSA while maintaining target CSA trough levels, and all 12 dogs had at least short-term resolution of clinical signs.[16] This reduced dose equalled a monetary saving of 35–71% when compared with the cost of treatment with CSA alone. Further studies in dogs with perianal fistulas had concurring results; a dose of KTZ of 10 mg/kg daily allowed for an 80% reduction of CSA administration, and doses of KTZ of 5.3–8.9 mg/kg twice daily enabled a reduction of CSA dose equalling a monetary saving of 70% compared with CSA alone.[15,17]

As CSA is a lipophilic drug, it distributes widely in tissue and has been reported in the skin at concentrations up to 10 times higher than blood concentrations in humans.[19,20] An abstract of an unpublished study in dogs dosed with CSA at 3.8 mg/kg once daily for 14 days found that skin levels of CSA were 2.5–6.4 times higher than the whole blood CSA levels, and that depletion of CSA is slower from the skin than from the blood.[21] Studies examining tissue levels of CSA are sparse and are primarily toxicological or post-mortem studies.

Concurrent use of KTZ and CSA for treatment of CAD has been suggested by veterinary dermatologists at continuing education meetings in North America.[22–26] However, we are not aware of any published studies that have evaluated the effects of KTZ on CSA skin levels in dogs, or any published clinical trials of the efficacy of this combination of drugs for the treatment of CAD. The specific aims of this study were to determine skin and whole blood CSA concentrations when CSA was administered alone at a recommended (5.0 mg/kg/day) and a subtherapeutic dose (2.5 mg/kg/day) and when administered at a subtherapeutic dose (2.5 mg/kg/day) concurrently with KTZ at two different doses (2.5 or 5.0 mg/kg/day). We hypothesized that when CSA was administered alone at the recommended dose (5.0 mg/kg/day), the skin and whole blood CSA concentrations would not differ significantly from those obtained with subtherapeutic CSA dosing (2.5 mg/kg/day) concurrently with either dose (2.5 or 5.0 mg/kg/day) of KTZ.

Materials and methods

The experimental protocol was approved by the Institutional Animal Use and Care Committee (IACUC) of The Ohio State University.

Animals

Six clinically normal adult laboratory dogs (foxhounds) 1–4 years of age were used in this study. All dogs had complete blood counts and serum biochemical profiles prior to study enrolment. Dogs were housed in the laboratory research facility at the veterinary college and were under the care of the University Laboratory Animal Resources (ULAR) staff. The animals were housed indoors, in individual concrete runs, in a temperature- and humidity-controlled environment. They were maintained on a diet of Iams Mini Chunks (The Iams Company, Cincinnati, OH, USA) or Teklad 25% Lab Dog Diet (Harlan Laboratories, Indianapolis, IN, USA), fed once a day, with occasional dog treats, and water *ad libitum*. During the study periods, food was available from 14.00 to 07.30 h.

All treatments (CSA and CSA + KTZ) were administered at 09.30 h to comply with the Atopica® label recommendation that the drug should be administered at least 2 h before or after feeding because the bioavailability is better in fasted animals.[27] Vomiting for more than two consecutive dosing periods (48 h) was deemed a criterion for withdrawal from the study, as were signs of systemic illness (lethargy, fever, changes in complete blood counts or chemistry values above or below the reference range). Anti-emetics were not permitted because most of these agents are also metabolized by (or affect) the cytochrome P450 enzyme system.[11] The dogs were visually monitored daily, and any adverse events (including vomiting or diarrhoea/soft stool, as well as erythema, swelling or discharge from biopsy sites) were recorded. Biopsy sites that became infected were to be treated topically with chlorhexidine gluconate solution 2% (Phoenix™ Pharmaceutical Inc., St Joseph, MO, USA) and Triple antibiotic ointment® (E. Fougera and Co., Melville, NY, USA) twice daily until completion of the study period, and then with 5.0–10.0 mg/kg generic cefpodoxime (Proxetil Putney Inc., Portland, ME, USA) once daily until resolution of the infection. Antibiotic administration was not permitted during the study period to avoid increasing the likelihood of vomiting or diarrhoea.

Sample collection

Whole blood samples for CSA analysis (1.0 mL) were collected via cephalic, lateral saphenous or jugular venipuncture with a 22-gauge needle. The blood was placed into a lavender-topped tube (EDTA tube) and gently mixed, then transferred to Eppendorf tubes (VWR International, Radnor, PA, USA) and stored frozen at −80°C until analysis.

Skin samples were collected from the dorsal or dorsolateral neck. These sites were chosen for ease of access and maximal skin thickness for sample analysis. Local anaesthesia was performed by injecting 0.5 mL of 2% lidocaine (Butler Schein™ Animal Health, Dublin, OH, USA) subcutaneously with a 25-gauge needle. After 5 min, the skin sample was collected with an 8 mm biopsy punch (Medichoice® Tru Punch Disposable Biopsy Punch; Owens & Minor, Mechanicsville, VA, USA), and the site was closed with a single cruciate suture using 3–0 absorbable monofilament (3–0 PDS, Ethicon©; Novartis Animal Health, Greensboro, NC, USA). All subcutaneous tissue was trimmed from the skin sample, and the skin was placed in an Eppendorf tube and stored frozen at −80°C until analysis.

Study design

Prior to commencement of the study, whole blood and skin samples were taken for CSA analysis to ensure that each dog was beginning with CSA levels below the limit of detection. Completion of each of the four treatment periods detailed below was followed by a 14-day washout, at which time whole blood and skin samples were collected for CSA analysis to ensure that all CSA concentrations were below the level of detection prior to entering the next treatment period. Complete blood counts and serum biochemical profiles were performed on all dogs within 90 days prior to study enrollment, as well as prior to (day 0) and immediately following completion (day 8) of Treatments 3 and 4.

The six dogs were randomly assigned via a computer-generated list (using the dog's research number) into two groups of three dogs each. One group was administered CSA at 5 mg/kg orally once daily for 7 days (Treatment 1), and the other group was administered CSA at 2.5 mg/kg orally once daily for 7 days (Treatment 2). Ciclosporin was administered as Atopica®, which is available as 10, 25, 50 and 100 mg capsules. Combinations of these capsule sizes were used to dose the dogs as closely as possible to 2.5 and 5.0 mg/kg/day. After the first, fourth and seventh dose of CSA, a skin sample was collected at 4 h (estimated peak skin concentration) and at 24 h (estimated trough skin concentration) to determine skin CSA levels.[21] After the first, fourth and seventh dose of CSA, a whole blood sample was collected at 1.4 h (peak whole blood concentration) and at 24 h (trough whole blood concentration) to determine whole blood CSA levels.[28] Peak concentration samples were thus collected on days 1, 4 and 7, while trough concentration samples were collected on days 2, 5, and 8.

Following a 14-day washout period, the same two groups of three dogs were then randomly assigned to receive either CSA at 2.5 mg/kg and KTZ at 5.0 mg/kg orally once daily for 7 days (Treatment 3) or CSA at 2.5 mg/kg and KTZ at 2.5 mg/kg orally once daily for 7 days (Treatment 4). Ketoconazole (Teva, Sellersville, PA, USA) was administered in the generic form of 200 mg tablets (or part thereof) or as a compounded solution of the tablets per Trissel's formulary (prepared by the facility's pharmacy) in order to ensure dosing as close to 2.5 or 5.0 mg/kg as possible.[29] The compounded solution was not used for the 5.0 mg/kg KTZ dose owing to the large volume required. The CSA and the KTZ were administered concurrently. After the first, fourth and seventh dose of CSA and KTZ, a skin sample was collected at 4 h (estimated peak skin concentration) and at 24 h (estimated trough skin concentration) to determine skin tissue CSA levels. After the first, fourth and seventh dose of CSA and KTZ a whole blood sample was collected at 1.4 h (peak whole blood concentration) and at 24 h (trough whole blood concentration) to determine whole blood CSA levels. Peak concentration samples were thus collected on days 1, 4 and 7, while trough concentration samples were collected on days 2, 5 and 8.

Cross-over

After a 14-day washout period, the two groups of dogs then followed a full cross-over study design. Thus, at completion of the study each of the six dogs had received each of the four treatments in random order.

Ciclosporin analysis

Skin and whole blood samples were shipped overnight on dry ice to iC42 Bioanalytics (UC Denver, Denver, CO, USA) for analysis. Samples were shipped and analysed in two batches; the first sent halfway through the study and the second at study completion.

Ciclosporin in EDTA whole blood and tissue was quantified using high-performance liquid chromatography–tandem mass spectrometry (HPLC-MS/MS) following the procedures as previously described. [30] All tissues were weighed. Tissues were pulverized under liquid nitrogen, and 100 mg of the frozen tissue powder was measured into 1 mL of the 0.5 mol/L potassium phosphate buffer (pH 7.4) and homogenized. Homogenates were prepared as 200 μL aliquots for extraction.

For protein precipitation, 800 μL of $ZnSO_4{\cdot}7H_2O$ (17.28 g/L) in 30:70 (v/v) HPLC grade water/methanol containing the deuterated internal standard ciclosporin-D4 (50 ng/mL) was added to 200 μL aliquots of EDTA whole blood and tissue homogenates. Samples were vortexed for 2.5 min and then centrifuged at 13,000***g*** for 10 min at 4°C. The supernatant was transferred into glass HPLC vials for analysis.

The extracts were analysed using an LC/LC-MS/MS system (HPLC Agilent 1100 Series, Applied Biosystems and Sciex API 4000 triple quadruple mass spectrometer, Carlsbad, CA, USA). For on-line sample clean-up, 20 μL supernatant was loaded and cleaned on a 4.6 mm × 12.5 mm, 5 μm, Eclipse XDB-C8 column (Agilent, Santa Clara, CA, USA) using a mobile phase of 20% methanol and 80% 0.1% formic acid at a flow rate of 5 mL/min for 1 min. Then the column switching valve (Rheodyne, Cotati, CA,USA) was activated and the analytes were back-flushed onto the analytical column (4.6 mm × 150 mm, 5 μm, Eclipse Zorbax XDB -C8, Agilent), which was kept at 65°C. A gradient was used from 87% methanol and 13% 0.1% formic acid to 100% methanol in 2.0 min at a flow rate of 1mL/min and held at 100% for 1.5 min. The mass spectrometer was run in the positive MRM (multiple reaction monitoring) mode. The declustering potential (DP) was set to 131 V. Detection of the ions was performed by monitoring the transitions of *m/z* 1224.6 → 1112.4 for ciclosporin $[M+Na^+]$ and *m/z* 1228.6 → 1112.4 for the deuterated internal standard ciclosporin-D4 $[M+Na^+]$. The collision energy (CE) was 85 eV.

The lower limit of quantification for ciclosporin in EDTA whole blood was 5.0 ng/mL, and for tissues 25 ng/g (0.025 ng/mg). The assay was linear over three orders of magnitude. The interassay accuracy was between 85 and 115%, and total imprecision was ≤17%. There were no matrix interferences, carry-over or ion suppression. Both batches of samples were reported with assay specific quality control data and calculated interassay accuracy.

Sample size estimation

A pilot study with two dogs was performed prior to the study. Results from the pilot study were used for a power calculation, using a power of 80% and significance level of 0.05, which indicated that six dogs would be needed in order to detect a significant difference in CSA concentrations in skin using the trough value from day 8 between treatment groups 1 and 2. The preliminary data suggested that differences when comparing the additional treatment groups were greater, and would require less than six dogs to achieve statistical significance (Stata 10; Stata Corp., College Station, TX, USA).

Statistical analysis

Daily CSA blood and skin concentrations were considered the outcomes in the data analyses using a repeated measures approach with PROC MIXED in SAS (version 9.2; SAS Institute Inc., Cary, NC, USA). Compound symmetry covariance structure was used to account for the nonindependence of the repeated observations from individual dogs. The effects of day, treatment and order of treatments on skin and blood CSA concentrations were initially assessed and then treatment–day interaction was also tested. If the treatment–day interaction was significant, analyses were further stratified by treatment; and blood and skin CSA concentrations between the days were compared within each treatment, separately for days with presumed peak (days 1, 4 and 7) and trough values (days 2, 5 and 8). Pairwise comparisons between days and between treatments were performed by obtaining least squares means and using Tukey–Kramer adjustment to account for multiple comparisons. The correlation between skin CSA and blood CSA values was assessed using Spearman correlation coefficients. For all analyses, values of $P \leq 0.05$ were considered statistically significant.

Results

All treatments were administered as intended (Table 1) except for one dog (no. 38), that received medications in ~15 g (1 tablespoon) of canned food because the dog was resistant to manual pilling. The interassay accuracy of the CSA HPLC-MS/MS according to comparison with internal quality controls was reported for the two batches of samples, with each batch containing samples of skin and whole blood from all four treatment groups. The first batch analysis showed that blood CSA detection accuracy ranged from 98.3 to 104%, and skin accuracy ranged from 95.7 to 115%. The second batch showed that blood CSA detection accuracy ranged from 86.7 to 102%, and skin accuracy ranged from 93.6 to 117%. None of the skin and whole blood samples collected prior to entry into the study or prior to each treatment (following the 14-day washout period) had detectable levels of CSA.

Descriptive statistics for the measured (unadjusted) whole blood and skin CSA concentrations for all treatment groups by day are presented in Table 2. Using the repeated measures model and evaluating for fixed effects, the treatment (Treatment 1, 2, 3 or 4), the day (day 1, 2, 4, 5, 7, 8) and the treatment–day interaction each had a significant effect on skin and whole blood CSA concentrations (*F*-test, $P < 0.0001$). However, the order in which treatments were received did not have a significant effect on whole blood or skin CSA concentrations (*F*-test, $P = 0.854$ and *F*-test, $P = 0.756$, respectively).

The adjusted mean whole blood CSA concentration across all days for Treatment 1 (307.5 ng/mL) was not significantly different from the adjusted mean whole blood CSA concentration for Treatment 2 (169.41 ng/mL, Tukey–Kramer, $P = 0.14$) or Treatment 4 (417.74 ng/mL, Tukey–Kramer, $P = 0.136$), when evaluated with a mixed-model approach considering treatment, day and treatment–day interaction. However, the adjusted mean whole blood CSA concentration for Treatment 1 was significantly lower than the adjusted mean whole blood CSA concentration for Treatment 3 (644.83 ng/mL, Tukey–Kramer, $P = 0.0002$). The adjusted mean whole blood CSA concentration for Treatment 3 was significantly higher than the adjusted mean whole blood CSA concentration for Treatment 4 (Tukey–Kramer, $P = 0.0081$), and the adjusted mean whole blood CSA concentration for Treatment 2 was significantly lower than that for Treatments 3 and 4 (Tukey–Kramer, $P < 0.0001$ and $P = 0.0040$, respectively).

Utilizing least squares means obtained from the mixed models, the daily mean peak whole blood CSA concentrations did not differ significantly from each other within any treatment group (Table 3). Likewise, the daily mean trough whole blood CSA concentrations were not significantly different within Treatment 3; however, they were lower on day 2 compared with day 5 and on day 2 when compared with day 8 in Treatments 1, 2 and 4 (Table 3).

Using the mixed-model approach considering treatment, day and treatment–day interaction, the adjusted mean skin CSA concentration for Treatment 1 (0.61 ng/mg) was significantly higher than the adjusted mean skin CSA concentrations for Treatment 2 (0.262 ng/mg, Tukey–Kramer, $P = 0.05$), not significantly different from the adjusted mean skin CSA concentration for Treatment 4 (0.697 ng/mg, Tukey–Kramer, $P = 0.895$), but was significantly lower than the adjusted mean skin CSA concentration for Treatment 3 (1.236 ng/mg, Tukey–Kramer, $P = 0.0006$). The adjusted mean skin CSA concentration for Treatment 3 was also significantly higher than the adjusted mean skin CSA concentration for Treatment 4 (Tukey–Kramer, $P = 0.0024$), and the adjusted mean skin CSA concentration for Treatment 2 was significantly lower than that of Treatments 3 and 4 (Tukey–Kramer, $P < 0.0001$ and $P = 0.0129$, respectively).

Utilizing least squares means obtained from the mixed models, the mean daily peak skin CSA concentrations on day 4 were significantly higher than day 1 mean daily peak CSA concentrations in Treatments 1, 2 and 3, while day 7 mean daily peak CSA concentrations were significantly higher than those of day 1 within all four treatments (Table 4). The mean trough CSA concentrations on day 5 were significantly higher than those on day 2 for Treatments 1 and 4; day 8 mean trough CSA concentrations were significantly higher than day 2 mean trough CSA concentrations for Treatments 1, 2 and 4; and day 8 mean trough CSA concentrations were significantly higher than those of day 5 only for Treatment 4 (Table 4).

The correlation between whole blood and skin CSA concentrations combining values from all treatments was moderate (Spearman correlation coefficient, $r^2 = 0.6689$). The correlation of whole blood and skin CSA values within each treatment group were moderate for Treatments 1 and 2 (Spearman correlation coefficient of 0.786 and 0.6881, respectively) and for Treatments 3 and 4

Table 1. Target and measured dosage range of ciclosporin administered alone or in combination with ketoconazole to six healthy dogs

	Treatment 1 (mg/kg)	Treatment 2 (mg/kg)	Treatment 3 (mg/kg)	Treatment 4 (mg/kg)
Ciclosporin				
Target dosage	5.0	2.5	2.5	2.5
Administered dosage (range)	5.0–5.3	2.5–2.9	2.5–2.9	2.5–2.9
Ketoconazole				
Target dosage	—	—	5.0	2.5
Measured dosage (range)			5.0–5.3	2.5

Treatment 1, 5.0 mg/kg of ciclosporin (CSA) once daily; Treatment 2, 2.5 mg/kg of CSA once daily; Treatment 3, 2.5 mg/kg of CSA and 5.0 mg/kg of ketoconazole (KTZ) once daily; Treatment 4, 2.5 mg/kg of CSA and 2.5 mg/kg of KTZ once daily.

Table 2. Descriptive statistics for ciclosporin concentrations in whole blood and skin

	Day 1	Day 2	Day 4	Day 5	Day 7	Day 8
Treatment 1						
Blood	544 (0–895)	34.5 (0–73.2)	682.3 (447–798)	87.0 (44.4–199)	710 (191–160)	94.8 (47.9–182)
Skin	0.27 (0–0.53)	0.27 (0.54)	1.21 (0.78–1.96)	0.69 (0.33–1.03)	1.06 (0.84–1.32)	0.78 (0.39–1.19)
Treatment 2						
Blood	338.5 (144–422)	18.7 (10.3–33.5)	412 (309–553)	31.6 (14.6–57.5)	347 (53.1–586)	380 (112–814)
Skin	0.16 (0.12–0.25)	0.19 (0.08–0.61)	0.44 (0.26–0.66)	0.24 (0.12–0.41)	0.43 (0.25–0.59)	0.36 (0.16–0.75)
Treatment 3						
Blood	738.7 (371–1420)	699.9 (423–1470)	981.4 (22.2–2130)	249.9 (95.1–522)	1451.3 (848–1950)	392.7 (112–814)
Skin	0.48 (0.19–0.94)	0.37 (0.17–0.60)	1.68 (0.98–2.91)	1.16 (0.96–1.57)	2.37 (1.25–4.57)	2.59 (1.26–8.11)
Treatment 4						
Blood	821 (574–1010)	42.6 (21.7–65.9)	813.3 (151–1190)	102 (66.5–179)	1013.7 (710–1270)	131.6 (68.8–206)
Skin	0.36 (0.20–0.49)	0.30 (0.20–0.40)	0.84 (0.51–1.05)	0.82 (0.52–1.31)	1.37 (0.97–2.44)	1.18 (0.78–1.42)

Values are expressed as means (range). Blood concentrations are reported in nanograms per millilitre, whereas skin concentrations are reported in in nanograms per milligram. Days 1, 4 and 7 represent peaks, while days 2, 5 and 8 represent troughs.

Table 3. Least squares means obtained from the mixed models for daily peak and trough whole blood ciclosporin (CSA) concentrations for six healthy dogs

	Peak blood CSA			Trough blood CSA		
	Day 1	Day 4	Day 7	Day 2	Day 5	Day 8
Treatment 1	544.00	710.00	682.33	$34.47^{a,b}$	87.02^{a}	94.83^{b}
Treatment 2	338.50	412.00	347.02	$18.70^{c,d}$	31.63^{c}	38.02^{d}
Treatment 3	738.67	981.37	1451.33	699.93	249.85	392.67
Treatment 4	821.00	813.33	1013.67	$42.53^{e,f}$	101.98^{e}	131.63^{f}

Blood concentrations are reported in nanograms per millilitre. The same superscripts on the daily peak or trough values within a treatment indicate a significant difference between the days, with the Tukey–Kramer adjusted *P*-values given, as follows: $^{a}P = 0.003$, $^{b}P = 0.012$, $^{c}P = 0.011$, $^{d}P = 0.007$, $^{e}P = 0.0008$ and $^{f}P < 0.0001$.

Table 4. Least squares means obtained from the mixed models for daily peak and trough skin ciclosporin (CSA) concentrations for six healthy dogs

	Peak skin CSA			Trough skin CSA		
	Day 1	Day 4	Day 7	Day 2	Day 5	Day 8
Treatment 1	$0.27^{a,b}$	1.21^{a}	1.06^{b}	$0.27^{i,j}$	0.68^{i}	0.78^{j}
Treatment 2	$0.16^{c,d}$	0.44^{c}	0.43^{d}	0.19^{k}	0.24	0.36^{k}
Treatment 3	$0.48^{e,f}$	1.68^{e}	2.37^{f}	0.36	1.16	2.58
Treatment 4	0.36^{g}	0.84^{h}	$1.37^{g,h}$	$0.30^{l,m}$	$0.82^{l,n}$	$1.19^{m,n}$

Skin concentrations are reported in nanograms per milligram. The same superscripts on the daily peak or trough values within a treatment indicate a significant difference between the days, with the Tukey–Kramer adjusted *P*-values given, as follows: $^{a}P < 0.0001$, $^{b}P = 0.0001$, $^{c}P = 0.0008$, $^{d}P = 0.0011$, $^{e}P = 0.023$, $^{f}P = 0.0013$, $^{g}P = 0.0006$, $^{h}P = 0.035$, $^{i}P = 0.0010$, $^{j}P = 0.0002$, $^{k}P = 0.0083$, $^{l}P = 0.0002$, $^{m}P < 0.0001$ and $^{n}P = 0.0030$.

(Spearman correlation coefficient of 0.5623 and 0.5766, respectively).

One dog (no. 38) exhibited higher skin CSA concentrations than other animals, especially for the day-7 peak and day-8 trough of Treatment 3. Figures 1 and 2 show the whole blood CSA (Figure 1) and skin CSA concentrations (Figure 2) for dog no. 38 (red), as well as the concentrations for the other five dogs obtained during Treatment 3. Statistical significance was not affected by these values.

Adverse events

Chemistry profile values and complete blood counts for all dogs were within the normal reference range for the laboratory prior to study commencement and remained within the reference ranges following completion of Treatments 3 and 4. Gastrointestinal upset was the most commonly noted adverse event and was generally sporadic. Four of six dogs vomited during the study period; two dogs vomited once, one dog vomited three times, and one dog vomited four times. Only one dog (no. 97) vomited for two consecutive dosing periods (48 h) during Treatment 1, but did not continue vomiting and thus was not withdrawn from the study. Six of the nine vomiting episodes occurred during Treatment 1. Soft stool was reported from one dog on two occasions during Treatment 1, and two dogs experienced diarrhoea on four and five total separate occasions during Treatments 1, 3 and 4.

Discussion

In this study, we have established the skin concentrations of CSA that are achieved in normal research dogs when administered CSA at 5.0 and 2.5 mg/kg orally once daily,

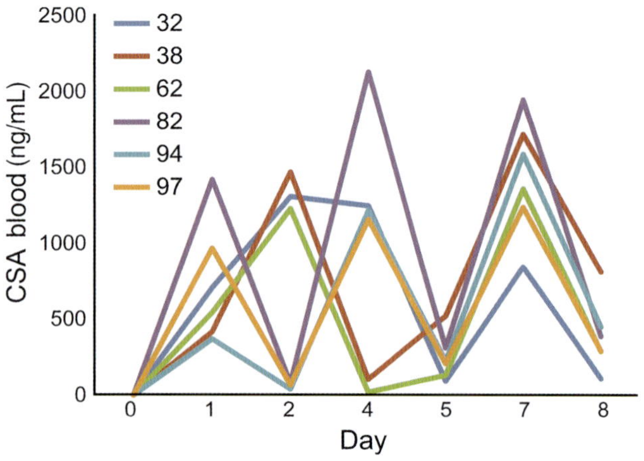

Figure 1. Ciclosporin (CSA) concentrations in whole blood for six healthy dogs (nos 32, 38, 62, 82, 94 and 97) treated with 2.5 mg/kg of CSA and 5.0 mg/kg of ketoconazole once daily (Treatment 3). Days 1, 4 and 7 represent peaks, while days 2, 5 and 8 represent troughs.

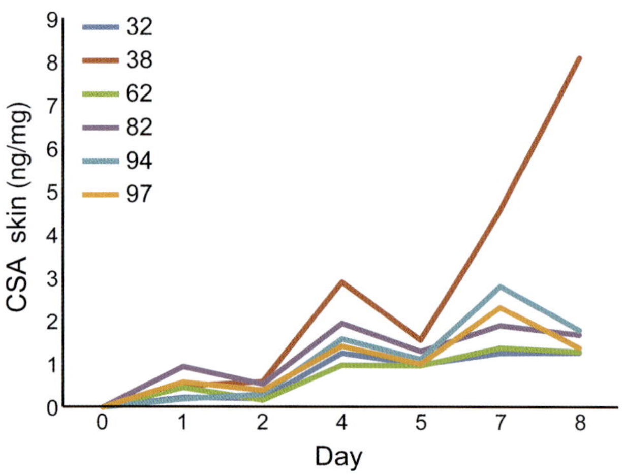

Figure 2. Ciclosporin concentrations in skin for six healthy dogs (nos 32, 38, 62, 82, 94 and 97) treated with 2.5 mg/kg of CSA and 5.0 mg/kg of ketoconazole once daily (Treatment 3). Days 1, 4 and 7 represent peaks, while days 2, 5 and 8 represent troughs.

as well as skin CSA concentrations achieved when CSA is administered at 2.5 mg/kg orally once daily with concurrent KTZ at either 2.5 or 5.0 mg/kg. The results from this study provide a baseline for comparison of CSA levels in skin and blood at two clinically relevant CSA dosages (5.0 and 2.5 mg/kg). They also provide evidence that concurrent administration of a CYP 450 inhibitor (KTZ) significantly elevates CSA levels in skin as well as blood.

Whole blood peak and trough concentrations of CSA when administered at 5.0 mg/kg in this study were within the range of those documented in previous studies.[10,28] Although 2 h blood CSA concentrations in humans are predictive of acute rejection and clinical outcome in solid organ transplantation, a study of 97 dogs with AD treated with CSA at a mean dose of 4.6 mg/kg orally once daily for 28 days found no significant correlation between clinical improvement and whole blood CSA concentrations.[27,28,31,32] As skin is likely to be the target organ for treatment of atopic dermatitis, the concentration of CSA achieved in the skin may be important in determining the clinical response to CSA therapy. This is further exemplified by the moderate correlation between skin and whole blood CSA concentrations in our study, which indicates that whole blood concentrations do not accurately predict CSA concentrations in the skin. Additionally, skin concentrations in Treatment 2, a dosage of CSA known to be ineffective for the control of CAD, were significantly lower than those found in Treatment 1.[6] The lack of significant difference in whole blood concentrations between Treatment groups 1 and 2 provides further support that skin concentrations may be more representative of the concentration of CSA required for clinical efficacy. Skin concentrations achieved in Treatment 4 were not different from those obtained in Treatment 1. It would be a fair expectation that clinically, treatment of CAD with either treatment regimen would yield similar results. Treatment 4 would offer a considerable (50%) reduction in cost of CSA administration. However, as it is not yet known whether skin CSA concentrations are correlated with clinical efficacy, identical treatment outcomes cannot be assumed and should be verified in atopic dogs. While Treatment group 1 establishes anticipated skin CSA concentrations, CSA concentrations in dogs clinically affected with CAD may differ from those found in research (normal) dogs, and may differ in clinically affected versus nonaffected skin. The skin levels established in this study were those found in the dorsal neck, which may differ from those sites typically affected by CAD, such as the inguinal and axillary regions, face, ears and ventral neck.

The highest CSA skin concentrations were obtained during Treatment 3, and were significantly higher than those found in both Treatment 1 and Treatment 4. If skin concentrations are in fact correlated with clinical efficacy, the higher CSA skin concentrations found with Treatment 3 may provide additional clinical effect for the control of CAD. However, it is possible that the degree of elevation of CSA paired with 5.0 mg/kg of KTZ may provide higher concentrations of CSA than necessary for control of CAD. Although the margin of safety for CSA administration in canines is much greater than that in humans, adverse effects from CSA have generally been observed to be dose dependent, supporting the importance of using the lowest effective dose. Although a recent retrospective analysis of the adverse effects of KTZ in dogs did not indicate that dose was a factor in the number or severity of adverse effects for KTZ, it has been shown that vomiting occurred more often with co-administration of CSA and KTZ.[7,33] Vomiting in the present study, however, occurred more frequently during Treatment 1. Additionally, inhibition of the CYP 450 enzymes by KTZ has been shown to be dose dependent, which was supported in the present study, with blood and skin CSA concentrations obtained in Treatment 3 being higher than those in Treatment 4.[18] As KTZ inhibition of CYP 450 can affect the metabolism of many other drugs and would be a lifelong therapeutic when paired with CSA for treatment of CAD, it may be important to use the lowest effective KTZ dose to limit the potential degree of interaction with other drugs.[9] Furthermore, it should be noted that in the present study, CSA and KTZ were administered for only 7 days, and the long-term effect of this drug combination on the whole blood and skin CSA concentrations is unknown.

The significant increases in mean skin CSA peaks on days 4 and 7 when compared with day 1, as well as significant increases in the mean skin CSA troughs on days 5 and 8 when compared with day 2, concur with previous studies indicating that CSA accumulates in skin after repeated administration.[34,35] It appears that skin CSA concentrations may have been approaching a steady state in Treatments 1, 2 and 3 after 7 days of drug administration, because there were no significant differences in the skin CSA concentration between days 4 and 7, or between days 5 and 8. However, this does not appear to be the case in Treatment 4, where day 4 peak skin CSA concentrations were significantly less than those on day 7, and day 5 trough skin CSA concentrations were significantly less than those on day 8. Further studies on CSA skin concentration after continuous daily treatment for more than 7 days are necessary in order to establish accurately when true skin CSA steady state is achieved. The accumulation or storage of CSA in skin may be a factor explaining why every other day or even every 3 day administration of CSA can control signs of CAD, and may be associated with the time of drug administration required to observe a clinical effect for treatment of CAD. As CSA does accumulate in the skin with repeated administration and the skin is not a true compartment for drug distribution when considering pharmacokinetics, it is unlikely that skin CSA levels have a clearly defined peak or time of maximal concentration. The time of maximal concentration is likely to be variable, depending on the duration of treatment, dose, co-administration of drugs affecting CSA metabolism (such as KTZ) and individual patient factors. Four hours was chosen as an estimated time for peak skin CSA concentration in this study based on previous reports.[21,35]

The degree of interindividual variability in whole blood CSA concentrations was comparable to those reported in previous studies.[10,28] Interindividual variation in whole blood CSA concentrations is a well-recognized phenomenon in humans and is associated with a variety of factors, such as age, race and comorbidities.[36] The genetic expression of a functional polymorphism of the CYP 450 enzyme responsible for CSA metabolism as well as *ABCB1* genotypes have been the focus of recent research on the interindividual variation of CSA concentration in humans.[37–39] *ABCB1* genotypes are important because CSA is a substrate of the P-glycoprotein system. *ABCB1* genetic polymorphisms have been identified in dogs, although not in the context of CSA administration.[40,41] One dog (no. 38) did have very high skin CSA concentrations, particularly during Treatment 3, even though this dog's blood CSA concentrations taken at the same time point fell within the normal range. Interestingly, this is the dog that received medications in a small amount of food (owing to difficulty in administration of the oral medications), which has been shown to increase variability in CSA concentrations.[28] However, there is no obvious explanation for why only the skin CSA concentrations were so significantly elevated, with a normal blood CSA concentration. It is possible that certain dogs may accumulate CSA in their skin at higher than expected levels, which could be correlated with the degree of clinical efficacy, the time taken to see clinical effect, the ability to reduce CSA dosing or adverse effects.

In conclusion, in the present study we have established skin CSA concentrations in normal research dogs when administered CSA at 5.0 mg/kg/day, the known therapeutic dose for treatment of CAD, and at 2.5 mg/kg/day, a known subtherapeutic dose for treatment of CAD. Additionally, skin and whole blood CSA concentrations when 2.5 mg/kg/day of CSA was administered with 2.5 or 5.0 mg/kg of KTZ were established. As there was no significant difference in mean blood or skin CSA concentrations when CSA was dosed at 5.0 mg/kg once daily (Treatment 1) when compared with CSA dosed at 2.5 mg/kg once daily with 2.5 mg/kg of KTZ once daily (Treatment 4), it is anticipated that administration of CSA and KTZ concurrently at 2.5 mg/kg/day may be as effective as CSA alone at 5.0 mg/kg/day for treatment of CAD. As the highest skin CSA concentrations were achieved with CSA dosed at 2.5 mg/kg concurrently with KTZ at 5 mg/kg, the possibility that this dosing regimen may translate into increased clinical efficacy in the treatment of CAD deserves further investigation. However, this dosing regimen may result in higher levels of CSA than needed for control of CAD, and caution is warranted because this combination of CSA and KTZ was also associated with significantly higher whole blood CSA concentrations, which may result in increased risk of adverse effects.

Acknowledgements

The authors would like to thank Wendy Lorch, Natalie Tabacca and Michele Fox for their assistance and support.

References

1. Animal Health, US, Inc. Atopica® (Cyclosporine capsules, USP) modified [package insert]. Greensboro, NC: Novartis Animal Health, US, Inc., 2008. NADA 141–218.
2. Matsuda S, Koyasu S. Mechanisms of action of cyclosporine. *Immunopharmacology* 2000; 47: 119–125.
3. Ferraccioli GF, Tomietto P, De Santis M. Rationale for T cell inhibition by cyclosporin A in major autoimmune diseases. *Ann N Y Acad Sci* 2005; 1051: 658–665.
4. Steffan J, Favrot C, Mueller R. A systematic review and meta-analysis of the efficacy and safety of cyclosporin for the treatment of atopic dermatitis in dogs. *Vet Dermatol* 2006; 17: 3–16.
5. Steffan J, Alexander D, Brovedani F *et al.* Comparison of cyclosporine A with methylprednisolone for treatment of canine atopic dermatitis: a parallel, blinded, randomized controlled trial. *Vet Dermatol* 2003; 14: 11–22.
6. Olivry T, Steffan J, Fisch RD *et al.* Randomized controlled trial of the efficacy of cyclosporine in the treatment of atopic dermatitis in dogs. *J Am Vet Med Assoc* 2002; 221: 370–377.
7. Radowicz SN, Power HT. Long-term use of cyclosporine in the treatment of canine atopic dermatitis. *Vet Dermatol* 2005; 16: 81–86.
8. Kuroha M, Kuze Y, Shimoda M *et al.* In vitro characterization of the inhibitory effects of ketoconazole on metabolic activities of cytochrome P-450 in canine hepatic microsomes. *Am J Vet Res* 2002; 63: 900–905.

9. Aidasani D, Zaya MJ, Malpas PB *et al.* In vitro drug-drug interaction screens for canine veterinary medicines: evaluation of cytochrome P450 reversible inhibition. *Drug Metab Dispos* 2008; 36: 1512–1518.
10. Daigle JC, Hosgood G, Foil CS *et al.* Effect of cimetidine on pharmacokinetics of orally administered cyclosporine in healthy dogs. *Am J Vet Res* 2001; 62: 1046–1050.
11. Radwanski NE, Cerundolo R, Shofer FS *et al.* Effects of powdered whole grapefruit and metoclopramide on the pharmacokinetics of cyclosporine in dogs. *Am J Vet Res* 2011; 72: 687–693.
12. Amatori FM, Meucci V, Giusiani M *et al.* Effects of grapefruit juice on the pharmacokinetics of cyclosporine in dogs. *Vet Rec* 2004; 154: 180–181.
13. D'mello A, Venkataramanan R, Satake M *et al.* Pharmacokinteics of the cyclosproine-ketoconazole interaction in dogs. *Res Commun Chem Pathol Pharmacol* 1989; 64: 441–454.
14. Dahlinger J, Gregory C, Bea J. Effect of ketoconazole on cyclosporine dose in healthy dogs. *Vet Surg* 1998; 27: 64–68.
15. Mouatt JG. Cyclosporin and ketoconazole interaction for treatment of perianal fistulas in the dog. *Aust Vet J* 2002; 80: 207–211.
16. Patricelli AJ, Hardie RJ, McAnulty JF. Cyclosporine and ketoconazole for the treatment of perianal fistulas in dogs. *J Am Vet Med Assoc* 2002; 220: 1009–1016.
17. O'Neill T, Edwards GA, Holloway S. Efficacy of combined cyclosporine A and ketoconazole treatment of anal furunculosis. *J Small Anim Pract* 2004; 45: 238–243.
18. Myre SA, Schoeder TJ, Grund VR *et al.* Critical ketoconazole dosage range for ciclosporin clearance inhibition in the dog. *Pharmacology* 1991; 43: 233–241.
19. Fisher GJ, Duell EA, Nickoloff BJ *et al.* Levels of cyclosporin in epidermis of treated psoriasis patients differentially inhibit growth of keratinocytes cultured in serum free versus serum containing media. *J Invest Dermatol* 1988; 91: 142–146.
20. Ellis CN, Fradin MS, Messana JM *et al.* Cyclosporine for plaque-type psoriasis. *New Eng J Med* 1991; 324: 277–284.
21. Steffan J, Maurer M, Rohlfs A. Cyclosporine concentration in the skin following oral administration, in *Proceedings. 18th Ann ESVD-ECVD Cong* 2002; 222.
22. Yu A. Dermatologic pearls: what's new in the diagnosis and treatment of skin disease, *in Proceedings. 80th Annu West Vet Conf*, V78, 2008, Available at: http://www.vin.com/Members/proceedings/Proceedings.plx?CID=WVC2008&Category=3183&PID=19908&O=VIN. Accessed April 7, 2012.
23. Ihrke P. The management of canine atopic dermatitis, in *Proceedings. Can Med Symp* 2009, Available at: http://www.vin.com/Members/Proceedings/Proceedings.plx?CID=UCDCMC2009&Category=&PID=32508&O=VIN. Accessed April 7, 2012.
24. MacDonald J. Treating the atopic dog: options to keep the pet owner happy, in *Proceedings. Atlantic Coast Vet Conf* 2007, Available at: http://www.vin.com/Members/Proceedings/Proceedings.plx?CID=ACVC2007&Category=&PID=19052&O=VIN. Accessed April 7, 2012.
25. Merchant S. Diagnosis and management of the pruitic dog, in *Proceedings. Atlantic Coast Vet Conf* 2009, Available at: http://www.vin.com/Members/Proceedings/Proceedings.plx?CID=acvc2009&PID=pr53372&O=VIN. Accessed April 7, 2012.
26. Marsella R. Medical management of pruritus: non-specifictherapy for management of the pruritic dog or cat, in *Proceedings. Atlantic Coast Vet Conf* 2008, Available at: http://www.vin.com/Members/proceedings/Proceedings.plx?CID=ACVC2008&Category=&PID=25941&O=VIN. Accessed April 7, 2012.
27. Lindholm A, Kahan BD. Influence of cyclosporine pharmacokinetics, trough concentrations, and AUC monitoring on outcome after kidney transplantation. *Clin Pharmacol Ther* 1993; 54: 205–218.
28. Steffan J, Strehlau G, Maurer M *et al.* Cyclosporin A pharmacokinetics and efficacy in the treatment of atopic dermatitis in dogs. *J Vet Pharmacol Ther* 2004; 27: 231–238.
29. Trissel LA. Trissel's stability of compounded formulations. In: *Trissel's Stability of Compounded Formulations.* 2nd edn. Washington, DC: American Pharmacists Association, 2000;206–207.
30. Christians U, Jacobsen W, Serkova N *et al.* Automated, fast and sensitive quantification of drugs in blood by liquid chromatography–mass spectrometry with on-line extraction: immunosuppressants. *J Chromatog B Biomed Sci Appl* 2000; 748: 41–53.
31. Levy G, Burra P, Cavallari A *et al.* Improved clinical outcomes for liver transplant recipients using cyclosporine monitoring based on 2-hr post-dose levels (C2)1. *Transplantation* 2002; 73: 953–959.
32. Pollard SG. Pharmacologic monitoring and outcomes of cyclosporine. *Transplant Proc* 2004; 36: S404–S407.
33. Mayer UK, Glos K, Schmid M *et al.* Adverse effects of ketoconazole in dogs – a retrospective study. *Vet Dermatol* 2008; 19: 199–208.
34. Niederberger W. Distribution and binding of cyclosporine in blood and tissues. *Transplant Proc* 1983; 15: 2419–2421.
35. Wagner O, Shcreier E, Heitz F *et al.* Tissue distribution, disposition, and metabolism of cyclosporine in rats. *Am Soc Pharmacol Exp Ther* 1987; 15: 377–385.
36. Pollard SG, Nashan B, Johnston A *et al.* A pharmacokinetic and clinical review of the potential clinical impact of using different formulations of cyclosporin A. *Clin Ther* 2003; 25: 1654–1669.
37. Cattaneo D, Ruggenenti P, Baldelli S *et al. ABCB1* genotypes predict cyclosporine-related adverse events and kidney allograft outcome. *J Am Soc Nephrol* 2009; 20: 1404–1415.
38. Zhu HJ, Yuan SH, Fang Y *et al.* The effect of CYP3A5 polymorphism on dose-adjusted cyclosporine concentration in renal transplant recipients: a meta-analysis. *Pharmacogenomics J* 2011; 11: 237–246.
39. Anglicheau D. CYP3A5 and MDR1 genetic polymorphisms and cyclosporine pharmacokinetics after renal transplantation. *Clin Pharmacol Ther* 2004; 75: 422–433.
40. Mealey KL. Therapeutic implications of the MDR-1 gene. *J Vet Pharmacol Ther* 2004; 27: 257–264.
41. Culmsee K, Gruber AD, von Samson-Himmelstjerna G *et al.* Quantification of MDR-1 gene expression in canine tissues by real-time reverse transcription quantitative polymerase chain reaction. *Res Vet Sci* 2004; 77: 223–229.

To cite this article, please use DOI: 10.1111/j.1365-3164.2012.01103.x

4.4

In vitro antiseptic susceptibilities for *Staphylococcus pseudintermedius* isolated from canine superficial pyoderma in Japan

Nobuo Murayama*, Masahiko Nagata*, Yuri Terada*, Mio Okuaki*, Noriyuki Takemura†, Hidemasa Nakaminami† and Norihisa Noguchi†

*ASC Dermatology Service, 1-3-2 Jindaijihigashi Chofu, Tokyo 182-0012, Japan
†Department of Microbiology, School of Pharmacy, Tokyo University of Pharmacy and Life Sciences, 1432-1 Horinouchi Hachioji, Tokyo 192-0932, Japan

Correspondence: Nobuo Murayama, ASC Dermatology Service, 1-3-2 Jindaijihigashi Chofu, Tokyo 182-0012, Japan. E-mail: muragon@d1.dion.ne.jp

Background – Topical therapy, particularly with chlorhexidine, is becoming increasingly common as a treatment option for canine pyoderma; however, there are limited studies on the susceptibility of *Staphylococcus pseudintermedius* to chlorhexidine compounds.

Objectives – To determine the *in vitro* susceptibility of both meticillin-resistant and meticillin-susceptible *S. pseudintermedius* isolates to chlorhexidine and other antiseptic agents and the presence of multidrug efflux pump genes.

Samples – One hundred *S. pseudintermedius* isolates from 23 initial and 77 recurrent cases of canine pyoderma.

Methods – After bacterial identification and *mecA* testing, minimal inhibitory concentrations (MICs) of antiseptic agents were determined. Multidrug efflux pump genes, including *qacA*, *qacB* and *smr*, were identified.

Results – Of the 100 isolates, 57 were identified as meticillin-resistant *S. pseudintermedius*. The MIC_{90} of chlorhexidine acetate, chlorhexidine gluconate, acriflavine, ethidium bromide and benzalkonium chloride were 1, 1, 2, 0.5 and 2 μg/mL, respectively. Multidrug efflux pump genes *qacA*, *qacB* and *smr* were not detected in any of the isolates.

Conclusions and clinical importance – The MICs for chlorhexidine and other antiseptics remain low, and multidrug efflux pump genes were not found in the tested isolates.

Introduction

Canine superficial pyoderma is a common skin disease of dogs, and the primary pathogen is *Staphylococcus pseudintermedius*.[1] In addition to addressing the underlying cause, treatment of superficial pyoderma includes the use of systemic antimicrobials and topical therapy. Following the emergence of multidrug-resistant *mecA*-positive *S. pseudintermedius*, there has been increased interest in the use of topical antiseptics as sole or adjuvant therapy. In previous studies, we demonstrated the efficacy of 2% chlorhexidine acetate (Nolvasan® Surgical Scrub; Fort Dodge Animal Health, Fort Dodge, IA, USA) as monotherapy for canine superficial pyoderma associated with meticillin-resistant (MR) *S. pseudintermedius* group (SIG), but not in all cases.[2–4] In those studies, 2–4% chlorhexidine acetate resulted in a positive clinical response in 60–70% of the dogs.[2–4] In humans, there are reports of topical treatment with chlorhexidine not being successful in eliminating meticillin-resistant *Staphylococcus aureus* (MRSA),[5] and a low level of resistance to chlorhexidine is a concern.[6] A possible explanation is the existence of multidrug efflux pump genes, which have been detected in *S. aureus* isolates, that confer resistance to antiseptic agents, including chlorhexidine, quaternary ammonium compounds (e.g. benzalkonium chloride) and dyes (e.g. acriflavine and ethidium bromide).[7–10] The aims of this study were to assess the *in vitro* susceptibilities of both meticillin-resistant and meticillin-susceptible (MS) *S. pseudintermedius* to chlorhexidine acetate, as well as other antiseptics, and to determine whether multidrug efflux pump genes (*qacA*, *qacB* and *smr*) were present.

Accepted 10 July 2012
Sources of Funding: This study was self-funded.
Conflict of Interest: No conflicts of interest have been declared.

Materials and methods

Bacterial isolates

One hundred clinical isolates were obtained from dogs with either a first occurrence of pyoderma (n = 23) or recurrent pyoderma (n = 77) between May 2009 and September 2010. Samples were collected from dogs presented to the ASC Dermatology Service, Tokyo, Japan. These samples have been used in previous studies.[2–4] Pyoderma was confirmed based on clinical signs, cytological findings and bacterial culture. Samples for bacterial culture and susceptibility testing were collected from skin lesions compatible with pyoderma. Swabs (Sterile BBL CultureSwab; Becton, Dickinson and Co., Franklin Lakes, NJ, USA) were rubbed vigorously against the sampling site and stored at 4°C, and were processed within 7 days. Each swab was inoculated onto blood agar (Nissui Pharmaceutical Co., Ltd, Tokyo, Japan) and mannitol salt agar (Nissui Pharmaceutical Co., Ltd), and incubated aerobically at 37°C for 18–24 h. Staphylococcal isolates were putatively identified using colony morphology, the ability to grow on mannitol salt agar, Gram-stain characteristics and coagulase reaction. The strains were stored in skimmed milk at −80°C until further use.

Identification of *S. pseudintermedius*

Bacterial speciation was performed as previously described using a multiplex PCR method.[11] (See Table S1 in Supplementary material for primers).

Determination of meticillin resistance by detection of *mecA*

Primers for *mecA* PCRs, mA1 (5′-TGCTATCCACCCTCAAACAGG-3′) and mA2 (5′-AACGTTGTAACCACCCCAAGA-3′), were used in the present study with a previously published method.[12] All results were confirmed by at least two independent experiments.

Antimicrobial and antiseptic susceptibility testing

Antimicrobial susceptibility testing was used to identify MR and MS staphylococci. The minimal inhibitory concentrations (MICs) of antimicrobial and antiseptic agents were determined by the standard agar plate dilution method according to the Clinical and Laboratory Standards Institute (CLSI) document M31-A3.[13] Isolates with a MIC for oxacillin ≥0.5 μg/mL or positive for *mecA* by PCR were regarded as MR strains.[14] The antiseptic agents tested included chlorhexidine acetate and chlorhexidine gluconate, acriflavine, ethidium bromide and benzalkonium chloride.

Determination of multidrug efflux pump genes, including *qacA*, *qacB* and *smr*

A search for *qacA/B* and *smr* genes was performed by multiple PCRs with the following sets of primers: 5′-GCAGAAAGTGCAGAGTTCG-3′ and 5′-CCAGTCCAATCAGCCTG-3′ for *qacA/B* (product size 361 bp);[15] and 5′-GCCATAAGTACTGAAGTTATTGGA-3′ and 5′-GACTACGGTTGTTAAGACTAAACCT-3′ for *smr* (product size 195 bp).[16] The PCR assays were performed using the modified colony direct method described by Tsuchizaki *et al.*[17] *Staphylococcus aureus* JCM16555 (TS77) in *qacA/B* and *S. aureus* JCM16554 (L20A) in *smr* were used as reference strains in the phenotypic and genotypic tests. All results were confirmed by at least two independent experiments.

Statistical analysis

The chi-square test was used to analyse differences between *mecA* presence in initial and recurrent cases. Noncontinuous and categorical, matched-pair Mann–Whitney *U*-tests were used to analyse differences in susceptibility to chlorhexidine between *mecA*-positive and *mecA*-negative *S. pseudintermedius*. Values of $P < 0.05$ were considered statistically significant. All analyses were performed using the software package Stata® version 11 (StataCorp LP, College Station, TX, USA).

Results

Species identification and detection of *mecA*

All 100 isolates were identified as *S. pseudintermedius*. Of these, 57 of 100 were *mecA* positive. The *mecA* was detected in 13 isolates from 23 dogs with first-time pyoderma and in 44 of 77 isolates from dogs with recurrent pyoderma. There was no significant difference between *mecA* presence in initial and recurrent cases ($P = 0.96$).

Antiseptic susceptibility testing

The MICs of antiseptic agents are shown in Table 1. The MIC_{90} of chlorhexidine acetate, chlorhexidine gluconate, acriflavine, ethidium bromide and benzalkonium chloride was 1, 1, 2, 0.5 and 2 μg/mL, respectively, for all 100 isolates. There were no significant differences in MICs of chlorhexidine acetate ($P = 0.32$) and chlorhexidine gluconate ($P = 0.54$) between *mecA*-positive and *mecA*-negative *S. pseudintermedius*. (See Table S2 in Supplementary material for details of antimicrobial susceptibility testing for the 100 isolates).

Detection of multidrug efflux pump genes

Multidrug efflux pump genes, including *qacA*, *qacB* and *smr*, were not detected in any isolates.

Discussion

Staphylococcus aureus can develop antiseptic resistance by multidrug efflux pumps in the bacterial cell membrane, which are encoded by some antiseptic resistance genes.[7–10] Two major groups of resistance genes, one group including *qacA* and *qacB* and another including *smr*, which is identical to *qacC*, *qacC9*, *qacD* or *ebr*, are associated with high-level and low-level resistance to antiseptics, respectively.[8] The multidrug efflux pump genes are more frequently isolated in MRSA than in MS *S. aureus* (MSSA).[18,19] Apart from *S. aureus* strains isolated from humans, multidrug efflux pump genes have been found in equine, bovine and feline staphylococcal strains, as well as in staphylococcal strains from unpasteurized milk from dairy cattle and dairy goat herds.[20–23] In the present study, *qacA*, *qacB* and *smr* were evaluated in 100 isolates of *S. pseudintermedius* from dogs, and none of these efflux pump genes was identified in either MS or MR *S. pseudintermedius*. Of the strains, 57 of 100 were *mecA*-positive and 50 of 57 were multidrug-resistant, i.e. they were resistant to at least three classes of antimicrobials in addition to the β-lactams (see Table S2 in Supplementary material).

Table 1. Minimal inhibitory concentrations (MICs) of antiseptic agents for meticillin-susceptible *Staphylococcus pseudintermedius* (MSSP) and meticillin-resistant *S. pseudintermedius* (MRSP) strains

	CHA		CHG		AF		EB		BKC	
MIC (μg/ml)	MSSP (*n*)	MRSP (*n*)	MSSP (*n*)	MRSP (*n*)	MSSP (*n*)	MRSP (*n*)	MSSP (*n*)	MRSP (*n*)	MSSP (*n*)	MRSP (*n*)
0.5	23	26	19	21	31	28	43	57	0	0
1	18	25	22	34	6	18	0	0	1	18
2	2	4	0	2	6	11	0	0	40	32
4	0	2	2	0	0	0	0	0	2	7

Abbreviations: AF, acriflavine; BKC, benzalkonium chloride; CHA, chlorhexidine acetate; CHG, chlorhexidine gluconate; EB, ethidium bromide.

One of the most commonly used topical antiseptics in small animal dermatology is chlorhexidine. The MICs of chlorhexidine are reportedly different in MRSA and MSSA, although no MIC standardization for chlorhexidine has yet been proposed.[24] The MIC of chlorhexidine for MSSA is considered to be 1 μg/mL,[7] but other sources cite 4 in MRSA or 8 μg/mL in MSSA.[25,26] In the present study, four isolates had a MIC of 4 μg/mL for chlorhexidine, although MIC standardization for chlorhexidine has yet to be proposed for *S. pseudintermedius*. Previous studies have shown that 2–4% chlorhexidine is an effective treatment for superficial pyoderma in some, but not all, dogs.[2–4,27] There are a number of possible explanations for discrepancies between *in vivo* antiseptic efficacy and *in vitro* susceptibility. Chlorhexidine might not have good penetration into the skin. Its concentration at 100 μm depth following 2 and 30 min exposure to human skin was reportedly 0.157 ± 0.047 and 0.077 ± 0.015 μg/mg, respectively.[28] Thus chlorhexidine might fail to reach the deeper skin layers and the hair follicles. Another explanation for lack of response may be related to biofilm development, which has been found in cases of *S. aureus* impetigo and furuncles in humans.[29] *Staphylococcus aureus* within a biofilm reportedly decreases the efficacy of chlorhexidine as a disinfectant.[30] A recent report suggests that *S. pseudintermedius* has the potential to form a biofilm.[31] Another explanation could be related to the fact that organic matter decreases the efficacy of disinfectants, including chlorhexidine.[32] In the case of skin disease, it might be less efficacious due to poor penetration into papules, pustules, crusts and/or exudate. Prewashing patients to remove gross debris may increase its efficacy. Finally, the most important factors for unsuccessful topical therapy are likely to be a lack of owner compliance and underlying or concurrent primary skin diseases which favour the persistence of pyoderma.[33] Further investigation will be warranted to identify whether clinical chlorhexidine resistance exists in some dogs with pyoderma.

References

1. Sasaki T, Kikuchi K, Tanaka Y *et al.* Reclassification of phenotypically identified *Staphylococcus intermedius* strains. *J Clin Microbiol* 2007; 45: 2770–2778.
2. Nagata M, Murayama N, Shibata K. Efficacy of Nolvasan Surgical Scrub containing 2% chlorhexidine acetate in topical management of canine superficial pyoderma: a randomized, double-blinded, controlled study. *Jpn J Vet Dermatol* 2006; 12: 1–6.
3. Murayama N, Nagata M, Terada Y *et al.* Efficacy of a surgical scrub including 2% chlorhexidine acetate for canine superficial pyoderma. *Vet Dermatol* 2010; 21: 586–592.
4. Murayama N, Terada Y, Okuaki M *et al.* Dose assessment of 2% chlorhexidine acetate for canine superficial pyoderma. *Vet Dermatol* 2011; 22: 449–453.
5. Pearman JW, Christiansen KJ, Annear DI *et al.* Control of methicillin-resistant *Staphylococcus aureus* (MRSA) in an Australian metropolitan teaching hospital complex. *Med J Aust* 1985; 21: 103–108.
6. Lee AS, Macedo-Vinas M, Francois P *et al.* Impact of combined low-level mupirocin and genotypic chlorhexidine resistance on persistent methicillin-resistant *Staphylococus aureus* carriage after decolonization: a case-control study. *Clin Infect Dis* 2011; 52: 1422–1430.
7. McDonnell G, Russell AD. Antiseptic and disinfectants: activity, action, and resistance. *Clin Microbiol Rev* 1999; 12: 147–179.
8. Alam MH, Kobayashi N, Uehara N *et al.* Analysis on distribution and genomic diversity of high-level antiseptic resistance genes *qacA* and *qacB* in human clinical isolates of *Staphylococcus aureus*. *Microb Drug Resist* 2003; 9: 109–121.
9. Mitchell BA, Brown MH, Skurray R. *QacA* multidrug efflux pump from *Staphylococcus aureus*: comparative analysis of resistance to diamidines, biguanidines, and guanylhydrazones. *Antimicrob Agents Chemother* 1998; 42: 475–477.
10. Tennent JM, Lyon BR, Midgley M *et al.* Physical and biochemical characterization of the *qacA* gene encoding antiseptic and disinfectant resistance in *Staphylococcus aureus*. *J Gen Microbiol* 1989; 135: 1–10.
11. Sasaki T, Tsubakishita S, Tanaka Y *et al.* Multiplex-PCR method for species identification of coagulase-positive staphylococci. *J Clin Microbiol* 2010; 48: 765–769.
12. Kawakami T, Shibata S, Murayama N *et al.* Antimicrobial susceptibility and methicillin resistance in *Staphylococcus pseudintermedius* and *Staphylococcus schleiferi* subsp. *coagulans* isolated from dogs with pyoderma. *J Vet Med Sci* 2010; 72: 1615–1619.
13. Clinical and Laboratory Standards Institute. *Performance Standards for Antimicrobial Disk and Dilution Susceptibility Tests for Bacteria Isolated From Animals; Approved Standard*, 3rd edition. CLSI document M31-A3 Wayne, PA: CLSI, 2008.
14. Papich MG. Proposed changes to clinical laboratory standards institute interpretive criteria for methicillin-resistant *Staphylococcus pseudintermedius* isolated from dogs. *J Vet Diagn Invest* 2010; 22: 160.
15. Rouch DA, Cram DS, DiBerardino D *et al.* Efflux-mediated antiseptic gene *qacA* from *Staphylococcus aureus*: common ancestry with tetracycline- and sugar-transport proteins. *Mol Microbiol* 1990; 4: 2051–2062.
16. Sasatsu M, Shima K, Shibata Y *et al.* Nucleotide sequence of a gene that encodes resistance to ethidium bromide from a transferable plasmid in *Staphylococcus aureus*. *Nucleic Acids Res* 1989; 17: 10103.
17. Tsuchizaki N, Ishikawa J, Hotta K. Colony PCR for rapid detection of antibiotic resistance genes in MRSA and enterococci. *Jpn J Antibiot* 2000; 53: 422–439.
18. Mayer S, Boos M, Beyer A *et al.* Distribution of the antiseptic resistance gene *qacA*, *qacB* and *qacC* in 497 methicillin-resistant and -susceptible European isolates of *Staphylococcus aureus*. *J Antimicrob Chemother* 2001; 47: 893–905.
19. Smith K, Gemmell CG, Hunter IS. The association between biocide tolerance and the presence or absence of *qac* genes among hospital-acquired and community-acquired MRSA isolates. *J Antimicrob Chemother* 2008; 61: 78–84.
20. Anthonisen IL, Sunde M, Steinum TM *et al.* Organization of antiseptic resistance gene *qacA* and Tn*552*-related β-lactamase gene in multidrug-resistance *Staphylococcus haemolyticus* strains of animal and human origins. *Antimicrob Agents Chemother* 2002; 46: 3606–3612.
21. Bjorland J, Steinum T, Kvitle B *et al.* Widespread distribution of disinfectant resistance genes among *Staphylococci* of bovine and caprine origin in Norway. *J Clin Microbiol* 2005; 43: 4363–4368.
22. Bjorland J, Steinum T, Sunde M *et al.* Novel plasmid-borne gene *qacJ* mediates resistance to quaternary ammonium compounds in equine *Staphylococcus aureus*, *Staphylococcus simulans*, and *Staphylococcus intermedius*. *Antimicrob Agents Chemother* 2003; 47: 3046–3052.
23. Bjorland J, Sunde M, Waage S. Plasmid-borne *smr* gene causes resistance to quaternary ammonium compounds in bovine *Staphylococcus aureus*. *J Clin Microbiol* 2001; 39: 3999–4004.
24. Lambert RJW. Comparative analysis of antibiotic and antimicrobial biocide susceptibility data in clinical isolates on methicillin-sensitive *Staphylococcus aureus*, methicillin-resistant *Staphylococcus aureus* and *Pseudomonas aerginosa* between 1989 and 2000. *J Appl Microbiol* 2004; 97: 699–711.

25. Sheng WH, Wang JT, Laderdale TL *et al.* Epidemiology and susceptibilities of methicillin-resistant *Staphylococcus aureus* in Taiwan: emphasis on chlorhexidine susceptibility. *Diagn Microbiol Infect Dis* 2009; 63: 309–313.
26. Koburger T, Hübner NO, Braun M *et al.* Standard comparison of antiseptic efficacy of triclosan, PVP-iodine, octenidine dihydrochloride, polyhexanide and chlorhexidine digluconate. *J Antimicrob Chemother* 2010; 65: 1712–1719.
27. Loeffler A, Cobb MA, Bond R. Comparison of a chlorhexidine and benzoyl peroxide shampoo as sole treatment in canine superficial pyoderma. *Vet Rec* 2011; 169: 249–253.
28. Karpanen TJ, Worthington T, Conway BR *et al.* Penetration of chlorhexidine into human skin. *Antimicrob Agents Chemother* 2008; 52: 3633–3636.
29. Akiyama H, Ueda M, Kanazaki H *et al.* Biofilm formation of *Staphylococcus aureus* strains isolated from impetigo and furuncle: role of fibrinogen and fibrin. *J Dermatol Sci* 1997; 16: 2–10.
30. Xing M, Shen F, Liu L *et al.* Antimicrobial efficacy of the alkaloid harmaline alone and in combination with chlorhexidine digluconate against clinical isolates of *Staphylococcus aureus* grown in planktonic and biofilm cultures. *Lett Appl Microbiol* 2012; 54: 475–482.
31. Osland AM, Vestby LK, Fanuelsen H *et al.* Clonal diversity and biofilm-forming ability of methicillin-resistant *Staphylococcus pseudintermedius*. *J Antimicrob Chemother* 2012; 67: 841–848.
32. Pitten F-A, Werner H-P, Kramer A. A standardized test to assess the impact of different organic challenges on the antimicrobial activity of antiseptics. *J Hosp Infect* 2003; 55: 108–115.
33. Rosenkrantz WS. Shampoo therapy. In: Bonagura JD, Twedt DC, eds. *Kirk's Current Veterinary Therapy XIV*. St Louis: Saunders Elsevier, 2009; 410–415.

Supporting Information

Additional Supporting Information may be found in the online version of this article:

Table S1. Oligonucleotide primers for multiplex-PCR for species identification of coagulase-positive staphylococci and *S. schleiferi* subsp. *schleiferi*.

Table S2. Antimicrobial susceptibility of meticillin-susceptible *Staphylococcus pseudintermedius* (MSSP) and meticillin-resistant *S. pseudintermedius* (MRSP) strains.

To cite this article, please use DOI: 10.1111/j.1365-3164.2012.01112.x

4.5

Photodynamic therapy for pythiosis

Layla Pires*, Sandra de M. G. Bosco†, Nelson F. da Silva Junior‡ and Cristina Kurachi*

*Physics Institute of São Carlos and †Instituto de Biociências de Botucatu, Univ Estadual Paulista, Campus Botucatu, Departamento de Microbiologia e Imunologia, Distrito de Rubião Júnior, S/N, 18618-970, Botucatu-SP, Brazil ‡Escola de Engenharia de São Carlos, University of São Paulo, Avenida Trabalhador São-Carlense, 400, Parque Arnold Schimidt, 13566-590, São Carlos-SP, Brazil

Correspondence: Layla Pires, Physics Institute of São Carlos, University of São Paulo, Avenida Trabalhador São-Carlense, 400, Parque Arnold Schimidt, 13566-590, São Carlos-SP, Brazil. E-mail: laylabtu@gmail.com

Background – Pythiosis is a life-threatening disease caused by *Pythium insidiosum*. Photodynamic therapy (PDT) is an alternative treatment to surgery that uses the interaction of a photosensitizer, light and molecular oxygen to cause cell death.

Objectives – To evaluate the effect of PDT on the *in vitro* growth of *P. insidiosum* and in an *in vivo* model of pythiosis.

Methods – For *in vitro* studies, two photosensitizers were evaluated: a haematoporphyrin derivative (Photogem®) and a chlorine (Photodithazine®). Amphotericin B was also evaluated, and the control group was treated with sterile saline solution. All experiments (PDT, porphyrin, chlorine and light alone, amphotericin B and saline solution) were performed as five replicates. For *in vivo* studies, six rabbits were inoculated with 20,000 zoospores of *P. insidiosum*, and an area of 1 cm^3 was treated using the same sensitizers. The PDT irradiation was performed using a laser emitting at 660 nm and a fluence of 200 J/cm^2. Rabbits were clinically evaluated daily and histopathological analysis was performed 72 h after PDT.

Results – For *in vitro* assays, inhibition rates for PDT ranged from 60 to 100% and showed better results in comparison to amphotericin B. For the *in vivo* assays, after PDT, histological analysis of lesions showed a lack of infection up to 1 cm in depth.

Conclusions and clinical importance – *In vitro* and *in vivo* studies showed that PDT was effective in the inactivation of *P. insidiosum* and may represent a new approach to treating pythiosis.

Introduction

Pythium insidiosum is a fungus-like organism from the Stramenopila Kingdom, Phylum Oomycota.[1] Several factors differentiate it from true fungi. Firstly, there is an absence of ergosterol in the cell membrane, which is the main target of antifungal drugs and explains why antifungal drugs are not very effective.[2] Secondly, oomycetes do not have chitin in their cell wall; their cell structure includes cellulose, which is difficult for drugs to penetrate.[3] Finally, the life cycle begins with parasitism of aquatic grasses by hyphae followed by the development of a sporangium, which matures and releases infective zoospores that encyst in plant or animal tissues.[4]

Pythiosis is a life-threatening disease that occurs mainly in tropical and subtropical areas of the world. Infections have been described in humans, some domestic and wild animals and recently in an aquatic bird.[5–12] The most commonly affected animal is the horse, for which no breed, age or sex predilection has been documented. Lesions are tumour like, with serosanguinous exudate, ulceration, pruritus and odour. The disease is endemic in the Brazilian Pantanal, which potentially may have the highest incidence in the world.[11] The literature describes more than 90 cases, but the true number is undoubtedly higher because this is not a notifiable disease. Dogs are the second most commonly affected species, presenting with both skin and gastrointestinal lesions. Over 100 cases of canine pythiosis (both forms) have been described in the USA alone.[13,14]

Surgery (aggressive surgical excision and amputation) is the most common treatment. Unfortunately, complete surgical excision is not possible due to the location of many lesions (e.g. distal limb of a horse), resulting in a high rate of local recurrence. Because of this, surgical excision is often coupled with concurrent antifungal drugs and immunotherapy.[15–17]

Photodynamic therapy (PDT) is a type of treatment where a dye reacts with a specific wavelength of light, resulting in the production of molecular oxygen in the target environment. The dye, termed the photosensitizer, absorbs light and starts photochemical reactions that transfer energy to molecular oxygen that in turn forms reactive oxygen species, which are highly toxic to cells, promoting their death.[18,19.]

This treatment has been widely used to treat cancer, multidrug-resistant strains of bacteria and other infectious diseases.[18] Photodynamic therapy has been used to treat

Accepted 13 July 2012

Sources of Funding: Fundação de Amparo à Pesquisa do Estado de São Paulo – FAPESP (grants 2008/03511-8 and 2010/02890-5) and FUNDUNESP (grant 42/11).

Conflict of Interest: No conflicts of interest have been declared.

chromoblastomycosis[20] and onychomycosis.[21] Treatment of caries, denture disinfection and biofilm formation with PDT have been investigated in various studies.[22–27] Hamblin *et al.*[19] used PDT to treat experimentally infected wounds and reported success without damage to the surrounding healthy tissue. Photosensitizers are selective, because they accumulate in microbial cells and not in healthy host tissues.[22,25]

Pythiosis is a challenging disease to treat. There is little response to conventional or available antimicrobial therapies. Experimental therapies often appear promising *in vitro*, but when tested *in vivo* the results are less promising with relapses occurring when treatment is discontinued. This is an important equine disease and newer treatments are needed.[13–16] The goal of this study was to evaluate the use of PDT on the *in vitro* growth of *P. insidiosum* and in an *in vivo* model of pythiosis to determine whether this is a potentially viable treatment option.

Material and methods

In vitro assays

Pythium isolation and culture.
An isolate of *P. insidiosum* was obtained from a horse diagnosed with pythiosis at São Paulo, School of Veterinary Medicine and Animal Science at Universidade Estadual Paulista, UNESP/Botucatu, Brazil. Cultures were maintained on Sabouraud dextrose agar (SDA; Difco, Sparks, MD, USA), incubated at 37°C aerobically and recultured weekly. For experimental purposes, standardized fragments 5 mm in diameter were obtained from the borders of the culture and subcultured onto SDA. Five replicates were performed for each assay (saline solution, chlorine alone and porphyrin alone, amphotericin B, light alone and PDT) and plates were incubated at 37°C for 30 days.

Light source.
The light source was a light-emitting diode (LED)-based system capable of emitting light at 530 nm for haematoporhyrin trials and at 660 nm for chlorine trials, developed by the Technological Support Laboratory of the University of São Paulo – LAT/USP. The intensity was 65 mW/cm^2.

Photosensitizers.
Two photosensitizers were used in this study at three different concentrations as follows: porphyrin (Photogem®; Photogem LLC Co., Moscow, Russia) at concentrations of 10, 15 and 25 mg/mL; and chlorine (Photodithazine®; VETA-GRAND Company, Moscow, Russia) at concentrations of 0.7, 1.0 and 1.3 mg/mL.

Treatment groups.
The control group consisted of standardized fragments treated with sterile saline solution cultured on SDA and incubated at 37°C.

For the amphotericin B group, 10 μL of amphotericin B (Eurofarma, Sao Paulo, Brazil) at a concentration of 100 μg/mL was added to standardized fragments of *P. insidiosum* cultured on SDA and incubated at 37°C. Amphotericin B was used in order to compare a common antifungal drug used in pythiosis treatment with photodynamic therapy.

The effect of dyes alone was evaluated at maximum concentrations of 25 mg/mL for porphyrin and 1.3 mg/mL for chlorine. Ten microlitres of each sensitizer concentration was added to standardized fragments of the Pythium cultured on SDA and incubated at 37°C. No washing was done after incubation.

In the light only group, fragments were exposed to light with a fluence of 30 J/cm^2 and irradiated for 461 s at 530 and 660 nm.

For photodynamic treatment, the standardized fragments of the Pythium culture were placed in Petri dishes with SDA and treated with either haematoporphyrin (10, 15, and 25 mg/mL) or chlorine (0.7, 1.0 and 1.3 mg/mL) and incubated in the dark for 20 min at 37°C. This was followed by the light irradiation. For porphyrin and chlorine, a wavelength of 530 and 660 nm was used, respectively. Irradiation lasted for 461 s, and immediately afterwards the plates were incubated at 37°C.

Analysis.
Petri dishes with treated fragments of *P. insidiosum* were viewed 48 h after each treatment. The growth area was measured using the software ImageJ® (image processing and analysis in JAVA; http://rsb web.nih.gov/ij/), and the inhibition rate was calculated as follows:

$$\text{Inhibition rate}(\%) = \left(1 - \frac{T}{C}\right)100$$

where T represents the growth area of fragments from the treatment group and C the growth area of fragments from the control group. Cultures were incubated at 37°C for 30 days after PDT, to look for a possible growth recovery. After 30 days, the fragments treated with PDT as described above and control fragments were submitted for analysis by scanning electron microscopy.

Statistical analyses were performed using Kruskal–Wallis and Dunn's tests to compare the treatment groups. A P-value of <0.05 was considered significant.

In vivo assays

This study was approved by the Ethical Committee of the Universidade Estadual Paulista 'Júlio de Mesquita Filho', UNESP/Botucatu, Brazil.

Lesion induction.
Experimental infections were induced by subcutaneous injection of 1 mL (20,000 zoospores/mL) of *P. insidiosum* into the dorsal thoracic region of six New Zealand rabbits. This resulted in a large lesion of approximately 10–30 cm^2 in size and 4–5 cm in depth. During this time rabbits were examined daily to ensure that the experimental infection was not resulting in a loss of body condition or causing signs of illness other than skin lesions. Investigators were prepared to administer pain medication or euthanize any rabbit if the infection caused suffering. For the study, a randomly selected area of 1 cm^2 within the main lesion was used for irradiation. As the mean light penetration for 660 nm is approximately 1 cm, it was estimated that the volume of tissue treated was 1 cm^3.

One of the rabbits was randomly selected as an infected, untreated control animal. Skin biopsy specimens from treated animals and the control animal were collected 72 h after treatment.

Light source.
A homogeneous optical fibre coupled to laser equipment emitting at 660 nm was used for chlorine assays. The intensity was set at 150 mW/cm^2 with a fluence of a 200 J/cm^2 obtained by 1333 s of exposure. For porphyrin assays, a LED device was used, emitting at 630 nm, with an intensity of 150 mW/cm^2 and fluence of 200 J/cm^2, as for chlorine.

Photosensitizer.
Chlorine at 1.0 mg/kg and porphyrin at 1.5 mg/kg was administered by intravenous injection into the auricular vein. Intravenous administration was chosen in order to obtain adequate distribution of photosensitizer in the lesion, given that topical application of the photosensitizer may not penetrate the lesion.

Photodynamic therapy treatment.
Rabbits were sedated with a combination of ketamine hydrochloride (Dopalen®; Vetbrands, Paulínia/SP, Brazil) and xylazine hydrochloride (Rompum®; Bayer, São Paulo/SP, Brazil), at a dose of 5 mg/kg of each agent, and anaesthetized with 1.7% isoflurane in oxygen using a mask. Four hours after administration of the photosensitizer, rabbits were anaesthetized and the skin lesion was irradiated. Dye photobleaching was monitored through fluorescence spectroscopy as previously described.[28] (Successful photobleaching

means that the photosensitizer is completely degraded and no fluorescence is observed after PDT.)

Analysis.
Three days (72 h) after treatment, the animals were euthanized and tissue biopsy specimens were collected, fixed in 10% neutral buffered formalin and routinely processed. Tissues were stained with haematoxylin and eosin or Gomori-Grocott's methenamine silver stain.

Results

In vitro assays

As noted in the Material and methods, the inhibition rate was calculated 48 h post-PDT and plates were incubated for 30 days post-treatment to look for evidence of regrowth.

Figure 1 shows the inhibition rates for the three concentrations of porphyrin (10, 15 and 25 mg/mL) with light and dye controls and amphotericin B. For porphyrin, PDT resulted in inhibition rates of more than 60% for all three concentrations; however, the greatest inhibition was found using 10 mg/mL of porphyrin, because all fragments were inactivated. In the 15 and 25 mg/mL groups, one of five fragments showed recovery growth in 7 days. Light alone and dye control (25 mg/mL) showed discrete inhibition rates in the first 48 h, but regrowth was noted in 7 days. A porphyrin PDT group (10 mg/mL) showed statistically significant inhibition rates compared with the untreated controls, light and dye only and Amphotericin B. The 10 mg/mL group showed statistically significant more inhibition compared with the amphotericin B group. No statistically significant difference was found between untreated controls, the dye only, light and amphotericin B groups.

Figure 2 shows the inhibition rates for the three concentrations of chlorine (0.7, 1.0 and 1.3 mg/mL) with light and dye controls, untreated controls (saline) and amphotericin B. For chlorine, PDT resulted in inhibition rates of

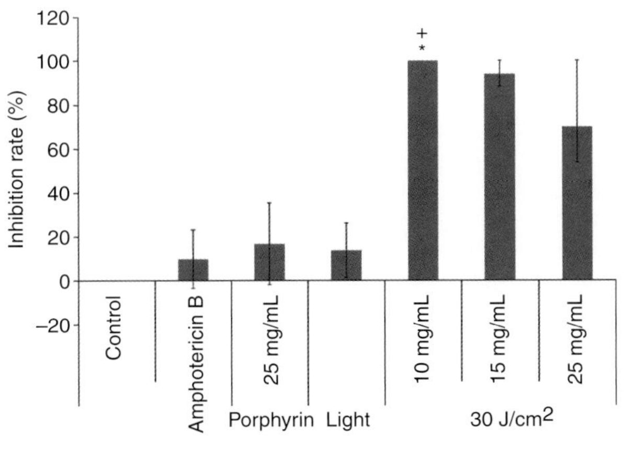

Figure 1. *In vitro* analyses of inhibition rates of hyphal growth with porphyrin at 48 h after each treatment. The group treated with the lower concentration of porphyrin showed a higher inhibition rate when compared with the two other concentrations evaluated. The photodynamic therapy (PDT) treatment also showed best results when compared with the amphotericin B group. *Groups for which $P < 0.05$ the inhibition rate showed statistical significance when compared with the untreated control group; and + groups that showed statistical significance when compared with the Amphotericin B group ($P < 0.05$).

between 80 and 100% (Figure 2). In the 1.0 and 1.3 mg/mL groups, one of five fragments showed recovery growth 48 h after treatment. In addition, the dye only control group showed a small rate of inhibition and recovery growth was noted within 7 days after treatment; the light only control group showed an increased effect.

There was no significant difference in inhibition rates among the dye only, light only and amphotericin B, when compared with the untreated saline control group. All chlorine PDT groups had significantly higher inhibition rates when compared with untreated control. The 0.7 mg/mL chlorine group showed statistical significance when compared with amphotericin B.

Scanning electron microscopy.
Figure 3 shows a fragment of hyphae from the control group. Figure 4 shows a fragment of hyphae after being treated with PDT using chlorine as the sensitizer. The surface is ill defined and replaced by amorphous material.

In vivo assays

Rabbits were observed daily postinoculation. For the first 10 days, the only noticeable finding was erythema and swelling that did not affect the animal's behaviour or appear to be pruritic or painful. At approximately 20 days postinoculation, tumour-like lesions developed and enlarged over time. By 40 days postinoculation well-circumscribed, firm circular lesions measuring 10–30 cm^2 in diameter and 4–5 cm in depth were noted. Rabbits were normophagic and normodipsic, did not lose body condition and appeared to be healthy except for the experimental local infection. A randomly selected site within the lesions measuring 1 cm^2 was selected for PDT to obtain 1 cm^3 of treated tissue.

The first experiment was performed using porphyrin and chlorine as sensitizers. Laser-induced fluorescence spectroscopy revealed an absence of porphyrin in the lesion after an incubation period of 4 h (pretreatment). Similarly, no bleaching was observed (post-treatment; Figure 5). For chlorine, an intensity emission peak at

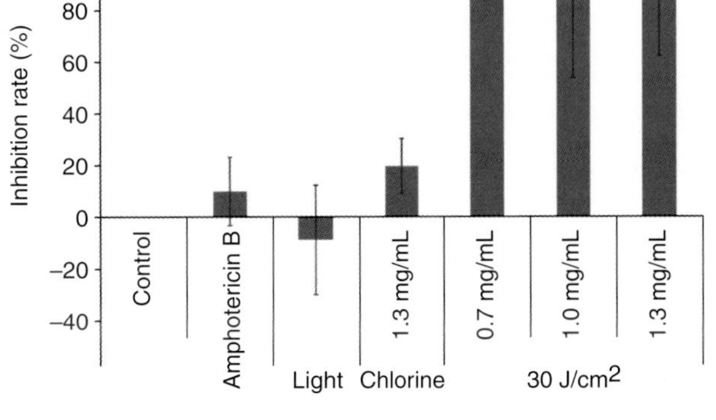

Figure 2. Inhibition rates obtained with chlorine at 48 h after each treatment. Best results were obtained for PDT with 0.7 mg/mL of chlorine. *Groups for which the inhibition rate showed statistical significance ($P < 0.05$) when compared with the untreated control group; and + groups that showed statistical significance ($P < 0.05$) when compared with the Amphotericin B group.

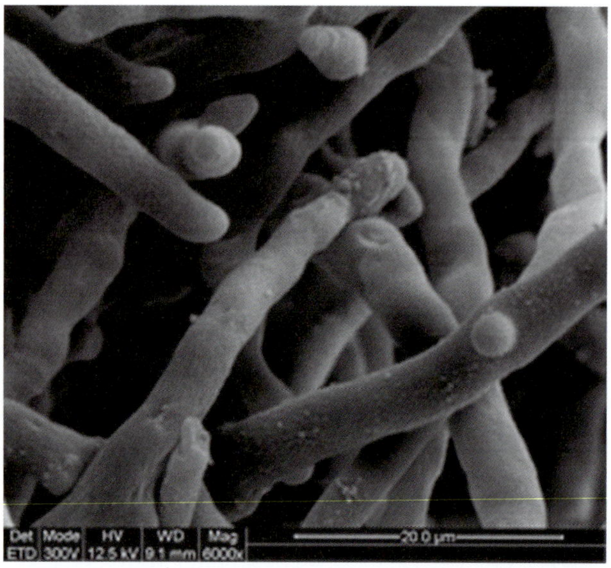

Figure 3. Scanning electron microscopy of a fragment of *Pythium insidiosum* from the control group. Cylindrical and broad hyphae, characteristic of *P. insidiosum*, can be observed.

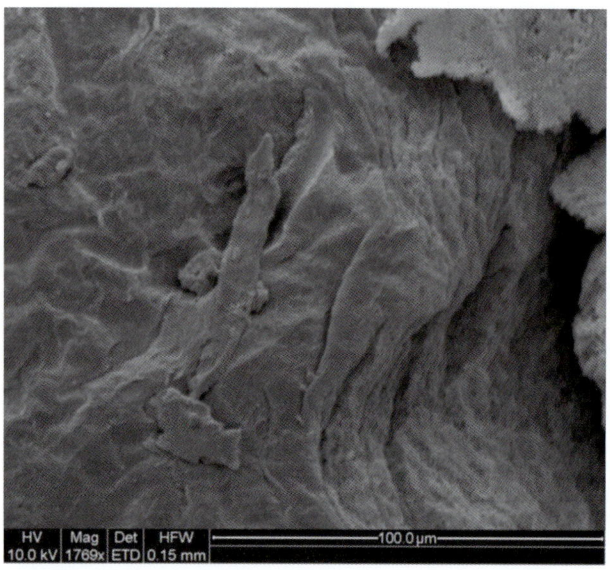

Figure 4. Scanning electron microscopy of a fragment of *Pythium insidiosum* treated with photodynamic therapy using chlorine as a sensitizer. The surface structure is ill defined and amorphous material is seen, possibly due to rupture of the cell wall and cell death.

660 nm, typical of the fluorescence emission of chlorine was observed, indicating the presence of this sensitizer in the lesion (pretreatment). After irradiation, photosensitizer fluorescence was absent, i.e. the sensitizer was photobleached, thereby indicating a response to photodynamic therapy. Thus, chlorine was chosen for *in vivo* experiments (Figure 6).

After the sessation of PDT with chlorine, the lesion was noticeably softer on palpation. Tissue biopsy specimens were collected at 72 h post-treatment.

The untreated control tissue biopsy specimens showed a severe inflammatory infiltrate, with fibrogranulomas and an irregular collagen fibre arrangement consistent with fibrosis (Figure 7). Gomori–Grocott methenamine staining

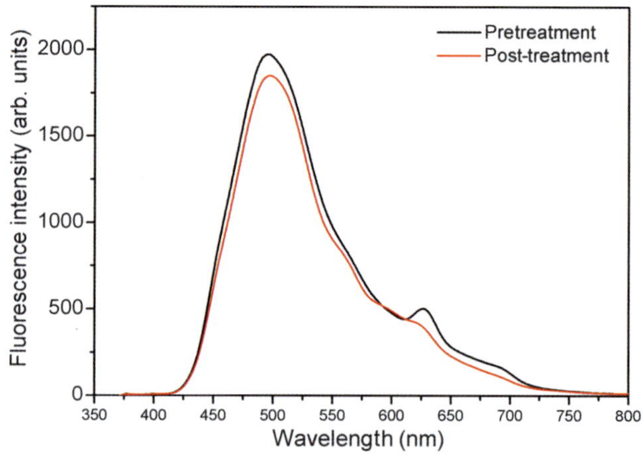

Figure 5. Fluorescence spectroscopy of pythiosis lesions 4 h after administration of porphyrin. In black, it is posible to observe the lesion spectrum before PDT, and in red, the lesion spectrum after PDT. The absence of an intensity peak at 614 nm demonstrates the lack of porphyrin in the lesion.

revealed the presence of hyphae, surrounded by an inflammatory process typical of pythiosis (Figure 8).

Histological examination of tissue biopsy specimens post-PDT showed normal epidermal cells and an intense inflammatory infiltrate at the dermo-epidermal junction, which is a characteristic finding of PDT. Blood vessels, dermal collagen and sebaceous glands were noted as normal (Figure 9). Gomori-Grocott methenamine silver staining showed a normal arrangement of collagen fibres and the absence of hyphae (Figure 10).

Discussion

In this study, both *in vitro* and *in vivo* evidence shows that PDT is a viable treatment option for *P. insidiosum. In vitro* studies demonstrated chlorine at lower concentrations to be most effective. Scanning electron microscopy showed an ill-defined surface of the hyphae, suggesting destruction of the pathogen. Photosensitizers and Amphotericin B groups showed some inhibition of growth in the first few days, but regrowth within 7 days was consistently seen in the absence of PDT. In the *in vivo* studies, lesions in rabbits showed signs of improvement within 72 h post-treatment; lesions treated were softer than the lesion in the untreated control rabbit. Moreover, histopathological analysis showed the absence of hyphae in the treated group.

Several studies have evaluated the effect of different antimicrobial drugs on *in vitro* and *in vivo* growth of *P. insidiosum*, with varying results. Pereira *et al.*[17] evaluated the activity of caspofungin *in vitro* and *in vivo* against Brazilian isolates of *P. insidiosum. In vitro* testing showed inhibition rates, but *in vivo* studies revealed relapse of the lesions once treatment was stopped. Dykstra *et al.*[14] reported 15 cases of cutaneous pythiosis in dogs, in which immunotherapy or antifungal therapy using amphotericin B, liposomal nystatin, itraconazole or ketoconazole were all unsuccessful.

In the present study, amphotericin B was ineffective when tested *in vitro*. This study found no statistically

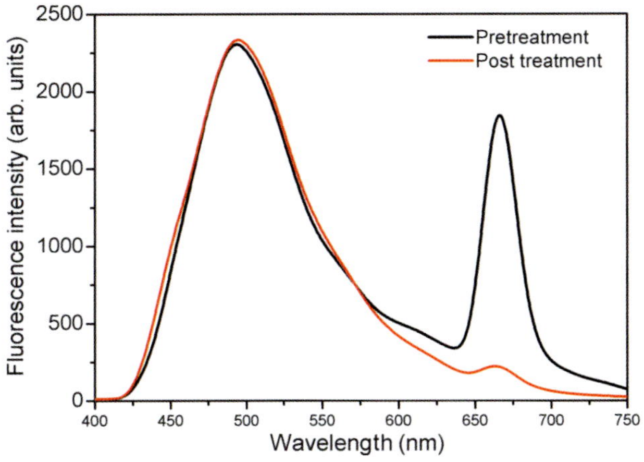

Figure 6. Laser-induced fluorescence spectroscopy of pythiosis lesions after a drug–light interval of 4 h. One can see lesion spectrum before and after PDT, in black and in red, respectively. The peak at 660 nm is characteristic of the presence of chlorine and photobleaching after PDT.

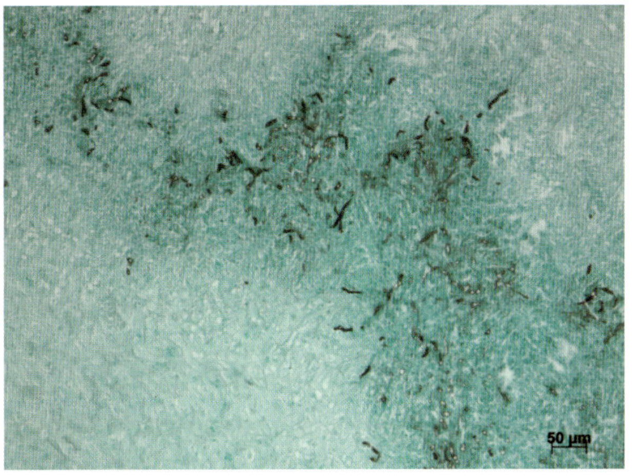

Figure 8. Gomori-Grocott methenamine silver staining of a biopsy from the control group, showing the presence of hyphae, coloured in black and dark brown, surrounded by an inflammatory process, as expected for pythiosis.

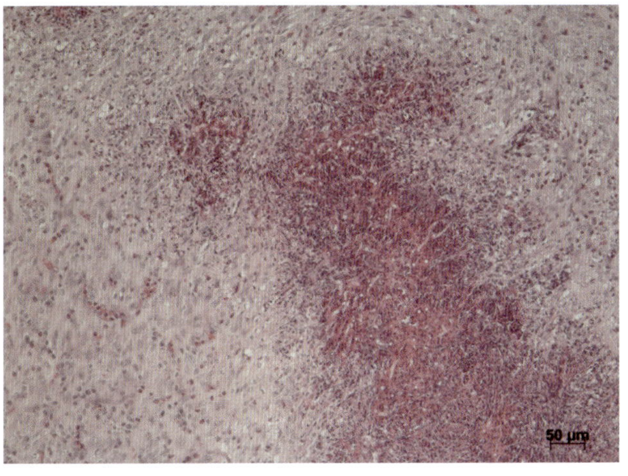

Figure 7. A biopsy from the control group reveals a severe inflammatory infiltrate and the presence of fibrogranulomas, characteristic of pythiosis, and fibrosis (haematoxylin and eosin stain).

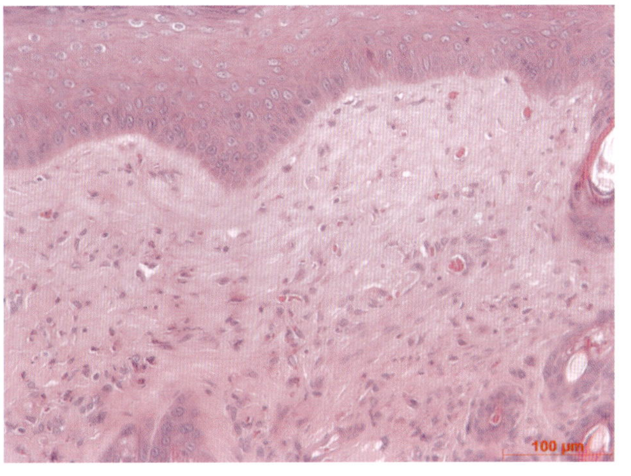

Figure 9. Haematoxylin and eosin staining of a skin biopsy collected after photodynamic therapy. One can observe epidermal cells regularly arranged. At the dermo-epidermal junction an inflammatory infiltrate can be seen, which is a characteristic outcome of PDT. Vessels with erythrocytes and a normal arrangement of collagen fibres are also noted.

significant difference among untreated controls, the dye only, light and amphotericin B groups. This raises further speculation about the usefulness of this drug.

Photodynamic therapy differs from antifungal drugs because in PDT there are a large number of potential targets for oxidative destruction, such as proteins, enzymes and unsaturated lipids, so the development of cell resistance is unlikely to occur.[25] This is an important advantage when treating micro-organisms because it is more difficult to develop resistance when a technique affects many cell targets.

In this study, *in vitro* experiments demonstrated a high efficiency for the chlorine used when compared with porphyrin. In order to obtain a similar inhibition rate it was necessary to use a higher concentration of porphyrin when compared with chlorine. Photostimulation of the *P. insidiosum* fragments was observed at 660 nm (chlorine), but not for porphyrin at 530 nm. One explanation is that biostimulation mechanisms that affect *P. insidiosum* differ for these wavelengths.[30] Sensitizer groups (dye controls of porphyrin and chlorine) showed inhibition at 48 h, but normal growth returned after 7 days. Further evidence of the effect of PDT was the undefined morphology of hyphae. Photogem® is a haematoporphyrin derivative with a molar extinction coefficient of 1170 M^{-1} cm^{-1}, while Photodithazine® is a chlorine e6 modified by the addition of *N*-methyl-D-glycosamine with a molar extinction coefficient of 3.82×10^4 M^{-1} cm^{-1}.[31] The molar extinction coefficient of chlorine is more than 30 times higher than for porphyrin.[31] Thus, concentrations evaluated for porphyrin were higher than those used for chlorine. The increased porphyrin concentration decreased the inhibition rate of the culture isolate. This probably occurred because at high concentrations photosensitizer molecules aggregated, making them less effective at transferring the absorbed energy to molecules of oxygen. Given that the *in vitro* study showed

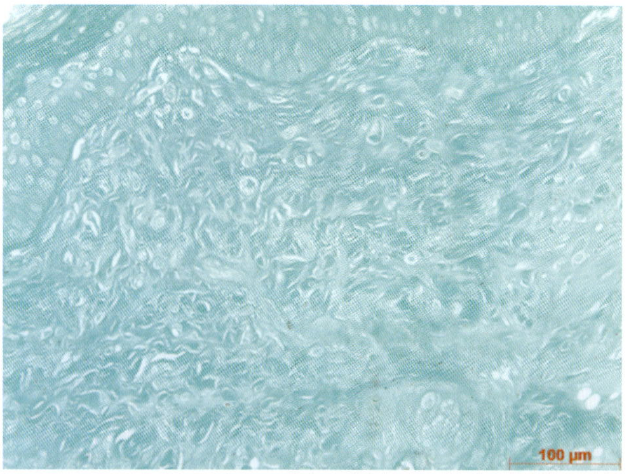

Figure 10. Gomori-Grocott methenamine silver staining of the lesion after PDT shows normal arrangement of collagen fibres and the absence of hyphae.

superior results, combined with the fluorescence spectroscopy analysis, chlorine was selected as the dye agent for the *in vivo* studies.

Fluorescence spectroscopy indicated an affinity of the sensitizer to damaged tissue and the organism. At the 660 nm emission, the fluorescence spectrum of the lesion showed accumulation of chlorine in the lesion, which is highly desirable for PDT treatment.

Histological examination of tissues showed the effects of PDT on *P. insidiosum* hyphae. Lesions in the experimental pythiosis model were tumour like and nonulcerative. The infection was localized inside the dermal fibrogranuloma, which protected it and acted as a barrier, preventing light penetration. In contrast, naturally infected lesions are usually fibrogranulomatous and ulcerative; therefore, light can interact directly with the infected tissue and, in these conditions the response to PDT might be improved, because the availability of oxygen is higher.

The advantages of using PDT as localized treatment are that it can be repeated as many times as needed, it is effective against *P. insidiosum* and the tissue response does not depend on the health of the animal. A disadvantage of the technique is the limited light penetration, meaning that surgical debulking is necessary prior to treatment.

In conclusion, results obtained from this study show a unique application of PDT. As it is a local treatment, repeated treatments can be performed as necessary. In this study, lower concentrations of chlorine were more successful in inactivating the pathogen. *In vitro* and *in vivo* studies have supported the potential of the technique to inactivate *P. insidiosum* and PDT may be an effective treatment option for cutaneous pythiosis.

References

1. De Cock AW, Mendoza L, Padhye AA *et al.* *Pythium insidiosum* sp. nov., the etiologic agent of pythiosis. *J Clin Microbiol* 1987; 25: 344–349.
2. Ghannoum MA, Rice LB. Antifungal agents: mode of action, mechanisms of resistance, and correlation of these mechanisms with bacterial resistance. *Clin Microbiol Rev* 1999; 12: 501–517.
3. Alexopoulos CJ, Mims CW, Blackwell M. Phylum Oomycota. Chapter 23. In: *Introductory Mycology*. New York: John Wiley & Sons Inc., 1996; 683–737.
4. Mendoza L, Hernandez F, Ajello L. Life cycle of the human and animal oomycete pathogen *Pythium insidiosum*. *J Clin Microbiol* 1993; 31: 2967–2973.
5. Pupaibool J, Chindamporn A, Patrakul K *et al.* Human pythiosis. *Emerg Infect Dis* 2006; 12: 517–518.
6. Rakich PM, Grooters AM, Tang KN. Gastrointestinal pythiosis in two cats. *J Vet Diagn Invest* 2005; 17: 262–269.
7. Pérez RC, Luis-León JJ, Vivas JL *et al.* Epizootic cutaneous pythiosis in beef calves. *Vet Microbiol* 2005; 109: 121–128.
8. Santurio JM, Monteiro AB, Leal AT *et al.* Cutaneous Pythiosis insidiosi in calves from the Pantanal region of Brazil. *Mycopathologia* 1998; 141: 123–125.
9. Videla R, van Amstel S, O'Neill SH *et al.* Vulvar pythiosis in two captive camels (*Camelus dromedarius*). *Med Mycol* 2012; 50: 219–224.
10. Pesavento PA, Barr B, Riggs SM *et al.* Cutaneous pythiosis in a nestling white-faced ibis. *Vet Pathol* 2008; 45: 538–541.
11. Sallis ESV, Pereira DIB, Raffi MB. Pitiose cutânea em equinos: 14 casos. *Cienc. Rural, Santa Maria* 2003; 33: 899–903.
12. Santurio JM, Leal AT, Leal AB *et al.* Three types of immunotherapics against pythiosis insidiosi developed and evaluated. *Vaccine* 2003; 21: 2535–2540.
13. Berryessa NA, Marks SL, Pesavento PA *et al.* Gastrointestinal pythiosis in 10 dogs from California. *J Vet Intern Med* 2008; 22: 1065–1069.
14. Dykstra M, Sharp NJH, Olivry T *et al.* A description of cutaneous-subcutaneous pythiosis in fifteen dogs. *Med Mycol* 1999; 37: 427–433.
15. Mendoza L, Newton JC. Immunology and immunotherapy of infection caused by *Pythium insidiosum*. *Med Mycol* 2005; 43: 477–486.
16. Mendoza L, Mandy W, Glass R. An improved *Pythium insidiosum*-vaccine formulation with enhanced immunotherapeutic properties in horses and dogs with pythiosis. *Vaccine* 2003; 21: 2797–2804.
17. Pereira DI, Santurio JM, Alves SH *et al.* Caspofungin *in vitro* and *in vivo* activity against Brazilian *Pythium insidiosum* strains isolated from animals. *J Antimicrob Chemother* 2007; 60: 1168–1171.
18. Wilson BC, Patterson MS. The physics, biophysics and technology of photodynamic therapy. *Phys Med Biol* 2008; 53: 61–109.
19. Hamblin MR, Hasan T. Photodynamic therapy: a new antimicrobial approach to infectious disease? *Photochem Photobiol Sci* 2004; 3: 436–450.
20. Lyon JP, Pedroso e Silva Azevedo Cde M, Moreira LM *et al.* Photodynamic antifungal therapy against chromoblastomycosis. *Mycopathologia* 2011; 172: 293–297.
21. Gilaberte Y, Aspiroz C, Martes MP *et al.* Treatment of refractory fingernail onychomycosis caused by nondermatophyte molds with methylaminolevulinate photodynamic therapy. *J Am Acad Dermatol* 2011; 65: 669–671.
22. Pereira CA, Romeiro RL, Costa AC *et al.* Susceptibility of *Candida albicans*, *Staphylococcus aureus*, and *Streptococcus mutans* biofilms to photodynamic inactivation: an in vitro study. *Lasers Med Sci* 2011; 26: 341–348.
23. Quiroga ED, Alvarez MG, Durantini EN. Susceptibility of *Candida albicans* to photodynamic action of 5,10,15,20-tetra(4-*N*-methylpyridyl) porphyrin in different media. *FEMS Immunol Med Microbiol* 2010; 60: 123–131.
24. Teichert MC, Jones JW, Usacheva MN *et al.* Treatment of oral candidiasis with methylene blue-mediated photodynamic therapy in an immunodeficient murine model. *Oral Surg Oral Med Oral Pathol Oral Radiol Endod* 2002; 93: 155–160.
25. Wainwright M. Photodynamic antimicrobial chemotherapy (PACT). *J Antimicrob Chemother* 1998; 42: 13–28.
26. Strakhovskaya MG, Zhukhovitskii VG, Mironov AF *et al.* Fungicidal activity of khlorin photosensitizers. *Dokl Biochem Biophys* 2002; 384: 155–158.

27. Pereira Gonzales F, Maisch T. Photodynamic inactivation for controlling *Candida albicans* infections. *Fungal Biol* 2012; 116: 1–10.
28. Vollet-Filho JD, Menezes PFC, Moriyama LT *et al.* Possibility for a full optical determination of photodynamic therapy outcome. *J Appl Phys* 2009; 105: 7 pp, 102038 (online).
29. Miller RI. Treatment of equine phycomycosis by immunotherapy and surgery. *Aust Vet J* 1981; 57: 377–382.
30. Karu T. Laser biostimulation: a photobiological phenomenon. *J Photochem Photobiol, B* 1989; 3: 638–640.
31. Detty MR, Gibson SL, Wagner SJ. Current clinical and preclinical photosensitizers for use in photodynamic therapy. *J Med Chem* 2004; 47: 3897–3915.

Part 5

Infectious Diseases

To cite this article, please use DOI: 10.1111/j.1365-3164.2012.01076.x

5.1

The canine and feline skin microbiome in health and disease

J. Scott Weese

Department of Pathobiology, Centre for Public Health and Zoonoses, Ontario Veterinary College, University of Guelph, Guelph, Ontario, Canada N1G 2W1.

Correspondence: J. Scott Weese, Department of Pathobiology, Centre for Public Health and Zoonoses, Ontario Veterinary College, University of Guelph, Guelph, Ontario, Canada N1G 2W1. E-mail: jsweese@uoguelph.ca

The skin harbours a diverse and abundant, yet inadequately investigated, microbial population. The population is believed to play an important role in both the pathophysiology and the prevention of disease, through a variety of poorly explored mechanisms.

Early studies of the skin microbiota in dogs and cats reported a minimally diverse microbial composition of low overall abundance, most probably as a reflection of the limitations of testing methodology. Despite these limitations, it was clear that the bacterial population of the skin plays an important role in disease and in changes in response to both infectious and noninfectious diseases.

Recent advances in technology are challenging some previous assumptions about the canine and feline skin microbiota and, with preliminary application of next-generation sequenced-based methods, it is apparent that the diversity and complexity of the canine skin microbiome has been greatly underestimated. A better understanding of this complex microbial population is critical for elucidation of the pathophysiology of various dermatological (and perhaps systemic) diseases and to develop novel ways to manipulate this microbial population to prevent or treat disease.

Introduction

In many ways, the skin represents an inhospitable site for micro-organisms, as a relatively cool, dry, high-salt, hydrophobic and acidic environment that is covered with antibacterial peptides and constantly shedding superficial layers.[1] Yet, despite these challenges, the skin harbours a large and complex microbial population, with estimates of 1 million to 1 billion bacteria per square centimetre of skin in humans.[2,3] This population of micro-organisms (the microbiota), particularly the bacterial component, has an intimate relationship with the host and plays a role in both protection and development of disease. Despite the recognition of the importance of the skin microbiota and the sum of its genetic components (the microbiome), understanding of this complex microbial environment is superficial, and approaches to modifying it (e.g. antimicrobials) have been rather crude.

Assessment of microbial populations

Understanding the structure and function of a microbial population requires methods to study the individual components of that population, something that can be challenging with large, complex microbial ecosystems. Traditionally, bacterial and fungal populations are assessed through conventional culture methods. While useful, culture has significant limitations in determining the overall microbiota because of the variable ability to culture different bacteria and limitations in the depth of study, which hamper investigation of locations that may contain millions to billions of bacteria from a variety of diverse genera. Even organisms that grow using conventional methods may be missed or underestimated when they are part of a complex population that includes other bacteria that grow readily in standard conditions (e.g. staphylococci). Accordingly, culture-based studies inherently lead to underestimation of the diversity and abundance, and overestimation of the presence of certain species or groups.[2]

Recognition of limitations in conventional culture and the need for methods that provide more depth of study led to development of culture-independent methods. These have been best explored in the gastrointestinal tract, and the shift towards nonculture-dependent methodologies has led to a revolution in our understanding of the body's microbial composition. A variety of culture-independent methods are available, each with advantages and disadvantages,[4,5] but most efforts are now focused on the use of high-throughput next-generation sequencing methods that are able to differentiate large numbers of individual sequences from complex mixtures. While still prone to some biases, particularly if inadequate quality control and data cleaning methods are used, this approach is providing tremendous new insight into our knowledge of microbiomes.

Accepted 18 May 2012
Sources of Funding: This study was self funded.
Conflict of Interest: No conflicts of interest have been declared.

The human skin

The human skin has been the most intensively studied skin microbiome, albeit with a fraction of the effort dedicated to the gastrointestinal tract. Classically, the skin microbiota is divided into two groups, the resident flora and the transient flora. The resident flora comprises the core microbiota that is relatively consistent and stable, and which repopulates itself rapidly after disruption.[6,7] This group is considered the true commensal microbiota. In contrast, the transient flora is an ever-changing population of temporary inhabitants that arise from the individual's environment or other external contacts and only persist on the skin for hours to days.[2,6] Properly defining resident and transient populations is dependent on the quality of the laboratory technique used, and therefore current information is at best incomplete, but the concept of a common, abundant and stable population living with a transient, dynamic and variable population is likely to be valid. Both groups can contain a range of harmless commensals and potential pathogens, yet disease occurs uncommonly despite the relative abundance of many well-adapted opportunistic pathogens. Given the proper circumstances, pathogenic members of both the resident and the transient microbiota can cause disease, and status as a member of the transient or resident microbiota is not necessarily an indication of the virulence of a micro-organism.

The bacterial microbiota: culture-based investigation

Early culture-based studies of the skin microbiota provided what is known to be rather superficial, yet critical, information.[8,9] Staphylococci were identified as predominant components of human skin, particularly *Staphylococcus epidermidis* and other coagulase-negative species. *Staphylococcus aureus* was recognized as an important cause of skin infection but also a relatively common inhabitant of healthy skin, indicating the complex, multifactorial nature of skin infections. Other commonly identified organisms included *Corynebacterium*, *Propionibacterium*, *Brevibacterium*, *Streptococcus* and *Micrococcus* spp., with variable results between studies based, in part, on the relative difficulties in isolating some of these organisms.

While less intensively studied, it was also recognized that a commensal fungal microbiota existed, predominantly involving *Malassezia* spp. in sebaceous regions, along with a limited parasitic population (i.e. *Demodex* spp.).[10,11] Very few studies on commensal viruses have been done, probably due to limitations and difficulties of broad viral screening, yet it is likely that a population of commensal mammalian viruses and bacteriophages exists on the skin.

The bacterial microbiome: culture-independent investigation

With the use of next-generation sequencing, it has become clear that the human skin microbiome is complex, diverse and abundant. For example, a study of the hands of 51 young healthy adults identified an astounding diversity, with hands typically containing >150 different bacterial species.[12] Remarkably, the overall bacterial diversity on the hands was reported to match or exceed that found in the mouth, oesophagus and even some small intestinal sites.[12] Therefore, while the skin certainly harbours fewer overall micro-organisms per unit of space than the gut, this numerically smaller microbiome can be equally diverse.

Four main bacterial phyla predominate on human skin, Actinobacteria, Firmicutes, Bacteroidetes and Proteobacteria (Tables 1 and 2). Remarkable, interindividual variation is present, probably reflecting differences in local conditions (e.g. temperature, acidity, pH, moisture, hair coverage, nutritional sources), as well as differences in exposure to micro-organisms from the environment, other individuals or other body sites on the same individual. Indeed, the variation between different body sites means that the microbiome from a site on one person's body is more likely to be similar to the same site on another person than a different ecological niche on the same person (e.g. the microbiome of a person's forehead is more similar to another person's forehead than the same person's hand). Despite this intraperson variation, contralateral sites on the same person tend to be more similar than the corresponding site of a different person (e.g. the left and right hand microbiomes on the same person are more similar to each other than the corresponding hand of another individual).[2] The relatively unique nature of an individual's hand microbiome has even led to investigation of the use of metagenomics for forensic purposes. Comparison of the skin-associated microbiome from objects to the skin microbiome of a person has been used to identify the individual who touched the object, albeit with mixed results.[13,14]

Marked variation can also occur within an individual over very close distances.[2] For example, hair follicles and sebaceous glands are relatively anoxic environments and can therefore support anaerobes that would have little chance to flourish or even survive only millimetres away. *Propionibacterium* spp. (Actinobacteria phylum) tend to dominate in sebaceous regions, while *Staphylococcus* spp. (Firmicutes phylum) and *Corynebacterium*

Table 1. Examples of genera belonging to selected phyla

Phylum	Common genera
Actinobacteria	*Propionibacterium*
	Corynebacterium
	Micrococcus
	Microbacterium
Bacteroidetes	*Bacteroides*
	Porphyromonas
	Sphingobacterium
	Chryseobacterium
Firmicutes	*Staphylococcus*
	Clostridium
	Streptococcus
	Lactobacillus
	Enterococcus
	Bacillus
Proteobacteria	*Escherichia*
	Pseudomonas
	Serratia
	Enterobacter
	Campylobacter
	Stenotrophomonas
	Delftia
	Comamonas

Table 2. Genus-level composition of the bacterial skin microbiome in humans

Skin site	Composition	Reference
Right axilla	*Staphylococcus**, 60% *Propionibacterium*†, 14% *Corynebacterium*†, 12% *Anaerococcus**, 5.7%	69
Back, abdomen, chest, limbs and neck	*Streptococcus**, 26% *Staphylococcus**, 16%	70
Hands	*Propionibacterium*†, 32% *Streptococcus**, 17% *Staphylococcus**, 8.3% *Corynebacterium*†, 4.3% *Lactobacillus**, 3.1%	12
Combined body sites	*Corynebacterium*†, 23% *Propionibacterium*†, 23% *Staphylococcus**, 17%	71
Forehead	*Propionibacterium*†, 73% *Staphylococcus**, 16%	22
Forearm	*Propionibacterium*†, 20% *Staphylococcus**, 13% *Corynebacterium*†, 10%	22

Symbols indicate bacterial phyla that correspond to the cited genera, as follows: *Firmicutes and †Actinobacteria.

(Actinobacteria phylum) are most common in moist regions.[2] Interestingly, dry regions are the most diverse, perhaps reflecting a location less amenable to specific bacterial adaptation and more representative of the multitude of micro-organisms to which the skin may be exposed.

Evaluation of bacterial diversity of different sites raises interesting questions about factors that influence intra- and interindividual variation. In one study, the microbial diversity was higher on the hands of women compared with men, with the microbiome also influenced by the time since hands were last washed and by handedness (i.e. left or right).[12] Additionally, while the bacterial diversity may be the same between dominant and nondominant hands, the composition of the microbiome varies.[12] The impact of handedness is interesting and probably represents different types of environmental and body site exposure between dominant and nondominant hands. The role of gender is less clear and might relate to the fact that men tend to have a more acidic skin environment,[15,16] because increased acidity has been linked to decreased microbial diversity in other ecological environments.[17,18] However, this is rather speculative, and other factors, such as sweat and sebum production, use of moisturizers or cosmetics, skin thickness, hormones, environmental contacts and frequency of handwashing, could all play a role.

Variation can also occur based on age. The skin microbiome is established shortly after birth, with vaginally delivered infants acquiring a microbiome similar to their mother's vagina and infants delivered by Caesarean section acquiring a microbiome most similar to the mother's skin.[19] Not surprisingly, the composition of the microbiome develops gradually over time, with increased relative abundance and evenness of the community developing with age.[20] Infants also have different phylum distributions compared with adults, with streptococci and staphylococci accounting for up to 40% of the total microbiome in young infants, and the abundance of the initially low-predominance genera increasing with age.

In addition to the concept of transient and resident flora, the core microbiome needs to be considered. The core microbiome can be defined as 'the suite of members shared among microbial consortia from similar habitats'.[21] In skin microbiome assessment, this represents the micro-organisms that are found in most or all samples from similar sites in different individuals. The core microbiome is presumably rather analogous to the resident microbiome, and it is assumed to be the group of micro-organisms that are critical for proper function of the community. In other ecological niches, the core microbiome tends to consist of a limited number of species or genera that comprise a large proportion of sequences, although by definition core components of the microbiome only need to be common amongst different individuals, not abundant within individuals. There has been limited evaluation of the core skin microbiome, and this population is currently ill defined. A study of forearm and forehead skin determined that 4.5% of genera (*Propionibacterium*, *Staphylococcus* and *Corynebacterium*) and 1.5% of species-level sequences were found in all subjects,[22] although as a cloning-based study the overall number of sequences studied was limited, something that may have affected the ability to define members of the core microbiome that were present at low abundances.

Even with the wealth of information generated by broad-range sequence-based studies, methodological limitations need to be considered. For skin, a major variable may be sampling technique. Skin swabs are commonly used because they are easy and noninvasive; however, it must be considered whether they adequately sample the skin microbiome, particularly bacteria that are resident in deep regions such as hair follicles.[3] It has been estimated that skin swabs collect approximately 10^5 bacteria/cm^2, while scrapings collect 5×10^5 bacteria/cm^2 and skin biopsy specimens 10^6 bacteria /cm^2.[3] Relative numbers are less important than differences in the organisms identified, and a study of human skin reported marked similarity in microbial composition data obtained using those three methods, with operational taxon units (groups of similar sequences) found by all three methods accounting for 97% of the overall sequences.[3] While some sequences were only found by individual sampling methods, these were low-abundance sequences that may be of limited concern when studying the microbiome. These data need confirmation for other body sites and other species, yet they suggest that easy-to-obtain skin swabs may be adequate.

The fungal microbiome

Minimal investigation of the fungal microbiome has been reported beyond targeted prevalence studies of specific organisms. The *Malassezia* microbiota has been assessed most thoroughly, with gender, body site, time of year and age identified as affecting prevalence and distribution.[23,24] The composition, diversity, abundance and variability of other fungal groups require further investigation.

The canine and feline skin bacterial microbiota: culture-dependent studies

Skin microbiota

The assessment of the canine skin microbiota is inadequate. It is widely cited that the canine skin harbours less than 350 bacteria/cm^2, based on a culture-dependent study of healthy dogs.[25] The same study reported a significantly larger population (859 bacteria/cm^2) on clinically normal skin sites on dogs with seborrhoea, with even larger numbers (16,150 bacteria/cm^2) from seborrhoeic skin lesions. A study that focused on *Micrococcus* spp., *Streptococcus* spp., *Bacillus* spp. and aerobic Gram-negative bacteria[26] reported counts of up to 180,000 bacteria per sample. Comorbidities may affect bacterial abundance, as demonstrated by the presence of 347,114 aerobic organisms/cm^2 in dogs with suspected hypothyroidism and a decrease to 994 bacteria/cm^2 after treatment.[27] Sampling method and site probably accounted for some of the variation between quantitative studies, with additional variation based on the culture method. Thus, the often-cited 350 bacteria/cm^2 is almost certainly a massive underestimate, and large numbers of bacteria are undoubtedly present at various skin sites.

Along with small numbers of bacteria, early studies also reported minimal bacterial diversity. 'Coagulase-negative cocci' (presumably coagulase-negative staphylococci) predominated in a study of healthy dogs, being present in all dogs as 89% of the microflora.[25] However, coagulase-negative cocci were found in only 33 and 38% of clinically normal and affected skin sites on seborrhoeic dogs, respectively, suggesting an alteration in this 'normal' microbiota in response to noninfectious disease. 'Aerobic diphtheroids' were the only other aerobes detected in healthy dogs, with *Clostridium* spp. being found in 60%. '*Staphylococcus aureus*' was found in healthy and diseased skin 62–63% of seborrhoeic dogs and, when present, accounted for 90–97% of the microflora. Aerobic diphtheroids and Gram-negative rods were also found, although Gram-negative rods accounted for less than 0.1% of the microflora present. This paper was published[25] after *S. intermedius* was first reported (1976),[28] but there was no information about how *S. aureus* was identified, and *S. intermedius* is not mentioned anywhere in the paper, so it is likely that '*S. aureus*' was in fact *Staphylococcus pseudintermedius*.

Similar data were obtained in a comparison of dogs' skin with suspected hypothyroidism pre- and post-thyroid hormone supplementation.[27] '*Staphylococcus aureus*' dominated prior to treatment, accounting for the entire microbiota in most animals, while after treatment, 'coagulase-negative cocci' were the sole or predominant bacteria isolated in most dogs.

A more comprehensive culture-based study of healthy dogs investigated seven different skin sites,[7] identifying greater microbial diversity. '*Staphylococcus aureus*' and *S. epidermidis* (a coagulase-negative species) were common, in contrast to the study,[25] where *S. aureus* was found on only diseased skin, yet the commonness of coagulase-negative staphylococci is consistent between the two studies. *Micrococcus* spp., streptococci and the Gram-negative *Acinetobacter* spp. were also quite common, while *Escherichia coli*, *Proteus mirabilis*, *Corynebacterium* sp. and *Bacillus* spp. were detected, but rare. This suggests that *Micrococcus* spp., *S. aureus*, α-haemolytic streptococci and *Acinetobacter* spp. comprised the resident microbiota, while Gram-negative organisms, *Bacillus* spp., *Corynebacterium* spp. and β-haemolytic streptococci comprised the transient microbiota.[7]

Two later studies provided more information and challenged some of those assumptions. The first study, which investigated skin and hair-shaft samples from 15 sites of clinically normal dogs reported isolation of *S. intermedius* (presumably *S. pseudintermedius*) from hair samples from 77% of dogs, with none harbouring *S. aureus*.[29] Furthermore, coagulase-negative staphylococci were found in all dogs at counts of up to 10 million bacteria per hair sample. Similar results, with commonness of *S. intermedius*, absence of *S. aureus* and ubiquity of coagulase-negative staphylococci, were found on skin swabs and punch biopsies. This study also suggested that there may be two populations of *S. intermedius*; one that resides within pilosebaceous units and one at mucocutaneous junctions that results in contamination of the distal hair shaft. It is possible that colonization of mucous membranes represents the main source of coagulase-positive staphylococci on skin, particularly considering the high mucosal colonization rates in dogs.[30,31] This subject is becoming increasingly important as rates of mucosal colonization with meticillin-resistant staphylococci increase.

A second, related, study[26] identified *Micrococcus* spp. as the most consistently recovered bacteria from different dogs and different sites, with Gram-negative bacteria also having a distribution consistent with resident organisms, in contrast with *Bacillus* spp. In that study, micrococci were equally, or more commonly found on the skin or proximal hair shaft compared with the distal hair shaft, leading to the suggestion that these could truly represent resident microbiota, because transient contaminants would plausibly be more common on the distal aspects of hair. This may appear to be in conflict with an *in vitro* study that reported poor adherence of micrococci to canine and feline corneocytes,[32] but the *Micrococcus* sp used in that study was of human origin, so it is hard to evaluate the meaning of those data.

Predominance of *S. aureus* (*S. pseudintermedius*) was also reported in a study of 10 dogs with atopic dermatitis, contact dermatitis or seborrhoeic dermatitis.[33] *Acinetobacter* spp., *Micrococcus* spp., α-haemolytic streptococci and *S. epidermidis* were also common, with lower prevalences of a range of bacteria, including *Alcaligenes* sp., *Cloaca (Enterobacter)* spp., *E. coli*, *Flavobacterium* spp., *Hafnia* spp., *Klebsiella* spp., *Moraxella* spp., *Proteus mirabilis*, *Pseudomonas* spp., *Bacillus* spp., *Corynebacterium* spp. and group B β-haemolytic streptococci (probably *Streptococcus canis*).

Assessment of these culture-based studies is hampered by differences in methodologies, small sample sizes and inherent limitations in bacterial culture, but some common and important findings are apparent. The most common cause of skin infections, coagulase-positive staphylococci, tend to be uncommon residents of the skin, and seeding from colonized mucosal sites may be a key aspect of the pathogenesis of skin infections in the presence of underlying risk factors. The commonness of coagulase-negative staphylococci on healthy skin is widely reported, and it is likely that a wide range of coagulase-negative species are part of the resident microbiota. However, limited information is available about individual species present. This probably relates to the effort required to speciate coagulase-negative staphylococci and limited incentive to do so in clinical studies because coagulase-negative species are generally considered to be of limited virulence. Some targeted studies have been performed, such as a study of *Staphylococcus sciuri* that identified this coagulase-negative species in 46% of 122 dogs.[34] Interest in coagulase-negative species has increased recently through recognition of the potentially disproportionate involvement of some species in skin and ear infections, particularly *Staphylococcus schleiferi schleiferi* and *S. epidermidis*.[35,36]

While limited information is available about canine skin microbiota, even less is known about cats. A culture-based study of multiple sites of 10 healthy cats reported a predominance of *Micrococcus* spp., *Acinetobacter* spp. and streptococci, with lesser representation of staphylococci.[7] *Escherichia coli*, *Proteus mirabilis*, *Pseudomonas* spp., *Alcaligenes* sp. and *Bacillus* sp. were also identified, albeit rarely. Of note was the inability to isolate any bacteria from almost 50% of sites. This was attributed to the 'cleanliness of the feline species', but it is highly unlikely that those sites were indeed sterile, and the inability to isolate bacteria is probably from a combination of sampling methods, culture methods and lower overall bacterial abundance. Broad microbiota assessment is lacking, and the staphylococcal population and dynamics of feline skin are not adequately described. It is known that *S. pseudintermedius* and *S. aureus* are less adept at adhering to feline corneocytes compared with canine cells *in vitro*,[32,37] something that probably may relate to the lesser incidence of staphylococcal skin infections in cats.

As with humans, the skin microbiota varies between different body sites in animals, presumably because of differences in local environment (e.g. hair coat, secretions, oxygen tension, temperature, pH, wetness, available bacterial binding sites) and bacterial exposure (e.g. environmental contact, grooming activities, contact with mucous membranes). One culture-based study reported the prevalence of different organisms from different body sites of 10 healthy dogs and 10 healthy cats.[7] While no abundance data were reported and no statistical analysis performed, results suggested some regional variation, with micrococci being more common over the parietal region of the head and a subjective assessment that the microbiota was 'poorest' in the lumbar region. Other studies that have included sampling of different sites likewise provided unclear information about relative differences in the microbiota between body sites.[29,38] As in humans,[2] there may be major differences in bacterial abundance and distribution over very short distances because of large variations in local environment between adjacent sites such as hair follicles, sebaceous glands and the stratum corneum.[39] The highest culturable bacterial population densities have been reported in the hair follicles,[39] which is probably a testament to the protected, moist, nutrient-rich conditions that are present.

Most recent investigations of canine and feline skin micro-organisms have focused on the conventional culture of pathogenic (or potentially pathogenic) species, such as staphylococci, *Malassezia pachydermatis* and dermatophytes. However, focusing solely on the pathogenic component (or any specific micro-organism by itself) results in a failure to appreciate and investigate the multifactorial nature of skin disease and has neglected the commensal microbial population, which presumably has a significant, if underappreciated, role in health.[2] Therefore, while understanding of pathogens is clearly important, proper evaluation of the skin microbiota requires detailed assessment of the overall microbial community of the skin, how this community contributes to health and disease and how the community is altered, both in disease and in response to treatment.

Canine and feline ear microbiota

The bacterial microbiota of the ear has been investigated, with most studies focusing on the prevalence of staphylococci, *Pseudomonas* and *Malasezzia* in dogs with otitis.[40–45] Broader studies have assessed groups of culturable bacteria identified in the ears of healthy dogs and dogs with otitis externa. In one study, *S. pseudintermedius*, *S. canis*, *Bacillus* spp., *Proteus* spp., coagulase-negative staphylococci, viridans streptococci, *Corynebacterium* spp. and *E. coli* were most common, with high prevalences of *S. pseudintermedius*, *S. schleiferi coagulans*, *Streptococcus canis*, nonhaemolytic streptococci, *E. coli*, *Proteus* spp. and *Pseudomonas aeruginosa* and a lower prevalence of coagulase-negative staphylococci in dogs with otitis externa compared with healthy dogs.[46] Likewise, another study reported finding *Pseudomonas* spp. and *Proteus* spp. only in dogs with otitis externa; however, this study did not identify a higher prevalence of coagulase-positive staphylococci in dogs with otitis externa and, in contrast to the previously cited study, found a higher prevalence of coagulase-negative staphylococci in affected dogs.[47] Other species that have been reported from canine ears include *Micrococcus* spp., *Enterococcus* spp., *Klebsiella* spp. and *Pasteurella multocida*.[46,47] Not surprisingly, a higher overall bacterial abundance has also been reported in dogs with otitis externa compared with healthy dogs.[47]

A study of the ear microbiota in feral cats reported a predominance of coagulase-negative staphylococci, which accounted for 67% of isolates.[41] However, it is noteworthy that no bacteria were recovered from 61% of ear swabs, indicating the insensitivity of culture-based methods or inadequate sampling techniques.

Canine and feline fungal and viral skin microbiota

Many studies have described the prevalence of selected potentially pathogenic organisms, particularly dermatophytes and *Malassezia*, on skin or in ears,[45,47–49] but there are fewer broad culture-based studies. One study described the predominance of *Penicillium* spp. in the ears of healthy dogs, with common detection of *M. pachydermatis* and less common identification of others, such as *Aspergillus* spp., *Spirodiobolus johnsonii*,

Bipolaris spp., *Curvularia* spp. and *Fusarium* spp.[50] A similar range of fungi can be found in the ears of dogs with atopy and otitis, albeit potentially in different relative proportions.[50] In a different study, *M. pachydermatis* was the most commonly found fungal organism, accounting for virtually all fungi isolated from dogs both with and without otitis externa.[46] In that study, *Candida* spp. and *Aspergillus fumigatus* were also identified. It is likely that culture methods greatly influenced these culture-dependent studies, and culture-independent investigation is likely to be required.

As with other species, broad-range viral studies are lacking, but canine papillomavirus can be found on the skin of healthy dogs.[51] Presumably, a variety of other viruses, predominantly bacteriophages, are also present, but data are not yet available.

The canine and feline skin microbiomes: culture-independent studies

Unlike in humans, there has been limited use of next-generation sequencing to investigate the canine and feline skin microbiomes. A preliminary study of the canine skin microbiome reported a complex and diverse microbiome, with 38–110 different species identified per sample.[52] However, these data indicated a very different composition of the skin microbiome compared with humans and, while there were some basic similarities to culture-based canine studies, numerous differences in diversity and abundance were apparent. The Firmicutes phylum was predominant, with large populations of staphylococci and lactobacilli. A large staphylococcal population is expected, but the high prevalence of lactobacilli is in contrast to culture-based studies and an example of an abundant organism that was overlooked because of its poor growth in standard aerobic culture conditions. *Propionibacterium* and *Streptococcus*, two common genera on human skin, were uncommon, while many bacterial genera that had not previously been reported on canine skin were identified, sometimes at high abundances. Proteobacteria were uncommon, in contrast to the situation in humans. The canine ear appears to have a less diverse microbiome, dominated by Firmicutes, particularly lactobacilli. Culture-independent studies of the feline skin microbiome are currently lacking.

Role of the skin microbiome in health and disease

A role of the skin as a source of opportunistic pathogens is beyond doubt and has been known for years; however, the overall role of the skin microbiome in health and disease is still poorly understood. While there is clear evidence regarding opportunistic infections, determining how the microbiome changes and whether microbiome changes reflect cause versus effect may be difficult. Perhaps even more challenging is discerning the role of microbiome modification in the pathophysiology of what are considered classically noninfectious diseases. The skin has abundant exposure to antigens and plays an important role in the host immune response. The skin microbiome and immune system are not completely separate entities, because they presumably work in concert and are influenced by each other.

Most of the available data regarding alterations of the skin microbiome in disease come from humans, with examples presented in Table 3. Beyond skin infections, there is increasing interest in the role of the microbiome in noninfectious skin diseases, such as atopic dermatitis, rosacea, psoriasis and acne.[3] Information pertaining to companion animals is limited and focuses mainly on isolation of staphylococci, dermatophytes, *Malassezia pachydermatis* or Enterobacteriaceae from skin or ear infections.[40,53–58] Broader study of the skin microbiome in disease is limited to a few culture-dependent studies. As cited above (Skin microbiota), there were differences in the culturable skin microbiota in dogs with seborrhoea compared with healthy control dogs,[25,27] and thyroid hormone supplementation in seborrhoeic dogs altered the skin microbiota, restoring it to what was considered a more normal population.[27] Greater overall bacterial 'density' was reported on healthy skin of dogs with furunculosis compared with healthy control dogs, consistent with some underlying factor that resulted in bacterial overgrowth.[59] Likewise, greater *S. aureus* (presumably *S. pseudintermedius*) density was reported from 'eczematous' skin sites of dogs with atopic dermatitis, contact dermatitis or seborrhoeic dermatitis compared with clinically normal sites on the same dogs,[33] providing more evidence of at least numerical alterations in the microbiota with those conditions. An increased prevalence of 'Gram-negative transients' has also been reported on 'eczematous' skin in dogs.[33] As in humans, there are changes to the staphylococcal skin population in dogs with atopic dermatitis. For example, a greater prevalence of *S. intermedius*-group colonization was identified in atopic dogs (88%) versus healthy dogs (37%),[30] numbers that are similar to *S. aureus* prevalence data in humans with the same condition.[8] This is perhaps unsurprising, given that *S. pseudintermedius* has shown more adherence to corneocytes from canine atopic skin versus skin from healthy dogs.[60–62] A poorly defined bacterial overgrowth syndrome has also been described,[63] with higher staphylococcal counts on affected dogs versus healthy

Table 3. Examples of alternations in the skin microbiome with different disease states in humans

Condition	Microbiome alteration	Reference
Atopic dermatitis	Increased *Staphylococcus aureus* and *Staphylococcus epidermidis* abundance and loss of bacterial diversity during flares	72
	Increases in streptococci, *Propionibacterium* spp. and *Corynebacterium* spp. after treatment	
Atopic dermatitis	Increased non-*Malassezia* yeast microbiota diversity (more species) in affected individuals	73
Psoriasis	Increased bacterial diversity, increased streptococcal populations and decreased *Propionibacterium acnes*	74
Psoriasis	Decreased relative abundance of Actinobacteria, with decreases in propionibacteria and staphylococci	70

dogs, and from affected skin sites versus clinically normal skin sites on the same dogs.[63]

Clearly, modifications of the skin microbiota (or at least certain components of it) occur in both infectious and noninfectious skin diseases. The clinical relevance of these changes, whether they represent cause or effect, and various other important aspects remain unanswered, as do the reasons for the changes. Therefore, while these studies provide important evidence of alterations in selected components of the skin microbiota in response to various conditions, the failure to assess the microbiota limits the conclusions that can be made.

Perhaps even more difficult to assess is interaction of different components of the skin microbiota, something that may be of relevance. This potential relevance has been highlighted by a recent study that demonstrated increased pathogenicity of *S. aureus in vitro* and *in vivo* in mice when grown with the common human skin commensal *Propionibacterium acnes*.[64] Considering the number of different micro-organisms in the skin microbiome, it is certainly plausible that various interactions, both positive and negative, could occur. Accordingly, clear understanding of the composition of the skin microbiome is important but is only one step in the process of understanding its role in health and disease. Assessment of potentially complex interactions between different components of the bacterial microbiome, between bacterial and other micro-organisms and between the overall microbiome and the immune system (and perhaps other aspects of host–pathogen interaction) is required.

Manipulation of the skin microbiome

If disruption of the microbiome is a trigger or consequence of disease, restoration or stabilization of the microbiome are logical goals to treat or prevent disease. The traditional approach for elimination of skin infection in animals has been to attempt to target the offending agent with antimicrobials. In reality, elimination of the offending skin pathogen is probably uncommon, because clinical cure and microbiological cure are not the same and because the main causes of bacterial infections are the same organisms that are often found on healthy skin. Therefore, antimicrobial therapy should probably be more appropriately considered as a means to reduce the numbers of the offending agent to allow the body's own defenses (and perhaps the other components of the skin microbiome) to suppress the pathogen adequately. This is certainly not a new concept, because it is recognized by clinicians that failure to address underlying risk factors increases the likelihood of treatment failure or disease recurrence when managing skin infections. While rather crude, antimicrobial therapy is typically effective, although the widespread dissemination of multidrug-resistant organisms, such as meticillin-resistant staphylococci, is certainly compromising the effectiveness of traditional antimicrobial-based approaches.[53,65,66] Furthermore, as more information is obtained about the commensal skin microbiome, questions should be raised about whether such a nonspecific approach is ideal. While the core skin microbiome of dogs is yet to be defined and its antimicrobial susceptibility determined, it is likely that the antimicrobials that are commonly used in the treatment of pyoderma have efficacy against much of the core microbiome and therefore may suppress both pathogenic and beneficial components. The potential role of the skin microbiome in disease beyond pyoderma should also lead to increased thought about 'optimizing' the skin microbiome as opposed to 'killing' micro-organisms in a rather nontargeted manner.

When considering manipulation of the microbiome, there are three main areas to consider: 'protection' of the core microbiome from alteration, 'improvement' of the core microbiome to confer increased resistance to change or disease and 'restoration' of an altered microbiome. Defining what these mean and how they are achieved is difficult based on the paucity of baseline information. However, at a basic level, this could include measures that modify the local skin environment (e.g. essential fatty acid supplementation[67], hair coat management), targeted vaccination (i.e. *Staphylococcus* bacteriophage lysate[68]), topical bacteriophage therapy, oral probiotic administration or even topical administration of core bacterial components. Modification of current practices, such as antimicrobial administration, topical biocide administration, dietary management and bathing might also be useful for modification of the skin microbiome. At this time, there is little information to guide these approaches; however, this remains an interesting and potentially important area of study.

Conclusion

While still largely unexplored, the skin microbiome represents a complex microbial population that is likely to play a critical role in health and disease of the host. With better understanding of the composition of the microbiome, how it changes in response to various influences, how it interacts with the immune system, how it is altered during disease and the impact of current therapeutic practices, new insights into the pathophysiology, diagnosis, treatment and prevention of disease may be obtained.

References

1. Percival SL, Emanuel C, Cutting KF *et al.* Microbiology of the skin and the role of biofilms in infection. *Int Wound J* 2012; 9: 14–32.
2. Kong HH, Segre JA. Skin microbiome: looking back to move forward. *J Invest Dermatol* 2012; 132: 933–939.
3. Grice EA, Kong HH, Renaud G *et al.* A diversity profile of the human skin microbiota. *Genome Res* 2008; 18: 1043–1050.
4. O'Sullivan DJ. Methods for analysis of the intestinal microflora. *Curr Issues Intest Microbiol* 2000; 1: 39–50.
5. Sekirov I, Russell SL, Antunes LCM *et al.* Gut microbiota in health and disease. *Physiol Rev* 2010; 90: 859–904.
6. Kong HH. Skin microbiome: genomics-based insights into the diversity and role of skin microbes. *Trends Mol Med* 2011; 7: 320–328.
7. Krogh HV, Kristensen S. A study of skin diseases in dogs and cats. II. Microflora of the normal skin of dogs and cats. *Nord Vet Med* 1976; 28: 459–463.

8. Leyden JJ, Marples RR, Kligman AM. *Staphylococcus aureus* in the lesions of atopic dermatitis. *Br J Dermatol* 1974; 90: 525–530.
9. Marples MJ. Life on the human skin. *Sci Am* 1969; 220: 108–115.
10. Soria X, Carrascosa JM. Normal cutaneous flora and secondary bacterial infection. *Actas Dermosifiliogr* 2007; 98(Suppl 1): 15–21.
11. Erbağci Z, Ozgöztaşi O. The significance of *Demodex folliculorum* density in rosacea. *Int J Dermatol* 1998; 37: 421–425.
12. Fierer N, Hamady M, Lauber CL *et al.* The influence of sex, handedness, and washing on the diversity of hand surface bacteria. *Proc Natl Acad Sci USA* 2008; 105: 17994–17999.
13. Fierer N, Lauber CL, Zhou N *et al.* Forensic identification using skin bacterial communities. *Proc Natl Acad Sci USA* 2010; 107: 6477–6481.
14. Tims S, van Wamel W, Endtz HP *et al.* Microbial DNA fingerprinting of human fingerprints: dynamic colonization of fingertip microflora challenges human host inferences for forensic purposes. *Int J Legal Med* 2010; 124: 477–481.
15. Kim M-K, Patel RA, Shinn AH *et al.* Evaluation of gender difference in skin type and pH. *J Dermatol Sci* 2006; 41: 153–156.
16. Dao H, Kazin RA. Gender differences in skin: a review of the literature. *Gend Med* 2007; 4: 308–328.
17. Fierer N, Jackson RB. The diversity and biogeography of soil bacterial communities. *Proc Natl Acad Sci USA* 2006; 103: 626–631.
18. Fierer N, Morse JL, Berthrong ST *et al.* Environmental controls on the landscape-scale biogeography of stream bacterial communities. *Ecology* 2007; 88: 2162–2173.
19. Dominguez-Bello MG, Costello EK, Contreras M *et al.* Delivery mode shapes the acquisition and structure of the initial microbiota across multiple body habitats in newborns. *Proc Natl Acad Sci USA* 2010; 107: 11971–11975.
20. Capone KA, Dowd SE, Stamatas GN *et al.* Diversity of the human skin microbiome early in life. *J Invest Dermatol* 2011; 131: 2026–2032.
21. Shade A, Handelsman J. Beyond the Venn diagram: the hunt for a core microbiome. *Environ Microbiol* 2012; 14: 4–12.
22. Staudinger T, Pipal A, Redl B. Molecular analysis of the prevalent microbiota of human male and female forehead skin compared to forearm skin and the influence of make-up. *J Appl Microbiol* 2011; 110: 1381–1389.
23. Akaza N, Akamatsu H, Sasaki Y *et al.* Cutaneous *Malassezia* microbiota of healthy subjects differ by sex, body part and season. *J Dermatol* 2010; 37: 786–792.
24. Sugita T, Suzuki M, Goto S *et al.* Quantitative analysis of the cutaneous *Malassezia* microbiota in 770 healthy Japanese by age and gender using a real-time PCR assay. *Med Mycol* 2010; 48: 229–233.
25. Ihrke PJ, Schwartzman RM, McGinley K *et al.* Microbiology of normal and seborrheic canine skin. *Am J Vet Res* 1978; 39: 1487–1489.
26. Harvey RG, Lloyd DH. The distribution of bacteria (other than staphylococci and *Propionibacterium acnes*) on the hair, at the skin surface and within hair follices of dogs. *Vet Dermatol* 1995; 6: 79–84.
27. Ihrke PJ, Schwartzman RM, Halliwell RE. Effects of hormonal therapy on the microbiology of seborrheic dogs. *Am J Vet Res* 1979; 40: 1495–1497.
28. Hajek V. *Staphylococcus intermedius,* a new species isolated from animals. *Int J Syst Bacteriol* 1976; 26: 401–408.
29. Harvey RG, Lloyd DH. The distribution of *Staphylococcus intermedius* and coagulase-negative staphylococci on the hair, skin surface, within the hair follicles and on the mucous membranes of dogs. *Vet Dermatol* 1994; 5: 75–81.
30. Fazakerley J, Nuttall T, Sales D *et al.* Staphylococcal colonization of mucosal and lesional skin sites in atopic and healthy dogs. *Vet Dermatol* 2009; 20: 179–184.
31. Hartmann FA, White DG, West SE *et al.* Molecular characterization of *Staphylococcus intermedius* carriage by healthy dogs and comparison of antimicrobial susceptibility patterns to isolates from dogs with pyoderma. *Vet Microbiol* 2005; 108: 119–131.
32. Lu Y-F, McEwan NA. Staphylococcal and micrococcal adherence to canine and feline corneocytes: quantification using a simple adhesion assay. *Vet Dermatol* 2007; 18: 29–35.
33. Kristensen S, Krogh HV. A study of skin diseases in dogs and cats. III. III. Microflora of the skin of dogs with chronic eczema. *Nord Vet Med* 1978; 30: 223–230.
34. Stepanović S, Dimitrijević V, Vuković D *et al.* Staphylococcus sciuri as a part of skin, nasal and oral flora in healthy dogs. *Vet Microbiol* 2001; 82: 177–185.
35. Penna B, Varges R, Medeiros L *et al.* Species distribution and antimicrobial susceptibility of staphylococci isolated from canine otitis externa. *Vet Dermatol* 2010; 21: 292–296.
36. Cain CL, Morris DO, Rankin SC. Clinical characterization of *Staphylococcus schleiferi* infections and identification of risk factors for acquisition of oxacillin-resistant strains in dogs: 225 cases (2003–2009). *J Am Vet Med Assoc* 2011; 239: 1566–1573.
37. Woolley K, Kelly R, Fazakerley J *et al.* Reduced *in vitro* adherence of *Staphylococcus* species to feline corneocytes compared to canine and human corneocytes. *Vet Dermatol* 2008; 19: 1–6.
38. Allaker RP, Lloyd DH. Occurrence of *Staphylococcus intermedius* on the hair and skin of normal dogs. *Res Vet Sci* 1992; 52: 174–176.
39. Lloyd D. The canine skin microbiota: habitats, acquisition, interactions and exchange. *Eur J Compan Anim Pract* 2008; 18: 61–67.
40. Cafarchia C, Gallo S, Capelli G *et al.* Occurrence and population size of Malassezia spp. in the external ear canal of dogs and cats both healthy and with otitis. *Mycopathologia* 2005; 160: 143–149.
41. Hariharan H, Coles M, Poole D *et al.* Update on antimicrobial susceptibilities of bacterial isolates from canine and feline otitis externa. *Can Vet J* 2006; 47: 253–255.
42. Igimi S, Takahashi E, Mitsuoka T. *Staphylococcus schleiferi* subsp. *coagulans* subsp. nov., isolated from the external auditory meatus of dogs with external ear otitis. *Int J Syst Bacteriol* 1990; 40: 409–411.
43. Lilenbaum W, Veras M, Blum E *et al.* Antimicrobial susceptibility of staphylococci isolated from otitis externa in dogs. *Lett Appl Microbiol* 2000; 31: 42–45.
44. McKay L, Rose CD, Matousek JL *et al.* Antimicrobial testing of selected fluoroquinolones against *Pseudomonas aeruginosa* isolated from canine otitis. *J Am Anim Hosp Assoc* 2007; 43: 307–312.
45. Oliveira LC, Leite CA, Brilhante RS *et al.* Comparative study of the microbial profile from bilateral canine otitis externa. *Can Vet J* 2008; 49: 785–788.
46. Lyskova P, Vydrzalova M, Mazurova J. Identification and antimicrobial susceptibility of bacteria and yeasts isolated from healthy dogs and dogs with otitis externa. *J Vet Med A Physiol Pathol Clin Med* 2007; 54: 559–563.
47. Yoshida N, Naito F, Fukata T. Studies of certain factors affecting the microenvironment and microflora of the external ear of the dog in health and disease. *J Vet Med Sci* 2002; 64: 1145–1147.
48. Dizotti CE, Coutinho SD. Isolation of *Malassezia pachydermatis* and *M. sympodialis* from the external ear canal of cats with and without otitis externa. *Acta Vet Hung* 2007; 55: 471–477.
49. Kennis RA, Rosser EJ, Olivier NB *et al.* Quantity and distribution of *Malassezia* organisms on the skin of clinically normal dogs. *J Am Vet Med Assoc* 1996; 208: 1048–1051.
50. Campbell JJ, Coyner KS, Rankin SC *et al.* Evaluation of fungal flora in normal and diseased canine ears. *Vet Dermatol* 2010; 21: 619–625.
51. Lange CE, Zollinger S, Tobler K *et al.* Clinically healthy skin of dogs is a potential reservoir for canine papillomaviruses. *J Clin Microbiol* 2011; 49: 707–709.
52. Sturgeon A, Costa MC, Weese JS. Preliminary evaluation of the bacterial microbiome of the skin and ear in dogs. *Vet Dermatol* 2012; 23 (Suppl) 68 (abstract).

53. Beck KM, Waisglass SE, Dick HLN *et al.* Prevalence of meticillin-resistant *Staphylococcus pseudintermedius* (MRSP) from skin and carriage sites of dogs after treatment of their meticillin-resistant or meticillin-sensitive staphylococcal pyoderma. *Vet Dermatol* 2012; 23: 369–e67.
54. Griffeth GC, Morris DO, Abraham JL *et al.* Screening for skin carriage of methicillin-resistant coagulase-positive staphylococci and *Staphylococcus schleiferi* in dogs with healthy and inflamed skin. *Vet Dermatol* 2008; 19: 142–149.
55. Morris DO, Mauldin EA, O'Shea K *et al.* Clinical, microbiological, and molecular characterization of methicillin-resistant *Staphylococcus aureus* infections of cats. *Am J Vet Res* 2006; 67: 1421–1425.
56. Crespo MJ, Abarca ML, Cabañes FJ. Occurrence of *Malassezia* spp. in the external ear canals of dogs and cats with and without otitis externa. *Med Mycol* 2002; 40: 115–121.
57. Mancianti F, Nardoni S, Cecchi S *et al.* Dermatophytes isolated from symptomatic dogs and cats in Tuscany, Italy during a 15-year-period. *Mycopathologia* 2002; 156: 13–18.
58. Prado MR, Brilhante RS, Cordeiro RA *et al.* Frequency of yeasts and dermatophytes from healthy and diseased dogs. *J Vet Diagn Invest* 2008; 20: 197–202.
59. Quadros E. Furunculosis in dogs. Aetiology, pathogenesis and treatment. A clinical study. *Acta Vet Scand Suppl* 1974; 52: 1–114.
60. McEwan NA, Kalna G, Mellor D. A comparison of adherence by four strains of *Staphylococcus intermedius* and *Staphylococcus hominis* to canine corneocytes collected from normal dogs and dogs suffering from atopic dermatitis. *Res Vet Sci* 2005; 78: 193–198.
61. McEwan NA, Mellor D, Kalna G. Adherence by *Staphylococcus intermedius* to canine corneocytes: a preliminary study comparing noninflamed and inflamed atopic canine skin. *Vet Dermatol* 2006; 17: 151–154.
62. Simou C, Thoday KL, Forsythe PJ *et al.* Adherence of *Staphylococcus intermedius* to corneocytes of healthy and atopic dogs: effect of pyoderma, pruritus score, treatment and gender. *Vet Dermatol* 2005; 16: 385–391.
63. Pin D, Carlotti D-N, Jasmin P *et al.* Prospective study of bacterial overgrowth syndrome in eight dogs. *Vet Rec* 2006; 158: 437–441.
64. Lo C-W, Lai Y-K, Liu Y-T *et al.* *Staphylococcus aureus* hijacks a skin commensal to intensify its virulence: immunization targeting β-hemolysin and CAMP factor. *J Invest Dermatol* 2011; 131: 401–409.
65. Kania SA, Williamson NL, Frank LA *et al.* Methicillin resistance of staphylococci isolated from the skin of dogs with pyoderma. *Am J Vet Res* 2004; 65: 1265–1268.
66. Loeffler A, Linek M, Moodley A *et al.* First report of multiresistant, *mecA*-positive *Staphylococcus intermedius* in Europe: 12 cases from a veterinary dermatology referral clinic in Germany. *Vet Dermatol* 2007;18:412–421.
67. Olivry T, Deboer DJ, Favrot C *et al.* Treatment of canine atopic dermatitis: 2010 clinical practice guidelines from the International Task Force on Canine Atopic Dermatitis. *Vet Dermatol* 2010; 21: 233–248.
68. DeBoer DJ, Moriello KA, Thomas CB *et al.* Evaluation of a commercial staphylococcal bacterin for management of idiopathic recurrent superficial pyoderma in dogs. *Am J Vet Res* 1990; 51: 636–639.
69. Egert M, Schmidt I, Höhne H-M *et al.* rRNA-based profiling of bacteria in the axilla of healthy males suggests right–left asymmetry in bacterial activity. *FEMS Microbiol Ecol* 2011;77:146–153.
70. Fahlén A, Engstrand L, Baker BS *et al.* Comparison of bacterial microbiota in skin biopsies from normal and psoriatic skin. *Arch Dermatol Res* 2012; 304: 15–22.
71. Grice EA, Kong HH, Conlan S *et al.* Topographical and temporal diversity of the human skin microbiome. *Science* 2009; 324: 1190–1192.
72. Kong HH, Oh J, Deming C *et al.* Temporal shifts in the skin microbiome associated with atopic dermatitis disease flares and treatment. *Genome Res* 2012; 22: 850–859.
73. Zhang E, Tanaka T, Tajima M *et al.* Characterization of the skin fungal microbiota in patients with atopic dermatitis and in healthy subjects. *Microbiol Immunol* 2011; 55: 625–632.
74. Gao Z, Tseng CH, Strober BE *et al.* Substantial alterations of the cutaneous bacterial biota in psoriatic lesions. *PLoS One* 2008; 3: e2719.

To cite this article, please use DOI: 10.1111/j.1365-3164.2012.01104.x

5.2

Ulcerated and nonulcerated nontuberculous cutaneous mycobacterial granulomas in cats and dogs

Richard Malik*, Bronwyn Smits†, George Reppas‡, Caroline Laprie§, Carolyn O'Brien¶ and Janet Fyfe**

*Centre for Veterinary Education, Conference Centre B22, The University of Sydney, Sydney, NSW, Australia
†Gribbles Veterinary, 57 Sunshine Avenue, Hamilton, New Zealand
‡Vetnostics, 60 Waterloo Road, North Ryde, Sydney, NSW, Australia
§Laboratoire Vet-Histo, 13008 Marseille, France
¶Faculty of Veterinary Science, The University of Melbourne, Parkville, Victoria, Australia
**Victorian Infectious Diseases Reference Laboratory, 10 Wreckyn Street, North Melbourne, Victoria, Australia

Correspondence: Richard Malik, Centre for Veterinary Education, Conference Centre B22, The University of Sydney, Sydney, NSW 2006, Australia. E-mail: richard.malik@sydney.edu.au

Background – Mycobacterial granulomas of the skin and subcutis can be caused by one of a number of pathogens. This review concentrates on noncultivable species that cause diseases characterized by focal granuloma(s), namely leproid granuloma (in dogs) and feline leprosy (in cats). Clinically indistinguishable lesions can be caused by tuberculous organisms (*Mycobacterium bovis* and *Mycobacterium microti*) and members of the *Mycobacterium avium* complex. Rapidly growing mycobacterial species that cause infection of the subcutaneous panniculus associated with draining tracts are not discussed. Disease caused by *Mycobacterium ulcerans* is an important emerging differential diagnosis for ulcerated cutaneous nodules in certain localized regions.

Clinical lesions – Lesions comprise one or multiple nodules in the skin/subcutis. These are generally firm and well circumscribed, and typically become denuded of hair. They may or may not ulcerate, depending on the virulence of the causal organisms and the immune response of the host.

Diagnosis – The most inexpensive, noninvasive means of diagnosis is by submission of methanol-fixed, Romanowsky-stained smears to a Mycobacterium Reference Laboratory after detecting negatively stained or acid-fast bacilli on cytological smears. Scrapings of material from slides usually provide sufficient mycobacterial DNA to enable identification of the causal organism using sequence analysis of amplicons after PCR using specific mycobacterial primers.

Therapy – Therapy relies upon a combination of marginal resection of easily accessible lesions and treatment using two or three drugs effective against slowly growing mycobacteria, choosing amongst rifampicin, clarithromycin, clofazimine and pradofloxacin/moxifloxacin.

Introduction

Canine leproid granuloma (CLG)[1–8] and the feline leprosy syndromes (FLS)[9–13] are relatively uncommon nodular dermatoses caused by species of saprophytic mycobacteria that are extremely fastidious and generally uncultivable in the laboratory. Infection may be self-limiting, particularly in dogs with CLG,[2] although it is impossible to predict which cases will have lesions that regress spontaneously. In addition, as differential diagnoses for cutaneous nodules include potentially life-threatening, progressive conditions (e.g. neoplasia and tuberculosis), it is critical to make a definitive diagnosis. These conditions can be diagnosed in general practice (especially with the assistance of a Mycobacterium Reference Laboratory), but definitive diagnosis may be challenging without a high degree of suspicion and experience with the respective entities.

Accepted 11 July 2012
Sources of Funding: Richard Malik was supported by the Valentine Charlton Bequest of the Centre of Veterinary Education of the University of Sydney.
Conflict of Interest: No conflicts of interest have been declared.

Canine leproid granuloma (canine leprosy)

Canine leproid granuloma is a cutaneous or subcutaneous, typically self-limiting, nodular mycobacteriosis caused by a single, novel mycobacterium yet to be characterized fully. This condition was first described in Rhodesia.[1] The causal organism is distributed worldwide and is especially common in Australia and Brazil. Cases have also been reported in the USA, particularly from the central valley of California (Figure S1).[5]

Aetiology

The route of inoculation is not known, but it is believed that biting flies, midges, mosquitoes or other arthropods may introduce mycobacteria into the patient from an environmental niche. Circumstantial evidence supporting this hypothesis includes the observation of potential vectors in the presence of affected dogs, lesions occurring at sites favoured by such vectors [e.g. the dorsal fold of the ears (Figure 1) and the head] and the prevalence of the condition in short-coated breeds and in dogs housed outdoors.[1,2,5,6] Traumatic wounds (e.g. from sharp vegetation) subsequently contaminated with the CLG organism represent a potential, though less likely, route of infection. Occasionally, multiple animals in a kennel develop CLG, possibly due to a combination of seasonal factors and the presence of abundant mechanical vectors. Such case clusters have occurred in New Zealand, Australia (Victoria) and the USA (Georgia).[8]

Signalment and clinical findings

The condition occurs almost exclusively in short-coated breeds, with boxer dogs and boxer crossbred dogs remarkably overrepresented. Staffordshire bull terriers, foxhounds and doberman pinchers are also commonly affected.[2,5,8] The finding of characteristic lesions in typical locations and in a short-coated breed is strongly suggestive of CLG.

Canine leproid granuloma presents as single or multiple, firm, well-circumscribed nodules in the skin or subcutis (2–50 mm in diameter). Nodules typically are located on the head, particularly the dorsal fold of the ears, but may be located elsewhere, e.g. the trunk, rump or limbs. Nodules tend to occur on anatomical prominences. Larger lesions may ulcerate, generally late in the clinical course (probably as a result of effective cell-mediated immunity, rather than a mycobacterial toxin). Affected dogs are otherwise healthy, with no signs of systemic involvement. Extension of the infection to lymph nodes, nerves and internal organs does not occur. Lesions are typically painless but may be pruritic, particularly when secondary infection with *Staphylococcus pseudintermedius* occurs.

Diagnosis

Haematology and serum biochemistry profiles demonstrate nonspecific changes and are not necessary to support a diagnosis. The differential diagnosis includes infectious, inflammatory and neoplastic diseases of the subcutis and skin, such as actinomycosis, nocardiosis, bacterial pseudomycetoma associated with *S. pseudintermedius*, cutaneous leishmaniosis, eumycotic mycetoma, phaeohyphomycosis, canine nodular dermatophytosis, cryptococcosis, parasitosis (e.g. neosporosis, cutaneous dirofilariosis), cutaneous foreign body, canine histiocytic disorders, canine sterile pyogranuloma syndrome or neoplasia (e.g. histiocytomas, basal cell tumours and mast cell tumours). Solitary lesions must be distinguished from mast cell tumours and other neoplasms that can have an aggressive clinical course.

When collecting samples, it is important first to wipe the skin surface twice or more with 70% ethanol, because environmental mycobacteria may be present on the epidermis and can cause erroneous results for both culture and PCR studies. When collecting samples for biopsy, some tissue should be preserved in 10% neutral buffered formalin, while fresh tissue should be stored in a sterile specimen jar at approximately 5°C to facilitate microbial culture, molecular studies, or both.

Cytological findings

Mycobacteria appear as negatively stained bacilli (NSB) in routine cytology preparations because their lipid cell wall prevents penetration by Romanovsky-type stains (e.g. Diff-Quik® Lab Aids, Sydney, Australia; Figure 2b). Mycobacterial rods can be positively stained using a modified acid-fast procedure, such as the Ziehl–Neelsen (ZN) stain, where the bacilli take up the carbol fuchsin to appear pink, resulting in the name of acid-fast bacilli (AFB; Figure 2a). In smears, CLG is characterized by the presence of numerous, often spindle-shaped, macrophages, variable numbers of lymphocytes and plasma cells, lower numbers of neutrophils and variable numbers of medium-length AFB, either intracellularly (within macrophages or giant cells) or extracellularly.[3] While some reports

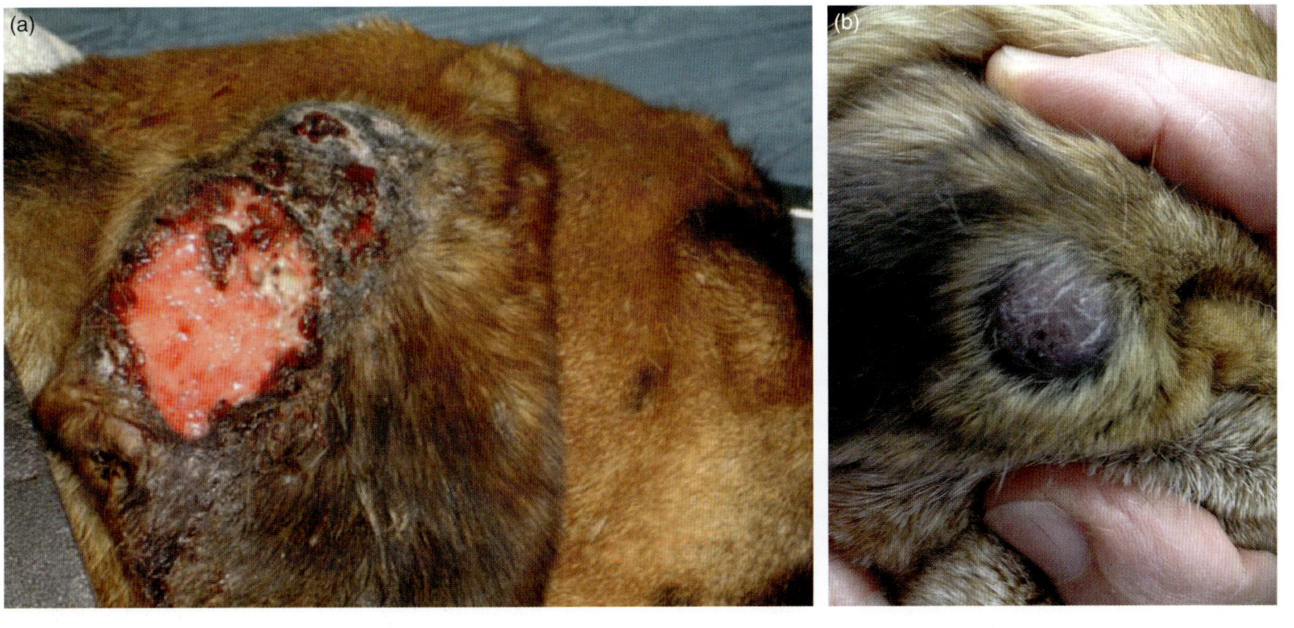

Figure 1. (a) Foxhound with severe leproid granuloma lesion on the dorsal ear fold after cleansing. Early in the disease course, lesions are nodular rather than ulcerated. Photograph courtesy of Richard Willis. (b) Early leproid granuloma lesion on the ear of a British bulldog. Photograph courtesy of Kim Barrett.

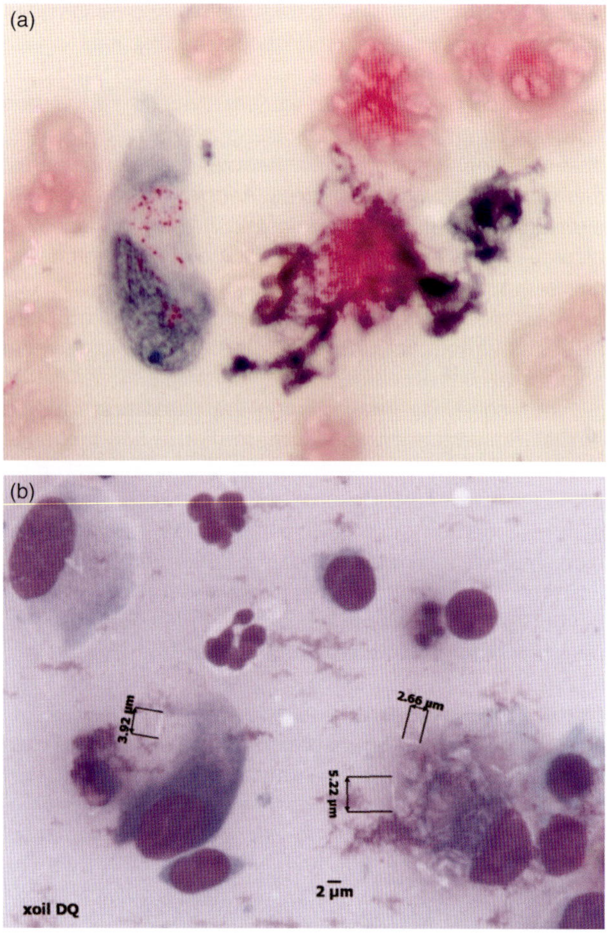

Figure 2. Cytology of canine leproid granulomas from a fine needle aspirate. In (a), a smear stained with modified Ziehl–Neelsen (ZN) method, the intracellular mycobacteria take up the stain in an irregular manner, giving rise to beaded acid-fast bacilli within macrophages. Photomicrographs courtesy of George Reppas. In (b), note the intracellular negative staining bacilli; the length of these is highly variable in Diff-Quik®-stained smears.

suggest that AFB are easy to locate in lesions, organisms can be extremely difficult to find in some instances, depending on the stage of the infection. Cytological preparations negative for AFB do not rule out CLG and should prompt examination of histological sections or submission of material for PCR. Lesions with scant AFB must be distinguished carefully from sterile granulomatous disease, for which corticosteroids are indicated, because these drugs have the potential to exacerbate CLG lesions.

Histological findings

Lesions within the dermis and subcutis consist of pyogranulomas composed of epithelioid macrophages, Langerhans-type giant cells with scattered neutrophils, plasma cells and small lymphocytes. The number and morphology of AFB in ZN-stained tissue sections is highly variable. Bacteria range from long, slender filaments in parallel sheaves to short, variably beaded bacilli or highly beaded to coccoid forms. Morphology may be more uniform in Diff-Quik®-stained smears than in fixed tissue sections. Sections may require a lengthy search, even by experienced pathologists, to locate foci in which AFB are evident.[3]

Culture

Culture of the CLG organism *in vitro* is not possible because its growth requirements have not been determined. The inability to culture this mycobacterial species has thus far prevented the full gamut of chemotaxonomy-based analyses and next-generation sequencing of the whole mycobacterial genome. Experimental transmission studies have not been attempted to date. Poorly collected specimens may be contaminated by rapidly growing mycobacteria; culture of such organisms on routine media can confound the diagnosis. Other organisms may be cultured, particularly *S. pseudintermedius*, which represents secondary infection of the lesions.

Polymerase chain reaction

Despite the organism associated with CLG being uncultivable, molecular studies have identified a mycobacterial species closely resembling members of the *Mycobacterium simiae*-related group, which contains many slow-growing saprophytic species.[2,4] A definitive diagnosis is made by amplifying regions of the bacterial 16S rRNA gene,[4] 16S–23S internal transcribed spacer region or a region within the *hsp*65 gene,[9] using mycobacterium-specific primers. Species identification is made via nucleotide sequence analysis of the amplified DNA fragment and comparison with known sequences in the GenBank database. Although PCR testing is more sensitive when performed on DNA extracted from fresh tissue, published PCR protocols are generally successful even when used on formalin-fixed, paraffin-embedded tissue.[4–6] False-negative results may occur, however, due to DNA degradation secondary to fixation, especially when contact time with formalin is over 48 h. Recently, one of the authors (J.F.) has developed a real-time PCR (qPCR) for the CLG organism that is sensitive, specific and improves the availability and accuracy of molecular diagnostics (Janet Fyfe, unpublished data). There is sufficient mycobacterial DNA in methanol-fixed slides stained with Diff-Quik® for this qPCR to be applied to material scraped from glass microscope slides and thus to arrive at a molecular diagnosis noninvasively.

Feline leprosy syndromes

Feline leprosy refers to a group of cutaneous or subcutaneous granulomas caused by mycobacteria that generally do not grow on routine laboratory media.[9–13] Cases occur worldwide, although certain mycobacterial species have strong geographical predilections. Critically, FLS lesions cannot be distinguished clinically or microscopically from lesions caused by tuberculosis bacteria (*Mycobacterium bovis* and *Mycobacterium microti*) and members of *Mycobacterium avium* complex (MAC).[14–17] Historically, FLS was sometimes included under the umbrella term 'cutaneous atypical mycobacteriosis'; however, this terminology is confusing and now redundant.

Aetiology

The location of lesions on cats suggests inoculation of organisms through insect bites, rodent bites or (most probably) fight wounds. Fight wounds are ascribed to cats, but may include injuries from prey species, such as

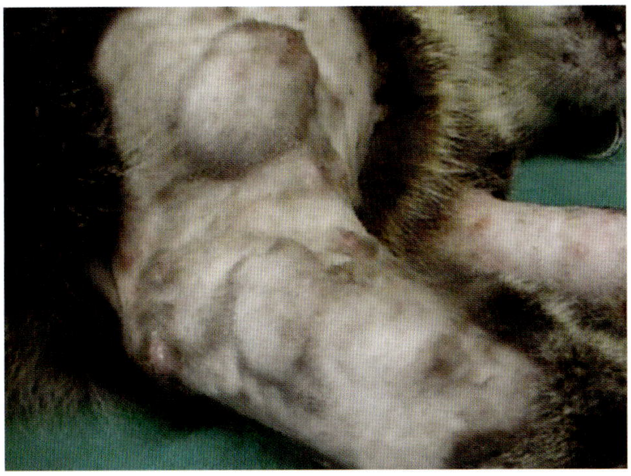

Figure 3. Cat from central France with feline leprosy due to *Mycobacterium lepraemurium* infection. The distribution of lesions suggests that the cat was inoculated by rat bites on the proximal thoracic limbs. Photograph courtesy of Caroline Laprie.

rats or possums. Mycobacterial species associated with feline leprosy include *Mycobacterium lepraemurium* (Figure 3),[18,19] *Mycobacterium visibile*,[11] *Mycobacterium* sp. strain Tarwin (Figure 4)[9] and a novel species found in New Zealand and the East coast of Australia.[12] Recent work suggests that this novel East coast species is genetically heterogeneous (Janet Fyfe and Carolyn O'Brien, unpublished data), similar to what was suggested for *Mycobacterium visibile*. *Mycobacterium lepraemurium* infections have been reported from the UK, the Netherlands, France, Greece, Australia, New Zealand the USA (including the island of Hawaii).[18,19]

The development of disease is due to a complex and incompletely understood interaction between the organism and the immune response of the host. Some organisms (e.g. *M.* sp. strain Tarwin) are associated with localized disease in an immunocompetent host, while others (e.g. the novel East coast species) are associated with haematogenously disseminated disease (usually limited to the skin) in an immunodeficient host.[9,10,12] Recent work has shown that cats with the novel East coast species can have internal organ involvement in addition to multifocal cutaneous lesions, as has been long suspected (Carolyn Obrien, personal observations).

Signalment and clinical findings

Feline leprosy syndrome is seen in cats with access to outdoors. Young male cats are overrepresented in some studies, probably because of their tendencies to fight and hunt. Cats may present with single or multiple cutaneous nodules ranging from 2 to 40 mm in diameter (Figure 4), typically accompanied by peripheral lymphadenomegaly. In cats with focal disease, lesions are often found on the face, head, limbs or trunk, areas that are vulnerable to penetrating injury. At the turn of the century, FLS was divided into the following two syndromes: (i) one in young cats (<4 years old) that initially developed localized, ulcerated, nodular lesions on the limbs (typically associated with tuberculoid pathology, paucibacillary disease and *M. lepraemurium*); and (ii) another in older cats (>9 years old) that developed generalized, nonulcerated and much less rapidly progressive skin lesions (associated with

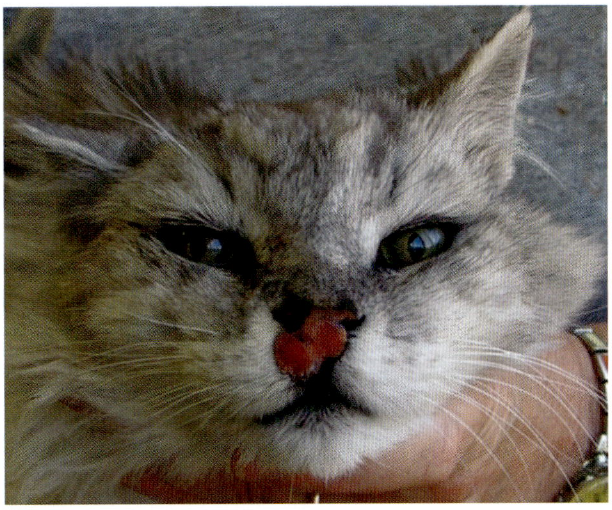

Figure 4. Mycobacterial granuloma (*Mycobacterium* sp. strain Tarwin) on the nasal planum and adjacent skin of a cat from rural Victoria, Australia. This organism is largely localized to a restricted geographical region in Tarwin, Mornington peninsula and the Eastern, North Eastern and South Eastern suburbs of Melbourne. Photograph courtesy of Dr Robert Hilton, Yarrambat, Australia.

lepromatous pathology, multibacillary disease and either the novel East coast species or *M. visibile*).[10] This schema has been questioned by Davies *et al.*,[13] who noted both tuberculoid and lepromatous histology in cats of all ages. Rarely, MAC infections can result in solitary or multifocal cutaneous granulomas in cats, resembling FLS. In the UK and Europe, tuberculosis due to *M. bovis* or *M. microti* can also produce similar skin lesions, with or without internal organ involvement in the chest or abdomen.[13–17]

Although infection with certain species (e.g. *M. lepraemurium* and *M.* sp. strain Tarwin) is linked with tuberculoid pathology, this is not absolute. Perhaps a better way to think about the pathological process is that lepromatous pathology is associated with immunodeficiency, as it is in human patients. Thus, certain mycobacterial species (*M. visibile* and the novel East coast species) are strongly associated with haematogenously disseminated disease consequent to inadequate cell-mediated immunity.

Unlike CLG, FLS typically has a progressive and occasionally aggressive clinical course, depending on the causal species, the size of the infective inoculum(s) and the immunological response of the host. In some instances, widespread lesions can develop. Large tuberculoid lesions may ulcerate. Infection can recur following incomplete surgical excision of lesions and after insufficiently long medical therapy.

Diagnosis

Haematology and serum biochemistry demonstrate nonspecific changes, but are worth pursuing, especially in older cats, because comorbidities such as liver or kidney disease can impact treatment choices and prognosis. Testing for feline immunodeficiency virus and feline leukaemia virus should be considered, although feline immunodeficiency virus positivity does not preclude successful treatment. Major differential diagnoses are similar to those described for CLG, although many of the listed conditions are rare or not observed in cats. In the UK and Europe, tuberculous skin disease (due to *M. bovis* and *M. microti*) and poxvirus infections are additional diagnostic possibilities, and accurate diagnosis is of public health significance.[14–17] In New Zealand, *M. bovis* infection must be excluded.

When collecting biopsy specimens, some tissue should be preserved in formalin and transported rapidly to the laboratory for routine histology, while fresh tissue should be stored in a sterile specimen jar at 5 or −20°C for mycobacterial culture or PCR studies, respectively.

Cytological examination

Cytologically, Diff-Quik®-stained needle aspirates from FLS lesions demonstrate large to enormous numbers of NSB, either within macrophages and giant cells or extracellularly. Acid-fast bacilli are easily seen in ZN-stained smears from needle aspirates of lesions.

Histological findings

Lesions are characterized by pyogranulomatous inflammation, with macrophages containing large to enormous numbers of AFB in sections stained with ZN or Fite's stain. Two histopathological patterns are described, although there is a spectrum between these extremes. The lepromatous form is characterized by a granulomatous reaction, with epithelioid macrophages containing numerous AFB. The tuberculoid form is characterized by lymphoid cells and macrophages surrounding necrotic foci containing small to moderate numbers of extracellular AFB.[9–11,13]

Histologically, FLS is not distinguishable from potentially zoonotic tuberculous infections. In cases due to *M. lepraemurium* and MAC, bacilli are not visible in haematoxylin and eosin-stained sections. In contrast, *M. visibile* (hence the name) and the novel East coast species can be seen in haematoxylin and eosin-stained sections because they take up the haematoxylin weakly.[10,11,13] Despite this distinguishing feature, histological features should not be relied on to predict aetiology, the specific organism involved or the prognosis. Indeed, it is desirable to instruct the veterinary laboratory to forward tissue specimens to a Mycobacterium Reference Laboratory for PCR and sequence analysis (to determine aetiology) and for attempted culture of mycobacteria and related organisms (e.g. *Nocardia* spp.).

Culture

Culture of cutaneous granulomas containing AFB typically are negative, even at the reference laboratory, although tuberculous mycobacteria (*M. bovis* and *M. microti*), MAC and, rarely, the novel East coast species may grow, the latter to only a very limited extent.[10] This may take as long as 2–3 months for tuberculous bacteria and MAC.[14–17] Although these fastidious, slow-growing mycobacteria do not readily grow on synthetic media, they may in the future be grown in cell lines in tissue culture, or within *Acanthomoeba* spp. in special media in the laboratory.

Polymerase chain reaction

As most organisms associated with FLS cannot be cultured, definitive diagnosis is made by the use of primers that amplify regions of the 16S rRNA gene and internal transcribed spacer region,[9,12] followed by sequence analysis of the resulting amplicon. The PCR testing is very sensitive even when used on formalin-fixed, paraffin-embedded tissues, as long as the contact time of the tissue specimen with formalin is <48 h. Recently, we have been able to utilize methanol-fixed smears of needle aspirates to amplify DNA in cases where NSB or AFB are abundant; this involves pippetting phosphate buffered saline (PBS; 500 μL) onto the stained glass slide using a disposable plastic filtered tip. The stained material adhering to the slide is scraped from its surface into the PBS using the pointed end of the same tip. The resulting suspension is then transferred to a 1.5 mL screw-capped plastic tube, followed by an appropriate DNA extraction procedure (Janet Fyfe, unpublished data). Indeed, this represents the most expedient and least invasive way to obtain a definitive diagnosis, where appropriate laboratory support is available.

Another strategy is to inoculate aspirates or tissue homogenates into liquid mycobacterial media (BACTEC™ MGIT™ 960 Mycobacterial Detection System; Becton Dickinson, Franklin Lakes, NJ, USA). It would seem that organisms may sometimes undergo limited multiplication in the media, which can then be used for DNA extraction.

Treatment of canine leproid granuloma and feline leprosy syndrome

The great majority of CLG infections are self-limiting, with spontaneous regression of lesions occurring within 1–3 months, regardless of treatment, most probably due to an effective adaptive cell-mediated immune response. This complicates assessment of efficacy of empirical antimicrobial regimes. In one study of CLG in dogs, 57% of cases recorded a favourable response to doxycycline, 63% had a favourable response to amoxicillin–clavulanic acid, while spontaneous regression occurred in 86% of untreated dogs.[2] Many clinicians believe drug therapy against secondary *S. pseudintermedius* is helpful, less expensive and has fewer adverse effects than drugs used for specific combination antimycobacterial therapy.

Persistence of lesions over a time frame exceeding that for which spontaneous regression commonly occurs (3–6 months) warrants further treatment. Cell-mediated immunity may be compromised in these patients, perhaps due to inherited immunodeficiency affecting major histocompatibility complex expression, innate immunity or the development of adaptive immunity. In this regard, it is of great interest that boxer dogs are at greatly increased risk for CLG, protothecosis, leishmaniosis and granulomatous (histiocytic ulcerative) colitis, diseases that may have in common insufficient innate or adaptive immunity.

In contrast, FLS generally have an unrelenting, progressive clinical course. Furthermore, lesions can recur following surgical excision, especially when inadequate margins are obtained and appropriate antimycobacterial agents are not given postoperatively. For this reason, medical treatment should be instituted immediately after diagnosis, because a delay may permit lesions to spread to contiguous skin, lymph nodes and even internal organs.

Surgical resection of nodules

In dogs with CLG, marginal surgical resection of nodules is typically curative, even if surgical excision is inadequate or margins of <2 mm are obtained. In some centers, lasers are used to vaporize the infected tissues. Although recurrence of lesions can occur in cats with early FLS lesions, this is rare when an appropriate combination of antimicrobials is administered before, during and after the procedure to ensure that therapeutic levels are present in blood and tissues intra- and postoperatively. In cases with large lesions or multifocal lesions, medical treatment alone may be a better first-line option.

Medical therapy

Treatment of mycobacterial disease presents several challenges. Antimicrobials must achieve therapeutic concentrations in a range of tissues, have minimal toxicity to the host and achieve intracellular concentrations within phagocytes. Furthermore, the drugs need to be efficacious even if there is an inadequate host immune response (defective innate or adaptive immunity, or both). Additionally, *Mycobacteria* spp. in general are known readily to develop antimicrobial-resistant clones. Therefore, combination antimicrobial therapy with agents known to be effective against slow-growing nontuberculous mycobacteria, such as rifampicin, clofazimine, clarithromycin and either moxifloxacin or pradofloxacin, may facilitate disease resolution.[20] Selection of appropriate antimicrobials is complicated by the fact that most slow-growing mycobacteria known to cause these diseases have yet to be cultured successfully on synthetic media or in tissue culture. Even those species that can be isolated on laboratory media take months to grow, which makes in vitro susceptibility testing exceeding difficult to perform.

Topical formulations of compounded clofazimine in petroleum jelly have been used as an adjunct to oral rifampicin and doxycycline to treat dogs with CLG successfully.[7] More recently, we have had good results with clofazimine compounded in silver sulphasalazine, with or without dimethyl sulfoxide.[8] Historically, radiation therapy was also found to be effective, although this is, of course, no longer recommended. A combination of rifampicin [10–15 mg/kg *per os* (p.o.) once daily] and clarithromycin (7.5–12.5 mg/kg p.o. two to three times a day) is recommended for treating severe or refractory CLG,[7] in concert with topical silver sulphasalazine. Some dogs with CLG develop lesions subsequent to therapy or self-cure, often some years later; it is not known whether the new lesions represent new infections or disease recrudescence.[2]

Feline leprosy syndromes can be treated with combinations of two to three drugs from Table 1, typically clarithromycin, pradofloxacin[21] and rifampicin or clofazimine.[9,10,20] Where pradofloxacin is unavailable, the human drug moxifloxacin[22] may be substituted at a dose of 10 mg/kg p.o. once daily; because of the large tablet size, this drug needs to be compounded for use in cats and small dogs.

Treatment of FLS should be continued until lesions have resolved completely, and ideally for a further 2–3 months after lesions have regressed, to reduce the risk of recurrence. Some cats with FLS may require lifelong treatment with clarithromycin to prevent recurrence of lesions. Some medications, for example rifampicin, may have serious adverse effects, specifically hepatotoxicity. Cats should be closely monitored for signs of liver dysfunction, including inappetence, vomiting or jaundice. Rifampicin hepatopathy can be fatal. A marked increase in serum alanine aminotransferase activity signifies the need to change therapy to a different drug, such as clofazimine. As clofazimine can cause

Table 1. Antimicrobials used in the treatment of canine leproid granuloma and feline leprosy syndromes

Drug	Dose for dogs (mg/kg)	Dose for cats (mg/kg)	Route of administration	Dosage interval (h)	Adverse effects
Pradofloxacin*	5 (tablets)	3 (suspension)	Oral	24	More effective than enrofloxacin, marbofloxacin and orbifloxacin against mycobacteria and is devoid of retinotoxicity even at high doses
Rifampicin	10–15 (maximum 600 mg total dose once daily)	10–15	Oral	24	Hepatotoxicity, induction of liver enzymes, generalized erythema and pruritus, dyspnoea, central nervous system signs, teratogenic
Clarithromycin	7.5–15	7.5–15 or 62.5–125 mg/cat/day	Oral Oral	12	Pinnal erythema, generalized erythema, hepatotoxicity
Clofazimine	Not assessed	4–10 or 25–50 mg/cat/day	Oral Oral	24 24–48	Hepatotoxicity, gastrointestinal signs, photosensitization, pitting corneal lesions
Doxycycline monohydrate	5–7.5	5–7.5	Oral	12	Gastrointestinal signs, oesophagitis
Amikacin	10–15	10–15	Intravenous, subcutaneous or intramuscular injection	24	Nephrotoxicity, ototoxicity

A combination of rifampicin (10–15 mg/kg orally once daily) and clarithromycin (7.5–12.5 mg/kg orally two to three times a day) is recommended for treating severe or refractory canine leproid granuloma,[7] in concert with topical silver sulphasalazine. Feline leprosy syndromes can be treated with combinations of two or three drugs from the table above, typically clarithromycin, pradofloxacin and rifampicin or clofazimine.
*Where pradofloxacin is unavailable, the human drug moxifloxacin may be substituted at a dose of 10 mg/kg orally once daily; because of the large tablet size, this drug needs to be compounded for use in cats and small dogs. Occasionally, it can cause vomiting.

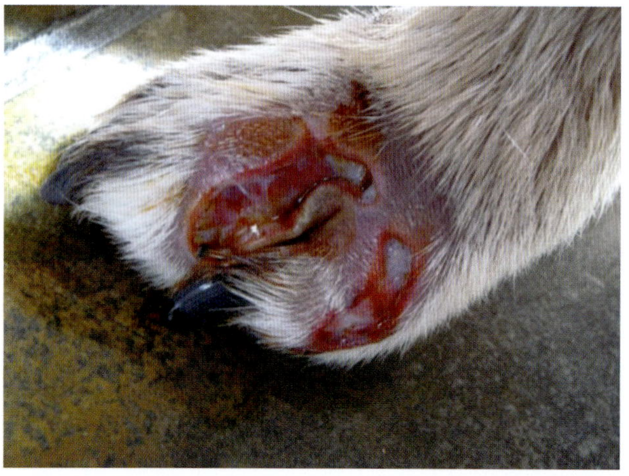

Figure 5. 'Cookie cutter-like' punched-out ulcerated lesion on the foot of an Australian kelpie attributable to *Mycobacterium ulcerans*. The patient was a working dog from a highly focal, endemic area in coastal Victoria, Australia.

photosensitization, cats should be housed indoors for the duration of therapy. When using either rifampicin or clofazimine, it is therefore prudent to monitor routine blood chemistries after 2 weeks of therapy, and perhaps on a monthly basis.

Treatment protocols will be refined as further investigations yield information about the ecological niche of mycobacteria involved in CLG and FLS, as well as growth and susceptibility of these organisms.

Localized infections due to *Mycobacterium ulcerans*

Mycobacterium ulcerans is the causative agent of Buruli ulcer,[23–28] a chronic localized infection of the skin and subcutis of human patients typically associated with necrotizing skin ulcers with undermined edges. Pre-ulcerative lesions, such as small red papules or painless subcutaneous nodules, have also been described. *Mycobacterium ulcerans* is closely related to *M. marinum*, the 'fish tank or swimming pool bacillus', which also causes infections of the skin and subcutis of people when contact with contaminated water or soil occurs in association with penetrating injury or skin maceration.[23] The extensive tissue destruction characteristic of ulcerative *M. ulcerans* infections is caused by mycolactone, a polyketide-derived macrolide with cytotoxic and immunosuppressive properties. The genes encoding the mycolactone biosynthetic pathway are located on a 174 kb plasmid likely to have been acquired by horizontal gene transfer during evolution.[23] While infections due to *M. marinum* occur in almost all geographical locations around the world, disease due to *M. ulcerans* is restricted to certain highly localized geographical regions. Presumably, this is because the organism has a restricted environmental niche, yet to be determined.

The disease is most prevalent in West Africa, where it is referred to as Buruli ulcer, whereas in Australia it occurs mainly in regions of coastal Victoria and Queensland, where it is known as Bairnsdale or Daintree ulcer, respectively. Nonhuman cases of *M. ulcerans* infection have only been reported from Victoria, mainly in marsupial species, such as koalas,[24] ringtail possums and a long-footed potoroo.[25] Two cases have been observed in alpacas (Carolyn O'Brien, personal communication). Recently, *M. ulcerans* has been diagnosed in a cat,[26] two horses,[27] more than five dogs (Figure 5)[28] and numerous brush-tailed and ring-tailed possums.[25] Polymerase chain reaction is exceedingly helpful for rapid diagnosis, although the organism grows slowly on synthetic media. Treatment involves judicious excision of infected tissues, followed by combination therapy using rifampicin and clarithromycin or a third-generation fluoroquinolone. In one horse, cryotherapy proved to be effective in resolving the lesion in the absence of systemic therapy.[27]

Zoonotic implications

The mycobacterial infections described in this review are by and large caused by saprophytic organisms, although the environmental niche of these organisms is generally not well recognized. Although it is conceivable that they may give rise to human infections via traumatic inoculation into the subcutis following penetrating injury (such as a bite or scratch), no such cases have been reported in the literature to the best of our knowledge. *Mycobacterium lepraemurium* is not considered to be a zoonosis.[19] The tuberculous organisms *M. bovis* and *M. microti* can potentially cause human disease, although the risk of contagion from infected cats to in-contact immunocompetent human patients is thought to be slight. Despite the very limited risk of zoonotic spread, it is prudent to wear disposable plastic gloves while treating wounds or medicating cats and dogs with mycobacterial infections or when manipulating the patients for other reasons, e.g. documenting lesions via photography.

Acknowledgements

Anne Fawcett was very helpful in assembling the material contained in this review.

References

1. Smith RLE. Canine skin tuberculosis. *Rhod Vet J* 1973; 3: 63–64.
2. Malik R, Love DN, Wigney DI *et al.* Mycobacterial nodular granulomas affecting the subcutis and skin of dogs (canine leproid granuloma syndrome). *Aust Vet J* 1998; 76: 403–407.
3. Charles J, Martin P, Wigney DI *et al.* Cytology and histopathology of canine leproid granuloma syndrome. *Aust Vet J* 1999; 77: 799–803.
4. Hughes MS, James G, Ball N *et al.* Identification by 16S rRNA gene analyses of a potential novel mycobacterial species as an etiological agent of canine leproid granuloma syndrome. *J Clin Microbiol* 2000; 38: 953–959.
5. Foley JE, Borjesson D, Gross TL *et al.* Clinical, microscopic, and molecular aspects of canine leproid granuloma in the United States. *Vet Pathol* 2002; 39: 234–239.
6. Conceição LG, Acha LM, Borges AS *et al.* Epidemiology, clinical signs, histopathology and molecular characterization of canine leproid granuloma: a retrospective study of cases from Brazil. *Vet Dermatol* 2011; 22: 249–256.

7. Malik R, Martin P, Wigney D *et al.* Treatment of canine leproid granuloma syndrome: preliminary findings in seven dogs. *Aust Vet J* 2001; 79: 30–36.
8. Smits B, Willis R, Studdert V *et al.* Case clusters of 'leproid granulomas' in foxhounds in New Zealand and Australia. *Vet Dermatol* 2012; 23: 465–e88.
9. Fyfe JA, McCowan C, O'Brien CR *et al.* Molecular characterization of a novel fastidious mycobacterium causing lepromatous lesions of the skin, subcutis, cornea, and conjunctiva of cats living in Victoria, Australia. *J Clin Microbiol* 2008; 46: 618–626.
10. Malik R, Hughes MS, James G *et al.* Feline leprosy: two different clinical syndromes. *J Feline Med Surg* 2002; 4: 43–59.
11. Appleyard GD, Clark EG. Histologic and genotypic characterisation of a novel *Mycobacterium* species found in three cats. *J Clin Microbiol* 2002; 40: 2425–2430.
12. Hughes MS, James G, Taylor MJ *et al.* PCR studies of feline leprosy cases. *J Feline Med Surg* 2004; 6: 235–243.
13. Davies JL, Sibley JA, Myers S *et al.* Histological and genotypical characterization of feline cutaneous mycobacteriosis: a retrospective study of formalin-fixed paraffin-embedded tissues. *Vet Dermatol* 2006; 17: 155–162.
14. Rüfenacht S, Bögli-Stuber K, Bodmer T *et al. Mycobacterium microti* infection in the cat: a case report, literature review and recent clinical experience. *J Feline Med Surg* 2011; 13: 195–204.
15. Gunn-Moore DA, McFarland SE, Brewer JI *et al.* Mycobacterial disease in cats in Great Britain: I. Culture results, geographical distribution and clinical presentation of 339 cases. *J Feline Med Surg* 2011; 13: 934–944.
16. Gunn-Moore DA, McFarland SE, Schock A *et al.* Mycobacterial disease in a population of 339 cats in Great Britain: II. Histopathology of 225 cases, and treatment and outcome of 184 cases. *J Feline Med Surg* 2011; 13: 945–952.
17. Gunn-Moore D, Dean R, Shaw S. Mycobacterial infections in cats and dogs. *In Pract* 2010; 32: 444–452.
18. Courtin F, Huerre M, Fyfe J *et al.* A case of feline leprosy caused by *Mycobacterium lepraemurium* originating from the island of Kythira (Greece): diagnosis and treatment. *J Feline Med Surg* 2007; 9: 238–241.
19. Rojas-Espinosa O, Løvik M. *Mycobacterium leprae* and *Mycobacterium lepraemurium* infections in domestic and wild animals. *Rev Sci Tech* 2001; 20: 219–251.
20. Mendoza-Aguilar M, Almaguer-Villagrán L, Jiménez-Arellanes A, *et al.* The use of the microplate alamar blue assay (MABA) to assess the susceptibility of *Mycobacterium lepraemurium* to anti-leprosy and other drugs. *J Infect Chemother* 2012; 18: 652–661.
21. Govendir M, Norris JM, Hansen T *et al.* Susceptibility of rapidly growing mycobacteria and *Nocardia* isolates from cats and dogs to pradofloxacin. *Vet Microbiol* 2011; 153: 240–245.
22. Govendir M, Hansen T, Kimble B *et al.* Susceptibility of rapidly growing mycobacteria isolated from cats and dogs, to ciprofloxacin, enrofloxacin and moxifloxacin. *Vet Microbiol* 2010; 147: 113–118.
23. Yip MJ, Porter JL, Fyfe JA *et al.* Evolution of *Mycobacterium ulcerans* and other mycolactone-producing mycobacteria from a common *Mycobacterium marinum* progenitor. *J Bacteriol* 2007; 189: 2021–2029.
24. McOrist S, Jerrett IV, Anderson M *et al.* Cutaneous and respiratory tract infection with *Mycobacterium ulcerans* in two koalas (*Phascolarctos cinereus*). *J Wildl Dis* 1985; 21: 171–173.
25. Fyfe JA, Lavender CJ, Handasyde KA *et al.* A major role for mammals in the ecology of *Mycobacterium ulcerans. PLoS Negl Trop Dis* 2010; 4: e791.
26. Elsner L, Wayne J, O'Brien CR *et al.* Localised *Mycobacterium ulcerans* infection in a cat in Australia. *J Feline Med Surg* 2008; 10: 407–412.
27. van Zyl A, Daniel J, Wayne J *et al. Mycobacterium ulcerans* infections in two horses in south-eastern Australia. *Aust Vet J* 2010; 88: 101–106.
28. O'Brien CR, McMillan E, Harris O *et al.* Localised *Mycobacterium ulcerans* infection in four dogs. *Aust Vet J* 2011; 89: 506–510.

Supporting information

Additional Supporting Information may be found in the online version of this article:

Figure S1. Diagrammatic representation of noncultivable mycobacterial infections of cats and dogs based on geography. Canine leproid granulomas are encountered in many locations (a), although the infection seems especially common in Australia and Brazil. *Mycobacterium ulcerans* has only been reported in animals from Australia, and only in animals in a tightly constrained geographic area, principally coastal Victoria (b). *Mycobacterium* sp. strain Tarwin is also seen in a geographically restricted region (c), although it was isolated from one cat residing near Lane Cove National Park in Sydney. The novel East coast species is encountered in a wider range of environments (d) in Queensland, New South Wales and Victoria; it has also been isolated from a single patient in Adelaide and in New Zealand.

To cite this article, please use DOI: 10.1111/j.1365-3164.2012.01051.x

5.3

Prevalence of and risk factors for isolation of meticillin-resistant *Staphylococcus* spp. from dogs with pyoderma in northern California, USA

Nicole G. Eckholm*, Catherine A. Outerbridge†, Stephen D. White† and Jane E. Sykes†

*William R. Pritchard Veterinary Medical Teaching Hospital and †Department of Medicine and Epidemiology, University of California, Davis, CA 95616, USA

Correspondence: Jane E. Sykes, Department of Medicine and Epidemiology, University of California, Davis, CA 95616, USA. E-mail: jesykes@ucdavis.edu

Background – Canine pyodermas associated with meticillin-resistant *Staphylococcus* spp. (MRS) have increased in prevalence over the past decade.

Hypothesis/Objectives – To compare the prevalence of MRS isolation from dogs with superficial pyoderma at a primary care clinic (PCC) and those at a tertiary care facility (VMTH) in California, USA, and identify associated risk factors.

Animals – Client-owned dogs from the VMTH (80 dogs) and the PCC (30 dogs).

Methods – Aerobic bacterial culture and antibiotic susceptibility were performed on swab specimens collected from dogs, and meticillin resistance was determined using microdilution methods according to Clinical and Laboratory Standards Institute guidelines. A *mecA* gene PCR assay was used to confirm meticillin resistance when possible.

Results – Of 89 staphylococcal isolates from the VMTH, 34 (38.2%) were meticillin resistant. In 31 dogs, pyoderma persisted, and one or more follow-up isolates were obtained. The species isolated and drug susceptibility changed unpredictably during treatment. Of 33 PCC isolates, nine (27.3%) were meticillin resistant. Multiple drug resistance was identified in 41 of 53 (77.3%) MRS isolates from the VMTH and five of nine from the PCC. The sensitivity and specificity of PCR for the detection of meticillin resistance was 34 of 39 (87%) and 86 of 87 (99%), respectively. Risk factors for meticillin resistance for both sites were antibiotic treatment within the last year ($P = 0.001$), and for VMTH, hospitalization of dogs within the last year ($P = 0.001$).

Conclusions and clinical importance – The prevalence of meticillin resistance was not different between VMTH and PCC isolates ($P = 0.29$). Previous antimicrobial therapy was an important risk factor for the isolation of MRS at both sites.

Introduction

In the past decade, skin infections caused by meticillin-resistant coagulase-positive *Staphylococcus* spp., particularly meticillin-resistant *Staphylococcus pseudintermedius* (MRSP), have become increasingly widespread in dogs.[1–4] Meticillin resistance results from presence of the *mecA* gene, which encodes penicillin binding protein 2a and confers resistance to all β-lactam antimicrobial drugs. The *mecA* gene exists on a large mobile genetic element (the staphylococcal cassette chromosome or SCC) and is passed on through clonal spread of *mecA*-positive bacteria.[5]

Prevalence rates ranging from 0.58 to 30% of meticillin-resistant *Staphylococcus* spp. isolated from dogs have been reported; however, comparison of these studies is difficult because of differences in the populations sampled (healthy versus diseased, hospitalized versus outpatients) and in the sites of specimen collection.[3,6–10] Risk factors for MRSP infection in dogs identified thus far include previous antimicrobial therapy, previous hospitalization, living in an urban environment and older age of the affected animal.[8]

Together with the increase in the prevalence of MRSP infections, there has been an increase in the number of all multidrug-resistant staphylococcal infections in dogs.[1] Multidrug resistance (MDR) is typically defined as resistance to three or more drug classes.[11,12] Staphylococci are capable of development of resistance not only to β-lactam antimicrobials but also to many other classes of antimicrobials.[1,13,14] The emergence of MDR in veterinary medicine has led to a limited range of treatment options, with increases in morbidity, mortality and cost of treatment.

Both MRSP and meticillin-resistant *Staphylococcus aureus* (MRSA) can cause pyoderma in dogs, but infections with MRSP are more prevalent.[15,16] As MRSA prefers to colonize humans, canine pyoderma caused by MRSA is of

Accepted 14 March 2012
Sources of Funding: This study is self-funded.
Conflict of Interest: No conflicts of interest have been declared.

greater zoonotic concern than pyoderma caused by MRSP.[17] Nevertheless, reports of MRSP infections in humans have been documented in the literature.[18–22]

The purpose of this study was to compare the prevalence of meticillin-resistant *Staphylococcus* (MRS) isolation from dogs with first-time or recurrent pyoderma from a primary care facility with those from a tertiary care facility, and to identify risk factors that might be associated with isolation of MRS. We hypothesized that a higher prevalence of MRS would be found in dogs seen at a tertiary care facility than in dogs seen at a primary care facility.

Materials and methods

Inclusion criteria

All dogs enrolled in the study were required to have both clinical and cytological evidence of superficial pyoderma. Pyoderma could be newly diagnosed or recurrent. Clinical abnormalities consistent with superficial pyoderma included epidermal collarettes, crusts, papules or pustules. All dogs included in the study were client-owned animals, and the study design was approved by the William R. Pritchard Veterinary Medical Teaching Hospital clinical trial review board at the University of California, Davis. Dogs with evidence of superficial pyoderma were not excluded from the study for any reason, including concurrent illness or current/previous medical therapy such as corticosteroids, antihistamines and antimicrobials. At the time of the initial appointment, owners were required to fill out a questionnaire regarding their dog's age, breed, sex, history of current and previous antibiotic administration, concurrent systemic and/or dermatological disease, previous hospitalizations, previous surgeries, bathing frequency (at home or by a professional groomer), and whether there were other pets in the household that were receiving antibiotics. In regards to humans sharing the household with the dog, the following factors were noted: whether any humans in the household were receiving or had a history of receiving antibiotics, and whether there were immunocompromised individuals, school-age athletes, healthcare workers or humans with a diagnosis of MRSA infections.

Specimen collection

Swab specimens were collected prospectively for aerobic bacterial culture and antibiotic susceptibility testing from dogs diagnosed with superficial pyoderma at their first appointment with the Dermatology Service of the William R. Pritchard Veterinary Medical Teaching Hospital, University of California, Davis (VMTH-UCD) between August 2010 and June 2011. Over the same time period, specimens were also collected from dogs diagnosed with superficial pyoderma at their first appointment by general practice veterinarians at a large general private practice in northern California. A sterile cotton swab was used to collect specimens from lesions consistent with superficial pyoderma.[23] Specimens were collected from pustules, beneath crusts and/or at the margin of epidermal collarettes. The same brand of cotton swab (BD BBL™ CultureSwab™ Plus Amies Gel without Charcoal, Double Swab; Franklin Lakes, NJ, USA) was used for collection at both the VMTH and the primary care clinic. Samples from the primary care clinic and the VMTH were submitted to the VMTH microbiology diagnostic laboratory within 24 h of collection.

Dogs seen at the VMTH-UCD were managed for the underlying cause(s) of superficial pyoderma, and systemic antimicrobial drug treatment was initiated for 30 days based on results of the bacterial culture and susceptibility. All dogs from the VMTH were treated with systemic antimicrobial therapy with the exception of one dog, which was treated with topical therapy alone. Some dogs were also treated with topical antimicrobial therapy in the formulation of shampoo, spray and/or wipe. Follow-up examination and, if clinical and cytological evidence of pyoderma persisted, skin aerobic bacterial culture and susceptibility testing, were recommended on a monthly basis after initiation of antimicrobial therapy. Whether and at what time re-evaluation occurred were dependent on owner compliance with these recommendations. For dogs that did have follow-up cultures performed, the time of follow-up after the initial visit and the results of culture and susceptibility were recorded.

Bacterial isolation

Swabs were inoculated within 24 h of collection onto 5% (v/v) sheep blood agar and MacConkey agar (Hardy Diagnostics, Santa Maria, CA, USA) and incubated at 37°C for 24–48 h. Primary identification of staphylococci was based on colony morphology, Gram staining and the conventional catalase test. Isolates were further identified using a panel of conventional biochemical tests including tube coagulase, haemolysis and acetoin production (maltose, mannitol, trehalose and arginine dihydrolase).[24] *Staphylococcus schleiferi* ssp. *coagulans* was differentiated from other coagulase-positive staphylococci, using standard biochemical methods, including the Voges–Proskauer, tube and slide coagulase assays.[25] Coagulase-negative staphylococci (CNS), including *S. schleiferi* ssp. *schleiferi*, were not identified to the species level. Coagulase-positive staphylococci with biochemical reaction patterns that did not clearly classify them as *S. intermedius*, *S. aureus*, *S. pseudintermedius* or *S. schleiferi* were designated as '*S. intermedius* group' (SIG) organisms.

Antimicrobial susceptibility testing

An automated microdilution method (Sensititre® Autoinoculator; Trek Diagnostic Systems, Clevland, OH, USA) was used for minimal inhibitory concentration (MIC) determination for 22 antimicrobial drugs according to Clinical and Laboratory Standards Institute (CLSI) guidelines.[26] The panel of antimicrobials tested included amikacin, amoxicillin–clavulanic acid, ampicillin, cefazolin, cefovecin, cefoxitin, cefpodoxime, ceftiofur, chloramphenicol, clindamycin, doxycycline, enrofloxacin, erythromycin, gentamicin, imipenem, marbofloxacin, oxacillin + 2% NaCl, penicillin, rifampicin, ticarcillin–clavulanic acid, ticarcillin and trimethoprim sulfamethoxazole. The isolates were characterized as susceptible, intermediate or resistant on the basis of cut-off MIC values published by the CLSI.[26] Isolates were classified as meticillin resistant if MIC values for oxacillin + 2% NaCl were above the MIC breakpoint published by the CLSI for that antimicrobial. Multidrug resistance was characterized as resistance to three or more different antimicrobial classes.[11,12]

mecA gene PCR assay

Quantitative PCR assay design

Primers and the probe used for *mecA* (penicillin binding protein 2a gene) were published previously.[27] Briefly, the forward primer sequence was 5′-CATTGATCGCAACGTTCAATTT-3′, the reverse primer sequence was 5′-TGGTCTTTC TGCATTCCTGGA-3′, and the probe was modified as a minor groove binder probe (Applied Biosystems, Life Technologies Corporation, Carlsbad, CA, USA) with the sequence 5′-FAM-AGTTAGATTGGGATCATAGC-BHQ-3′. The quantitative PCR systems were validated using twofold dilutions of genomic DNA that contained the *mecA* gene. The dilutions were analysed in triplicate, and a standard curve was plotted against the dilutions. The slope of the standard curve was used to calculate amplification efficiencies using the formula $E = 10^{1/-s} - 1$, where E is efficiency and s is slope of the curve with assay efficiency at 97.4%. All PCRs were carried out with a positive control. Water was used as a negative control.

Sample collection and automated nucleic acid preparation

Colonies were selected randomly and were scraped into 200 μL of PBS and vortexed for 20 s. Total nucleic acid was extracted from 200 μL of cell suspension using an automated nucleic acid extraction system (QiaX-tractor; Qiagen, Valencia, CA, USA) according to the manufacturer's recommendations.

PCR conditions

The PCR assays contained a final concentration of 400 nM for each primer and 80 nM for the probe. The PCR was performed using 1 μL bacterial genomic DNA, 4 μL water and a commercially available PCR mastermix (TaqMan Universal PCR Mastermix; Applied Biosystems, Carlsbad, CA, USA) containing 10 mM Tris–HCl (pH 8.3), 50 mM KCl, 5 mM $MgCl_2$, 2.5 mM deoxynucleotide triphosphates, 0.625 units AmpliTaq Gold DNA polymerase per reaction and 0.25 units AmpErase uracil-*N*-glycosylase per reaction in a final volume of 12 μL. The samples were placed in 384-well plates, amplified in an automated fluorometer (AB PRISM 7900 HT FAST; Applied Biosystems, Foster City, CA, USA) and run with the *mecA* gene assay along with a panbacterial assay designed to detect bacterial 16S DNA for extraction quality control (PanBakt assay; University of California, Davis molecular core facility, Davis, CA, USA). This assay utilizes two forward primers (5′-AACTCAAAGGAATTG-ACGGGG-3′ and 5′-AAACTCAAATGAATTGACGGGG-3′). The reverse primer sequence was 5′-GCTCGTTGCGGGACTTA-3′, and the minor groove binder probe 5′-FAM-TGTCGTCAGCTCGTG-BHQ-3′. Standard amplification conditions were used, as follows: 2 min at 50°C, 10 min at 95°C, 40 cycles of 15 s at 95°C and 60 s at 60°C. Fluorescence signals were collected during the annealing temperature and cycle threshold (*Ct*) values exported with a threshold of 0.1 and baseline values of 3–10. Any *Ct* value <40 was considered positive.

Statistical analysis

A two-tailed Fisher's exact test was used to compare prevalence between groups for categorical variables. The chi-squared test was used for comparisons that involved more than two groups. A *P* value of <0.05 was considered significant.

Results

VMTH cases

Animals and bacterial isolates

Eighty dogs were included in the study. Dogs ranged in age from 1 to 15 years (median 5.5 years, mean 6.4 years). There were 35 female dogs and 45 male dogs. A total of 89 staphylococcal isolates were obtained from the 80 dogs at their initial appointment at the VMTH (visit one). Thirty-four (38.2%) were meticillin resistant. The distribution of staphylococcal species isolated and prevalence of meticillin resistance for each species are shown in Table 1. There was no statistical difference in the prevalence of meticillin resistance between staphylococcal species.

Fifty-nine (73.8%) of 80 dogs presented for a follow-up examination at the VMTH. Resolution of pyoderma occurred in 28 of 59 (47.5%) dogs, while 31 of 59 (52.5%) dogs had clinical abnormalities supportive of persistent superficial pyoderma. Of those 31 dogs, visit two occurred at 1 month (25 dogs), 2 months (five dogs) and 4 months (one dog) after initial examination. All of these 31 dogs had a least one follow-up culture, with 24 (77.4%) having only a single follow-up culture performed, six (19.4%) having two follow-up cultures and one (3.2%) having three follow-up cultures.

The initial (visit one) cultures yielded 31 isolates from the 31 dogs that had a follow-up culture performed (Table 1). At visit two, 35 isolates were obtained from these 31 dogs. The distribution of staphylococcal species isolated and prevalence of meticillin resistance for each species are shown in Table 1. There was no difference in the prevalence of meticillin resistance among isolates obtained from visit one and visit two. For the 15 dogs from which an MRS was isolated at visit one, at visit two an MRS was again isolated from nine dogs, an MRS and a meticillin-susceptible staphylococcus (MSS) was isolated from one dog, and an MSS was isolated from five dogs. Of the 16 dogs that were infected with an MSS at visit one, at visit two an MSS was isolated from 10 dogs, an MRS from five dogs, and an MRS and MSS from one dog (Table 2).

Of the seven dogs that had a third culture performed (visit three), seven isolates were obtained (Table 1). Two of the three dogs from which an MRS was isolated at visit three originally tested positive for an MSS at visits one and two, and the remaining dog tested positive for an MSS on visit one and then again MRS on visit two. Two of four dogs from which an MSS was isolated at visit three also tested positive for an MSS at visits one and two, and two tested positive for an MRS at both time points. One dog had a fouth culture performed at visit four and tested positive for an MSS. This dog had an MSS isolated on visit one and visit two, and an MRS at visit three.

Different staphylococcal species were isolated over time for 11 of 31 (35.4%) dogs (Table 2), which included six of 25 (24%) dogs from which *S. pseudintermedius* was initially isolated, two of three dogs from which coagulase-negative staphylococci were initially isolated, two of two dogs from which *S. schleiferi* ssp. *coagulans* was initially isolated, and the dog from which a SIG organism was isolated.

Multidrug resistance was identified in 41 (31.6%) of all 132 staphylococcal isolates and 41 (77.3%) of the 53 MRS isolates from the VMTH ($P < 0.001$). Multidrug-resistant isolates comprised 28 of 93 (30.1%) *S. pseudintermedius*, nine of 25 (36.0%) CNS, two of eight *S. schleiferi* ssp. *coagulans*, and two of six SIG organisms. There was no difference in the prevalence of MDR among staphylococcal species ($P = 0.42$). All 53 MRS isolates were resistant to the β-lactam antimicrobial class, 38 were resistant to the lincosamides, 34 to the fluoroquinolones, 31 to the macrolides, 28 to the sulfona-

Table 1. Prevalence of meticillin resistance (number of meticillin-resistant isolates/total number of isolates) among different staphylococcal species presenting to tertiary and primary care clinics with pyoderma

Population	Visit number	SP (%)	CNS	SSC	SIG	SA	All species (%)
All VMTH dogs	1	25/67 (37.3)	7/12	2/7	0/3	n.a.	34/89 (38.2)
VMTH dogs with follow-up	1	11/25 (44)	2/3	2/2	0/1	n.a.	15/31 (48.3)
	2	10/20 (50)	5/12	0/1	0/1	1	16/35 (45.7)
	3	1/4	1/1	0	1/2	n.a.	3/7
Primary care	1	5/24	2/2	2/3	0/3	0/1	9/33 (27.3)

Abbreviations: CNS, coagulase-negative *Staphylococcus* species; n.a., not applicable; SA, *Staphylococcus aureus*; SIG, *Staphylococcus intermedius* group; SP, *Staphylococcus pseudintermedius*; SSC, *Staphylococcus schleiferi* ssp. *coagulans*; and VMTH, Veterinary Medical Teaching Hospital.

Table 2. Temporal changes in staphylococcal species isolated and meticillin resistance among dogs re-examined at a tertiary referral clinic for pyoderma

	Staphylococcal species				Meticillin resistance			
Number of dogs	Visit 1	Visit 2	Visit 3	Visit 4	Visit 1	Visit 2	Visit 3	Visit 4
1	CNS	SP	—	—	MRS	MRS	—	—
1	CNS	CNS	—	—	MRS	MRS	—	—
1	CNS	SIG	—	—	MSS	MSS	—	—
1	SIG	SP	—	—	MSS	MSS	—	—
1	SSc	SP	—	—	MRS	MSS	—	—
1	SSc	SA	—	—	MRS	MRS	—	—
1	SP	CNS	SIG	—	MRS	MRS	MSS	—
2	SP	CNS	—	—	MRS	MSS	—	—
1	SP	CNS + SSc	—	—	MRS	MRS + MSS	—	—
4	SP	SP	—	—	MRS	MRS	—	—
1	SP	SP	SP	—	MRS	MRS	MSS	—
1	SP	SP	—	—	MRS	MSS	—	—
2	SP	CNS	—	—	MSS	MRS	—	—
2	SP	CNS	—	—	MSS	MSS	—	—
1	SP	SP	CNS	SP	MSS	MSS	MRS	MSS
1	SP	SP + CNS	SIG	—	MSS	MSS + MSS	MRS	—
2	SP	SP	SP	—	MSS	MSS	MSS	—
1	SP	SP	SP	—	MSS	MRS	MRS	—
2	SP	SP	—	—	MSS	MRS	—	—
2	SP	SP	—	—	MSS	MSS	—	—
1	SP	SP + CNS	—	—	MSS	MRS + MSS	—	—
1	SP	SP + CNS	—	—	MSS	MSS + MSS	—	—

Abbreviations: CNS, coagulase-negative *Staphylococcus* species; MRS, meticillin-resistant *Staphylococcus*; MSS, meticillin-susceptible *Staphylococcus*; SA, *S. aureus*; SIG, *S. intermedius* group; SP, *S. pseudintermedius*; and SSc, *S. schleiferi* ssp. *coagulans*.

mides, 10 to the aminoglycosides, four to chloramphenicol, and three to the tetracyclines; however, intermediate resistance to tetracyclines was identified in 29 of the isolates. The prevalence of MDR was not different between the MRS isolates from visit one and those from follow-up visits.

Antimicrobial therapy prescribed after visit one culture

Of the 48 dogs from which an MSS was isolated at visit one (day 0), 26 were treated with cefalexin, 15 with cefpodoxime, four with lincomycin, two with doxycycline, and one with marbofloxacin. Of the 32 dogs from which an MRS was isolated at visit one, 16 were treated with doxycycline, seven with clindamycin, five with chloramphenicol, two with marbofloxacin, one with enrofloxacin, and one with a topical 4% chlorhexidine spray (Trizchlor 4% Spray™; Dermapet, Potomac, MD/Dechra, Overland Park, KS, USA).

Of the 16 dogs with follow-up cultures from which an MSS was isolated at visit one (day 0), eight were treated with cefalexin, four with cefpodoxime, two with lincomycin, one with marbofloxacin, and one with doxycycline. Of the eight dogs treated with cefalexin, five were culture positive for an MRS at visit two. Of the four dogs treated with cefpodoxime, one was culture positive for an MRS at visit two. There was no difference in the proportion of dogs infected with an MRS at visit two between dogs treated with cefalexin and dogs treated with cefpodoxime ($P = 0.54$). None of four dogs treated with non-β-lactam drugs was culture positive for an MRS at visit two. There was no difference in the proportion of dogs from which an MRS was isolated at visit two when dogs treated with non-β-lactam drugs and dogs treated with β-lactams ($P = 0.23$) or cefalexin alone ($P = 0.08$) were compared.

Of the 15 dogs with follow-up cultures that were culture positive for an MRS at visit one (day 0), 10 were subsequently treated with doxycycline, two with chloramphenicol, one with enrofloxacin, one with clindamycin, and one with 4% chlorhexidine topical spray. All dogs except for four of the dogs treated with doxycycline and the dog treated with clindamycin remained culture positive for an MRS at visit two. The one dog from which a clindamycin-susceptible and erythromycin-susceptible MRSP was isolated was treated with clindamycin; subsequently, a clindamycin- and erythromycin-resistant, meticillin-susceptible *S. pseudintermedius* (MSSP) was isolated from this dog. Chloramphenicol-susceptible MRS species were isolated from two dogs (one *S. pseudintermedius* and the other a CNS), and in both cases treatment with chloramphenicol was followed by isolation of chloramphenicol-resistant *S. pseudintermedius* MRS isolates.

No statistical associations between antimicrobial use and persistence of MRS isolates could be made.

Isolates from primary care visits

Animals and bacterial isolates

A total of 33 dogs were enrolled in the study from the primary care clinic. The dogs ranged in age from 8 weeks to 13 years (median 6 years, mean 5.6 years). There were 16 females and 17 males. A total of 33 staphylococcal isolates were obtained from the 33 dogs at their initial visit to the primary care practice. Nine (27.3%) were meticillin resistant. There was no difference in the distribution of staphylococcal species from dogs seen at tertiary and primary care clinics (Table 1). The prevalence of meticillin resistance among staphylococci was not different among

VMTH isolates when compared with that among isolates from primary care visits ($P = 0.29$).

Multidrug resistance was identified in five (15.2%) of the 33 isolates, these being five (55.5%) of the nine MRS isolates. Of the nine MRS isolates, nine were resistant to the β-lactam antimicrobial class, four to the lincosamides, four to the fluoroquinolones, two to the macrolide class, two to the aminoglycosides, one to the sulfonamides, one to chloramphenicol, and none to the tetracyclines; however, intermediate resistance to the tetracyclines was identified in two of the nine isolates. The prevalence of MDR among all staphylococci from the primary care clinic was not significantly different from that among isolates from the tertiary referral clinic ($P = 0.08$).

Analysis of risk factors

An identifiable underlying disease was present in 66 (82.5%) of the 80 dogs seen at the tertiary referral hospital. Fifty-nine dogs had allergic skin disease, five had endocrine disease, one had a skin-related immune-mediated disease and one had neoplasia (splenic haemangiosarcoma). Of the 32 dogs from which an MRS was isolated on the initial visit, 31 (96.8%) had an identifiable underlying disease. At the primary care clinic, an underlying disease was identified in 11 (33.3%) of 33 cases, which included the nine dogs from which an MRS was isolated. Eight dogs were identified as having allergic skin disease, three had endocrine diseases, and for 22 dogs an underlying disease was not identified. Analysis of risk factors for dogs from both facilities showed that those receiving antibiotics at presentation, those that had received antibiotics in the last year, and those that were hospitalized in the last year were more likely to be culture positive for an MRS (Table 3). No other variables analysed were significantly associated with meticillin resistance.

mecA gene PCR

One hundred and twenty-six isolates were available for *mecA* gene PCR, which included 39 (62.9%) of the 62 MRS isolates and 87 MSS. Meticillin-resistant species included 28 *S. pseudintermedius*, six CNS, three *S. schleiferi*, one *S. aureus* and one SIG organism. Meticillin-susceptible species included 67 *S. pseudintermedius*, seven SIG organisms, seven *S. schleiferi*, five CNS and one *S. aureus*. The panbacterial PCR assay was positive for all isolates (median *Ct* value 17.60; range 14.11–23.86). All except five MRS isolates (three *S. pseudintermedius*, one *S. aureus* and a coagulase-negative staphylococcal species) tested positive for the *mecA* gene (median *Ct* value 19.05; range 15.84–23.19). One MSSP tested positive for the *mecA* gene (*Ct* value 20.72). Thus, using phenotypic (conventional biochemical) testing as the gold standard, the sensitivity and specificity of the assay were 87 and 99%, respectively.

Discussion

This study examined the prevalence of MRS isolation from dogs with superficial pyoderma in a tertiary referral hospital and compared it with that seen in a primary care practice. The prevalence of MRS isolation in dogs with first time or recurrent pyoderma seen at primary care facilities has not previously been reported, to our knowledge. In our study, we found that 38.2% of staphylococcal isolates from the VMTH and 27.3% of isolates from the primary care facility were MRS species. The prevalence of meticillin resistance among staphylococci in the study reported here appeared to be higher than that reported recently for dogs with pyoderma seen at veterinary teaching hospitals in Spain (10.4%) and Korea (17.6%), but lower than that reported for dogs with pyoderma in Japan, where the prevalence of meticillin resistance among *S. pseudintermedius* and *S. schleiferi* isolates as determined using PCR was 66.5 and 30%, respectively.[7,13,28] However, direct comparisons are difficult to make owing to differences in the populations of dogs studied and specimen collection methods used. In a recent study from the University of Pennsylvania, USA, 57% of 225 *S. schleiferi* isolates were meticillin resistant.[29]

In the study reported here, we found no significant difference in the prevalence of meticillin resistance in dogs with pyoderma between a primary care facility and a tertiary referral hospital. This contrasted with our initial hypothesis that the prevalence of MRS isolation would be lower in dogs from a primary care clinic. Likewise, we found that there was no difference in the prevalence of MDR between primary care and tertiary referral clinics, although the lack of an association was less strong ($P = 0.08$). If the prevalence of meticillin resistance in dogs seen for pyoderma at other primary care clinics is similar to that found in this study, it could support the need for culture of skin lesions from all dogs with newly diagnosed pyoderma.

As found in other studies of dogs with pyoderma and/or studies that examined MRS colonization, a his-

Table 3. Analysis of risk factors for isolation of meticillin-resistant staphylococci in 80 dogs with pyoderma from a tertiary referral hospital

	VMTH			Primary care			All dogs		
Variable	MRS	MSS	*P*-value	MRS	MSS	*P*-value	MRS	MSS	*P*-value
Treated with antibiotics at presentation	11/17	6/17	0.026	1/4	3/4	1	12/21	9/21	0.042
Not treated with antibiotics at presentation	21/63	42/63		8/29	21/29		29/92	63/92	
Antibiotics in the last year	32/34	32/34	<0.001	9/12	3/12	<0.001	41/76	35/76	<0.0001
No antibiotics in the last year	0/16	16/16		0/21	21/21		0/37	37/37	
Hospitalized in the last year	14/19	5/19	0.001	4/8	4/8	0.17	18/27	9/27	<0.001
Not hospitalized in the last year	18/61	43/61		5/25	20/25		23/86	63/86	
Owned by/lived with healthcare worker	6/16	10/16	1	1/4	3/4	1	7/20	13/20	1
Not living with a healthcare worker	26/64	38/64		8/29	21/29		34/93	59/93	

Significance was defined as $P < 0.05$. Abbreviations: MRS, meticillin-resistant *Staphylococcus*; MSS, meticillin-susceptible *Staphylococcus*; and VMTH, Veterinary Medical Teaching Hospital.

tory of antimicrobial drug therapy was the single most important risk factor for isolation of MRS in our study.[8,11,28,30,31] This was true for both dogs from primary care and those from tertiary referral clinics. In fact, all of the dogs from which MRS were isolated, from both clinics, had received antibiotics within the last year. In contrast, two-thirds of the dogs infected with an MSS seen at the tertiary referral clinic and fewer than 15% of the dogs with an MSS seen at the primary care clinic had received antibiotics within the last year. The exact time frame within the year in which each dog in this group had received antibiotics was not determined. A previous study found that most dogs treated with antimicrobials within the last 6 months were more likely to be colonized with MRSP.[30] A history of antimicrobial drug use has also been associated with the isolation of MDR bacteria in dogs.[11,32] We did not examine factors associated with MDR in this study.

The use of cephalosporins, carbapenems and fluoroquinolones are known risk factors for acquisition of MRSA in humans.[33,34] When examined prospectively, we were unable to find an association between the specific antimicrobial drug used at visit one and the development of meticillin resistance, but the numbers were too small for statistical significance to be identified. Five dogs from which an MSS was isolated (all *S. pseudintermedius*) that were treated with cefalexin or cefpodoxime subsequently became culture positive for an MRS isolate of the same or different (CNS) staphylococcal species within 1 month after initiating therapy, but other dogs treated with these antibiotics remained culture positive for an MSS isolate. Some dogs that were initially culture positive for an MRS became culture positive for an MSS within 1 month after initiating therapy with a variety of different antimicrobial drug classes. One dog from which a clindamycin-susceptible MRSP was isolated was treated with clindamycin; subsequently, a clindamycin-resistant but MSSP was isolated from this dog. Inducible clindamycin resistance has been reported in canine meticillin-resistant MRSP isolates.[35] As D-testing was not performed in the present study, we could not confirm that this was due to inducible clindamycin resistance. In two dogs, a chloramphenicol-susceptible MRS was isolated (*S. pseudintermedius* and a CNS), and in both dogs, treatment with chloramphenicol was followed by isolation of a chloramphenicol-resistant MRSP.

In the present study, MRS isolates were significantly more likely to be MDR than MSS isolates, both from primary care and from tertiary referral care facilities. There was no difference in the prevalence of MDR among staphylococcal species, but the number of isolates for some species, such as *S. schleiferi* and *S. aureus*, was probably too low for a difference to be detected. Numerous other studies have also shown an association between meticillin resistance and MDR.[1,5,6,13] Resistance among isolates from both the VMTH and the primary care facility was most commonly found to the β-lactam group, followed by the lincosamide, fluoroquinolone, macrolide and sulfonamide antimicrobial classes. There was a low prevalence of resistance to chloramphenicol, aminoglycosides and tetracyclines, although many isolates had intermediate resistance to tetracyclines, which might suggest questionable efficacy of tetracycline *in vivo*. A previous study showed that 69.9% of *S. pseudintermedius* isolates from dogs in Europe and North America carry the *tet K* or the *tet M* gene, respectively, which confer tetracycline resistance.[5]

Of interest, we found that both resistance patterns and the staphylococcal species isolated changed unpredictably with each follow-up culture after initiation of treatment. There were no significant patterns recognized with regard to the staphylococcal species isolated except that the most frequently cultured species was *S. pseudintermedius* on both initial and follow-up cultures. However, in some cases initial cultures grew *S. pseudintermedius*, and on follow-up a CNS or *S. schleiferi* ssp. *coagulans* was isolated, or vice versa. The reasons for this are unclear, but it may be related to selection of a particular species as a result of antibiotic pressure. Alternatively, more than one staphylococcal species may be present in different anatomical locations, and culture at different sites may account for variation in the species isolated. In some studies, more than one staphylococcal species was isolated from the same lesion in dogs with superficial bacterial folliculitis.[23,36–38] Therefore, it is possible that in some cases multiple staphylococcal species were present but only one was isolated. Finally, the detection of an organism at the site of a lesion does not necessarily imply pathogenicity, because only colonization may be present. This may also explain the isolation of CNS from dogs with pyoderma, which (apart from *S. schleiferi* ssp. *schleiferi*) are normally considered to be nonpathogenic. However, in this study, *S. schleiferi* ssp. *schleiferi* were not differentiated from other CNS.

In this study, we used a *mecA* gene PCR assay to confirm meticillin resistance in 126 of the165 isolates as documented using phenotypic methods. The *mecA* gene was detected in 87% of oxacillin-resistant isolates and is therefore likely to represent the primary means of acquiring resistance. Other mechanisms of resistance are also possible, such as production of oxacillin-specific β-lactamase.[1] This may explain the negative *mecA* gene PCR results for five of the MRS isolates. One MSS isolate was *mecA* positive. It has been suggested that some susceptible isolates that are *mecA* positive on PCR assay may contain a full-length copy of the *mecA* gene but are unable to express penicillin binding protein 2a as a result of a mutation in an open reading frame or promoter.[39] Alternatively, MSS isolates may have a fully functional gene that is transcriptionally downregulated. In both of these situations, the *mecA* gene would be detected using PCR, but isolates would be phenotypically negative for oxacillin resistance.

In the present study, we also evaluated risk factors that may be associated with MRS isolation. Risk factors for the development of MRSA have been studied extensively in human medicine and to some degree in veterinary medicine. Magalhaes *et al.*[40] found that the number of courses of antimicrobials, the number of days admitted to veterinary clinics and a history of surgical implants were important risk factors for isolation of MRSA from dogs.[40] In addition to previous antimicrobial therapy, we also found that dogs hospitalized within the last year were more likely to be culture positive for an MRS. We did not specifically examine the number of visits to a veterinary hospital for each dog. Other risk factors examined were not found to be significantly associated with MRS isolation, although the small sample size in this study for some groups may have limited our ability to identify some factors as important.

In conclusion, we found no significant difference in the prevalence of meticillin resistance of staphylococcal isolates among dogs with pyoderma seen at a tertiary referral hospital and a primary care facility in northern California, USA. We also found that the majority of MRS isolates were MDR, and the staphylococcal species isolated and drug susceptibility changed unpredictably with treatment in dogs that did not clear their infection. Finally, we also identified previous antimicrobial therapy and hospitalization within the last year as important risk factors in the development of an MRS pyoderma. These findings may support the need for culture-based antimicrobial therapy and, if possible, the use of topical antibacterial therapy in lieu of systemic antimicrobials for the treatment of superficial pyoderma in dogs.

Acknowledgements

The authors thank Casey Stepnik, Samantha Crothers, Nina Toebe and Judy Schettler for sample collection. Special thanks are due to Eileen Samitz for her invaluable expertise in sample identification.

References

1. Jones RD, Kania SA, Rohrhach BW *et al.* Prevalence of oxacillin- and multidrug-resistant staphylococci in clinical samples from dogs: 1,772 samples (2001–2005). *J Am Vet Med Assoc* 2007; 230: 221–227.
2. Yoo JH, Yoon JW, Young-Lee SY *et al.* High prevalence of fluoroquinolone and methicillin-resistant *Staphylococcus pseudintermedius* isolates from canine pyoderma and otitis externa in veterinary teaching hospital. *J Microbiol Biotechnol* 2010; 20: 798–802.
3. Griffeth GC, Morris DO, Abraham JL *et al.* Screening for carriage of methicillin-resistant coagulase-positive staphylococci and *Staphylococcus schleiferi* in dogs with healthy and inflamed skin. *Vet Dermatol* 2008; 19: 142–149.
4. De Lucia M, Moodley A, Latronico F *et al.* Prevalence of canine methicillin-resistant *Staphylococcus pseudintermedius* in a veterinary diagnostic laboratory in Italy. *Res Vet Sci* 2011; 91: 346–348.
5. Perreten V, Kadlec K, Schwarz S *et al.* Clonal spread of methicillin-resistant *Staphylococcus pseudintermedius* in Europe and North America: an international multicentre study. *J Antimicrob Chemother* 2010; 65: 1145–1154.
6. Ruscher C, Lubke-Becker A, Wleklinski CG *et al.* Prevalence of methicillin-resistant *Staphylococcus pseudintermedius* isolated from clinical samples of companion animals and equidaes. *Vet Microbiol* 2009; 136: 197–201.
7. Kawakami T, Shibata S, Murayama N *et al.* Antimicrobial susceptibility and methicillin resistance in *Staphylococcus pseudintermedius* and *Staphylococcus schleiferi* subsp. coagulans isolated from dogs with pyoderma in Japan. *J Vet Med Sci* 2010; 72: 1615–1619.
8. Nienhoff U, Kadlec K, Chaberny IF *et al.* Methicillin-resistant *Staphylococcus pseudintermedius* among dogs admitted to a small animal hospital. *Vet Microbiol* 2011; 150: 191–197.
9. Morris DO, Rook KA, Schofer FS *et al.* Screening of *Staphylococcus aureus*, *Staphylococcus intermedius*, and *Staphylococcus schleiferi* isolates obtained from small companion animals for antimicrobial resistance: a retrospective review of 749 isolates (2003–04). *Vet Dermatol* 2006; 17: 332–337.
10. Bemis DA, Jones RD, Frank LA *et al.* Evaluation of susceptibility test breakpoints used to predict *mecA*-mediated resistance in *Staphylococcus pseudintermedius* isolated from dogs. *J Vet Diagn Invest* 2009; 21: 53–58.
11. Pellerin JL, Bourdeau P, Sebbag H *et al.* Epidemiosurveillance of antimicrobial compound resistance of *Staphylococcus intermedius* clinical isolates from canine pyodermas. *Comp Immunol Microbiol Infect Dis* 1998; 21: 115–133.
12. Hoekstra KA, Paulton RJL. Clinical prevalence and antimicrobial susceptibility of *Staphylococcus aureus* and *Staph. intermedius* in dogs. *J Appl Microbiol* 2002; 93: 406–413.
13. Yoon JW, Lee KJ, Chae MJ *et al.* Antibiotic resistance profiles of *Staphylococcus pseudintermedius* isolates from canine patients in Korea. *J Microbiol Biotechnol* 2010; 20: 1764–1768.
14. Penna B, Varges R, Medeiros L *et al.* Species distribution and antimicrobial susceptibility of staphylococci isolated from canine otitis externa. *Vet Dermatol* 2009; 21: 292–296.
15. Hanselman BA, Kruth S, Weese SJ. Methicillin-resistant staphylococcal colonization in dogs entering a veterinary teaching hospital. *Vet Microbiol* 2008; 126: 277–281.
16. Weese JS, Van Duijkeren E. Methicillin-resistant *Staphylococcus aureus* and *Staphylococcus pseudintermedius* in veterinary medicine. *Vet Microbiol* 2010; 140: 418–429.
17. Paul NC, Moodley A, Ghibaudo G *et al.* Carriage of methicillin-resistant *Staphylococcus pseudintermedius* in small animal veterinarians: indirect evidence of zoonotic transmission. *Zoonoses Public Health* 2011; 58: 533–539.
18. Campanile F, Bongiorno D, Borbone S *et al.* Characterization of a variant of the SCC*mec* element in a bloodstream isolate of *Staphylococcus intermedius. Microb Drug Resist* 2007; 13: 7–10.
19. Kempker R, Mangalat D, Kongphet-Tran T *et al.* Beware of the pet dog: a case of *Staphylococcus intermedius* infection. *Am J Med Sci* 2009; 338: 425–427.
20. Stegmann R, Burnens A, Maranta CA *et al.* Human infection associated with methicillin-resistant *Staphylococcus pseudintermedius* ST71. *J Antimicrob Chemother* 2010; 65: 2047–2048.
21. Van Hoovels L, Vankeerberghan A, Boel A *et al.* First case of *Staphylococcus pseudintermedius* infection in a human. *J Clin Microbiol* 2006; 44: 4609–4612.
22. Chuang CY, Yang YL, Hsueh PR *et al.* Catheter-related bacteremia caused by *Staphylococcus pseudintermedius* refractory to antibiotic-lock therapy in a hemophilic child with dog exposure. *J Clin Microbiol* 2010; 48: 1497–1498.
23. White SD, Brown A, Chapman P *et al.* Aerobic bacterial culture of epidermal collarettes in dogs. *J Am Vet Med Assoc* 2005; 226: 904–908.
24. Jang SS, Hirsh DC, Biberstein EL. *A Diagnostic Manual of Veterinary Clinical Bacteriology and Mycology*,revised edn. Davis, CA: University of California Press, 2005.
25. Ljutov V. Technique of Voges-Proskauer test. *Acta Pathol Microbiol Scand* 1963; 58: 325–335.
26. CLSI. *Performance Standards for Antimicrobial Susceptibility Testing.* M100-S19 CLSI, Wayne, PA, (2005 and 2011), 2009.
27. Francois P, Pittet D, Bento M *et al.* Rapid detection of methicillin-resistant *Staphylococcus aureus* directly from sterile or nonsterile clinical samples by a new molecular assay. *J Clin Microbiol* 2003; 41: 254–260.
28. Huerta B, Maldonado A, Ginel PJ *et al.* Risk factors associated with the antimicrobial resistance of staphylococci in canine pyoderma. *Vet Microbiol* 2011; 150: 302–308.
29. Cain CL, Morris DO, Rankin SC. Clinical characterization of *Staphylococcus schleiferi* infections and identification of risk factors for acquisition of oxacillin-resistant strains in dogs: 225 cases (2003–2009). *J Am Vet Med Assoc* 2011; 239: 1566–1573.
30. Sasaki T, Kikuchi K, Tanaka Y *et al.* Methicillin-resistant *Staphylococcus pseudintermedius* in a veterinary teaching hospital. *J Clin Microbiol* 2007; 45: 1118–1125.
31. Penna B, Varges R, Medeiros L *et al.* Species distribution and antimicrobial susceptibility of staphylococci isolated from canine otitis externa. *Vet Dermatol* 2010; 21: 292–296.

32. Kunkle GA. New considerations for rational antibiotic therapy of cutaneous staphylococcal infection in the dog. *Semin Vet Med Surg (Small Anim)* 1987; 2: 212–220.
33. Westh H, Zinn CS, Rosdahl VT *et al.* An international multicenter study of antimicrobial consumption and resistance in *Staphylococcus aureus* isolates from 15 hospitals in 14 countries. *Microb Drug Resist* 2004; 10: 169–176.
34. Tacconelli E, De Angelis G, Cataldo MA *et al.* Antibiotic usage and risk of colonization and infection with antibiotic-resistant bacteria: a hospital population-based study. *Antimicrob Agents Chemother* 2009; 53: 4264–4269.
35. Rubin JE, Ball KR, Chirino-Trejo M. Antimicrobial susceptibility of *Staphylococcus aureus* and *Staphylococcus pseudintermedius* isolated from various animals. *Can Vet J* 2011; 52: 153–157.
36. Pinchbeck LR, Cole LK, Hillier A *et al.* Genotypic relatedness of staphylococcal strains isolated from pustules and carriage sites in dogs with superficial bacterial folliculitis. *Am J Vet Res* 2006; 67: 1337–1346.
37. Medleau L, Long RE, Brown J *et al.* Frequency and antimicrobial susceptibility of Staphylococcus species isolated from canine pyodermas. *Am J Vet Res* 1986; 47: 229–231.
38. Frank LA, Kania SA, Hnilica KA *et al.* Isolation of *Staphylococcus schleiferi* from dogs with pyoderma. *J Am Vet Med Assoc* 2003; 222: 451–454.
39. Kania SA, Williamson NL, Frank LA *et al.* Methicillin resistance of staphylococci isolated from the skin of dogs with pyoderma. *Am J Vet Res* 2004; 65: 1265–1268.
40. Magalhaes RJS, Loeffler A, Lindsay J *et al.* Risk factors for methicillin-resistant *Staphylococcus aureus* (MRSA) infection in dogs and cats: a case control study. *Vet Res* 2010; 41: 55.

To cite this article, please use DOI: 10.1111/j.1365-3164.2012.01100.x

5.4

Usefulness of cefovecin disk-diffusion test for predicting *mecA* gene-containing strains of *Staphylococcus pseudintermedius* and clinical efficacy of cefovecin in dogs with superficial pyoderma

Keita Iyori*, Yoichi Toyoda†, Kaori Ide†, Toshiroh Iwasaki† and Koji Nishifuji†

*Animal Medical Center, Tokyo University of Agriculture and Technology, Tokyo 183-8509, Japan
†Department of Veterinary Medicine, Faculty of Agriculture, Tokyo University of Agriculture and Technology, Tokyo 183-8509, Japan

Correspondence: Koji Nishifuji, Department of Veterinary Medicine, Faculty of Agriculture, Tokyo University of Agriculture and Technology, 3-5-8 Saiwai-cho, Fuchu, Tokyo 183-8509, Japan. E-mail: kojimail@cc.tuat.ac.jp

Background – Cefovecin has been widely used to treat skin infections in dogs. The relationship of the cefovecin disk-diffusion test results to the presence of the *mecA* gene and the clinical efficacy of cefovecin have not been fully evaluated.

Hypothesis/Objectives – To determine the usefulness of an *in vitro* cefovecin disk-diffusion test in predicting the presence of the *mecA* gene in *Staphylococcus pseudintermedius*, as well as the *in vivo* efficacy of cefovecin therapy in dogs with superficial pyoderma.

Methods – Twenty-six *S. pseudintermedius* strains isolated from 22 dogs with pyoderma were used. *In vitro* disk-diffusion test results of cefovecin were compared with agar-dilution test results, the presence of the *mecA* gene, and the improvement in clinical scores of dogs with superficial pyoderma at 14 days post treatment.

Results – There was a significant linear correlation ($r = -0.83$) between the diameter of the obvious zone of inhibition by disk diffusion and the minimal inhibitory concentration for cefovecin ($P < 0.0001$). Receiver operating characteristic analysis revealed that zone diameters between 25 and 27 mm exhibited better sensitivity (92.9%) and specificity (100.0%) for detection of strains carrying the *mecA* gene. The mean improvement in clinical scores in dogs carrying cefovecin-resistant strains was significantly lower than in dogs carrying cefovecin-susceptible strains ($P < 0.01$).

Conclusions and clinical importance – The cefovecin disk-diffusion test with a cut-off value estimated in this study was valuable for predicting *mecA* gene carriage in *S. pseudintermedius*, as well as the *in vivo* efficacy of cefovecin therapy in dogs with superficial pyoderma caused by *S. pseudintermedius*.

Introduction

Superficial pyoderma is a common bacterial disease in dogs.[1] *Staphylococcus pseudintermedius* is the major staphylococcal species isolated from lesions of canine superficial pyoderma.[2–4] Cephalosporins are commonly recommended as the first choice for the treatment of canine superficial pyoderma.[1] Cefovecin (Convenia®; Pfizer Animal Health, New York, NY, USA), a broad-spectrum and long-acting cephalosporin injectable antibiotic, has recently been approved for the treatment of skin infections in dogs. The pharmacokinetic and pharmacodynamic properties of cefovecin, which are characterized as having slow elimination and long-lasting antibacterial activity,[5] allow veterinarians to prescribe the drug at 14 day intervals for the treatment of cutaneous infections in dogs. Two studies demonstrated that cefovecin is as effective as oral cefadroxil or amoxicillin–clavulanate for improving the clinical signs in dogs with pyoderma.[6,7]

Meticillin-resistant or multidrug-resistant staphylococci are increasingly being isolated from dogs with superficial pyoderma and are a therapeutic problem.[3,8,9] Meticillin-resistant staphylococci express the penicillin-binding protein 2a (PBP2a), which is encoded by the *mecA* gene; thus, organisms possessing this gene show low affinity for all β-lactam antibiotics currently marketed for clinical use.[1,10–12] It is therefore important to determine the presence of the *mecA* gene in clinical isolates of staphylococci prior to the selection of an antibiotic for the treatment of canine pyoderma.

The disk-diffusion and agar-dilution tests are used to determine susceptibility of bacteria to antimicrobial drugs. Disk-diffusion susceptibility tests are used in clinical laboratories because of their rapid and uncomplicated pro-

Accepted 4 July 2012
Sources of Funding: This study was sponsored and test materials were supplied by Pfizer Japan Inc.
Conflict of Interest: No conflicts of interest have been declared.

cedures. Oxacillin-susceptibility tests have been used to determine whether isolates are sensitive or resistant to meticillin. Meanwhile, detection of the *mecA* gene or PBP2a is considered an alternative method to detect meticillin-resistant staphylococcal strains.[13,14] There is limited information on the correlation between disk-diffusion results and the presence of the *mecA* gene using clinical isolates from veterinary patients. The objectives of the present study were to determine the usefulness of an *in vitro* cefovecin disk-diffusion test for predicting the presence of the *mecA* gene in *S. pseudintermedius* and as a predictor of *in vivo* efficacy of cefovecin therapy in dogs with superficial pyoderma caused by *S. pseudintermedius*.

Materials and methods

Cases

Twenty-two client-owned dogs diagnosed with superficial pyoderma between September 2010 and July 2011 at Tokyo University of Agriculture and Technology Animal Medical Center, Japan, were enrolled in this study. The diagnosis of superficial pyoderma was made on the basis of compatible clinical signs (papules, erythema, scales, epidermal collarettes or a combination thereof) and cytological examination of skin lesions (infiltration of neutrophils with presence of extra- and intracellular cocci). After obtaining informed consent from owners, samples were obtained and cefovecin (8 mg/kg) was injected subcutaneously for the treatment of the superficial pyoderma. Dogs were excluded from the study if they had ectoparasitic infestations or fungal skin infections or were being treated with antiseptic shampoos during the cefovecin trial. Previous history of antibiotic use, underlying diseases and concurrent nonantibiotic therapy were also recorded for all study dogs. All studies were given ethical approval by Tokyo University of Agriculture and Technology as a sponsored research project with Pfizer Japan Inc.

Clinical evaluation of canine superficial pyoderma

Clinical signs of superficial pyoderma were evaluated before (day 0) and after the administration of cefovecin (day 14) in accordance with the guidelines of the Japanese Society of Antimicrobials for Animals.[15] Briefly, the severity and extent of erythema, papules or pustules, crusts and/or alopecia were scored using a scale from 0 (no visible lesions) to 4 (severe). The clinical score for each lesion type (e.g. erythema) was calculated by multiplying the lesion severity score by the lesion extent score. The total clinical score for each case was calculated as the sum of the clinical score for the four types of skin lesions. The improvement rate of the clinical score was calculated by the following formula: improvement score (%) = [(total clinical score at day 0 − total clinical score at day 14)/ total clinical score at day 0] × 100. Improvement scores were standardized as 0% in cases in which total clinical scores worsened after cefovecin therapy. Dogs with total clinical scores <10 at day 0 were excluded from this study, because in such cases the clinical efficacy of cefovecin treatment was difficult to evaluate.

Bacterial strains

Bacterial samples were collected using sterile swabs from skin lesions on days 0 and 14. If the skin lesions were absent on day 14, bacterial samples were collected from the skin sites sampled on day 0. Samples were inoculated onto sheep blood agar plates (Nissui Pharmaceutical, Tokyo, Japan) and incubated at 37°C for 24 h. Catalase-positive colonies were selected for additional diagnostic testing. Genomic DNA was isolated from bacterial colonies using the Ultra Clean Microbial Isolation kit (MO BIO, Carlsbad, CA, USA). Identification of *S. pseudintermedius* was determined by PCR after amplification of the thermonuclease gene (*nuc*) using a previously reported primer pair.[16] The PCR amplification was performed using AmpliTaq Gold 360 Master Mix (Applied Biosystems, Carlsbad, CA, USA) for 30 cycles of 30 s at 95°C, 30 s at 55°C and 60 s at 72°C. Polymerase chain reaction products were resolved by electrophoresis through 1.2% (w/v) agarose gels, and visualized using ultraviolet light after staining with ethidium bromide.

Disk-diffusion susceptibility test

Staphylococcus pseudintermedius strains were cultured in Luria-Bertani (LB) broth (Invitrogen, San Diego, CA, USA) and incubated at 37°C for 24 h. The culture was diluted in sterile saline, adjusted to 0.5 McFarland (McFarland Turbidity Standard No. 0.5; Becton, Dickinson and Co., Franklin Lakes, NJ, USA), and inoculated on Mueller–Hinton agar (Becton, Dickinson and Co.). An antimicrobial susceptibility disk containing 30 μg of cefovecin (Sensi-Disc®; Becton, Dickinson and Co.) was placed on culture plates, which were then incubated at 35°C for 16–18 h. Zone diameters with obvious growth inhibition were measured after culture.

Agar-dilution test

The minimal inhibitory concentrations (MICs) of cefovecin were determined by the agar-dilution test with Mueller–Hinton agar (Oxoid, Cambridge, UK) in accordance with the guidelines of the Clinical Laboratory Standards Institute: CLSI Ninteenth Informational Supplement, M100-S19.[17] The concentration range tested for cefovecin was 0.125–512 μg/mL.

Detection of *mecA*

The presence of the *mecA* gene in *S. pseudintermedius* isolates was detected by PCR analysis using a primer pair as previously reported.[18] DNA amplification was performed as described in the section of ''bacterial strains'' to amplify the *nuc* gene.

Statistical analysis

Pearson's correlation coefficient (two-tailed) test was used to confirm the correlation between inhibition zone diameters and MICs for cefovecin. Receiver operating characteristic (ROC) analysis was performed to estimate a breakpoint of the inhibition zone diameters for detection of the *mecA* gene. The Mann–Whitney *U*-test was used to compare the zone of inhibition diameters among *mecA*-positive and *mecA*-negative *S. pseudintermedius* isolates. Among dogs with pyoderma, Student's paired *t*-test and Fisher's exact test were used to compare the clinical efficacies of cefovecin therapy in dogs carrying *S. pseudintermedius* isolates with a zone of inhibition diameter above the estimated breakpoint and those below the breakpoint. All statistical analyses were carried out with STATVIEW software (version 5.0; Hulinks, Tokyo, Japan). A *P*-value of <0.05 was considered statistically significant.

Results

Dogs and clinical data

There were 17 male dogs (five neutered) and five females (four spayed) in this study (Table 1). The most common breed was the miniature dachshund (*n* = 5). Possible underlying diseases for pyoderma were identified in five of 22 cases (18.2%), as follows: atopic dermatitis (*n* = 3), hypothyroidism (*n* = 1) and concurrent atopic dermatitis with hypothyroidism (*n* = 1). Prior therapies were noted in 13 dogs and included cephalosporin [nine of 22 dogs (40.9%)], recombinant canine interferon-γ (dog no. 2), prednisolone (dog no. 12), ciclosporin (dog no. 16), and allergen-specific immunotherapy (dog no. 21). Concurrent medical therapies were unchanged in dogs during the study (see Table 1).

Correlation between inhibition zone diameters and MICs

Disk-diffusion susceptibility and agar-dilution tests for cefovecin were performed on 36 *S. pseudintermedius*

Table 1. Summary of dogs with superficial pyoderma

Case no.	Breed	Age (years)	Sex	Concurrent diseases	Medical history of antibiotic use	Concurrent therapy
1	French bulldog	7	M	—	—	—
2	Pug	8	M	Atopic dermatitis	Cefalexin	Recombinant canine interferon-γ
3	American cocker spaniel	5	FS	—	Cefalexin	—
4	Dalmatian	6	M	—	Enrofloxacin	—
5	French bulldog	10	MC	—	Cefcapene Amoxicillin	—
6	Golden retriever	5	F	Hypothyroidism	Cefalexin Cefovecin	—
7	Yorkshire terrier	10	M	—	—	—
8	Miniature dachshund	5	M	—	Cefalexin	—
9	Miniature dachshund	7	M	—	—	—
10	English springer spaniel	8	FS	—	—	—
11	Miniature dachshund	13	MC	—	—	—
12	Shih tzu	10	M	Atopic dermatitis	Cefalexin	Prednisolone
13	Miniature dachshund	6	M	—	—	—
14	Miniature dachshund	2	M	—	Cefalexin	—
15	Papillon	6	MC	—	Cefalexin	—
16	French bulldog	6	FS	Atopic dermatitis Hypothyroidism	—	Ciclosporin
17	Newfoundland	9	M	—	—	—
18	Tibetan spaniel	1	M	—	—	—
19	Shetland sheepdog	2	MC	—	—	—
20	Toy poodle	9	M	—	Cefalexin Enrofloxacin Minocycline	—
21	Shiba inu	8	FS	Atopic dermatitis	Enrofloxacin Minocycline	Allergen-specific immunotherapy
22	French bulldog	8	MC	—	—	—

Abbreviations: F, female; FS, female spayed; M, male; and MC, male castrated.

isolates cultured from the skin of the dogs (22 from day 0 and 14 from day 14; Table 2). The results of cefovecin disk-diffusion tests and MICs of 10 strains isolated on day 14 (SP nos. 23, 25, 27, 28, 29, 31, 32, 33, 34 and 36) were similar to 10 strains isolated on day 0 (SP nos 3, 5, 7, 8, 11, 15, 16, 19, 20 and 22) and were excluded from further statistical analysis; therefore, a total of 26 strains were characterized further. There was a significant linear correlation ($r = -0.83$) between the diameter of the zone of inhibition by disk diffusion and the MICs for cefovecin (Pearson's correlation coefficient, two-tailed, $P < 0.0001$; Figure 1). The range of zone diameters of inhibition for cefovecin was 6–39 mm (mean, 26.5 mm). The MICs of seven strains with zones of inhibition ≤6 mm were ≥512 μg/mL ($n = 5$), 256 μg/mL ($n = 1$) and 1 μg/mL ($n = 1$). The MICs of 13 strains whose zones of inhibition ≥30 mm were ≤0.25 μg/mL (Table 2).

Determination of a better breakpoint of the cefovecin disk-diffusion susceptibility test to predict the presence of the *mecA* gene in *S. pseudintermedius*

The PCR analyses revealed that 14 of 26 *S. pseudintermedius* isolates possessed the *mecA* gene (Table 2). The zone diameters associated with isolates that contained the *mecA* gene ($n = 14$; median, 11 mm; range, 6–35 mm) were significantly smaller than those in strains that did not contain the *mecA* gene ($n = 12$; median, 35.5 mm; range, 28–39 mm; Mann–Whitney *U*-test, $P < 0.0001$; Figure 2).

When *S. pseudintermedius* isolates with a zone diameter of ≤19 mm were interpreted as resistant strains, as previously reported,[5] the sensitivity for detection of the *mecA* gene was 57.1% (eight of 14). The disk diffusion test results were therefore subjected to ROC analysis to estimate a better breakpoint for detection of *mecA* gene carriage in *S. pseudintermedius*. A zone of inhibition of 24 mm resulted in a sensitivity of 85.7% and specificity of 100% for detecting the presence of *mecA*, whereas a zone diameter of 35 mm resulted in a sensitivity of 100% and a specificity of 50%. A zone diameter of 25–27 mm resulted in a sensitivity of 100% and a specificity of 92.9% (Figure 3). An inhibition zone diameter of 27 mm by cefovecin disk-diffusion assay was therefore regarded as a more accurate breakpoint for the detection of *S. pseudintermedius* strains possessing the *mecA* gene than previously advocated criteria.[5]

Use of the cefovecin disk-diffusion test for predicting clinical efficacy of cefovecin therapy in dogs with superficial pyoderma

The results of *in vitro* disk-diffusion tests using cefovecin were compared with the mean clinical improvement score for dogs receiving cefovecin therapy (Table 2). The clinical improvement score in dogs carrying *S. pseudintermedius* strains with an inhibition zone of ≤27 mm ($n = 9$) was 48.4 ± 48.4%, which was significantly lower than for dogs carrying strains with zone diameters of >27 mm (63.5 ± 36.5%; $n = 13$; Student's paired *t*-test, $P < 0.01$; Figure 4). An improvement score of >80% was achieved in 11 of 13 dogs carrying strains with zone diameters of >27 mm, which was significantly higher than for those carrying the strains with zone diameters of ≤27 mm (two

Table 2. Clinical improvement of superficial pyoderma, strain numbers, isolated skin lesions, disk diffusion zone diameter, and minimum inhibitory concentration (MIC) for cefovecinas associated with the presence of *mecA*-containing strains of *S. pseudintermedius*

	Clinical score			*S. pseudintermedius* isolated before cefovesin therapy (Day 0)				*S. pseudintermedius* isolated after cefovesin therapy (day 14)			
Case no.	Day 0	Day 14	Clinical improvement (%)	Strain No.	Disk diffusion zone diameter (mm)	MIC (µg/mL)	*mecA* gene	Strain no.	Disk diffusion zone diameter (mm)	MIC (µg/mL)	*mecA* gene
1	40	23	42.5	SP1	25	1	+	NI			
2	25	0	100	SP2	36	0.25	–	NI			
3	21	1	95.2	SP3	35	0.25	–	SP23	25	0.25	–
4	21	2	90.5	SP4	6 ≤	512	+	SP24	24	64	+
5	17	16	5.9	SP5	20	16	+	SP25	19	32	+
6	17	34	0	SP6	6 ≤	> 512	+	NI			
7	26	19	26.9	SP7	38	0.125	–	SP26	6≤	>512	+
								SP27	40	0.125	–
8	18	20	0	SP8	6 ≤	> 512	+	SP28	6 ≤	> 512	+
9	19	0	100	SP9	30	0.25	–	NI			
10	18	2	88.9	SP10	33	0.25	–	NI			
11	19	2	89.5	SP11	34	0.125	–	SP29	32	0.125	–
								SP30	6 ≤	1	+
12	21	26	0	SP12	6 ≤	256	+	NI			
13	16	0	100	SP13	39	0.25	–	NI			
14	20	2	90	SP14	36	0.25	–	NI			
15	28	20	28.6	SP15	36	0.25	–	SP31	34	0.125	–
16	16	13	18.8	SP16	22	128	+	SP32	25	256	+
17	17	3	82.4	SP17	33	0.125	–	NI			
18	18	0	100	SP18	35	0.125	+	NI			
19	31	1	96.8	SP19	22	256	+	SP33	22	256	+
20	34	3	91.2	SP20	36	0.25	–	SP34	41	0.25	–
21	22	4	81.8	SP21	28	0.125	–	SP35	6 ≤	> 512	+
22	40	14	65	SP22	16	256	+	SP36	20	256	+

Abbreviations: NI, not isolated.

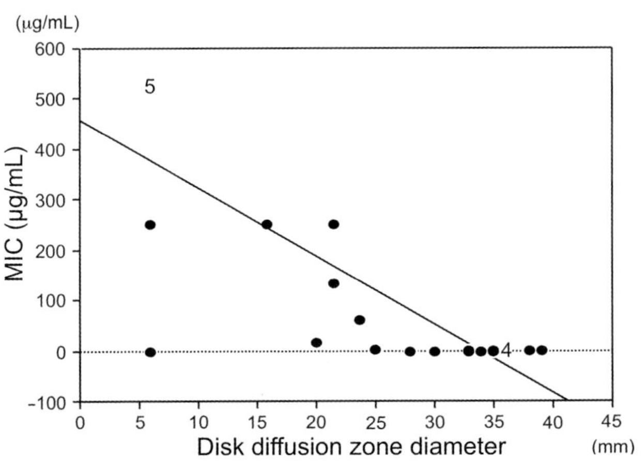

Figure 1. Zone of inhibition versus minimal inhibitory concentration (MIC) for cefovecin against *Staphylococcus pseudintermedius* isolated from dogs with superficial pyoderma. Zone diameters of obvious growth inhibition and MICs for cefovecin are plotted. There was a significant linear correlation ($r = -0.83$) between the disk-diffusion zone diameters and MICs for cefovecin (Pearson's correlation coefficient, two-tailed, $P < 0.0001$). Single dot indicates data from a single strain. The number indicates the number of strains that showed the same zone diameter and MIC.

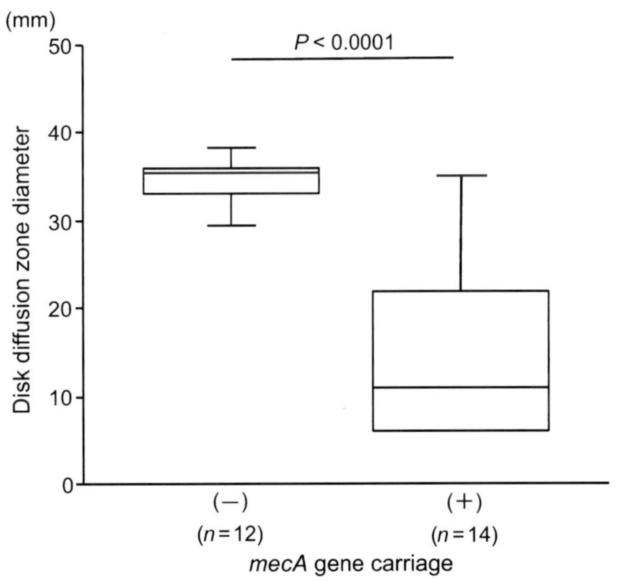

Figure 2. Comparison of zones of inhibition by disk-diffusion assay among *mecA* gene-positive and -negative isolates of *S. pseudintermedius*. The zone diameters of obvious growth inhibition by cefovecin in *mecA*-negative and -positive strains were compared. The diameters were significantly lower in *mecA* gene-positive strains than for *mecA* gene-negative strains (Mann–Whitney *U*-test, $P < 0.0001$). In the box and whisker plots, the bottom and top of the boxes represent the lower and upper quartiles, respectively, and the bands near the middle of the boxes represent medians. The lower and upper ends of the whiskers represent the minimum and maximum of all the data, respectively.

of nine dogs; Fisher's exact test, $P < 0.05$). Complete resolution of clinical signs of superficial pyoderma was achieved in only four dogs carrying the strains with zone diameters of >27 mm, while no improvement was seen in three dogs carrying the strains that exhibited inhibition zones of ≤27 mm. Moreover, in dogs with strains isolated

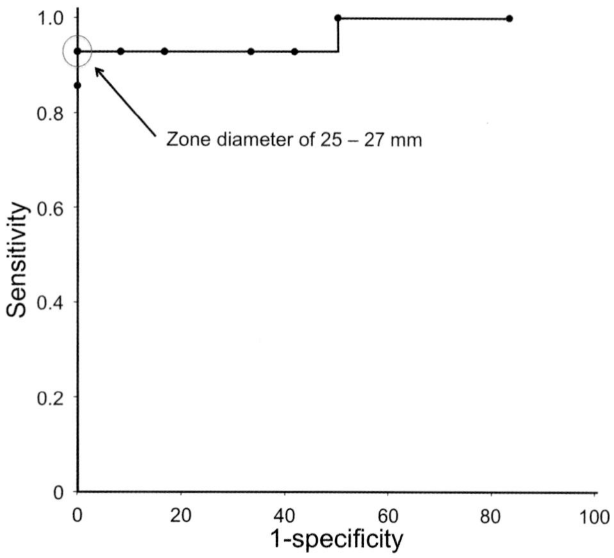

Figure 3. Receiver operating characteristic curve based on sensitivity and specificity of disk-diffusion test on cefovecin for *S. pseudintermedius* positive for the *mecA* gene. A zone diameter of 25–27 mm exhibited improved sensitivity (92.9%) and specificity (100%) compared with previously reported data.

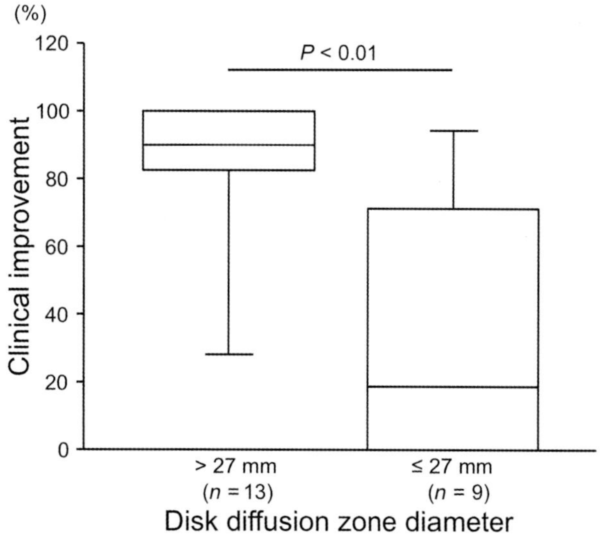

Figure 4. Comparison of the clinical improvement of superficial pyoderma after cefovecin therapy and disk-diffusion zone diameters for cefovecin. The improvement rates of the clinical scores in dogs carrying *S. pseudintermedius* strains with inhibition zone diameters of >27 mm were significantly lower than those for dogs carrying the strains with zone diameters of ≤27 mm (Student's paired *t*-test, $P < 0.01$). In the box and whisker plots, the bottom and top of the boxes represent the lower and upper quartiles, respectively, and the bands near the middle of the boxes represent medians. The lower and upper ends of the whiskers represent the minimum and maximum of the data, respectively.

on day 0 with zone diameters of ≤27 mm (66.7%; six of nine dogs), the isolation of *mecA*-carrying *S. pseudintermedius* strains on day 14 was significantly higher than in dogs with strains on day 0 with zone diameters >27 mm (15.4%; two of 13 dogs; Fisher's exact test, $P < 0.05$). These findings indicate that the cefovecin disk-diffusion test, using a breakpoint of 27 mm, is useful for predicting clinical efficacy of cefovecin therapy in dogs with superficial pyoderma.

Discussion

This study revealed a significant negative correlation between the diameter of the zone of inhibition by the cefovecin disk-diffusion assay and MICs for cefovecin for *S. pseudintermedius* isolated from dogs with superficial pyoderma. This suggests that the cefovecin disk-diffusion test could be a simple, accurate and reliable tool to determine the susceptibility of *S. pseudintermedius* strains to cefovecin. Using a breakpoint of 27 mm for the cefovecin disk-diffusion test, the specificity and sensitivity for predicting whether *S. pseudintermedius* strains contained the *mecA* gene were 92.9 and 100%, respectively. β-Lactam antibiotics should not be administered for infections caused by *mecA*-positive strains, even if a disk-diffusion test shows a susceptible strain, because these bacteria will obtain antimicrobial resistance when the strains contact the antibiotics.[17] Based on the findings of this study, the cefovecin disk-diffusion test with the breakpoint of >27 mm might also be useful for the selection of antibiotics for dogs with superficial pyoderma.

One isolate of *S. pseudintermedius* (SP no. 18) was shown by PCR analysis to contain the *mecA* gene and also to show susceptibility to cefovecin by disk-diffusion susceptibility and agar-dilution tests. The reason for this discrepancy is unknown. One of the possibilities is that mutations in the *mecA* gene open reading frame caused expression of inactivated PBP2a. Another possibility is that decreased translation of *mecA* gene caused decreased expression of PBP2a. Indeed, previous reports describe low-resistance strains that possess the *mecA* gene but express a low amount of PBP2a.[19,20] Considering these previous reports, it is conceivable that strain SP no. 18 was one of these low-resistance strains. Although the latex aggregation test has been reported to be a useful test for detecting PBP2a expression in *Staphylococcus aureus*,[21–23] it frequently exhibits false-positive reactions with *S. pseudintermedius*.[24] Further studies are needed to develop accurate detection methods for PBP2a in *S. pseudintermedius* at the protein level.

Our findings also revealed that the disk-diffusion test for cefovecin with a breakpoint of 27 mm might also be useful for predicting the *in vivo* efficacy of cefovecin therapy in dogs with superficial pyoderma caused by *S. pseudintermedius*. In the present study, we examined all eligible cases, regardless of a history of antibiotic therapy using β-lactam antibiotics, because the medical history and prior therapy might not affect the relationship between the results of the cefovecin disk-diffusion test and the clinical efficacy of cefovecin therapy. Among 13 dogs with strains that showed inhibition zones greater than the breakpoint on day 0, two dogs (dog nos. 7 and 15) did not show marked improvement of clinical signs of pyoderma. In dog no. 7, a *mecA*-positive *S. pseudintermedius* strain (SP no. 26) resistant to cefovecin was isolated after cefovecin therapy. Thus, treatment failure might be due to microbial substitution after cefovecin therapy. In contrast, strains that did not possess the *mecA* gene were isolated prior to and after cefovecin therapy in dog no. 15. The exact reasons for this discrepancy are unknown. Conversely, three of nine dogs for which isolated strains showed a zone of inhibition of ≤27 mm on day 0 (dog nos. 4, 18 and 19) showed an improvement rate of >80%, and the *mecA* gene was detected in those strains. The exact reasons for this discrepancy are also unknown, but might be due to the tissue concentration of cefovecin after injection exceeding the mutant prevention concentration threshold and being sufficient to kill antibiotic-resistant bacteria.

Previous reports demonstrated that the cefoxitin disk-diffusion test performed in accordance with the CLSI guidelines for coagulase-negative staphylococci underestimates the presence of the *mecA* gene in *S. pseudintermedius*;[10,25,26] however, the sensitivity for the detection of the *mecA* gene could be increased to 94% when the cut-off value was re-estimated by ROC analysis. Our findings also support the importance of optimizing breakpoints for disk-diffusion tests for *S. pseudintermedius* isolates by molecular comparisons for the presence of the *mecA* gene.

In conclusion, the cefovecin disk-diffusion susceptibility test with the breakpoint estimated in this study appeared to be useful for detecting *mecA*-positive *S. pseudintermedius* and for predicting the clinical efficacy of cefovecin in dogs with superficial pyoderma caused by *S. pseudintermedius* infection. Further studies to compare cefovecin- and oxacillin-susceptibility tests using a larger number of staphylococcal strains are needed to estimate the appropriate breakpoints to determine meticillin-resistant strains in clinical isolates.

Acknowledgements

The authors are grateful to Yutaka Tamura and Kanako Ishihara at Rakuno Gakuen University for performing the agar-dilution tests and to Pfizer Japan Inc. for financial support of this study.

References

1. Scott DW, Miller GH, Griffin CE. Bacterial skin disease. In: *Muller & Kirk's Small Animal Dermatology*. Philadelphia: W.B. Saunders Co., 2003; 274–335.
2. Bannoehr J, Ben Zakour NL, Waller AS *et al.* Population genetic structure of the *Staphylococcus intermedius* group: insights into *agr* diversification and the emergence of methicillin-resistant strains. *J Bacteriol* 2007; 189: 8685–8692.
3. Devriese LA, Vancanneyt M, Baele M *et al. Staphylococcus pseudintermedius* sp. nov., a coagulase-positive species from animals. *Int J Syst Evol Microbiol* 2005; 55: 1569–1573.
4. Sasaki T, Kikuchi K, Tanaka Y *et al.* Methicillin-resistant *Staphylococcus pseudintermedius* in a veterinary teaching hospital. *J Clin Microbiol* 2007; 45: 1118–1125.
5. Stegemann MR, Sherington J, Blanchflower S. Pharmacokinetics and pharmacodynamics of cefovecin in dogs. *J Vet Pharmacol Ther* 2006; 29: 501–511.
6. Six R, Cherni J, Chesebrough R. Efficacy and safety of cefovecin in treating bacterial folliculitis, abscesses, or infected wounds in dogs. *J Am Vet Med Assoc* 2008; 233: 433–439.
7. Stegemann MR, Coati N, Passmore CA *et al.* Clinical efficacy and safety of cefovecin in the treatment of canine pyoderma and wound infections. *J Small Anim Pract* 2007; 48: 378–386.
8. Griffeth GC, Morris DO, Abraham JL *et al.* Screening for skin carriage of methicillin-resistant coagulase-positive staphylococci and *Staphylococcus schleiferi* in dogs with healthy and inflamed skin. *Vet Dermatol* 2008; 19: 142–149.
9. Weese JS, Van Duijkeren E. Methicillin-resistant *Staphylococcus aureus* and *Staphylococcus pseudintermedius* in veterinary medicine. *Vet Microbiol* 2010; 140: 418–429.
10. Bemis DA, Jones RD, Frank LA *et al.* Evaluation of susceptibility test breakpoints used to predict *mecA*-mediated resistance in *Staphylococcus pseudintermedius* isolated from dogs. *J Vet Diagn Invest* 2009; 21: 53–58.
11. Berger-Bachi B, Rohrer S. Factors influencing methicillin resistance in staphylococci. *Arch Microbiol* 2002; 178: 165–171.
12. Loeffler A, Linek M, Moodley A *et al.* First report of multiresistant, *mecA*-positive *Staphylococcus intermedius* in Europe: 12 cases from a veterinary dermatology referral clinic in Germany. *Vet Dermatol* 2007; 18: 412–421.
13. Chambers HF. Methicillin resistance in staphylococci: molecular and biochemical basis and clinical implications. *Clin Microbiol Rev* 1997; 10: 781–791.
14. Brown DF. Detection of methicillin/oxacillin resistance in staphylococci. *J Antimicrob Chemother* 2001; 48(Suppl 1): 65–70.
15. Iwasaki T, Nagata M, Ohmuro T *et al.* Validation of a novel guideline for clinical trial of antimicrobials in canine bacterial pyoderma. *Jpn J Vet Dermatol* 2008; 14: 71–75.
16. Sasaki T, Tsubakishita S, Tanaka Y *et al.* Multiplex-PCR method for species identification of coagulase-positive staphylococci. *J Clin Microbiol* 2010; 48: 765–769.
17. Clinical and Laboratory Standards Institute. Performance standards for antimicrobial susceptibility testing; nineteenth informational supplement. 2009; CLSI: M100-S19.
18. Okuma K, Iwakawa K, Turnidge JD *et al.* Dissemination of new methicillin-resistant *Staphylococcus aureus* clones in the community. *J Clin Microbiol* 2002; 40: 4289–4294.
19. Hososaka Y, Hanaki H, Endo H *et al.* Characterization of oxacillin-susceptible *mecA*-positive *Staphylococcus aureus*: a new type of MRSA. *J Infect Chemother* 2007; 13: 79–86.
20. Liu H, Buescher G, Lewis N *et al.* Detection of borderline oxacillin-resistant *Staphylococcus aureus* and differentiation from methicillin-resistant strains. *Eur J Clin Microbiol Infect Dis* 1990; 9: 717–724.
21. Louie L, Matsumura SO, Choi E *et al.* Evaluation of three rapid methods for detection of methicillin resistance in *Staphylococcus aureus*. *J Clin Microbiol* 2000; 38: 2170–2173.
22. Sakoulas G, Gold HS, Venkataraman L *et al.* Methicillin-resistant *Staphylococcus aureus*: comparison of susceptibility testing methods and analysis of *mecA*-positive susceptible strains. *J Clin Microbiol* 2001; 39: 3946–3951.
23. Skov R, Smyth R, Clausen M *et al.* Evaluation of a cefoxitin 30 μg disc on Iso-Sensitest agar for detection of methicillin-resistant *Staphylococcus aureus*. *J Antimicrob Chemother* 2003; 52: 204–207.
24. Pottumarthy S, Schapiro JM, Prentice JL *et al.* Clinical isolates of *Staphylococcus intermedius* masquerading as methicillin-resistant *Staphylococcus aureus*. *J Clin Microbiol* 2004; 42: 5881–5884.
25. Bemis DA, Jones RD, Hiatt LE *et al.* Comparison of tests to detect oxacillin resistance in *Staphylococcus intermedius*, *Staphylococcus schleiferi*, and *Staphylococcus aureus* isolates from canine hosts. *J Clin Microbiol* 2006; 44: 3374–3376.
26. Schissler JR, Hillier A, Daniels JB *et al.* Evaluation of Clinical Laboratory Standards Institute interpretive criteria for methicillin-resistant *Staphylococcus pseudintermedius* isolated from dogs. *J Vet Diagn Invest* 2009; 21: 684–688.

To cite this article, please use DOI: 10.1111/j.1365-3164.2012.01099.x

5.5

Small *Demodex* populations colonize most parts of the skin of healthy dogs

Iván Ravera*, Laura Altet†, Olga Francino†, Armand Sánchez†, Wendy Roldán*, Sergio Villanueva*, Mar Bardagí* and Lluís Ferrer*

*Department of Animal Medicine and Surgery and †Servei Veterinari de Genètica Molecular, Veterinary School, Universitat Autònoma de Barcelona, 08193 Barcelona, Spain

Correspondence: Lluís Ferrer, Department of Clinical Sciences, Tufts Cumming's School of Veterinary Medicine, 200 Westboro Road, North Grafton, MA 01536, USA. E-mail: lluis.ferrer@tufts.edu

Background – It is unproven that all dogs harbour *Demodex* mites in their skin. In fact, several microscopic studies have failed to demonstrate mites in healthy dogs.

Hypothesis/Objectives – *Demodex canis* is a normal inhabitant of the skin of most, if not all, dogs. This hypothesis was tested using a sensitive real-time PCR to detect *Demodex* DNA in the skin of dogs.

Animals – One hundred dogs living in a humane society shelter, 20 privately owned and healthy dogs and eight dogs receiving immunosuppressive or antineoplastic therapy.

Methods – Hair samples (250–300 hairs with their hair bulbs) were taken from five or 20 skin locations. A real-time PCR that amplifies a 166 bp sequence of the *D. canis* chitin synthase gene was used.

Results – The percentage of positive dogs increased with the number of sampling points. When a large canine population was sampled at five cutaneous locations, 18% of dogs were positive for *Demodex* DNA. When 20 skin locations were sampled, all dogs tested positive for mite DNA. Our study indicates that *Demodex* colonization of the skin is present in all dogs, independent of age, sex, breed or coat. Nevertheless, the population of mites in a healthy dog appears to be small. *Demodex* DNA was amplified from all 20 cutaneous points investigated, without statistically significant differences.

Conclusions and clinical importance – Using a real-time PCR technique, *Demodex* mites, albeit in very low numbers, were found to be normal inhabitants of haired areas of the skin of healthy dogs.

Introduction

Understanding canine demodicosis remains one of the most difficult challenges in veterinary dermatology. Despite the prevalence and severity of the disease, many aspects of the pathogenesis of this entity remain obscure or poorly documented. Reference textbooks repeatedly make the following two statements:[1,2] (i) demodex mites are part of the normal fauna of the dog, and mites are present in the hair follicles of healthy dogs; and (ii) a genetically preprogrammed immunological defect is responsible for the exaggerated replication of mites in demodicosis.[1]

The 'fact' that all dogs harbour *Demodex* mites in the skin has not been proved using reproducible scientific methods. Most textbooks refer to the classic research done by Gaafar *et al.*, in which *Demodex* mites were found in the skin of 5.4% of healthy dogs.[3,4] The authors concluded that *Demodex* mites could be found in the skin of healthy dogs and that 'follicular mange' is a complex condition, but not that all dogs harbour mites in their skin. More recently, Fondati *et al.*,[5] using trichoscopy, could not detect *Demodex canis* mites in any of 78 dogs examined, and found a single *Demodex injai* mite in one dog. Furthermore, aspects such as the preferred anatomical location of the mites on the canine skin, the mite density, and the influence of age and breed on the *Demodex* mite population remain unknown. Recently, we have developed a highly sensitive real-time PCR to detect *D. canis* DNA.[6] In that study, we were able to amplify the DNA of *D. canis* in nine of 51 dogs (17.6%), after sampling only two points of the skin (lateral face and interdigital skin).[6] Interestingly, this is a much higher percentage than previously reported.[7,8]

The prevalence of *Demodex* mites in the skin of healthy humans is close to 100%, with a mean mite density of 0.7 mites/cm^2 (facial skin).[9–14] *Demodex* mites are assumed to be normal inhabitants of the skin of most mammals.[9,14,15] Therefore, considering data from other species and the biology of *Demodex* mites, the goal of the present study was to determine whether *D. canis* mites are normal inhabitants of the skin of most, if not all, dogs

Accepted 4 July 2012

Sources of Funding: I.R. received a PhD grant from the ECVD-ESVD.

Conflict of Interest: No conflicts of interest have been declared.

or if only a subset of the canine population harbours the mites, and these dogs serve as a reservoir of the parasite.

Materials and methods

Dogs

One hundred dogs living in a humane society shelter were used in this study. All were adult dogs, ranging in age from 9 months to 13 years, and included dogs of both sexes and of different breeds, with a large majority of dogs being of mixed breed. The shelter housed between 250 and 300 dogs, and only dogs with normal physical and dermatological examinations were used. As canine leishmaniosis is endemic in the region, serological testing was performed on all 100 dogs, and 17 tested positive. Dogs were sampled on three occasions, for experiments 1, 2 and 3. The Board of the Centre gave written permission for the study to be carried out, provided that that all sampling procedures were done under the supervision of the shelter veterinarians.

Twenty privately owned healthy adult dogs presented to the Veterinary Teaching Hospital for preventive medicine examinations and veterinary counselling were included in the study. In addition, eight dogs being treated at the Veterinary Medical Teaching Hospital for different diseases that required immunosuppressive or antineoplastic therapy for more than 2 months were also sampled. None of these eight dogs had skin lesions suggestive of demodicosis. All owners were informed of the nature of the study and gave their written consent.

Hair sampling and DNA extraction

Hair samples (n = 250–300) were obtained by gentle plucking of hair in the direction of the growth so as to include the hair bulb (root) in the sample. Each sample included 250–300 hairs. The number of sampling locations in each experiment is shown in Table 1. Hair samples were maintained in phosphate-buffered saline and stored at −20°C until DNA extraction. For the DNA extraction, samples were centrifuged in a microcentrifuge at maximal speed for 30 min; once the supernatant was removed, 200 μL of digestion buffer (50 mmol/L Tris–HCl, pH 8.5; and 1 mmol/L EDTA) and 4 μL of proteinase K solution (10 mg/mL) were added, and samples were incubated at 56°C overnight. After inactivation of the proteinase K for 10 min at 95°C, the samples were centrifuged for 10 min at maximal speed. Supernatant was transferred to a new tube and diluted 1:10 for PCR amplification.

Experiments

Five different sampling experiments were conducted (Table 1). Briefly, in experiment 1, 100 healthy dogs living in an animal shelter had hair samples collected from the following five cutaneous locations: head, dorsal area, foreleg, abdomen and hindleg. In experiment 2, 16 dogs with positive samples from experiment 1 and 30 dogs with negative samples were resampled 6 months after the initial sampling. In experiment 3, five healthy dogs living in the shelter were sampled from the following 20 cutaneous locations: lip and periocular skin (four points), perinasal skin, temporal area, chin, ventral and dorsal neck, dorsum (two points), sternum, abdomen (two points), thigh (two points) and interdigital area (four points, one on each foot). As shelter dogs may not be representative of a normal canine population, five healthy, privately owned dogs were sampled in a similar manner (experiment 4). Finally, in experiment 5, eight dogs receiving immunosuppressive or antineoplastic therapy were sampled from five cutaneous locations.

PCR technique to detect *Demodex* DNA in canine hairs

The technique has been described in detail elsewhere.[6] Real-time PCR was carried out in a final volume of 20 μL using FastStart Universal SYBR Green Master (Roche Diagnostics GmbH, Mannheim, Germany), 0.3 μmol/L of each primer and 4 μL of diluted DNA. Primer pairs used were as follows: *D. canis* forward, 5′-GATGAAGCGGCGAGTAATGTTC-3′; and *D. canis* reverse, 5′-GACTCCATCTTTTACGATGTCTGATTT-3′. They amplified a 166 bp fragment of the chitin synthase gene. The eukaryotic 18S RNA Pre-developed TaqMan Assay Reagent (Applied Biosystems, Foster City, CA, USA) was used as an internal reference for dog genomic DNA amplification to ensure suitability of each sample for PCR amplification and to be certain that negative results corresponded to true negative samples rather than to a problem with DNA loading, sample degradation or PCR inhibition. Water was used as a negative control for the PCR. Positive PCR controls were obtained from clinical samples that had previously been amplified and sequenced to confirm *Demodex*. The thermal cycling profile was 50°C for 2 min and 95°C for 10 min, followed by 40 cycles at 95°C for 15 s and 60°C for 1 min. Specificity assessment of the PCR was performed by adding a dissociation curve analysis at the end of the run. The product of the real-time PCR was sequenced using the BigDye Terminator Cycle Sequencing Ready Reaction Kit (Life Technologies Corp., Carlsbad, CA, USA) with the same primers, and the sequences obtained were compared with the GenBank database (http://blast.ncbi.nlm.nih.gov/Blast.cgi).

Statistical analyses

The chi-square test and the Saphiro–Francia normality test were used for the statisitical analysis of the results ('R' program; R Foundation for Statistical Computing, Vienna, Austria).

Results

The results of the five experiments are shown in Table 1. Briefly, the percentage of positive dogs increased with the number of sampling sites. When a large canine population (experiment 1) was sampled at five cutaneous locations, 18% of the dogs were positive for *Demodex* mites using PCR. No association between sex, age, type of coat or *Leishmania* seropositivity was found. The percentage of *Leishmania* seropositive dogs was similar in the two groups (22.2% in the positive group and 15.8% in the negative group; $P > 0.1$, chi-square test).

This relatively low percentage of positive dogs could indicate that only a subset of the canine population harbours *Demodex* mites, acting as a reservoir of the

Table 1. Dogs included in each experiment and results of the real-time PCR for *Demodex canis* DNA

Experiment no.	Number of dogs and origin	Sampling locations	Number of dogs testing positive in *Demodex* PCR (%)
Experiment 1	100 healthy dogs from a shelter	5	18 (18)
Experiment 2	16 dogs positive in experiment 1	5	3 (18.5)
	30 dogs negative in experiment 1		5 (20)
Experiment 3	5 healthy dogs from a shelter	20	5 (100)
Experiment 4	20 privately owned dogs from VTH-UAB	20	18 (90)
Experiment 5	8 dogs receiving immunosuppressive or antineoplastic therapy from the VTH-UAB	5	4 (50%)

Abbreviation: VTH-UAB, Veterinary Teaching Hospital – Universitat Autònoma de Barcelona.

parasite, as mentioned in the introduction. However, the low percentage could also be due to low diagnostic sensitivity of the technique used, which resulted in *Demodex* not being detected in some or most dogs. To resolve this dilemma, we repeated the sampling 6 months later (experiment 2), including dogs that tested positive and negative in the first trial, to verify that positive dogs (n = 16) remained positive and negative dogs (n = 30) remained negative. In this second experiment, only three of the 16 previously positive dogs tested positive (18.75%), but five of the 30 previously negative dogs (20%) tested positive at one or more sampled site. A possible explanation for this was low test sensitivity, resulting in some negative results being false negatives (i.e. some dogs had *Demodex* mites in their skin but the mites were probably not included in the samples). Experiment 3 was conducted to increase the number of sampling sites in order to determine whether the percentage of positive dogs also increased. When dogs were sampled at 20 skin locations, all five dogs tested positive in at least one location; increasing the sample size increased the sensitivity, as the percentage of positive dogs was 100% (five of five).

The results of experiment 4 (privately owned dogs) confirmed that the majority of the healthy dogs (18 of 20) harboured *Demodex* mites in the skin. In this last group of dogs, *Demodex* DNA could be amplified from all of the 20 skin locations in at least one of the dogs (range one to six positive dogs at each location). No individual sample site had significantly more positive outcomes than others ($P > 0.1$, Shapiro–Francia normality test).

Finally, we investigated a group of eight dogs receiving immunosuppressive or antineoplastic therapy (experiment 5). In this group, the percentage of positive dogs was clearly higher than in the general canine population. Four of the eight dogs (50%) were positive after sampling only five sites (general canine population 18%), and in three of the dogs three or more locations were positive (Table 2).

Table 2. Data of the dogs included in experiment 5 and results of the real-time PCR for *Demodex canis* DNA

Signalment and diagnosis	Treatment	Result of the *Demodex* PCR
Boxer dog, male, 2 years old; corticosteroid -responsive meningitis	Prednisone, 2 mg/kg/day; 2 months	Positive for 3 of 5 skin points
Mixed breed, female, 7 years old; immune -mediated haemolytic anaemia	Prednisone, 1–2 mg/kg/day; 2 months	Negative (only four points sampled)
Golden retriever dog, male, 10 years old; multiple myeloma	Melphalan, prednisone (1 mg/kg/day), famotidine 3 months	Negative
German shepherd dog, male, 4 years old; immune-mediated haemolytic anaemia	Prednisone, 1–2 mg/kg/day and azathioprine, 1 mg/kg 2 months	Negative
Labrador retriever dog, male, 5 years old; immune-mediated polyarthritis	Prednisone, 1–2 mg/kg/day and ciclosporin, 5 mg/kg >3 months	Positive for 1 of 5 skin points
Bull mastiff dog, female, 6 years old; lymphoma (stage IV)	Wisconsin–Madison protocol* (prednisone from 2 to 0.5 mg/kg/day, 6 weeks)	Positive for 5 of 5 skin points
Mixed breed, male, 9 years old; splenic haemangiosarcoma	Doxorubicin, chlorambucil 2 months	Positive for 3 of 5 skin points
German shepherd dog, female, 4 years old; lymphoma (stage IVb)	Wisconsin–Madison protocol* (prednisone from 2 to 0.5 mg/kg/day, 6 weeks)	Negative

*Wisconsin–Madison protocol includes L-asparaginase, vincristine, cyclophosphamide, doxorubicin and prednisone.

Discussion

From this study, it was difficult to demonstrate that *Demodex* mites lived in the skin of all dogs. However, we were able to amplify *D. canis* DNA from the skin of most healthy dogs. Therefore, *Demodex* can be considered a normal inhabitant of the canine skin. This seems to be the case for most mammals investigated so far.[14] In humans, for instance, the prevalence of *Demodex* mites on the facial skin, especially on the chin, is reported to be close to 100%.[9–11] Our study indicates that *Demodex* colonization of the skin is present in dogs, independent of age, sex, breed or coat.

Nevertheless, the population of mites in a healthy dog must be very small, for several reasons. First, in clinical practice positive skin scrapings and skin biopsy samples that identify *Demodex* mites are rare in healthy dogs. Second, exhaustive rigorous microscopic examination of 78 dogs failed to detect a single *D. canis* mite.[5] Third, even using a highly sensitive real-time PCR technique, we had to increase the number of sampling sites to be able to detect the parasite in a majority of dogs. In humans, however, the estimated mean mite density is as high as 0.7 to over 5 mites/cm^2 in some disease entities, such as rosacea and perioral dermatitis.[10,13] The current technique, unfortunately, does not allow quantification of the number of mites in the sample, although development of a modified quantitative technique is underway.

Interestingly, *Demodex* DNA was amplified from all the cutaneous locations investigated, without statistically significant differences. The chin and perilabial skin locations were positive more frequently than the interdigital and perianal skin, but the differences were not significant. This is in contrast with the situation in humans, where *Demodex* is located almost exclusively in some parts of the facial skin. These results also differ somewhat from those of the pioneering study of Greve and Gaafar,[4] who detected *D. canis* in all sampled areas of the skin, but more abundantly on the head and legs. According to our data, dogs harbour a very small population of *Demodex* mites in all sites of haired skin that were sampled, and these mites probably maintain nomadic behaviour on the skin surface. It is well known that *Demodex* mites move at a speed of 16 mm/h and move from one follicle to the next,[9] especially during the night due to their negative phototaxia.

The *Demodex* colonization of the skin of mammals seems to be an extraordinary example of adaptation of one organism to another. Some authors consider that rather than parasitism, this should be viewed as commensalism or a mutualistic relationship.[16] Our present knowledge suggests that *Demodex* mites normally have a symbiotic relationship with mammals. In normal circumstances, they appear to live as commensals, feeding on their host's sebum. It is possible in this role that they may even confer a mutualistic host benefit by ingesting bacteria or other organisms in the follicular canal.[16,17] The host's innate immune system appears to tolerate the presence of these mites, but it may have a 'culling' or inhibitory effect on mite proliferation, keeping numbers in the hair follicle under control without inducing an inflammatory response.[18,19] If mite numbers increase to a critical level (possibly causing physical distension of follicles with keratinocyte disruption), they could develop a pathogenic role, causing insult to the host.[16,18–20] Furthermore, in most mammals *Demodex* behaves as an opportunistic pathogen with the potential to change its status from commensal to parasite (the mites benefit but harm the host) if the host's cutaneous environment facilitates their proliferation.[16] In this context, the dog seems to be unique, with a small number of *Demodex* mites on healthy skin, but a high prevalence of cases of generalized and severe demodicosis in young dogs, without a primary or predisposing cause. The most plausible explanation is that canine generalized juvenile demodicosis is one of the negative traits associated with the creation of dog breeds.[21] This would explain the strong breed predisposition for demodicosis, with the odds ratios for some breeds being as high as 35.5 (American Staffordshire terrier), 17.1 (Staffordshire bull terrier), 7.2 (Chinese shar-pei) and 5 (French bulldog).[22] In addition, the genetic association between demodicosis and some alleles of the dog leukocyte antigen system has been reported.[23] The genetic aspects of canine demodicosis require urgent investigation.

Demodicosis in humans is associated with treatment with immunosuppressive drugs[13,24–26] and with some antineoplastic therapies, such as epidermal growth factor receptor inhibitor.[27] Furthermore, one of the main causes of generalized demodicosis in adult dogs is prolonged corticosteroid therapy. We therefore investigated the presence of *Demodex* DNA in the skin of a group of dogs receiving corticosteroid therapy or antineoplastic therapy. This preliminary study seems to demonstrate an increase in the presence of *Demodex* mites in these patients. Although these results must be confirmed in a larger study, they seem to suggest that some immunosuppressive therapies induce a progressive increase of the cutaneous *Demodex* populations resulting in clinical demodicosis.

In short, the present study formally demonstrates, by means of a real-time PCR technique, that *Demodex* mites, albeit in very low numbers, are normal inhabitants of hairy skin of healthy dogs.

Acknowledgements

The authors thank the veterinarians of the Centre d'Atenció d'Animals de Companyia del Maresme (Catalonia, Spain); Mar Alcalá and Belen Barrantes, and all the staff for their valuable help with the sampling of the dogs included in this study.

References

1. Scott DW, Miller WH, Griffin CE. Parasitic diseases. In: *Muller and Kirk's Small Animal Dermatology*, 6th edition. Philadelphia, PA: W.B. Saunders Co., 2001; 457–474.
2. Gross TL, Ihrke PJ, Walder EJ *et al.* Pustular and nodular diseases with adnexal destruction. In: *Skin Diseases of the Dog and Cat: Clinical and Histopathological Diagnosis*, 2nd edition, Oxford: Blackwell Publishing Ltd, 2005; 420–459.
3. Gaafar SM, Smalley HE, Turk RD. The incidence of *Demodex* species on skins of apparently normal dogs. *J Am Vet Med Assoc* 1958; 133: 122–132.
4. Greve JH, Gaafar SM. Natural transmission of *Demodex canis* in dogs. *J Am Vet Med Assoc* 1966; 148: 1043–1045.
5. Fondati A, De Lucia M, Furiani N *et al.* Prevalence of *Demodex canis*-positive healthy dogs at trichoscopic examination. *Vet Dermatol* 2010; 21: 146–151.
6. Ravera I, Altet L, Francino O *et al.* Development of a real-time PCR to detect *Demodex canis* DNA in different tissue samples. *Parasitol Res* 2011; 108: 305–308.
7. Rodriguez-Vivas RI, Ortega-Pacheco A, Rosado-Aguilar JA *et al.* Factors affecting the prevalence of mange-mite infestation in stray dogs of Yucatán, Mexico. *Vet Parasitol* 2003; 115: 61–65.
8. Tsai Y, Chung W, Wang L *et al.* The dog mite, *Demodex canis*: prevalence, fungal co-infection, reactions to light, and hair follicle apoptosis. *J Insect Sci* 2011; 11: 1–13.
9. Norn MS. The follicle mite (*Demodex folliculorum*). *Eye Ear Nose Throat Mon* 1972; 51: 187–191.
10. Forton F, Seys B. Density of *Demodex folliculorum* in rosacea: a case-control study using standardized skin-surface biopsy. *Br J Dermatol* 1993; 128: 650–659.
11. Forton F, Song M. Limitations of standardized skin surface biopsy in measurement of the density of *Demodex folliculorum*. A case report. *Br J Dermatol* 1998; 139: 697–700.
12. Askin Ü, Seckin D. Comparison of the two techniques for measurement of the density of *Demodex folliculorum*: standardized skin surface biopsy and direct microscopic examination. *Br J Dermatol* 2010; 162: 1124–1126.
13. Dolenc-Voljc M, Pohar M, Lunder T. Density of *Demodex folliculorum* in perioral dermatitis. *Acta Derm Venereol* 2005; 85: 211–215.
14. Nutting WB, Kettle PR, Tenquist JD *et al.* Hair follicle mites (*Demodex* spp.) in New Zealand. *New Z J Zool* 1975; 2: 219–222.
15. Scott DW. *Large Animal Dermatology*. Philadelphia, PA: W.B. Saunders Co.; 1988; 226–230
16. Lacey N, Raghallaigh S, Powell F. *Demodex* mites – commensals, parasites or mutualistic organisms? *Dermatology* 2011; 222: 128–130.
17. Kligman A, Christensen M. *Demodex folliculorum*: requirements for understanding its role in human skin disease. *J Invest Dermatol* 2011; 131: 8–10.
18. Forton FMN. Papulopustular rosacea, skin immunity and Demodex: pityriasis folliculorum as a missing link. *J Eur Acad Dermatol Venereol* 2012; 26: 19–28.
19. Yamasaki K, Gallo R. The molecular pathology of rosacea. *J Dermatol Sci* 2009; 55: 77–81.
20. Bevins CL, Liu F. Rosacea: skin innate immunity gone awry? *Nat Med* 2007; 8: 904–905.
21. Cruz F, Vila C, Webster M. The legacy of domestication: accumulation of deleterious mutations in the dog genome. *Mol Biol Evol* 2008; 25: 2331–2336.

22. Plant JD, Lund EM, Yang M. A case–control study of the risk factors for canine juvenile-onset generalized demodicosis in the USA. *Vet Dermatol* 2010; 20: 95–99.
23. It V, Barrientos L, López-Gappa J *et al.* Association of canine juvenile generalized demodicosis with the dog leukocyte antigen system. *Tissue Antigens* 2010; 76: 67–70.
24. Bøge-Rasmussen T, Christensen JD, Gluud B *et al. Demodex folliculorum hominis* (Simon): incidence in a normomaterial and in patients under systemic treatment with erythromycin or glucocorticoid. *Acta Derm Venereol* 1982; 62: 454–456.
25. Basta-Juzbasić A, Subić JS, Ljubojević S *et al. Demodex folliculorum* in development of dermatitis rosaceiformis steroidica and rosacea-related diseases. *Clin Dermatol* 2002; 20: 135–140.
26. Fujiwara S, Okubo Y, Irisawa R *et al.* Rosaceiform dermatitis associated with topical tacrolimus treatment. *J Am Acad Dermatol* 2010; 62: 1050–1052.
27. Gerber PA, Kukova G, Buhren BA *et al.* Density of *Demodex folliculorum* in patients receiving epidermal growth factor receptor inhibitors. *Dermatology* 2011; 222: 144–147.

Part 6

Oncology

To cite this article, please use DOI: 10.1111/j.1365-3164.2012.01107.x

6.1

Advances in the management of skin cancer

Pamela D. Martin and David J. Argyle

Royal (Dick) School of Veterinary Studies and Roslin Institute, Easter Bush, Midlothian EH25 9RG, UK

Correspondence: David J. Argyle, Royal (Dick) School of Veterinary Studies and Roslin Institute, Easter Bush, Midlothian EH25 9RG, UK. E-mail: david.argyle@ed.ac.uk

Skin cancer is one of the most commonly diagnosed cancers in the world today in both humans and our pet population. Advances in molecular techniques are now affording us an opportunity to develop therapeutics targeted at specific cancer-related cellular pathways. However, despite progress in conventional treatments, such as chemotherapy and radiation, and the new targeted therapies, some cancers, such as melanoma and cutaneous lymphoma, continue to cause significant mortality and morbidity.

This short synopsis is not complete but is aimed at providing an insight into current advanced treatments and horizon therapies for cutaneous malignancies in dogs and cats with comparative aspects.

Introduction

In human medicine, the term 'skin cancer' is often restricted to either cutaneous malignant melanoma or nonmelanoma 'skin cancers', which are a group largely made up of basal cell carcinoma and squamous cell carcinoma. Currently, between 2 and 3 million nonmelanoma skin cancers and 132,000 melanoma skin cancers occur globally each year. One in every three cancers diagnosed is a skin cancer.[1] As the molecular mechanisms of cutaneous neoplasias are elucidated, the similarities between the human and animal diseases become more apparent. Animal models can provide rich foundations for translational research, both *in vivo* and *in vitro*, into some of the most aggressive and devastating cancers affecting both humans and animals. Molecular targeted therapies have the general advantages of a more targeted cellular approach to the management of cancer, with the aims of better outcome and fewer adverse effects. In this short synopsis, we focus on the most current and horizon therapies for malignant cutaneous neoplasms in both human and animal patients.

Receptor tyrosine kinase inhibitors

One of the most significant advances in the management of cutaneous neoplasms in animal patients in recent years has been the introduction of receptor tyrosine kinase (RTK) inhibitors for veterinary use. Receptor tyrosine kinases are a large family of transmembrane receptors that, when stimulated by their cognate ligands (growth factors), trigger cytoplasmic and nuclear signalling, resulting in cell proliferation and differentiation.[2] These growth factor receptors are divided into 20 families according to their different extracellular ligand-binding domains. A vast array of cancer types in both humans and animals have demonstrated dysregulation of RTKs. Receptor tyrosine kinases have also been implicated in new blood vessel formation (angiogenesis) in tumours and the process of metastasis. The normal activity of RTKs – such as the platelet-derived growth factor receptor (PDGFR) or the vascular endothelial growth factor receptor (VEGFR) – may be utilized by the tumour stroma to maintain angiogenesis, promote metastasis and support the tumour niche environment.

Accepted 16 July 2012
Sources of Funding: This study was self-funded.
Conflict of Interest: No conflicts of interest have been declared.

The development of inhibitors of the RTK (RTKi) pathways has been a hotly contested arena in the pharmaceutical industry. The initial success of imatinib (Gleevec®; Novartis, Basel, Switzerland) in human leukaemia suggested that this approach to cancer therapy could be highly successful in a range of other cancers. Specific small-molecule tyrosine kinase inhibitors (RTKis) are able to block the activity of receptors by competitive inhibition of ATP binding (Figure 1). Recently, the following two RTKis were approved by the European Medicines Agency and the US Food and Drug Administration for use in mast cell tumours (MCTs) in dogs: (i) toceranib phosphate (Palladia®; Pfizer Inc., Manhattan, New York, NY, USA), approved for use in recurrent, nonresectable grade II/III MCTs;[3] and (ii) masitinib (Masivet®; AB Sciences, Paris, France), approved for use in nonresectable grade II/III MCTs with established c-KIT mutation, which should be confirmed before treatment.[4]

Both drugs were developed to target RTKs, in particular c-KIT on canine MCTs.[5,6] Toceranib also targets VEGFR2 and PDGFR, suggesting that the use of this drug would also target tumour stroma (through PDGFR) and neoangiogensis (through VEGFR2), perhaps having an additional effect on tumour metastasis. Both drugs have demonstrated efficacy as single agents in prospective clinical trials in dogs with mast cell tumours.[7,8] The initial clinical

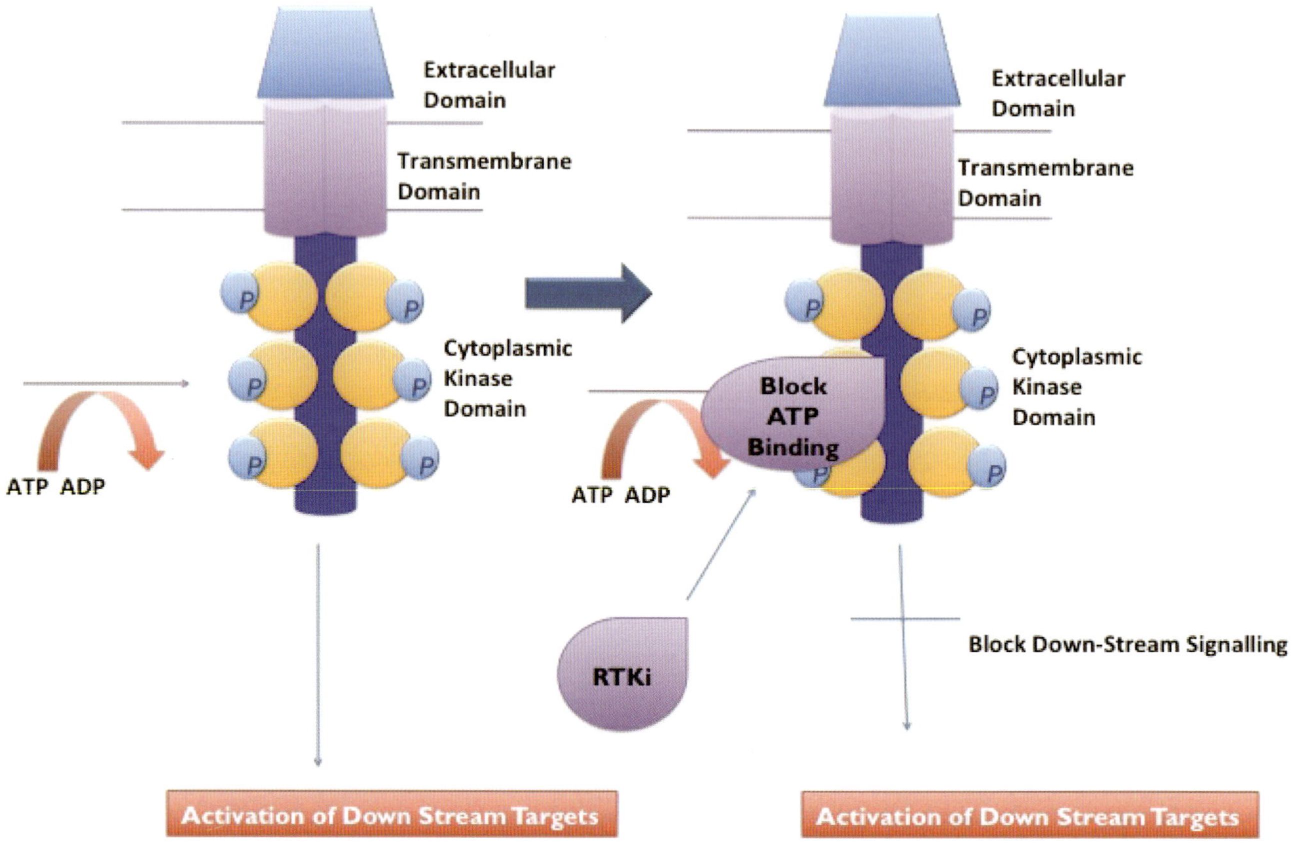

Figure 1. Mechanism of action of receptor tyrosine kinase (RTK) inhibitors. In normal cellular physiology, ligand binding to RTK causes phosphorylation of serine residues through the activity of ATP. Phosphorylation activates downstream proteins, ultimately affecting cellular proliferation. The RTK inhibitors (RTKi) block the ATP binding site, thereby preventing phosphorylation.

trials for toceranib revealed biological activity in a variety of tumour types, including carcinomas, sarcomas, melanomas and lymphomas, with the highest response rates in dogs with MCTs.[9] A recent retrospective study surveyed the biological activity of toceranib in other solid tumours, including apocrine gland anal sac adenocarcinoma, metastatic osteosarcoma, thyroid carcinoma, head and neck carcinoma and nasal carcinoma.[10] A response achieving clinical benefit (complete remission, partial remission or stable disease) was seen in 74% of treated dogs, indicating that further studies are needed to evaluate the efficacy of this drug for targeting other tumour types.

Mutations in *KIT* have been found to occur in approximately 15% of mucosal and 23% of acral melanomas in human studies.[11] Trials are currently underway to evaluate the RTKi imatinib in mucosal and acral melanomas with *KIT* mutations. A recent preliminary veterinary investigation found that buccal amelanotic melanomas showed strong positive staining for the c-KIT protein compared with melanotic melanomas.[12] These findings may provide the framework for future studies into the role of *KIT* in melanoma, using a canine model for human melanoma. The overall prognosis for metastatic melanoma remains grave for both human and veterinary patients, with future translational research having the potential to benefit both species.

Squamous cell carcinoma has been shown to express the RTK epidermal growth factor receptor (EGFR), which can be exploited for directed molecular targeted therapy. In a recent meta-analysis of cutaneous human head and neck squamous cell carcinoma (SCC), overexpression of EGFR was found in 56% of primary tumours and 58% of regional metastases.[13] Erlotinib (Tarceva®; OSI Pharmaceuticals, LLC, Farmingdale, New York, NY, USA) and gefitinib (Iressa®; AstraZeneca plc, London, UK) are EGFR inhibitors, previously approved to treat haematopoietic malignancies, which are now being tested in clinical trials of human patients with cutaneous SCC.[14] Overexpression of EGFR is also a feature of feline SCC, which generally has a poor to grave prognosis because most cases are presented in the advanced stages.[15] Epidermal growth factor receptor is not a target for either of the veterinary approved RTKis, toceranib or masitinib.[5] In our laboratory, we recently investigated the effects of the RTKi gefitinib on a feline SCC cell line.[16] Treatment with gefitinib resulted in decreased cell proliferation but ultimately the development of drug resistance. Resistance could be overcome with RNAi targeted to EGFR, and suggests that ultimately multimodal therapy may become important.

Veterinary studies combining RTKs with conventional chemotherapy drugs are currently lacking. However, Robat *et al.*[17] recently conducted a phase 1 clinical study to evaluate the safety of the combination of vinblastine and toceranib phosphate (Palladia®; Pfizer) in dogs with MCTs. In that study, the dose-limiting toxicity for the simultaneous combination was neutropenia, and the maximally tolerated combined doses were 1.6 mg/m^2 every other week (vinblastine) and 3.25 mg/kg orally, every other day (toceranib). This represents greater than a 50%

reduction in dose intensity for vinblastine (compared with single-agent use) and, as such, does not support this combination based on current chemotherapy combination paradigms. While a strict adherence to dose paradigms speaks against the combination, evidence of significant activity (71% objective response) and enhanced myelosuppression suggest additive or synergistic activity. A prospective randomized evaluation comparing this combination with standard single-agent treatments needs to be conducted to interrogate this possibility.

The use of RTKis (inhibitors) with radiotherapy, another proven treatment modality, has recently been investigated. A muticentre prospective trial was conducted to establish the tolerability of using toceranib phosphate in combination with palliative radiotherapy in nonresectable MCTs.[18] In that study, toceranib was administered for 1 week before initiation of radiotherapy consisting of a total of 24 Gy delivered in three or four fractions. The overall response rate was 76.4%, with 58.8% of dogs achieving a complete response and 17.6% a partial response. The median time to best response was 32 days, and the median progression-free interval was 316 days. The overall median survival time was not reached with a median follow-up of 374 days. These response rates and durations were higher than those reported for toceranib as a single-agent treatment for MCT, but the study did include the addition of prednisolone. Predictably, the most common toxicities were related to the gastrointestinal tract and the liver.

Subpopulations of T lymphocytes are often dysregulated in cancer, with decreases in numbers of effector T cells and increases in regulatory T cells. In murine models, T cells have been shown to have a direct suppressive effect on the immune response to tumours.[19] Additionally, regulatory T-cell numbers have been correlated with clinical outcome in both human and veterinary cancer patients.[20,21] A recent study conducted by Mitchell *et al.*[22] combined toceranib phosphate and metronomic dosing of cyclophosphamide in an attempt to improve tumour control by suppression of regulatory T cells and restoration of T-cell-mediated immune responses. In that study, 15 client-owned dogs with advanced tumours were entered into a prospective clinical trial. Results demonstrated that toceranib significantly decreased the number and percentage of regulatory T cells in the peripheral blood of dogs with cancer. Dogs receiving toceranib and cyclophosphamide demonstrated a significant increase in serum concentrations of interferon-γ, which was inversely correlated with regulatory T-cell numbers after 6 weeks of combination treatment. These data support an immunomodulatory function of RTKis in cancer.

Small-molecule tyrosine kinase inhibitors are a new and exciting class of drugs that give the veterinary practitioner a further readily accessible modality in treating MCTs. All the potential indications for this class of drugs are not yet known, but the number of cancers proving responsive to these agents is on the rise as our knowledge of cellular signalling pathways is exploited. The oral formulations would suggest that this class of drugs is easy to administer and monitor in clinical patients. It is essential, however, that the same precautions and considerations be given to using these drugs as we would for conventional cytotoxic therapy, because adverse drug-specific reactions have been described with both medications.

Retinoids

Retinoids, both naturally occurring compounds and synthetically derived substances, are derivatives of vitamin A. These are biological response modifiers, which have antineoplastic activities.[23] Retinoids act via activation of the nuclear retinoid receptors, retinoic acid receptor (RAR) and retinoid X receptor (RXR), each of which has three isoforms (α, β and γ). Antineoplastic effects of retinoids occur via suppression of cellular proliferation, induction of terminal differentiation and, ultimately, apoptosis.[24,25]

Retinoids have been used topically in human cutaneous T cell lymphoma (CETL) for more than 20 years [26,27] and, more recently, in canine and feline CETL with mixed results (40–50% response rate of 5–13 months).[28,29] Isotretinoin (Accutane®; Roche Pharmaceuticals, Basel, Switzerland) and etretinate (Tegison®; Roche Pharmaceuticals) have been removed from the North American human market due mutagenic and teratogenic effects, which persist even long after discontinuation of therapy. Acitretin (Soriatane®; Stiefel Laboratories, Inc., Research Triangle Park, NC, USA or Neotigason®; Actavis UK Ltd, Barnstaple, UK), a RAR agonist, is still commercially available; however, objective studies on efficacy are seriously lacking. Latterly, bexarotene (Targretin®; Eisai Co., Ltd, Tokyo, Japan), a synthetic RXR agonist, has been efficacious as a single agent in patients with CETL.[29] It has biological activity taken orally as well as applied topically and has shown efficacy in human patients with mycosis fungoides and Sézary syndrome.[30] The expression of retinoid receptors in normal canine lymphoid tissue and canine nodal lymphoma has been recently investigated.[31] Normal lymphoid tissue did not express retinoid receptors, whereas canine nodal lymphomas exhibited strong expression. Cutaneous T-cell lymphomas were shown to express both RARs and RXRs in 29 of 30 dogs with CETL, which suggests that retinoid therapy may be beneficial.[32] To date, however, there are no large-scale studies that have tested this hypothesis.

Toll-like receptor agonists

Toll-like receptors are a subset of pattern recognition receptors within the innate immune system that function to recognize pathogens.[33] Their expression results in production of immunoregulatory cytokines, such as tumour necrosis factor-α, interferon-α and interferon-γ, and increases in immune surveillance. Toll-like receptor agonists that mediate these effects in the immune system have been used clinically for several years to treat basal cell carcinoma and cutaneous lymphoma in humans.[34,35] Dendritic cells present in the dermis are key antigen-presenting cells for induction of adaptive antitumour immune responses. Imiquimod and resiquimod are Toll-like receptor agonists with promise as targeted therapies for CETL.[36,37] Imiquimod has shown limited potential as a sole agent due to variable bioavailability and may be more useful as an adjunct therapy. Resiquimod has markedly greater bioavailability with topical application and, consequently, the potential to induce systemic immune activation, resulting in targeting of tumour cells. These compounds have shown initial success both in terms of enhancing immune responses and in eliciting antitumour activity in human CETL patients.[38] Recently, Kim *et al.*[39] used *in situ* vaccination of CETL lesions with the Toll-like receptor 9 agonist CpG oligonucleotides in conjunction with local radiation, which led to regression of distant CETL lesions. These findings highlight the potential pivotal role that stimulation of the innate immune system with immunomodulatory agents can play in treatment of cancer and the need to explore more means of multimodal immunotherapy in both human and veterinary patients to provide enhanced disease control.

Histone deacetylase inhibitors

Dissection of the tumour kinome and exploration of key signalling pathways has identified new targets. Histones are small nuclear proteins responsible for packaging of DNA within nucleosomes. Transcription of DNA occurs in the acetylated state, whereas the hypoacetylated state results in compaction of DNA and repression of transcription. Abberant hypoacetylation is characteristic of some cancers suppressing cellular differentiation. Histone deacetylase (HDAC) inhibitors can activate both the death receptor and intrinsic apoptotic pathways and result in the reactivation of tumour suppressor gene transcription, leading to cytotoxicity and apoptosis.[40] In the human field, the HDAC inhibitors vorinostat (Zolinza®; Merck, Whitehouse Station, NJ, USA) and romidepsin (Istodax®; Celgene, Summit, NJ, USA) have been approved for use in CETL.[41,42] These drugs are generally very well tolerated and have little to no effects on normal cells. The activity of HDAC inhibitors appears to be multifactorial, and pathways include myc, JAK-STAT, B-Tumour Growth Factor and Bcl-6.[43,44] The HDAC inhibitors OSU-HDAC42 and SAHA have recently been investigated in canine tumour cell lines (including T-cell lymphosarcoma and MCT) and found to have potent histone acetylation activity at micromolar concentrations.[45] This represents an exciting potential therapeutic target for many canine solid tumours and a role for new drug development.

BRAF inhibitors

The Cancer Genome Project[46] brought to light an unanticipated pathway for induction of melanoma.[47] Mutations were identified in the *BRAF* oncogene, which is the serine/threonine kinase downstream of melanocyte-stimulating hormone. The high frequency of *BRAF* mutation in melanoma (50%) may be due to melanocyte biology. Ultraviolet B light causes upregulation of melanocyte-stimulating hormone, which in turn binds to its receptor, upregulating cyclic AMP and causing increased proliferation of melanocytes. This melanocyte-specific signalling pathway elucidates why there are higher numbers of *BRAF* mutations in melanoma compared with other cancers.

The BRAF inhibitor vemurafenib (Figure 2) was recently approved (2011) by the US Federal Drug Administration and European Medicines Agency for treatment of human metastatic melanoma.[48,49] This drug has a response rate of up to 78% in patients expressing the *BRAF*-V600E mutation, with no response in patients who lack this mutation. Despite excellent results, almost all patients develop progressive disease due to vemurafenib resistance. A variety of mechanisms of resistance have been described, precluding development of definitive subsequent treatment strategies.

Xenogeneic DNA vaccine for canine melanoma

Recent collaborative efforts on melanoma between human cancer researchers, veterinary investigators and industry resulted in the first commercially available veterinary cancer vaccine. The canine melanoma vaccine has been approved for use in the USA and is available in Europe to veterinary oncologists.[50] Dogs treated with vaccination in the trial achieved a median survival time of 389 days. In a recent retrospective study, Manley *et al.*[51] reviewed the outcome in a cohort of dogs with digital melanoma that received adjunctive xenogeneic melanoma vaccination following surgery. The overall median survival time was 476 days, with those dogs having the longest survival time being free of metastatic disease (105 versus 533 days). As opposed to vaccines that are cell based, this vaccine carries a xenogeneic DNA plasmid, which has been shown to elicit antitumour humoral and cellular immune responses. In theory, this should give a stronger immune response against the melanoma tyrosinase.[52] The vaccine is easy to administer but, despite many of the claims, it is still difficult to ascertain the true value of this approach. Overall, there is around a 20% response rate and, in the authors' opinion, these vaccines are only of value where there is minimal disease.

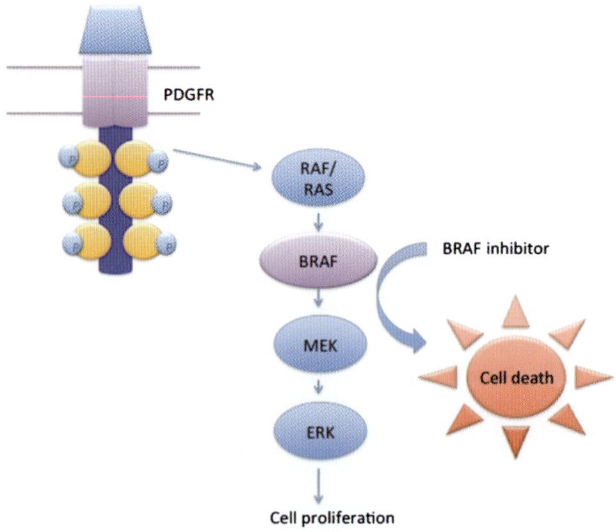

Figure 2. BRAF is a major protein intermediate in RAF/MEK.ERK signalling in normal cells but causes excessive proliferation in melanoma cells with *BRAF* mutations. The BRAF inhibitors cause cell death by apoptosis.

Monoclonal antibodies

Over the past 20–30 years, in parallel to the vast research efforts to map complex age-related diseases in mammals, revolutionary research has also developed in the field of monoclonal antibodies as therapeutics. Some of the top-line treatments of human disease include the use of monoclonal antibodies and, in the past 10 years, the area of human monoclonal therapeutics has become one of the fastest growing drug development markets, overtaking small molecules. Monoclonal antibodies are emerging as the market leaders in all cancer-based therapeutics, holding an 80% share of the US targeted cancer market. Monoclonal antibodies are antibodies cloned from a unique parent cell created by the fusion of an immunized cell with a myeloma cell. Monoclonal antibodies bind exclusively to the same epitope (part of an antigen recognized by the immune system). As well as being therapeutic themselves, monoclonal antibodies can also be used to deliver cytotoxic drugs or develop methods of sophisticated diagnostic imaging using radioisotopes (Figure 3). Monoclonal antibody-based therapeutics have been around for the last 20 years, with 30 immunoglobulins (IgGs) approved for a variety of conditions; some of the monoclonal antibodies are used to exploit our physiological knowledge of cell signalling and include receptors such as Vascular endothelial growth factor, epidermal growth factor receptor, *ERBB2* (v-erb-b2 erythroblastic leukemia viral oncogene homolog 2) CD20, CD33 and CD52. One major limitation of monoclonal antibody therapeutics is target selection that is clinically relevant. While many companies first selected the clinically validated targets in the literature, this area has become overcrowded. Companies are now developing second- and third-generation antibodies towards these same targets that are directed towards different epitopes, with longer half-lives or with different scaffolds.[53]

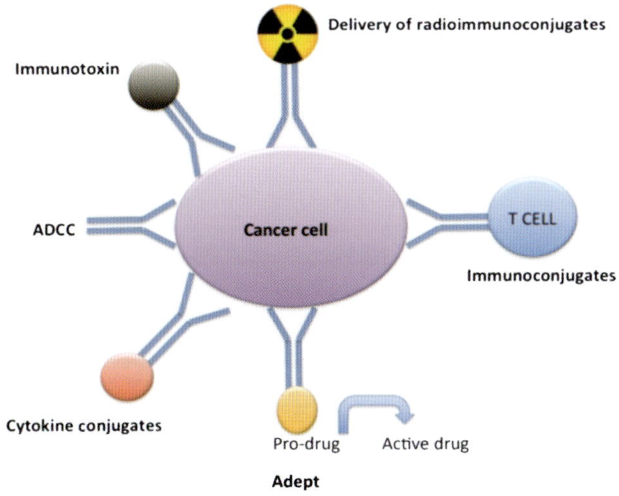

Figure 3. Monoclonal antibodies are becoming an exciting therapeutic modality. This figure demonstrates the multiple ways that antibodies can be used to kill cancers, including delivery of radionuclides, delivery of immune cells, delivery of cytokines, delivery of prodrugs (antibody-dependent enzyme prodrug therapy; ADEPT) and delivery of toxins, as well as simple antibody-mediated cellular cytotoxicity (ADCC).

Monoclonal antibodies in the treatment of skin cancer

Ipilimumab (Yervoy®; Bristol-Myers Squibb, New York, NY, USA) is a monoclonal antibody developed for the treatment of metastatic melanoma in human patients.[54] Its action, binding of cytotoxic T-lymphocyte antigen 4, leads to T-cell activation and expansion, resulting in tumour cell recognition and targeting for destruction by the immune system. A modest improvement in survival (45.6% 1 year survival rate) has been demonstrated with treatment. Currently, a phase I/II combinational study with vemurafenib (BRAF inhibitor) and ipilimumab is underway to investigate concurrent use of these agents in resistant metastatic melanoma.[55]

Vaccine therapy using antibodies to CD4 (zanolimumab) and CD52 (alemtuzumab) broadly targets T cells and has shown clinical responses ranging from 38 to 78% in patients with CETL.[56–58] However, vaccine immunotherapy for CETL is at an early stage. A scarcity of target antigens has hampered this work, but new antigens for these disorders are being detected by novel serological screens with use of tissue complementary DNA libraries. Studies in animals and humans of B-cell lymphoma suggest that dendritic cells pulsed with idiotype proteins (antigens) can elicit antitumour responses and tumour regression.[59–61] Cloning or synthesizing the unique T-cell receptor sequences expressed by cells of CETL, analogous to the B-cell idiotype, is technically feasible and can provide a unique tumour target for immunotherapy. An alternative strategy is to load autologous dendritic cells with tumour cells or lysates and inject them directly into a patient's lymph node. Geskin *et al.*[62] showed that administration of autologous tumour-loaded dendritic cells treated with T-helper 1-priming cytokines to heavily pretreated patients with sezary syndrome resulted in beneficial clinical responses.

Canine monoclonal IgE has been commercially available and used in allergy testing for more than 20 years. Recently, preliminary data were presented on an *in vitro* study exploiting the expression of FcεRIα IgE receptor present only on tissue mast cells and basophils. Recombinant IgE Fc and death receptor (TRAIL) fusion proteins were cloned from canine genomic DNA and shown to bind C2 mastocytoma cells expressing FcεRIα.[63] This effect was inhibited using a commercially available monoclonal IgE developed for allergen detection. This system could be explored for immunotherapeutic potential in cutaneous MCTs.

Identifying appropriate targets

Development of improved strategies for the diagnosis and treatment of sporadic cancers in animals such as dogs and cats presents the same fundamental problem as for humans: target selection, drug delivery and relapse or resistance. While the last decade has witnessed a large rise in the development of biologics entering the human oncology field, there has been little progress made in canine oncology.[64]

Commonly, many conventional anticancer drugs used to treat human cancers (e.g. doxorubicin) are also being used to treat animal patients. Recently, newer therapies, such as tyrosine kinase inhibitors and melanoma vaccination, have made inroads to molecular targeting of canine and feline cancers. Therapies such as monoclonal antibodies, in contrast, have not been brought forward for animal patients and cannot simply be used in different species. As a prototype example, the anti-CD20 'humanized' monoclonal antibody retuximab is used as a single agent or in combination therapy in non-Hodgkin's lymphoma and has proven efficacy. It cannot, however, be used in dogs for two reasons.[65] First of all, retuximab does not recognize the canine CD20 protein due to a single amino acid change in the extracellular domain of the CD20 monoclonal antibody epitope and, second, the canine immune system would clear the humanized antibody from its system before it could have an effect even if it did cross-react.[66] Since the development of rituximab in 1997 there have been a variety of second- and third-generation anti-CD20 antibodies designed to be more potent and have fewer adverse effects with reduced immunogenicity in human patients. Anti-human CD20 monoclonals are on their third generation, while there is yet to be a first-generation antibody for the treatment of canine lymphoma. Thus, there is a need for the development of monoclonal antibodies specifically for use in dogs and cats so that the therapeutic response to these antibodies for skin tumours and other cancers can be assessed.

The hurdles to clinical advancement

Evidence is mounting to support the idea of cancer as a stem cell disease.[67,68] Cell populations within solid tumours have been found to be heterogeneous, indicating that either not all tumour cells are derived from the same progenitor cell or that the progenitor cell has the capability of multilineage proliferation (cancer stem cell). Molecular targeted treatments of cancer have resulted in markedly improved response rates by some tumours. Resistance to these therapies appears to develop quickly, however, further promoting the idea that cancer stem cells are inherently resistant to chemotherapy and rapidly proliferate following killing of susceptible tumour cells. Alternative theories state that cancer cells are capable of rapid mutation, which may confer resistance to the tumour population, resulting in progressive disease following initial response. The characterization of cancer stem cells continues because future successes in therapy will rely on targeting the bulk cancer population as well as the small population of cancer stem cells that maintain the tumour population.[69]

Conclusions

Despite significant clinical advances over the past 10 years, numerous challenges remain to treating cancer in veterinary patients. Improvements in detecting the molecular mechanisms of neoplasia have provided the means to develop more effective therapies. Further work is necessary to understand the complex interactions among the various altered molecular pathways and how to translate this knowledge into meaningful therapeutics.

References

1. World Heath Organization website. Skin cancer information. Ultraviolet radiation and the INTERSUN Programme. Available at: http://www.who.int/uv/faq/skincancer/en/index1.html. Accessed July 9, 2012.
2. McGill MA, McGllade CJ. Cellular signaling. In: Tannock I, Hill R, Bristow R *et al.* eds. *The Basic Science of Oncology*. New York: McGraw-Hill Medical Publishing Division, 2005; 142–166.
3. London CA, Malpas PB, Wood-Follis SL *et al.* Multi-center, placebo-controlled, double-blind, randomized study of oral toceranib phosphate (SU11654), a receptor tyrosine kinase inhibitor, for the treatment of dogs with recurrent (either local or distant) mast cell tumor following surgical excision. *Clin Cancer Res* 2009; 15: 3856–3865.
4. Hahn KA, Ogilvie G, Rusk T *et al.* Masitinib is safe and effective for the treatment of canine mast cell tumors. *J Vet Intern Med* 2008; 22: 1301–1309.
5. Pryer NK, Lee LB, Zadovaskaya R *et al.* Proof of target for SU11654: inhibition of KIT phosphorylation in canine mast cell tumors. *Clin Cancer Res* 2003; 9: 5729–5734.
6. Dubreuil P, Letard S, Ciufolini M *et al.* Masitinib (AB1010), a potent and selective tyrosine kinase inhibitor targeting KIT. *PLoS One* 2009; 4: e7258.
7. London CA, Seguin B. Mast cell tumors in the dog. *Vet Clin North Am: Small Animl Pract* 2003; 33: 473–489.
8. Hahn KA, Legendre AM, Shaw NG *et al.* Evaluation of 12-and 24-month survival rates after treatment with masitinib in dogs with nonresectable mast cell tumors. *Am J Vet Res* 2010; 71: 1354–1361.
9. London CA, Hannah AL, Zadovoskaya R *et al.* Phase I dose-escalating study of SU11654, a small molecule receptor tyrosine kinase inhibitor, in dogs with spontaneous malignancies. *Clin Cancer Res* 2003; 9: 2755–2768.
10. London CA, Mathie T, Stingle N *et al.* Preliminary evidence for biologic activity of toceranib phosphate (Palladia) in solid tumours. *Vet Comp Oncol* 2012; 10: 194–205.
11. Beadling C, Jacobson-Dunlop E, Hodi FS *et al. KIT* gene mutations and copy number in melanoma subtypes. *Clin Cancer Res* 2008; 14: 6821–6828.
12. Teixeira TF, Dagli MLZ. c-KIT immunostaining differs in canine buccal melanotic and amelanotic melanomas. in *Proceedings*. 2nd World Veterinary Cancer Congress. 2012; 90.
13. Zhang S, Chen J, Jiang H *et al.* Anti-epidermal growth factor receptor therapy for advanced head and neck squamous cell carcinoma: a meta-analysis. *Eur J Clin Pharmacol* 2012; 68: 561–569.
14. Cranmer LD, Engelhardt C, Morgan SS. Treatment of unresectable and metastatic cutaneous squamous cell carcinoma. *Oncologist* 2010; 15: 1320–1328.
15. Sabatini S, Marconato L, Zoff A *et al.* Epidermal growth factor receptor expression is predictive of poor prognosis in feline cutaneous squamous cell carcinoma. *J Feline Med Surg* 2010; 12: 760–768.
16. Bergkvist GT, Argyle DJ, Pang LY *et al.* Studies on the inhibition of feline EGFR in squamous cell carcinoma enhancement of radiosensitivity and rescue of resistance to small molecule inhibitors. *Cancer Biol Ther* 2011; 11: 927–937.
17. Robat CS, London CA, Selting KA. Safety evaluation of combination vinblastine and toceranib phosphate (Palladia®) in dogs: a phase I dose-finding study. *J Vet Intern Med* 2011; 25: 745–746.
18. Carlsten KS, London CA, Haney S *et al.* Multicenter prospective trial of hypofractionated radiation treatment, toceranib, and prednisone for measurable canine mast cell tumors. *J Vet Intern Med* 2012; 26: 135–141.
19. Gallimore A, Godkin A. Regulatory T cells and tumour immunity – observations in mice and men. *Immunology* 2008; 123: 157–163.
20. Biller BJ, Guth A, Burton H *et al.* Decreased ratio of CD8+ T cells to regulatory T cells associated with decreased survival

in dogs with osteosarcoma. *J Vet Intern Med* 2010; 24: 1118–1123.

21. Boucek J, Mrkvan T, Chovanec M *et al.* Regulatory T cells and their prognostic value for patients with squamous cell carcinoma of the head and neck. *J Cell Mol Med* 2009; 14: 426–433.
22. Mitchell L, Thamm DH, Biller BJ. Clinical and immunomodulatory effects of toceranib combined with low-dose cyclophosphamide in dogs with cancer. *J Vet Intern Med* 2012; 26: 355–362.
23. Lansigan F, Foss FM. Current and emerging treatment strategies for cutaneous T-cell lymphoma. *Drugs* 2010; 70: 273–286.
24. Altucci L, Leibowitz MD, Ogilvie KM *et al.* RAR and RXR modulation in cancer and metabolic disease. *Nat Rev Drug Disc* 2007; 6: 793–810.
25. Fields AL, Soprano DR, Soprano KJ. Retinoids in biological control and cancer. *J Cell Biochem* 2007; 102: 886–898.
26. Apisarnthanarax N, Duvic M. Cutaneous T-cell lymphoma. New immunomodulators. *Dermatol Clin* 2001; 19: 737–748.
27. Apisarnthanarax N, Duvic M. Therapy options in cutaneous T-cell lymphoma. *Expert Rev Anticancer Ther* 2001; 1: 403–420.
28. White SD, Rosychuck RAW, Scott KV *et al.* Use of isotretinoin and etretinate for the treatment of benign cutaneous neoplasia and cutaneous lymphoma in dogs. *J Am Vet Med Assoc* 1993; 202: 387–391.
29. Breneman D, Duvic M, Kuzel T *et al.* Phase 1 and 2 trial of bexarotene gel for skin-directed treatment of patients with cutaneous T-cell lymphoma. *Arch Dermatol* 2002; 138: 325–332.
30. Kim EJ, Hess S, Richardson SK *et al.* Immunopathogenesis and therapy of cutaneous T cell lymphoma. *J Clin Invest* 2005; 115: 798–812.
31. Souza CH, Valli VE, Fan TM *et al.* Detection of retinoid receptor expression in canine normal lymph node and in nodal lymphoma. *Vet Comp Oncol* 2004; 2: 106–107.
32. Souza CH, Valli VE, Selting KA *et al.* Immunohistochemical detection of retinoid receptors in tumors from 30 dogs diagnosed with cutaneous lymphoma. *J Vet Intern Med* 2010; 24: 1112–1117.
33. Takeda K, Akira S. TLR signalling pathways. *Semin Immunol* 2004; 16: 3–9.
34. Daudén E, BASALE Study Group. Effectiveness and satisfaction with imiquimod for the treatment of superficial basal cell carcinoma in daily dermatological practice. *J Eur Acad Dermatol Venerol* 2011; 25: 1304–1310.
35. Wysocka M, Newton S, Benoit BM *et al.* Synthetic imidazoquinolines potently and broadly activate the cellular immune response of patients with cutaneous T-cell lymphoma: synergy with interferon-gamma enhances production of interleukin-12. *Clin Lymphoma Myeloma* 2007; 7: 524–534.
36. Suchin KR, Junkins-Hopkins JM, Rook AH. Treatment of stage IA cutaneous T-cell lymphoma with topical application of the immune response modifier imiquimod. *Arch Dermatol* 2002; 138: 1137–1139.
37. Wysocka M, Dawany N, Benoit B *et al.* Synergistic enhancement of cellular immune responses by the novel Toll receptor 7/8 agonist 3M-007 and interferon-γ: implications for therapy of cutaneous T-cell lymphoma. *Leuk Lymphoma* 2011; 52: 1970–1979.
38. Howman RA, Prince HM. New drug therapies in peripheral T-cell lymphoma. *Expert Rev Anticancer Ther* 2011; 11: 457–472.
39. Kim YH, Gratzinger D, Harrison C *et al.* *In situ* vaccination against mycosis fungoides by intratumoral injection of a TLR9 agonist combined with radiation: a phase 1/2 study. *Blood* 2012; 119: 355–363.
40. Zain J. Role of histone deacetylase inhibitors in the treatment of lymphomas and multiple myeloma. *Hematol Oncol Clin North Am* 2012; 26: 671–704.
41. Rangwala S, Zhang C, Duvic M. HDAC inhibitors for the treatment of cutaneous T-cell lymphomas. *Future Med Chem* 2012; 4: 471–486.
42. Marks PA. The clinical development of histone deacetylase inhibitors as targeted anticancer drugs. *Expert Opin Investig Drugs* 2010; 19: 1049–1066.
43. Dokmanovic M, Clarke C, Marks PA. Histone deacetylase inhibitors: overview and perspectives. *Mol Cancer Res* 2007; 5: 981–989.
44. Marks PA, Xu WS. Histone deacetylase inhibitors: potential in cancer therapy. *J Cell Biochem* 2009; 107: 600–608.
45. Kisseberth WC, Murahari S, London CA *et al.* Evaluation of the effects of histone deacetylase inhibitors on cells from canine cancer cell lines. *Am J Vet Res* 2008; 69: 938–945.
46. Wellcome Trust Sanger Institute Cancer Genome Project. Publications. BRAF Nature paper. Available at : http://www.sanger.ac.uk/genetics/CGP/Publications. Accessed July 5, 2012.
47. Davies H, Bignell GR, Cox C *et al.* Mutations of the *BRAF* gene in human cancer. *Nature* 2002; 417: 949–954.
48. Joseph EW, Pratilas CA, Poulikakos P *et al.* PLX4032, a selective inhibitor of RAF kinase activity, inhibits BRAF (V600E) tumor proliferation and MAPK signaling *in vitro* and *in vivo*. in *Proceedings*. American Association for Cancer Research Annual Meeting 2008;49: 815.
49. Joseph EW, Pratilas CA, Poulikakos P *et al.* The RAF inhibitor PLX4032 inhibits ERK signaling and tumor cell proliferation in a V600E BRAF-selective manner. *Proc Natl Acad Sci USA* 2010; 107: 14903–14908.
50. Bergman PJ, McKnight J, Novosad A *et al.* Long-term survival of dogs with advanced malignant melanoma after DNA vaccination with xenogeneic human tyrosinase: a phase I trial. *Clin Cancer Res* 2003; 9: 1284–1290.
51. Manley CA, Leibman NF, Wolchok JD *et al.* Xenogeneic murine tyrosinase DNA vaccine for malignant melanoma of the digit of dogs. *J Vet Intern Med* 2011; 25: 94–99.
52. Liao JC, Gregor P, Wolchok JD *et al.* Vaccination with human tyrosinase DNA induces antibody responses in dogs with advanced melanoma. *Cancer Immun* 2007; 6: 1–10.
53. Beck A, Wurch T, Bailly C *et al.* Strategies and challenges for the next generation of therapeutic antibodies. *Nat Rev Immunol* 2010; 10: 345–352.
54. Hodi FS, O'Day SJ, McDermott DF. Ipilimumab improves survival in metastatic melanoma patients. *Immunotherapy* 2011; 3: 928–929.
55. Memorial Sloan-Kettering Cancer Center website. Clinical trials information. A phase I/II study of vemurafenib plus ipilimumab in patients with V600 BRAF mutation-positive metastatic melanoma. Available at: http://www.mskcc.org/cancer-care/adult/melanoma/clinical-trials/11-148. Accessed May 30, 2012.
56. Alexandroff AB, Shpadaruk V, Bamford WM *et al.* Alemtuzumab-resistant Sézary syndrome responding to zanolimumab. *Br J Haematol* 2011; 154: 419–421.
57. Mayes S, Brown N, Illidge TM. New antibody drug treatments for lymphoma. *Expert Opin Biol Ther* 2011; 11: 623–640.
58. Parker E. Immune function may persist following alemtuzumab therapy for cutaneous T-cell lymphoma. *Expert Rev Clin Immunol* 2012; 8: 211.
59. Henson MS, Curtsinger JM, Larson VS *et al.* Immunotherapy with autologous tumour antigen-coated microbeads (large multivalent immunogen), IL-2 and GM-CSF in dogs with spontaneous B-cell lymphoma. *Vet Comp Oncol* 2011; 9: 95–105.
60. Hsu Fj, Caspar CB, Czerwinski D *et al.* Tumor-specific idiotype vaccines in the treatment of patients with B-cell lymphoma – long-term results of a clinical trial. *Blood* 1997; 89: 3129–3135.
61. Kwak LW, Campbell MJ, Czerwinski DK *et al.* Induction of immune responses in patients with B-cell lymphoma against the surface-immunoglobulin idiotype expressed by their tumors. *N Engl J Med* 1992; 327: 1209–1215.
62. Geskin L, Kingston A, Whiteside T *et al.* An engineered autologous dendritic cell therapy induces potent tumor specific T-cell activity and clinical response in a patient with end-stage cutaneous T-cell lymphoma (Proceedings of the 65th Annual meeting of the Society for Investigative Dermatology) *J Invest Dermatol* 2004; 122: A51 (abstract 301).

63. Elders R, Bains S, Holder A *et al.* Development of recombinant canine IgE Fc-based immunotherapy for canine mast cell tumours. in *Proceedings*. 2nd World Veterinary Cancer Congress 2012; 40.
64. Impellizeri JA, Howell K, McKeever KP *et al.* The role of rituximab in the treatment of canine lymphoma: an ex vivo evaluation. *Vet J* 2006; 171: 556–558.
65. Saini KS, Azim HA Jr, Cocorocchio E *et al.* Rituximab in Hodgkin lymphoma: is the target always a hit? *Cancer Treat Rev* 2011; 37: 385–390.
66. Binder M, Otto F, Mertelsmann R et al. The epitope recognized by rituximab. *Blood* 2006; 108: 1975–1978.
67. Argyle DJ, Blacking TM. From viruses to cancer stem cells: dissecting the pathways to malignancy. *Vet J* 2008; 177: 311–323.
68. Blacking TM, Wilson H, Argyle DJ. Is cancer a stem cell disease? Theory, evidence and implications. *Vet Comp Oncol* 2007; 5: 76–89.
69. Pang L, Argyle DJ. Using naturally occurring tumours in dogs and cats to study telomerase and cancer stem cell biology. *Biochim Biophys Acta* 2009; 1792: 380–391.

To cite this article, please use DOI: 10.1111/j.1365-3164.2012.01081.x

6.2

Kinase dysfunction and kinase inhibitors

Cheryl A. London

Department of Veterinary Biosciences, College of Veterinary Medicine, The Ohio State University, Columbus, OH 43214, USA

Correspondence: Cheryl A. London, Department of Veterinary Biosciences, The Ohio State University, 454 VMAB, 1925 Coffey Road, Columbus, OH 43210, USA. E-mail: cheryl.london@cvm.osu.edu

With recent advances in molecular biology, abnormalities in cancer cells that contribute to dysregulation of cell survival and proliferation are being characterized with greater precision. Through this process, key abnormalities in cancer cells involving proteins that regulate signal transduction, migration, mitosis and other critical processes have been identified. Such abnormalities often involve a class of proteins called kinases that act to phosphorylate other proteins in the cell, resulting in activation of these proteins in the absence of appropriate stimulation/regulation. Given their role in tumour biology, substantial effort has been directed at blocking the function of these proteins. Several approaches have been used, including monoclonal antibodies and small molecule inhibitors. While antibodies are primarily directed at cell surface proteins, small molecule inhibitors, also known as kinase inhibitors, target proteins throughout the cell.

A variety of kinase inhibitors have been approved for the treatment of human cancers. In some instances, these inhibitors have exhibited significant clinical efficacy, and it is likely that their biological activity will be further enhanced as combination regimens with standard treatment modalities are explored.

The use of kinase inhibitors in dogs and cats is relatively recent, although two inhibitors, toceranib (Palladia; Pfizer Animal Health, Madison, NJ, USA) and masitinib (Kinavet; Catalent Pharma Solutions, Somerset, NJ, USA) have been approved by the Federal Drug Administration (USA) for use in dogs. This article reviews the biology of protein kinase dysfunction in human and animal cancers, and the application of specific kinase inhibitors to veterinary cancer patients.

Protein kinases and normal cell biology

Protein kinases are critical regulators of normal cell signalling, because they control several key processes, such as cell survival, growth, differentiation and migration. The kinases act through phosphorylation of other proteins. They accomplish this by binding adenosine triphosphate (ATP) and using this to add phosphate groups to key amino acids on themselves (also known as autophosphorylation) and on other proteins, thereby promoting the transmission of cellular signals. This process usually occurs in response to stimuli generated by growth factors (GFs) or other substances outside of the cell that intiate the process. Protein kinases are termed tyrosine kinases (TKs) if they phosphorylate proteins on the amino acid tyrosine or serine/threonine kinases if they phosphorylate proteins on the amino acids serine and threonine. These kinases can be expressed on the cell surface, in the cytoplasm and in the nucleus.

Receptor tyrosine kinases (RTKs) are those TKs expressed on the cell surface that are stimluated by binding of GFs. Receptor tyrosine kinases are structured to contain an extracellular ligand binding domain, a transmembrane domain that anchors the RTK in the membrane, and a cytoplasmic kinase domain that positively and negatively regulates phosphorylation through inhibition of spontaneous dimerization.[1–3] Binding of a GF to the RTK induces dimerization of the receptor, thereby inducing a conformational change that allows ATP binding, autophosphorylation, and the initiation of a downstream signal through subsequent binding of adaptor proteins and additional TKs.[1] It is now understood that dysregulation of RTKs through mutation, overexpression or chromosomal translocation results in pathway activation and subsequent uncontrolled signalling. While the molecular aspects of these events have been extensively researched in human cancers, characterization of similar abnormalities in canine and feline cancers is just beginning. Examples of RTKs known to be dysregulated in human and canine cancers include KIT, MET, anaplastic lymphoma kinase (ALK) and epidermal growth factor receptor (EGFR).[4–8]

Receptor tyrosine kinase signalling is also an important driver of the process of new blood vessel growth, known as angiogenesis, which is essential for expansion of tumours beyond 1–2 mm in size. The RTKs involved in angiogenesis include vascular endothelial growth factor receptor (VEGFR), platelet-derived growth factor receptor (PDGFR), fibroblast growth factor receptor (FGFR), and Tie-1 and Tie-2 (receptors for angiopoietin).[9–12] Vascular endothelial growth factor receptors are expressed on new blood vessel cells, and signalling promotes migration and proliferation;[9] PDGFR is expressed on pericytes, pro-

Accepted 28 May 2012
Sources of Funding: This study was self funded.
Conflict of Interest: No conflicts of interest have been declared.

moting their maturation;[11,12] and FGFR is expressed on endothelial cells, enhancing expression of VEGF. [11] Both Tie-1 and Tie-2 are expressed on blood vessels in tumours and are important in the recruitment of pericytes and smooth muscle cells to the newly forming vascular channels.[13]

Kinases present in the cytoplasm act to transmit signals generated by RTKs to the nucleus through a series of intermediates that also become phosphorylated.[14] In cancer cells, two specific cytoplasmic pathways are known to be dysregulated with signficant frequency. The first includes members of the RAS–RAF–MEK–ERK/p38/JNK families,[15,16] most of which are serine/threonine kinases. Their activation results in ERK phosphorylation, translocation into the nucleus, and subsequent alteration of transcription factor and nuclear kinase activity important for controlling the cell cycle. Specific members known to be mutated in human tumours include RAS (lung cancer, colon cancer and several haematologic malignancies) and BRAF (melanomas, thyroid carcinomas and colon cancer).[16–18]

The second cytoplasmic pathway frequently altered in cancer includes phosphatidyl inositol-3 kinase (PI3K) and its downstream signal transducers AKT, nuclear factor κB and mTOR, among others.[19,20] Phosphatidyl inositol-3 kinase is activated by RTK stimulation and in turn phosphorylates AKT, which alters several additional proteins involved in the regulation of cell survival, cycling and growth.[21] AKT phosphorylates targets that promote apoptosis (BAD, procaspase-9 and Forkhead transcription factors) and activates nuclear factor κB, a transcription factor that regulates multiple cellular processes.[19–21] AKT also phosphorylates other proteins such as mTOR, p21, p27 and GSK3, resulting in redistribution of these proteins either in or out of the nucleus, ultimately inhibiting apoptosis while stimulating cell cycling.[19–21] Abnormalities of PI3K, including mutations and gene amplification, are found in many human cancers, including breast, colorectal, lung and ovarian carcinomas.[22] Another manner in which this pathway can become activated is through loss of activity of PTEN, a phosphatase that normally acts to regulate AKT and terminate signalling.[19,23,24] *PTEN* mutations and/or decreased PTEN expression occur in many human cancers (e.g. glioblastoma and prostate cancer)[22,23] and have been documented in canine cancers as well (osteosarcoma and melanoma).[25–27]

The act of signal transduction serves to influence cellular events by affecting gene transcription and multiple proteins that regulate cell cycling. The cyclins and their kinase partners [cyclin-dependent kinases (CDKs)] control progression of cells through various phases of the cell cycle.[28–30] Cyclins D and E and their CDK partners (CDK2, 4 and 6) are the primary regulators of entry into the cell cycle, as co-ordinated function of these is necessary for cells to progress from G1 into S phase. Signals generated by RTKs often induce expression and activation of cyclin D/CDK4,6 complexes that act to phosphorylate the tumour suppressor Rb, partly repressing its activity.[29,30] This is further enhanced by cyclin E/CDK complexes, thereby initiating the process of DNA replication necessary for cell division. Dysregulation of the cylins and CDKs occurs frequently in human cancers, with overexpression of cyclins D and E found in breast, pancreas, and head and neck carcinomas.[30]

Kinases and cancer cells

Dysfunction of protein kinases occurs frequently in human cancers, and recent data indicate that dog and cat cancers may also experience a similar level of dysfunction. Mutation, overexpression, the generation of fusion proteins and the presence of autocrine loops of activation are all mechanisms by which this may take place. Mutations often alter the structure of a kinase such that phosphorylation occurs in the absence of an appropriate stimulus. For example, a point mutation occurs in the *BRAF* gene in approximately 60% of human cutaneous melanomas[18,31,32] that induces a conformational change in the protein, resulting in constitutive activation, downstream ERK signalling, and promotion of cell growth and survival.[33,34] RAS is another kinase that is dysregulated through point mutation in several haematopoietic neoplasms, lung cancer, colon cancer and many others.[16,31,32]

KIT, an RTK normally expressed on haematopoietic stem cells, melanocytes, interstitial cells of Cajal, in the central nervous system and on mast cells, has been shown to be dysregulated in several cancers.[35] In approximately 25–30% of canine grade 2 and 3 mast cell tumours, mutations consisting of internal tandem duplications are found in the juxtamembrane domain of KIT, resulting in ligand-independent activation. These mutations are associated with a higher risk of local recurrence and metastasis.[36–38] Deletions in the juxtamembrane domain of KIT are found in approximately 50–80% of human patients with gastrointestinal stromal tumours and have been identified in canine gastrointestinal stromal tumours as well.[39–41] Other cancers in which *KIT* mutations have been identified include melanoma and acute myelogenous leukaemia. Other examples include *FLT3* internal tandem duplications in acute myelogenous leukaemia,[42–45] *EGFR* point mutations in lung carcinomas,[46,47] and *PI3Ka* mutations in several types of carcinomas.[22]

Overexpression of kinases often involves the RTKs and either promotes an enhanced response to normal levels of growth factor or, more commonly, induces spontaneous receptor dimerization in the absence of ligand binding. Perhaps the most well-described example is overexpression of the RTK HER2/Neu (a member of the EGFR family) in breast and ovarian carcinomas.[3,48,49] *EGFR* is also overexpressed in human lung, bladder, cervical, ovarian, renal and pancreatic cancers, and some tumours have as many as 60 copies of the gene per cell.[6] Fusion proteins are generated when a portion of the kinase becomes attached to another gene through chromosomal rearrangement, thereby disrupting the mechanisms that typically control protein function. One of the best-characterized fusion proteins is BCR-ABL, which is found in 90% of patients with chronic myelogenous leukaemia (CML).[50,51] This fusion induces constitutive activation of the cytoplasmic kinase ABL, contributing to malignant transformation. Other examples include TEL-PDGFRα in leukaemia and EML4-ALK in non-small-cell lung cancer.[52] Lastly, autocrine loops of activation primarily occur when tumour cells express both the RTK and the growth factor resulting in constitutive receptor activation.

Examples include coexpression of transforming growth factor β and EGFR in glioblastoma and squamous cell carcinoma, insulin-like growth factor (IGF) and its ligand, IGF-1R, in breast and colorectal cancer, and VEGF and VEGFR in melanoma and glioblastoma.[3,53–55] In canine cancers, possible autocrine loops have been documented in osteosarcoma (OSA, MET and HGF) and haemangiosarcoma (HSA, KIT and SCF).[56–58]

Kinase inhibitors

With the understanding that certain molecular events can act as drivers of uncontrolled cancer cell growth and survival, substantial effort has been directed at blocking the specific proteins that initiate this process either directly, at the level of the tumour cell, or indirectly, at the level of the tumour microenvironment. The two approaches most commonly used are monoclonal antibodies and small molecule inhibitors.

Technology now exists to engineer antibodies to recognize specific epitopes on a variety of proteins. This method has been successfully used to generate antibodies that can bind to the extracellular domains of RTKs or circulating growth factors, thereby inhibiting function of these proteins. One of the most successful examples is a humanized monoclonal antibody called trastuzumab (Herceptin; Genentech, South San Francisco, CA, USA) that targets HER2/Neu, which is overexpressed in approximately 30% of breast cancers, as well as other epithelial cancers.[59] In women with metastatic HER2-positive breast cancer, trastuzumab resulted in a response rate of approximately 25%[60] that improved to approximately 50% when trastuzumab was combined with chemotherapy.[61] When used in the adjuvant setting, multiple studies have demonstrated that trastuzumab markedly improves survival of women with HER2-positive breast cancer and, consequently, it is now part of the routine standard of care.[62,63] Other examples of monoclonal antibodies approved for use in human cancers include rituxumab (Rituxan; Genentech), which targets CD20 expressed in B-cell malignancies[64,65] and cetuximab (Erbitux; Bristol-Meyers Squibb, Princeton, NJ, USA), which targets ErbB1/EGFR overexpressed in several human carcinomas.[6,59,66]

The second major method for blocking the function of a protein is through the use of small molecule inhibitors. These work either by blocking the ATP binding site of kinases, essentially acting as competitive inhibitors, or by blocking protein–protein interactions, known as allosteric inhibition.[67] Those small molecule compounds that block ATP binding to the kinase prevent autophosphorylation, as well as downstream phosphorylation, thereby interrupting the survival/growth signal essential to the tumour cell, ultimately resulting in cell death. In contrast to the monoclonal antibodies, the small molecule inhibitors are often easy to synthesize in large quantities, are usually orally bioavailable and can readily enter cells to bind the intended target.

The first small molecule inhibitor to be approved for human use was imatinib (Gleevec; Novartis Oncology US, East Hanover, NJ, USA), an orally administered drug that binds the ATP pocket of ABL, as well as the RTKs KIT and PDGFRα.[68] As previously mentioned, BCR-ABL fusion proteins are present in over 90% of human patients with CML, making this a good target for therapy. The use of imatinib for treatment of patients with CML has been transformative, with significant biological activity resulting in the approval of this drug as standard of care for affected individuals.[69–74] In the chronic phase of CML, imatinib induces a remission rate of close to 95%, and most patients remain in remission for longer than 1 year. The activity of imatinib is much lower in patients with blast crisis (20–50%), often lasting <10 months. Resistance to therapy is primarily due to the development of mutations in *ABL* that preclude drug binding, although gene amplification has also been documented.[75,76] Through its ability to inhibit KIT, imatinib also has substantial single-agent activity against human gastrointestinal stromal tumours, in which up to 80% of the tumours have activating mutations in *KIT*.[77,78] Response rates of 50–70% have been reported to imatinib, far better than the 5% response rate seen with standard chemotherapy.[79,80]

There are now several small molecule inhibitors approved for use in the treatment of a variety of human cancers, and many more currently undergoing clinical investigation. A subset of people with non-small-cell lung cancer (NSCLC) have tumours with activating mutations in *EGFR* that respond to erlotinib (Tarceva; Genentech OSI Pharmaceuticals, Pharma Inc., Farmingdale, NY, USA) or gefitinib (Iressa; Astra-Zeneca, Wilmington, DE, USA), small molecule inhibitors of EGFR.[81] Response rates in patients with *EGFR* mutations can be as high as 80%, compared with <10–20% for those without. A small number of patients with NSCLC also exhibit activation of the RTK ALK through its fusion to EML4.[82] A small molecule inhibitor of ALK, crizotinib (Xalkori; Pfizer, New York, NY, USA) has demonstrated significant activity against patients whose tumours express the EML4-ALK translocation, with 56% of affected patients experiencing objective response to therapy and another 31% experiencing stable disease.[82,83] More recently, vemurafenib (Zelboraf; Genentech), a small molecule inhibitor of BRAF, has demonstrated substantial activity in human patients with malignant melanoma carrying B-RAF-activating mutation, with close to 50% meeting the criteria for objective response.[84] This compares to an objective response rate of only 5% in patients treated with the chemotherapeutic agent dacarbazine. Lastly, inhibition of mTOR has become of interest in several cancers, given the activation of the PI3K pathway and the critical role of mTOR in mediating its effects. While rapamycin, a drug used for many years as an immunosuppressive agent, is the prototypic mTOR inhibitor,[85,86] the more specific rapamycin analogues, temisorlimus and evorolimus, have been approved for use in patients with metastatic renal carcinoma; additional mTOR inhibitors are under investigation for their potential activity in soft tissue sarcomas and bone sarcomas.[85,86]

While the small molecule agents discussed above tend to block a restricted set of targets, there are other inhibitors that exhibit far broader activity. Sunitinib (Sutent; Pfizer) is a small molecule inhibitor of several RTKs, including VEGFR1,2, PDGFRα/β, KIT, FLT3, CSFR1 and RET.[87] The multitargeted nature of this inhibitor may be responsible for its observed activity in several types of cancer, including gastrointestinal stromal tumours, renal cell carcinoma, thyroid carcinoma and insulinoma.[87] While such agents often have significant clinical activity, they are usually associated with a more substantial range of toxicities that may limit their chronic use.

Kinase inhibitors: the veterinary experience

There are now two small molecule inhibitors approved for use in veterinary medicine. The first, toceranib phosphate (Palladia; Pfizer Animal Health, Madison, NJ, USA), is an orally bioavailable small molecule inhibitor that blocks a variety of RTKs, including VEGFR2, PDGFRα and KIT.[88] However, it is very closely related to the small molecule inhibitor sunitinib (Sutent; see above), suggesting that it is likely to be active against several other RTKs.[87] A recent kinome analysis (C. A. London, unpublished data) supports the broad activity of toceranib against the split kinase RTKs, RET and possibly JAK family members.

The first evaluation of toceranib in dogs was a phase I clinical trial in 57 dogs with a variety of cancers.[88] In this study, objective responses occurred in 16 dogs, consisting of six complete responses and 10 partial responses, with stable disease in an additional 15 dogs, for an overall biological activity of 54%. Responding tumours included sarcomas, carcinomas, melanomas, myeloma and mast cell tumours (MCTs). The highest response rate was in MCTs, with 10 of 11 dogs with *KIT* mutations exhibiting response to therapy. The maximal tolerated dose was established as 3.25 mg/kg every other day, and the adverse event profile was found to be primarily gastrointestinal in nature, including loss of appetite, diarrhoea and, less commonly, vomiting, although these toxicities were relatively well controlled with the addition of appropriate concomitant medications.

Based on the phase I trial results, a placebo-controlled randomized study of toceranib was subsequently performed in dogs with grade 2 and 3 MCTs.[89] During the blinded phase, the response rate in toceranib treated dogs (n = 86) was 37.2% (seven complete responses and 25 partial responses) versus 7.9% (five partial responses) in placebo-treated dogs (n = 63). Of 58 dogs that received toceranib following placebo escape, 41.4% (eight complete responses and 16 partial responses) experienced an objective response. The overall response rate for all 145 dogs was 42.8% (21 complete responses and 41 partial responses), with an additional 16 dogs experiencing stable disease. Dogs with MCT that had *KIT* mutations were more likely to respond to toceranib than those without (69 versus 37%).

Following its approval in 2009, toceranib was used to treat a variety of canine solid tumours, often in the setting of failed primary therapy or metastatic disease. A retrospective analysis of its off-label use provided evidence of biological activity in anal gland anal sac adenocarcinoma, metastatic osteosarcoma, thyroid carcinoma, head and neck carcinoma and nasal carcinoma.[90] Clinical benefit was observed in 63 of 85 (74%) dogs, including 28 of 32 anal gland anal sac adenocarcinomas (eight partial responses and 20 stable disease), 11 of 23 osteosarcomas (one partial response and 10 stable disease), 12 of 15 thyroid carcinomas (four partial responses and eight stable disease), seven of eight head and neck carcinomas (one complete response, five partial responses and one stable disease) and five of seven nasal carcinomas (one complete response and four stable disease). These data provided preliminary evidence that toceranib may have biological activity against certain solid tumours, although future prospective studies are necessary to define its true effects.

Given the use of non-steroidal anti-inflammatory drugs (NSAIDs) in veterinary medical oncology, there was interest in combining an NSAID with toceranib to treat solid tumours. Published data suggest that piroxicam, a mixed COX-1/COX-2 inhibitor, has activity in some canine cancers, particularly carcinomas. A phase I trial was therefore performed in tumour-bearing dogs to establish the safety of toceranib/piroxicam coadministration.[91] The combination of standard dosages of both drugs (toceranib at 3.25 mg/kg every other day and piroxicam at 0.3 mg/kg/day) was found generally to be safe, and several antitumour responses were noted. As the dogs were not monitored long term to assess whether gastrointestinal adverse effects occurred after continued drug coadministration, it is now recommended that piroxicam be given every other day, alternating with the toceranib to avoid potential gastrointestinal issues.

In order to begin to determine how best to combine toceranib with chemotherapeutic agents, a phase I clinical trial was performed to identify an appropriate dosing regimen, combining toceranib with vinblastine in canine MCT, where both drugs have single-agent activity.[92] The dose-limiting toxicity for the toceranib/vinblastine combination was found to be neutropenia, and the maximal tolerated dose of vinblastine was 1.6 mg/m^2 every other week with toceranib at 3.25 mg/kg every other day. The dose of vinblastine represented a 50% reduction in dose intensity necessitated by the enhanced myelosuppression when combined with toceranib. Despite this, the overall response rate was 71% to the drug combination, superior to either drug alone. The significant biological activity and enhanced myelosuppression suggest the possibility of additive/synergistic effects of the drug combination, although a prospective study is needed to confirm this.

In addition to chemotherapy, there is interest in combining toceranib with radiation therapy. Mast cell tumours were used to evaluate this combination, because both treatment modalities have single-agent activity.[93] Dogs with nonresectable MCTs received prednisone, omeprazole, diphenhydramine and toceranib for 1 week prior to starting coarse fractionated radiation therapy (6 Gy given once per week for 4 weeks). The overall response rate was 76.4%, with 58.8% of dogs achieving complete response and 17.6% partial response. The overall median survival time was not reached with a median follow-up longer than 1 year. Importantly, there was no evidence of enhanced radiation-induced toxicities in this study, suggesting that combined toceranib/radiation therapy may achieve significant clinical activity in dogs without serious adverse effects.

The second small molecule inhibitor approved for use in dogs is masitinib (Kinavet; AB Science, Paris, France), which blocks the activity of KIT, PDGFRα/β and the cytoplasmic kinase Lyn. A large placebo-controlled clinical trial was performed in over 200 dogs with MCTs, in which masitinib significantly improved time to progression compared with placebo, and outcome was improved in dogs with MCTs possessing *KIT* mutations.[94] Subsequent follow-up of dogs treated with masitinib for 1–2 years identified an increased number of dogs with long-term disease control compared with those treated with placebo (40 versus 15% alive at 2 years).[95] Lastly, small studies have evaluated the efficacy of imatinib for the treatment of canine and feline MCTs.[96–98] Imatinib was well tolerated, and objective antitumour responses were observed in dogs with both mutant and wild-type *KIT*. Responses have also been observed in cats with MCTs that have *KIT* mutations.[99,100]

Resistance to therapy

The response of tumour cells to small molecule inhibitors in the presence of known protein dysregulation is often dramatic, with objective response rates often exceeding 50%, far higher than that typically observed with chemotherapy alone. Unfortunately, in most instances these responses are typically not durable, lasting from 6 to 18 months on average before relapse. The mechanisms that drive resistance to small molecule inhibitors have been well characterized for specific therapeutics, such as imatinib and erlotinib, but remain only partly understood for many others.[101] In general, more than one cellular alteration contributes to drug resistance, complicating strategies to prevent or circumvent this issue.

Perhaps the most intensively investigated mechanism of drug resistance is that associated with imatinib treatment of BCR-ABL-positive CML.[102,103] For patients who take imatinib, the primary cause for relapse is the development of point mutations in the kinase domain of BCR-ABL that often prevent imatinib binding. Several have been identified in the ATP binding loop, activation loop, imatinib contact sites outside the loop and other locations. Additionally, some patients develop resistance through upregulation of *BCR-ABL* mRNA, resulting in protein overexpression that overwhelms the ability of imatinib to block function.[104] Lastly, elevated P-glycoprotein expression and enhanced multidrug efflux, as well as activation of other growth factor pathways, have been documented in some patients.

For patients with mutations in *EGFR* that respond to the EGFR inhibitor erlotinib, resistance to therapy is known to be mediated by three different mechanisms.[105] The first is the generation of a second mutation in the EGFR ATP binding pocket (T790M) that sterically hinders drug binding. The second involves amplification of the gene encoding MET, which upregulates MET protein expression, causing phosphorylation through heterodimerization with ERBB3 (another EGFR family member) that sustains PI3K/AKT signalling downstream, thus circumventing the inhibition of EGFR signalling by erlotinib. Lastly, overexpression of HGF, the ligand for MET, has been documented in some patients who received erlotinib, resulting in MET phosphorylation and PI3K/AKT signalling that is independent of ERBB3 binding.

Other mechanisms of resistance to kinase inhibitors that are not as well characterized include epigenetic changes secondary to alterations in histone acetylation/deacetylation and chromatin and histone methylation.[101] These changes act to modify the expression of genes that regulate responsiveness to kinase inhibitors, thus promoting escape from therapy. Taken together, these observations reinforce the notion that drug-resistant cell populations may be selected via multiple mechanisms, making prevention and treatment of this resistance challenging.

Summary

Progress in molecular biology has permitted a greater understanding of how dysregulation of signal transduction in cancer cells contributes to uncontrolled growth and survival. This has translated into an entirely new approach to cancer therapy through the use of small molecule inhibitors, many of which have demonstrated substantial single-agent activity in a variety of human cancers. The use of such agents is only beginning to be explored in veterinary oncology, and this process has been accelerated through the approval of both toceranib and masitinib. Nevertheless, significant challenges remain, including the determination of how these therapies can be combined effectively with chemotherapy and radiation therapy to provide optimal anticancer efficacy without enhancing toxicity, and the identification of strategies that are less likely to result in drug resistance.

References

1. Lemmon MA, Schlessinger J. Cell signaling by receptor tyrosine kinases. *Cell* 2010; 141: 1117–1134.
2. Madhusudan S, Ganesan TS. Tyrosine kinase inhibitors in cancer therapy. *Clin Biochem* 2004; 37: 618–635.
3. Zwick E, Bange J, Ullrich A. Receptor tyrosine kinases as targets for anticancer drugs. *Trends Mol Med* 2002; 8: 17–23.
4. Barreca A, Lasorsa E, Riera L *et al.* Anaplastic lymphoma kinase in human cancer. *J Mol Endocrinol* 2011; 47: R11–R23.
5. Fletcher JA. Role of KIT and platelet-derived growth factor receptors as oncoproteins. *Semin Oncol* 2004; 31: 4–11.
6. Laskin JJ, Sandler AB. Epidermal growth factor receptor: a promising target in solid tumours. *Cancer Treat Rev* 2004; 30: 1–17.
7. Ma PC, Jagadeeswaran R, Jagadeesh S *et al.* Functional expression and mutations of c-Met and its therapeutic inhibition with SU11274 and small interfering RNA in non-small cell lung cancer. *Cancer Res* 2005; 65: 1479–1488.
8. Ma PC, Maulik G, Christensen J *et al.* c-Met: structure, functions and potential for therapeutic inhibition. *Cancer Metastasis Rev* 2003; 22: 309–325.
9. Thurston G, Gale NW. Vascular endothelial growth factor and other signaling pathways in developmental and pathologic angiogenesis. *Int J Hematol* 2004; 80: 7–20.
10. Eskens FA. Angiogenesis inhibitors in clinical development; where are we now and where are we going? *Br J Cancer* 2004; 90: 1–7.
11. Cherrington JM, Strawn LM, Shawver LK. New paradigms for the treatment of cancer: the role of anti-angiogenesis agents. *Adv Cancer Res* 2000; 79: 1–38.
12. McCarty MF, Liu W, Fan F *et al.* Promises and pitfalls of anti-angiogenic therapy in clinical trials. *Trends Mol Med* 2003; 9: 53–58.
13. Thurston G. Role of angiopoietins and tie receptor tyrosine kinases in angiogenesis and lymphangiogenesis. *Cell Tissue Res* 2003; 314: 61–68.
14. Blume-Jensen P, Hunter T. Oncogenic kinase signalling. *Nature* 2001; 411: 355–365.
15. Johnson GL, Lapadat R. Mitogen-activated protein kinase pathways mediated by ERK, JNK, and p38 protein kinases. *Science* 2002; 298: 1911–1912.

16. Downward J. Targeting RAS signalling pathways in cancer therapy. *Nat Rev Cancer* 2003; 3: 11–22.
17. Davies H, Bignell GR, Cox C *et al.* Mutations of the *BRAF* gene in human cancer. *Nature* 2002; 417: 949–954.
18. Mercer KE, Pritchard CA. Raf proteins and cancer: B-Raf is identified as a mutational target. *Biochim Biophys Acta* 2003; 1653: 25–40.
19. Fresno Vara JA, Casado E, de Castro J *et al.* PI3K/Akt signalling pathway and cancer. *Cancer Treat Rev* 2004; 30: 193–204.
20. Franke TF, Hornik CP, Segev L *et al.* PI3K/Akt and apoptosis: size matters. *Oncogene* 2003; 22: 8983–8998.
21. Mitsiades CS, Mitsiades N, Koutsilieris M. The Akt pathway: molecular targets for anti-cancer drug development. *Curr Cancer Drug Targets* 2004; 4: 235–256.
22. Markman B, Atzori F, Pérez-García J *et al.* Status of PI3K inhibition and biomarker development in cancer therapeutics. *Ann Oncol* 2010; 21: 683–691.
23. Simpson L, Parsons R. PTEN: life as a tumor suppressor. *Exp Cell Res* 2001; 264: 29–41.
24. Weng LP, Smith WM, Dahia PL *et al.* PTEN suppresses breast cancer cell growth by phosphatase activity-dependent G1 arrest followed by cell death. *Cancer Res* 1999; 59: 5808–5814.
25. Kanae Y, Endoh D, Yokota H *et al.* Expression of the *PTEN* tumor suppressor gene in malignant mammary gland tumors of dogs. *Am J Vet Res* 2006; 67: 127–133.
26. Koenig A, Bianco SR, Fosmire S *et al.* Expression and significance of p53, rb, p21/*waf-1*, p16/*ink-4a*, and PTEN tumor suppressors in canine melanoma. *Vet Pathol* 2002; 39: 458–472.
27. Levine RA, Forest T, Smith C. Tumor suppressor PTEN is mutated in canine osteosarcoma cell lines and tumors. *Vet Pathol* 2002; 39: 372–378.
28. Swanton C. Cell-cycle targeted therapies. *Lancet Oncol* 2004; 5: 27–36.
29. Ortega S, Malumbres M, Barbacid M. Cyclin D-dependent kinases, INK4 inhibitors and cancer. *Biochim Biophys Acta* 2002; 1602: 73–87.
30. Malumbres M, Barbacid M. To cycle or not to cycle: a critical decision in cancer. *Nat Rev Cancer* 2001; 1: 222–231.
31. Brose MS, Volpe P, Feldman M *et al. BRAF* and *RAS* mutations in human lung cancer and melanoma. *Cancer Res* 2002; 62: 6997–7000.
32. Malumbres M, Barbacid M. *RAS* oncogenes: the first 30 years. *Nat Rev Cancer* 2003; 3: 459–465.
33. Wan PT, Garnett MJ, Roe SM *et al.* Mechanism of activation of the RAF-ERK signaling pathway by oncogenic mutations of B-RAF. *Cell* 2004; 116: 855–867.
34. Dhillon AS, Kolch W. Oncogenic B-Raf mutations: crystal clear at last. *Cancer Cell* 2004; 5: 303–304.
35. Galli SJ, Zsebo KM, Geissler EN. The kit ligand, stem cell factor. *Adv Immunol* 1994; 55: 1–95.
36. Downing S, Chien MB, Kass PH *et al.* Prevalence and importance of internal tandem duplications in exons 11 and 12 of c-kit in mast cell tumors of dogs. *Am J Vet Res* 2002; 63: 1718–1723.
37. London CA, Galli SJ, Yuuki T *et al.* Spontaneous canine mast cell tumors express tandem duplications in the proto-oncogene c-*kit*. *Exp Hematol* 1999; 27: 689–697.
38. Zemke D, Yamini B, Yuzbasiyan-Gurkan V. Mutations in the juxtamembrane domain of c-*KIT* are associated with higher grade mast cell tumors in dogs. *Vet Pathol* 2002; 39: 529–535.
39. Demetri GD. Targeting the molecular pathophysiology of gastrointestinal stromal tumors with imatinib. Mechanisms, successes, and challenges to rational drug development. *Hematol Oncol Clin North Am* 2002; 16: 1115–1124.
40. Demetri GD. Differential properties of current tyrosine kinase inhibitors in gastrointestinal stromal tumors. *Semin Oncol* 2011; 38(Suppl 1): S10–S19.
41. Frost D, Lasota J, Miettinen M. Gastrointestinal stromal tumors and leiomyomas in the dog: a histopathologic, immunohistochemical, and molecular genetic study of 50 cases. *Vet Pathol* 2003; 40: 42–54.
42. Kondo M, Horibe K, Takahashi Y *et al.* Prognostic value of internal tandem duplication of the FLT3 gene in childhood acute myelogenous leukemia. *Med Pediatr Oncol* 1999; 33: 525–529.
43. Nakoa M, Yokota S, Iwai T *et al.* Internal tandem duplication of the flt3 gene found in acute myeloid leukemia. *Leukemia* 1996; 10: 1911–1918.
44. Yokota S, Kiyoi H, Nakao M *et al.* Internal tandem duplication of the FLT3 gene is preferentially seen in acute myeloid leukemia and myelodysplastic syndrome among various hematological malignancies. A study on a large series of patients and cell lines. *Leukemia* 1997; 11: 1605–1609.
45. Iwai T, Yokota S, Nakao M *et al.* Internal tandem duplication of the FLT3 gene and clinical evaluation in childhood acute myeloid leukemia. The Children's Cancer and Leukemia Study Group, Japan. *Leukemia* 1999; 13: 38–43.
46. Pao W, Chmielecki J. Rational, biologically based treatment of *EGFR*-mutant non-small-cell lung cancer. *Nat Rev Cancer* 2010; 10: 760–774.
47. Wen J, Fu J, Zhang W *et al.* Genetic and epigenetic changes in lung carcinoma and their clinical implications. *Mod Pathol* 2011; 24: 932–943.
48. Paik S, Hazan R, Fisher ER *et al.* Pathologic findings from the National Surgical Adjuvant Breast and Bowel Project: prognostic significance of erbB-2 protein overexpression in primary breast cancer. *J Clin Oncol* 1990; 8: 103–112.
49. Slamon DJ, Clark GM, Wong SG *et al.* Human breast cancer: correlation of relapse and survival with amplification of the HER-2/neu oncogene. *Science* 1987; 235: 177–182.
50. Melo JV, Hughes TP, Apperley JF. Chronic myeloid leukemia. *Hematology Am Soc Hematol Educ Program* 2003; 132–152.
51. Van Etten RA. Mechanisms of transformation by the *BCR-ABL* oncogene: new perspectives in the post-imatinib era. *Leuk Res* 2004; 28(Suppl 1): S21–S28.
52. Medves S, Demoulin JB. Tyrosine kinase gene fusions in cancer: translating mechanisms into targeted therapies. *J Cell Mol Med* 2012; 16: 237–248.
53. Sciacca L, Costantino A, Pandini G *et al.* Insulin receptor activation by IGF-II in breast cancers: evidence for a new autocrine/paracrine mechanism. *Oncogene* 1999; 18: 2471–2479.
54. Ekstrand AJ, James CD, Cavenee WK *et al.* Genes for epidermal growth factor receptor, transforming growth factor α, and epidermal growth factor and their expression in human gliomas *in vivo*. *Cancer Res* 1991; 51: 2164–2172.
55. Graeven U, Fiedler W, Karpinski S *et al.* Melanoma-associated expression of vascular endothelial growth factor and its receptors FLT-1 and KDR. *J Cancer Res Clin Oncol* 1999; 125: 621–629.
56. Fosmire SP, Dickerson EB, Scott AM *et al.* Canine malignant hemangiosarcoma as a model of primitive angiogenic endothelium. *Lab Invest* 2004; 84: 562–572.
57. MacEwen EG, Kutzke J, Carew J *et al.* c-Met tyrosine kinase receptor expression and function in human and canine osteosarcoma cells. *Clin Exp Metastasis* 2003; 20: 421–430.
58. Ferracini R, Angelini P, Cagliero E *et al.* MET oncogene aberrant expression in canine osteosarcoma. *J Orthop Res* 2000; 18: 253–256.
59. Harris M. Monoclonal antibodies as therapeutic agents for cancer. *Lancet Oncol* 2004; 5: 292–302.
60. Vogel CL, Cobleigh MA, Tripathy D *et al.* First-line Herceptin monotherapy in metastatic breast cancer. *Oncology* 2001; 61(Suppl 2): 37–42.
61. Slamon DJ, Leyland-Jones B, Shak S *et al.* Use of chemotherapy plus a monoclonal antibody against HER2 for metastatic breast cancer that overexpresses HER2. *N Engl J Med* 2001; 344: 783–792.
62. Arteaga CL, Sliwkowski MX, Osborne CK *et al.* Treatment of HER2-positive breast cancer: current status and future perspectives. *Nat Rev Clin Oncol* 2012; 9: 16–32.
63. Mukai H. Treatment strategy for HER2-positive breast cancer. *Int J Clin Oncol* 2010; 15: 335–340.

64. Cabanillas F. Front-line management of diffuse large B cell lymphoma. *Curr Opin Oncol* 2010; 22: 642–645.
65. Vidal L, Gafter-Gvili A, Salles G *et al.* Rituximab maintenance for the treatment of patients with follicular lymphoma: an updated systematic review and meta-analysis of randomized trials. *J Natl Cancer Inst* 2011; 103: 1799–1806.
66. Brand TM, Iida M, Wheeler DL. Molecular mechanisms of resistance to the EGFR monoclonal antibody cetuximab. *Cancer Biol Ther* 2011; 11: 777–792.
67. Zhang J, Yang PL, Gray NS. Targeting cancer with small molecule kinase inhibitors. *Nat Rev Cancer* 2009; 9: 28–39.
68. de Kogel CE, Schellens JH. Imatinib. *Oncologist* 2007; 12: 1390–1394.
69. Mauro MJ, Druker BJ. STI571: targeting BCR-ABL as therapy for CML. *Oncologist* 2001; 6: 233–238.
70. Kantarjian H, Sawyers C, Hochhaus A *et al.* Hematologic and cytogenetic responses to imatinib mesylate in chronic myelogenous leukemia. *N Engl J Med* 2002; 346: 645–652.
71. Beham-Schmid C, Apfelbeck U, Sill H *et al.* Treatment of chronic myelogenous leukemia with the tyrosine kinase inhibitor STI571 results in marked regression of bone marrow fibrosis. *Blood* 2002; 99: 381–383.
72. Druker BJ, Talpaz M, Resta DJ *et al.* Efficacy and safety of a specific inhibitor of the BCR-ABL tyrosine kinase in chronic myeloid leukemia. *N Engl J Med* 2001; 344: 1031–1037.
73. Druker BJ, Sawyers CL, Kantarjian H *et al.* Activity of a specific inhibitor of the BCR-ABL tyrosine kinase in the blast crisis of chronic myeloid leukemia and acute lymphoblastic leukemia with the Philadelphia chromosome. *N Engl J Med* 2001; 344: 1038–1042.
74. Sawyers CL. Rational therapeutic intervention in cancer: kinases as drug targets. *Curr Opin Genet Dev* 2002; 12: 111–115.
75. Weisberg E, Griffin JD. Resistance to imatinib (Glivec): update on clinical mechanisms. *Drug Resist Updat* 2003; 6: 231–238.
76. Nardi V, Azam M, Daley GQ. Mechanisms and implications of imatinib resistance mutations in BCR-ABL. *Curr Opin Hematol* 2004; 11: 35–43.
77. Duffaud F, Blay JY. Gastrointestinal stromal tumors: biology and treatment. *Oncology* 2003; 65: 187–197.
78. Heinrich MC, Rubin BP, Longley BJ *et al.* Biology and genetic aspects of gastrointestinal stromal tumors: KIT activation and cytogenetic alterations. *Hum Pathol* 2002; 33: 484–495.
79. Miettinen M, Sarlomo-Rikala M, Lasota J. Gastrointestinal stromal tumors: recent advances in understanding of their biology. *Hum Pathol* 1999; 30: 1213–1220.
80. Miettinen M, Sarlomo-Rikala M, Lasota J. Gastrointestinal stromal tumours. *Ann Chir Gynaecol* 1998; 87: 278–281.
81. Peled N, Yoshida K, Wynes MW *et al.* Predictive and prognostic markers for epidermal growth factor receptor inhibitor therapy in non-small cell lung cancer. *Ther Adv Med Oncol* 2009; 1: 137–144.
82. Bang YJ. The potential for crizotinib in non-small cell lung cancer: a perspective review. *Ther Adv Med Oncol* 2011; 3: 279–291.
83. Shaw AT, Yeap BY, Solomon BJ *et al.* Effect of crizotinib on overall survival in patients with advanced non-small-cell lung cancer harbouring *ALK* gene rearrangement: a retrospective analysis. *Lancet Oncol* 2011; 12: 1004–1012.
84. Chapman PB, Hauschild A, Robert C *et al.* Improved survival with vemurafenib in melanoma with BRAF V600E mutation. *N Engl J Med* 2011; 364: 2507–2516.
85. Markman B, Dienstmann R, Tabernero J. Targeting the PI3K/Akt/mTOR pathway – beyond rapalogs. *Oncotarget* 2010; 1: 530–543.
86. Vilar E, Perez-Garcia J, Tabernero J. Pushing the envelope in the mTOR pathway: the second generation of inhibitors. *Mol Cancer Ther* 2011; 10: 395–403.
87. Papaetis GS, Syrigos KN. Sunitinib: a multitargeted receptor tyrosine kinase inhibitor in the era of molecular cancer therapies. *BioDrugs* 2009; 23: 377–389.
88. London CA, Hannah AL, Zadovoskaya R *et al.* Phase I dose-escalating study of SU11654, a small molecule receptor tyrosine kinase inhibitor, in dogs with spontaneous malignancies. *Clin Cancer Res* 2003; 9: 2755–2768.
89. London CA, Malpas PB, Wood-Follis SL *et al.* Multi-center, placebo-controlled, double-blind, randomized study of oral toceranib phosphate (SU11654), a receptor tyrosine kinase inhibitor, for the treatment of dogs with recurrent (either local or distant) mast cell tumor following surgical excision. *Clin Cancer Res* 2009; 15: 3856–3865.
90. London C, Mathie T, Stingle N *et al.* Preliminary evidence for biologic activity of toceranib phosphate (Palladia®) in solid tumours(*). *Vet Comp Oncol* 2012; 10: 194–205.
91. Chon E, McCartan L, Kubicek LN *et al.* Safety evaluation of combination toceranib phosphate (Palladia®) and piroxicam in tumour-bearing dogs (excluding mast cell tumours): a phase I dose-finding study(*). *Vet Comp Oncol* 2012; 10: 184–193.
92. Robat C, London C, Bunting L *et al.* Safety evaluation of combination vinblastine and toceranib phosphate (Palladia®) in dogs: a phase I dose-finding study(*). *Vet Comp Oncol* 2012; 10: 174–183.
93. Carlsten KS, London CA, Haney S *et al.* Multicenter prospective trial of hypofractionated radiation treatment, toceranib, and prednisone for measurable canine mast cell tumors. *J Vet Intern Med* 2012; 26: 135–141.
94. Hahn KA, Ogilvie G, Rusk T *et al.* Masitinib is safe and effective for the treatment of canine mast cell tumors. *J Vet Intern Med* 2008; 22: 1301–1309.
95. Hahn KA, Legendre AM, Shaw NG *et al.* Evaluation of 12- and 24-month survival rates after treatment with masitinib in dogs with nonresectable mast cell tumors. *Am J Vet Res* 2010; 71: 1354–1361.
96. Isotani M, Ishida N, Tominaga M *et al.* Effect of tyrosine kinase inhibition by imatinib mesylate on mast cell tumors in dogs. *J Vet Intern Med* 2008; 4: 985–988.
97. Marconato L, Bettini G, Giacoboni C *et al.* Clinicopathological features and outcome for dogs with mast cell tumors and bone marrow involvement. *J Vet Intern Med* 2008; 4: 1001–1007.
98. Yamada O, Kobayashi M, Sugisaki O *et al.* Imatinib elicited a favorable response in a dog with a mast cell tumor carrying a *c-kit* c.1523A>T mutation via suppression of constitutive KIT activation. *Vet Immunol Immunopathol* 2011; 142: 101–106.
99. Isotani M, Tamura K, Yagihara H *et al.* Identification of a *c-kit* exon 8 internal tandem duplication in a feline mast cell tumor case and its favorable response to the tyrosine kinase inhibitor imatinib mesylate. *Vet Immunol Immunopathol* 2006; 114: 168–172.
100. Isotani M, Yamada O, Lachowicz JL *et al.* Mutations in the fifth immunoglobulin-like domain of kit are common and potentially sensitive to imatinib mesylate in feline mast cell tumours. *Br J Haematol* 2009; 148: 144–153.
101. Rosenzweig SA. Acquired resistance to drugs targeting receptor tyrosine kinases. *Biochem Pharmacol* 2012; 83: 1041–1048.
102. O'Hare T, Eide CA, Deininger MW. Bcr-Abl kinase domain mutations, drug resistance, and the road to a cure for chronic myeloid leukemia. *Blood* 2007; 110: 2242–2249.
103. O'Hare T, Eide CA, Deininger MW. Bcr-Abl kinase domain mutations and the unsettled problem of Bcr-AblT315I: looking into the future of controlling drug resistance in chronic myeloid leukemia. *Clin Lymphoma Myeloma* 2007; 7(Suppl 3): S120–S130.
104. Mahon FX, Deininger MW, Schultheis B *et al.* Selection and characterization of BCR-ABL positive cell lines with differential sensitivity to the tyrosine kinase inhibitor STI571: diverse mechanisms of resistance. *Blood* 2000; 96: 1070–1079.
105. Kosaka T, Yamaki E, Mogi A *et al.* Mechanisms of resistance to EGFR TKIs and development of a new generation of drugs in non-small-cell lung cancer. *J Biomed Biotechnol* 2011; 2011: 165214.

To cite this article, please use DOI: 10.1111/j.1365-3164.2012.01101.x

6.3

The contribution of stem cells to epidermal and hair follicle tumours in the dog

Chiara Brachelente*, Ilaria Porcellato*, Monica Sforna*, Elvio Lepri*, Luca Mechelli* and Laura Bongiovanni†

*Department of Biopathological Sciences and Hygiene of Animal and Alimentary Productions, Faculty of Veterinary Medicine, University of Perugia, Perugia, Italy

† Department of Comparative Biomedical Sciences, Faculty of Veterinary Medicine, University of Teramo, Teramo, Italy

Correspondence: Chiara Brachelente, Department of Biopathological Sciences and Hygiene of Animal and Alimentary Productions, Faculty of Veterinary Medicine, University of Perugia, Via San Costanzo, 4 – 06126 Perugia, Italy. E-mail:chiara.brachelente@unipg.it

Background – Although cutaneous stem cells have been implicated in skin tumourigenesis in humans, no studies have been conducted to elucidate the presence and the possible role of stem cells in hair follicle tumours in the dog.

Hypothesis – Stem cell markers are expressed in canine epidermal and follicular tumours and can be used to better understand the biology and origin of these tumours.

Animals and Methods – In the present study, normal skin sections and 44 follicular tumours were retrospectively investigated for the immunohistochemical expression of keratin 15 (K15) and nestin. In addition, 30 squamous cell carcinomas were evaluated for K15 expression.

Results – In normal skin, K15 and nestin were expressed in the outer root sheath cells of the isthmic portion of the hair follicle (bulge region), and K15 expression was also scattered in the basal cell layer of the epidermis. Infundibular keratinizing acanthomas, pilomatricomas and squamous cell carcinomas were mostly negative for K15, trichoblastomas were moderately to strongly positive, tricholemmomas were either negative or strongly positive, and trichoepitheliomas had heterogeneous staining. Nestin expression was generally faint in all follicular tumours.

Conclusions and clinical importance – Our results show that K15 can be a reliable marker for investigating the role of stem cells in hair follicle tumours of the dog, while nestin was judged to be a nonoptimal marker. Furthermore, our study suggests that hair follicle stem cells are present in the bulge region of hair follicles and could possibly play a role in tumourigenesis of canine tumours originating from this portion of the follicle, namely trichoblastomas, tricholemmomas and trichoepitheliomas. The loss of K15 expression in squamous cell carcinomas compared with normal skin suggests that this event could be important in the malignant transformation.

Introduction

During the last 30 years, stem cells have been the subject of many studies aimed at defining their location, biological activity and functions. A detailed explanation of the functions and biology of stem cells is beyond the scope of this paper; interested readers are referred to reviews in this area.[1–6] In human skin, adult stem cells are located in the hair follicle bulge, in the interfollicular areas of the surface epidermis and in the sebaceous glands.[1] As with other somatic stem cells, epidermal stem cells express well-defined markers,[7,8] and several studies have demonstrated the differential expression of stem cell markers in human hair follicles and interfollicular epidermis.[9–11] In dogs, CD34, nestin and keratin 15 (K15) have been found to be useful hair follicle stem cell markers.[12–15] In addition to studying the role of cancer stem cells in the development of tumours, the differential expression of stem cell markers has been used as a tool to classify or reclassify several neoplasias. Using morphology alone, it is often difficult to determine the cell of origin of skin tumours.[16,17] The more commonly used stem cell markers for these studies are CD34, K15 and nestin, which have been demonstrated in normal canine hair follicles.[12–15]

The goals of this study were as follows: (i) to investigate the expression of stem cell markers in canine epidermal and hair follicle tumours; and (ii) to clarify the origin of follicular tumours in the dog according to tumour immunophenotype.

Accepted 7 July 2012

Sources of Funding: This study was self-funded.

Conflict of Interest: No conflicts of interest have been declared.

Materials and methods

Tumour samples

Thirty cutaneous squamous cell carcinomas (SCCs) and 44 follicular tumours were selected from the archives of the Department of Biopathological Sciences and Hygiene of Animal and Alimentary Productions, Perugia and from the archives of the Department of Comparative Biomedical Sciences, Teramo. For the follicular tumours, four cases of tricholemmomas (TLs) and 10 cases each of infundibular keratinizing acanthomas (IKAs), trichoblastomas (TBs), pilomatricomas (PMs) and trichoepitheliomas (TEs) were used.

Histological examination

All specimens were routinely fixed in 10% neutral buffered formalin, paraffin embedded, and cut into 4- to 5-μm-thick sections. The slides were stained with haematoxylin and eosin (H&E) and examined by light microscopy.

Immunohistochemical examination

Immunohistochemistry was performed using a commercially available mouse monoclonal antibody against K15 (1:75 dilution; Keratin15 Ab-1, clone LHK15; Thermoscientific, Fremont, CA, USA) and a rabbit polyclonal antibody against nestin (1:500 dilution; ab7659; Abcam, Cambridge, UK). Formalin-fixed and paraffin-embedded tissue sections were deparaffinized, rehydrated, and washed in distilled water. Antigen retrieval was performed by microwave treatment for 20 min at the highest power in a preheated Tris–EDTA buffer solution (10 mmol/L Tris base and 1 mmol/L EDTA, pH 9.0) for the K15 antibody and in sodium citrate buffer (10 mmol/L sodium citrate, pH 6.0) for the nestin antibody. Endogenous peroxidase was blocked using 3% H_2O_2 for 5 min at room temperature. Slides were then washed for 10 min in TBS (Tris–phosphate-buffered saline) and incubated with primary antibodies for 1 h in a humidified chamber at room temperature. After incubation, slides were washed in TBS for 10 min and incubated with secondary biotinylated anti-rabbit, anti-mouse and anti-goat immunoglobulins in phosphate-buffered saline followed by sequential incubation with peroxidase-labelled streptavidin (LSAB+/System-HRP; Dakocytomation, Glostrup, Denmark). 3-Amino-9ethylcarbazole was used as the chromogen (AEC + Substrate-Chromogen Ready-to-use; Dakocytomation) and Carazzi's haematoxylin as the counterstain. Coverslips were mounted with Faramount Mounting Medium (Dakocytomation). Negative controls were treated in the same manner, omitting the primary antibody and incubating tissue sections with TBS.

In a preliminary phase of our experimental setting, we tested the bulge-specific expression of CD34 (biotinylated mouse anti-canine CD34; BD Biosciences, San Diego, CA, USA) in canine hair follicles, as previously described.[13] However, no reaction was observed in any of the control and tumour samples, for any dilution or antigen retrieval method used.

The expression of the K15 and nestin was evaluated by determining cytoplasmic reactivity. Any nuclear staining was considered a background artifact. The percentage of immunopositive neoplastic cells in the tumour mass showing cytoplasmic expression of K15 or nestin was semiquantitatively evaluated and scored as negative (score 0; <5% of positive tumour cells), mild (score 1; 6–25% of positive tumour cells), moderate (score 2; 26–50% of positive tumour cells) or high (score 3; >50% of positive tumour cells). The intensity of the reaction was also evaluated as absent (0), weak (1), moderate (2) or strong (3). For each tumour, the location of positive cells was also recorded (i.e. central lobules versus peripheral part of the tumour lobules; basal versus differentiated cells).

Data analysis

Data were analysed using descriptive statistics.

Results

Tumour samples and histopathological examination

Tumours were classified independently by two pathologists (C.B. and L.B.) according to Gross *et al.*[18] When applicable, tumours were subclassified into the subtypes recognized by the current classification.[18] When a discrepancy emerged in the assessment/reassessment of tumours, the two pathologists reviewed the cases and came to a final agreement. Of the follicular tumours, five cases were malignant (three trichoepitheliomas and two pilomatricomas). The remaining tumours were benign. The desmoplastic reaction, the degree of invasiveness into the surrounding tissue, the presence of ulceration and the degree of inflammatory reaction were recorded as additional features. See Table S1 for the signalment, location and stem cell marker results for individual tumours.

Immunohistochemical examination

Expression of K15 and nestin in normal epidermis and hair follicle.

Figure 1 shows K15 and nestin expression in the normal canine skin. Keratin 15 was detected in the cytoplasm of cells of the external root sheath of the hair follicle, in the isthmic region close to the insertion of the arrector pili muscle and multifocally in the basal layer of the epidermis of control dogs and in normal skin adjacent to tumours. Nestin expression was less pronounced, more diffuse, and confined to the middle portion of the hair follicle.

Expression of K15 and nestin in hair follicular tumours.

Figure 2 summarizes the suggested origin of follicular tumours from the different portions of the hair follicle, according to the differential expression of stem cell markers based on the findings of this study. Many follicular tumours showed areas of positive staining, and the immunolabelling score of K15 and nestin in neoplastic cells of follicular tumours is summarized in Figure 3. When present, the intensity of staining was generally higher in the peripheral cells of tumour nests and lobules.

Amongst infundibular keratinizing acanthomas, 90% of tumours were negative or mildly positive and only one of 10 tumours showed a high K15 expression score. All tumours were negative for nestin.

Trichoblastomas showed the highest percentage of K15-positive cells in comparison to all other tumour types examined, with 80% of tumours having moderate to high staining scores. In trabecular trichoblastomas, the reactivity was more prominent in the centre of tumour lobules and in small nests of cells compared with large lobular aggregates of cells, whereas in ribbon-type trichoblastomas the staining was more intense in the peripheral cells of tumour lobules and within the thin ribbons of neoplastic cells. Nestin was less pronounced, with six trichoblastomas showing less than 25% of positive cells and four between 26 and 50% of positive cells (Figure 4).

Trichoepitheliomas had a variable K15 expression (Figure 5). Two tumours were negative, three tumours showed mild positivity, three tumours were moderately positive and two had high K15 staining. When present, the strongest intensity was noted in paucicellular (up to about 30 cells) nests and lobules of the tumour. Areas with squamous differentiation were positive only in the peripheral cell layer, whereas the more differentiated cells towards the centre of lobules were negative. Of the three cases of malignant trichoepitheliomas in this study, two were mildly positive, while one showed a strong reactivity. Nestin was evident in a small percentage of tumour cells in two cases and in up to 50% of neoplastic

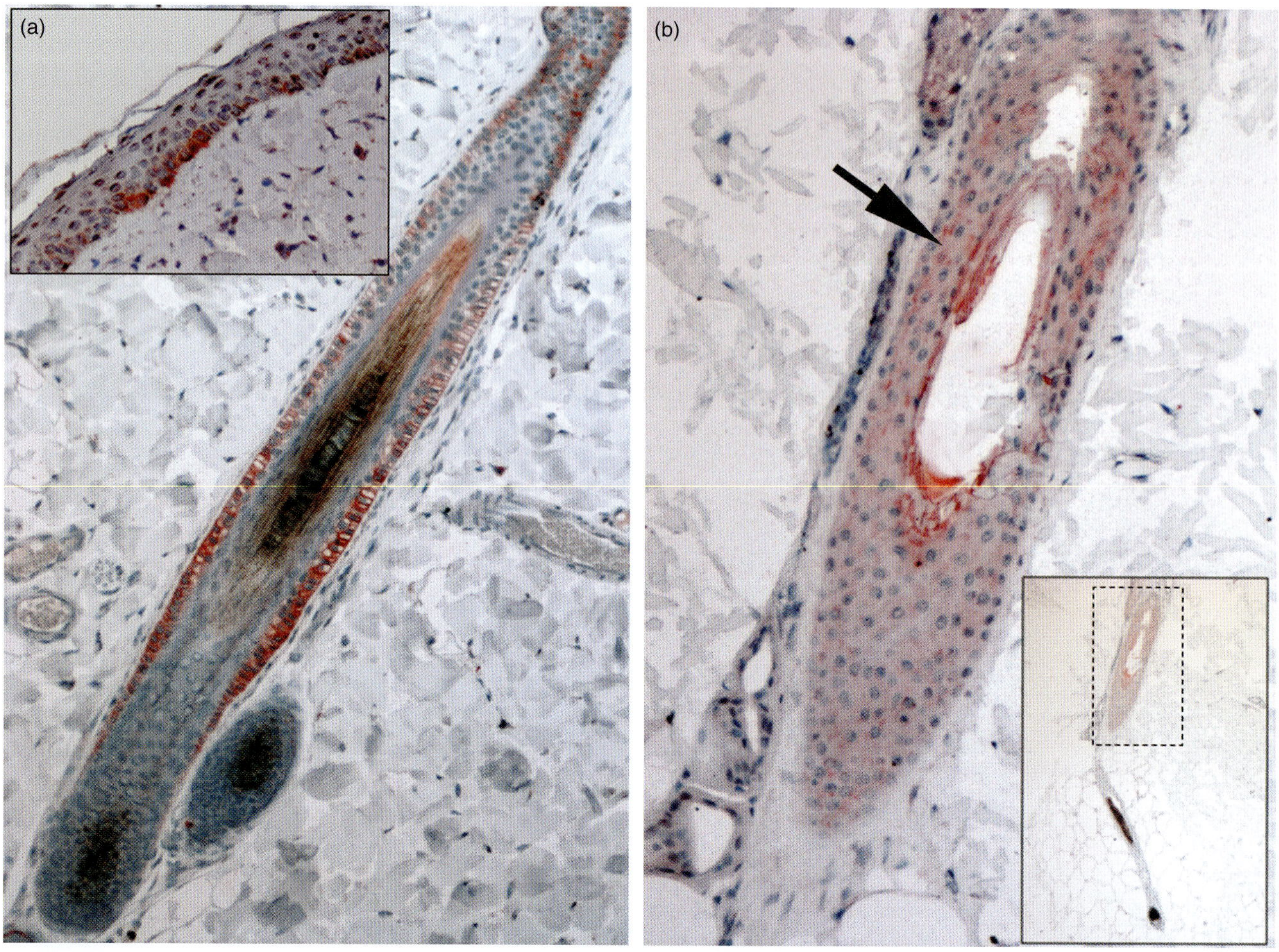

Figure 1. Expression of keratin 15 (K15) and nestin in normal skin. (a) Cytoplasmic labelling of K15 by immunohistochemistry in normal adult canine hair follicles is localized in the external root sheath cells of the isthmic region. Inset shows multifocal positive K15 staining in the basal layer of the epidermis. (b) Diffuse and mild cytoplasmic labelling of nestin by immunohistochemistry in normal adult canine hair follicle in the middle portion (isthmic region) of the hair follicle. Inset shows immunohistochemistry for nestin, illustrating the localization of the positive segment in the hair follicle.

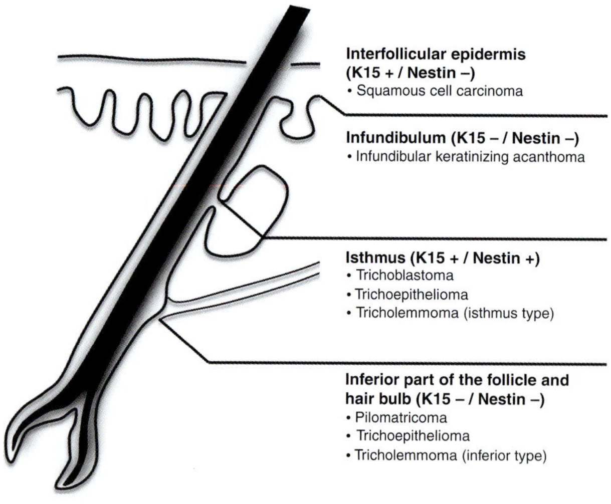

Figure 2. Suggested origin of follicular tumours from the different portions of the hair follicle, according to the differential expression of stem cell markers.

cells in two other cases, whereas the remaining six tumours were negative.

For tricholemmomas, two tumours scored negative and two strongly positive (score 3) for K15, and one tumour scored negative, one moderately positive and two strongly positive for nestin expression (Figure 6).

Of the pilomatricomas, only one tumour was moderately positive for K15, and the remaining nine were negative or mildly positive (including benign and malignant tumours). Nestin was negative in all pilomatricomas tested.

The analysis of the staining intensity of each marker did not reveal remarkable difference between the different types of tumours considered or between the different areas of tumour (i.e. peripheral versus central areas of the tumour mass).

Expression of K15 in squamous cell carcinomas.
Many SCCs (26 of 30; 87%) were negative for K15 or showed only a mild positivity; one tumour was moderately positive, while three cases were strongly positive.

For any of the follicular tumours and squamous cell carcinomas examined, K15/nestin expression or staining intensity of neoplastic cells was not influenced by the presence of additional features, such as tumour subtype, desmoplastic reaction, degree of invasiveness into the surrounding tissue, presence of ulceration, and inflammatory reaction around the tumour mass.

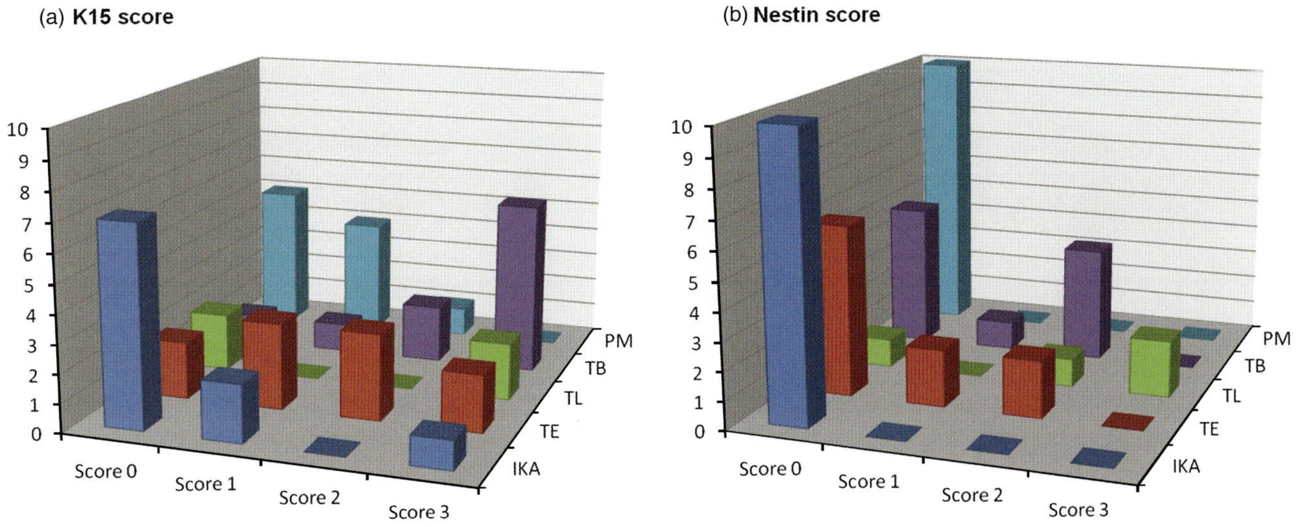

Figure 3. Keratin 15 and nestin expression in hair follicle tumours. Number of cases (*y*-axes) of follicular tumours showing different immunolabelling score classes (0 to 3, based on the percentage of positive cells, x-axes) for K15 (a) and nestin (b). Abbreviations: IKA, infundibular keratinizing acanthoma; PM, pilomatricoma; TB, trichoblastoma; TE, trichoepithelioma; and TL, tricholemmoma.

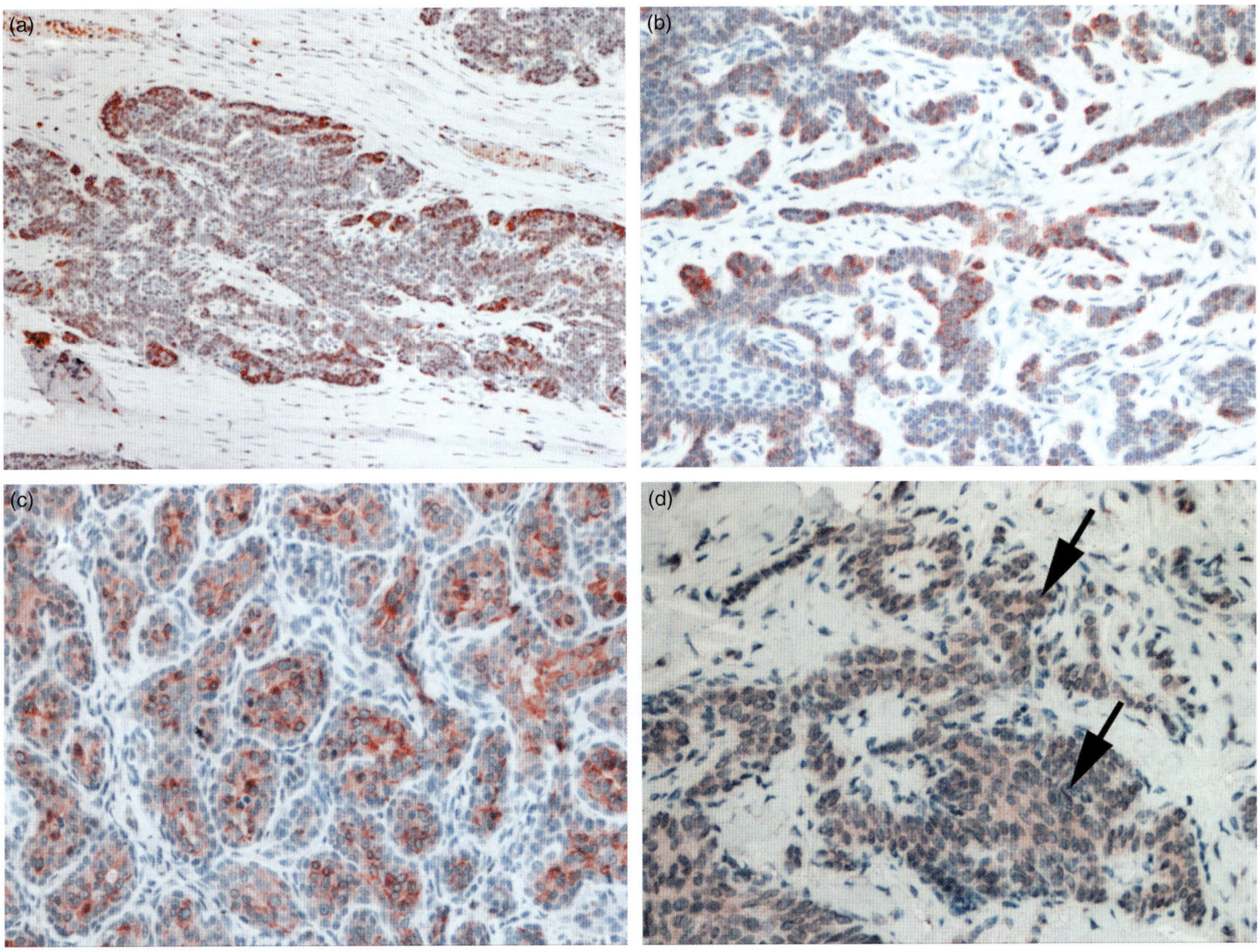

Figure 4. Expression of stem cell markers in trichoblastomas. (a and b) Ribbon trichoblastoma, showing K15 immunoreactivity located in the peripheral cells of growing neoplastic cords and ribbons. Immunohistochemistry for K15, at low (a) and higher power (b). (c) Trabecular trichoblastoma, showing K15 immunoreactivity located in the centre of the lobules and in the small nests of cells. (d) Trabecular trichoblastoma, showing neoplastic lobules with diffuse and mild nestin immunoreactivity (arrows).

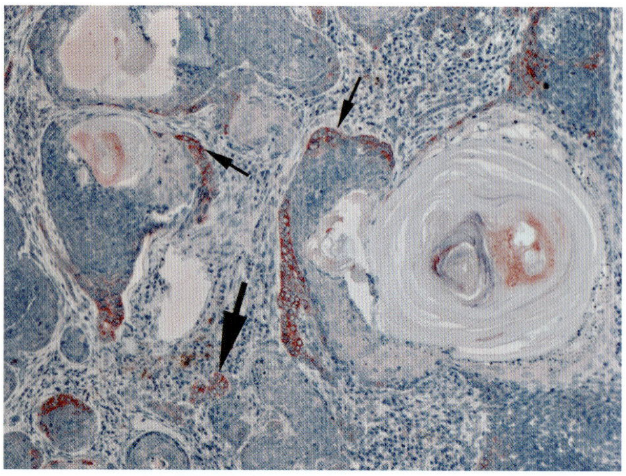

Figure 5. Expression of K15 in trichoepithelioma assessed by immunohistochemistry. K15 immunoreactivity is evident in cells of small tumour nests or lobules (large arrow). Areas with squamous differentiation show a cytoplasmic labelling only in the peripheral cell layer (small arrows).

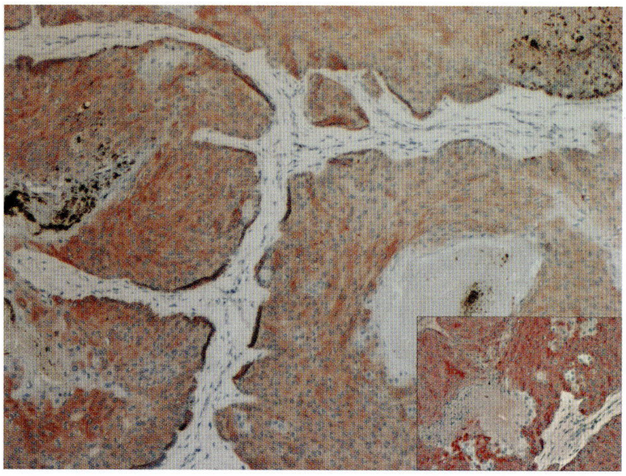

Figure 6. Expression of nestin in tricholemmoma assessed by immunohistochemistry. Nestin labelling is diffuse and involves almost all cells of the tumour, with areas of strong intensity (inset shows higher magnification).

Discussion

Other investigators have confirmed the presence of stem cells in canine hair follicles using the selective stem cell markers CD34, K15 and nestin.[12–15] After testing CD34 with inadequate results, we focused on K15 and nestin. K15 is recognized as a stem cell marker of the bulge region of the human and mouse hair follicle.[19,20] K15-positive cells have features of stem cells, such as being slowly cycling, self renewing and multipotent.[21] K15 expression is not restricted to the bulge region, but also involves cells of the outer root sheath of the isthmus region and is found multifocally scattered in the basal cell layer of the epidermis.[21] Nestin was originally identified as a marker for neuronal progenitor cells in the brain, but was subsequently found in the follicular bulge cells and in perifollicular spindle cells of the connective tissue sheath, where it seems to identify the mesenchymal stem cell component of the folliculo-sebaceous apocrine unit.[17] No nestin expression has been found in interfollicular epidermis.

In this study, K15 was used as a marker for epidermal and hair follicle stem cells and nestin as a marker for hair follicle stem cells. In agreement with the study of Kobayashi *et al.*,[15] our results demonstrated that in normal skin, K15 was expressed in the cytoplasm of cells of the basal layer of the epidermis and of the external root sheath in the isthmic region. Nestin expression was less pronounced and confined to the middle portion of the hair follicle. From the data obtained in the present study, K15 seems to be a better marker than nestin to study the expression of hair follicle stem cells in follicular tumours. The heterogeneity of K15 and nestin expression in the different tumours examined could be explained in several ways, as follows: (i) origin from different stem-cell-positive portions of the hair follicle; (ii) stem cell heterogeneity, a feature that has been demonstrated in hair follicle stem cells;[19] and/or (iii) loss of bulge-related marker expression during tumour progression.

Most cases of infundibular keratinizing acanthoma, in our study, did not show immunoreactivity for K15 and nestin, thereby confirming that the origin of these tumours is associated with the infundibular portion of normal hair follicles. The only positive case had a multifocal invasive growth pattern, which suggested squamous cell carcinoma as a differential diagnosis in the reassessment of the case for the purposes of this study. No data are available regarding the expression of K15 in skin tumours of the dog, but a comparison with a study on human keratoacanthomas (sharing histological features with infundibular keratinizing acanthomas of dogs) can be made, showing similar results.[22]

Trichoblastoma was the tumour class with the highest score of positive cells for K15. In humans, immunohistochemical studies have demonstrated the origin of trichoblastomas from follicular stem cells.[22–25] Our results seem to confirm the same origin in the dog, supporting the classification of these tumours among hair follicle tumours.[18] The peculiar distribution of positive cells in the different histotypes may suggest a role of stem cells in the propagation of the tumour (centrifugally in trabecular trichoblastomas and along ribbons in ribbon-type trichoblastomas), but further studies are needed to confirm this.

Trichoepitheliomas had the most heterogeneous expression of both nestin and K15. In general, areas with deep follicular differentiation were commonly positive, whereas in areas of squamous differentiation, only basal cells of the neoplastic lobules expressed K15. In the study of Jih *et al.*,[22] all trichoepitheliomas examined were positive, with a pattern of reaction that was in agreement with the results of our study. The heterogeneity in K15 staining of different portions of the tumour may be related to the origin of these tumours from all portions of follicular epithelium.[18] The mild immunoreactivity of the two malignant tumours studied in our series could be explained by the loss of expression of specific surface markers, typical of undifferentiated cells, although a higher number of malignant trichoepitheliomas should be assessed.

Tricholemmoma was the only group in which the highest nestin score was noted, in accordance with studies on human tricholemmomas.[26] Human tricholemmomas arise from the follicular infundibulum, although they differentiate towards the outer root sheath,[27] as confirmed by their origin from the nestin-positive/K15-positive outer root sheath cells from the middle portion of the hair follicle.[26] In the veterinary literature, two types of tricholemmomas are recognized (bulb type and isthmic type), originating from the outer root sheath cells of the hair bulb or of the isthmic segment of the hair follicle, respectively.[18] According to some morphological features and expression of stem cell markers, based upon the findings of the present study, this group of tumours may be more correctly classified as isthmic type tricholemmomas. However, no distinction is made in the human literature between the different subtypes of tricholemmomas, and we wonder whether the subclassification used in veterinary literature reflects a real biological difference.

The majority of pilomatricoma cases did not express K15 and nestin or expressed these markers in a low percentage of cells, confirming the origin of these tumours from bulb germ cells,[18] which are indeed negative for the stem cell markers used in this study.

Regarding the epidermal tumours, data obtained in SCC cases in the present study are similar to what is published in the human literature, where a progressive loss of K15 expression in infiltrative SCCs compared with *in situ* carcinomas and actinic keratosis has been described, suggesting that it may play a role in the malignant transformation of keratinocytes.[28] Unfortunately, the present study analysed only SCCs, and a comparison with proliferative, preneoplastic and neoplastic, non-invasive lesions should be performed in order to investigate this.

The results of this study progress our understanding of the biology and origin of epidermal and follicular tumours of the dog. At a later stage, the evaluation of the expression of stem cells markers could be correlated with the clinical features of epidermal and follicular tumours in order to evaluate the role of epidermal/follicular stem cells in skin carcinogenesis in the dog.

The present study is therefore considered to provide important insight, and the conclusions are summarized as follows: (i) some canine follicular tumours (trichoblastomas, trichoepitheliomas and tricholemmomas) show an expression of hair follicle stem cell markers; (ii) although further studies are needed, it could be suggested that these positive cells, having some features of stem cells, may play a role in tumour development; (iii) the follicular tumours staining negative for stem cells markers (infundibular keratinizing acanthomas and pilomatricomas) originate from portions of the hair follicle away from the bulge and are not expected to express bulge stem cell markers; (iv) no histological features, such as associated inflammation, malignant phenotype or tumour subtype, correlated with stem cell marker expression; and (v) the loss of K15 expression in SCCs compared with normal skin suggests that this event could play a role in the malignant transformation of epidermal tumours.

Acknowledgements

The authors would like to acknowledge E. Del Rossi, C.Ferracci, S. Leto, G. Ceccarani and L. Stefanelli for their work, efforts and support.

References

1. Lavker RM, Sun TT. Epidermal stem cells: properties, markers, and location. *Proc Natl Acad Sci U S A* 2000; 97: 13473–13475.
2. Watt FM, Lo Celso C, Silva-Vargas V. Epidermal stem cells: an update. *Curr Opin Genet Dev* 2006; 16: 518–524.
3. Watt FM, Hogan BL. Out of Eden: stem cells and their niches. *Science* 2000; 287: 1427–1430.
4. Owens DM, Watt FM. Contribution of stem cells and differentiated cells to epidermal tumours. *Nat Rev Cancer* 2003; 3: 444–451.
5. Cotsarelis G, Kaur P, Dhouailly D *et al.* Epithelial stem cells in the skin: definition, markers, localization and functions. *Exp Dermatol* 1999; 8: 80–88.
6. Kumar V, Abbas AK, Fausto N, *et al.* Tissue renewal, regeneration and repair. In: *Robbins and Cotran Pathologic Basis of Disease*, 8th edition. Philadelphia, PA: Saunders Elsevier, 2010; 79–110.
7. Ambler CA, Maatta A. Epidermal stem cells: location, potential and contribution to cancer. *J Pathol* 2009; 217: 206–216.
8. Ma DR, Yang EN, Lee ST. A review: the location, molecular characterisation and multipotency of hair follicle epidermal stem cells. *Ann Acad Med Singapore* 2004; 33: 784–788.
9. Jiang S, Zhao L, Purandare B *et al.* Differential expression of stem cell markers in human follicular bulge and interfollicular epidermal compartments. *Histochem Cell Biol* 2010; 133: 455–465.
10. Ohyama M. Hair follicle bulge: a fascinating reservoir of epithelial stem cells. *J Dermatol Sci* 2007; 46: 81–89.
11. Inoue K, Aoi N, Sato T *et al.* Differential expression of stem-cell-associated markers in human hair follicle epithelial cells. *Lab Invest* 2009; 89: 844–856.
12. Kobayashi T, Shimizu A, Nishifuji K *et al.* Canine hair-follicle keratinocytes enriched with bulge cells have the highly proliferative characteristic of stem cells. *Vet Dermatol* 2009; 20: 338–346.
13. Pascucci L, Mercati F, Gargiulo AM *et al.* CD34 glycoprotein identifies putative stem cells located in the isthmic region of canine hair follicles. *Vet Dermatol* 2006; 17: 244–251.
14. Mercati F, Pascucci L, Gargiulo AM *et al.* Immunohistochemical evaluation of intermediate filament nestin in dog hair follicles. *Histol Histopathol* 2008; 23: 1035–1041.
15. Kobayashi T, Iwasaki T, Amagai M *et al.* Canine follicle stem cell candidates reside in the bulge and share characteristic features with human bulge cells. *J Invest Dermatol* 2010; 130: 1988–1995.
16. Sellheyer K, Atanaskova-Mesinkovska N, Nelson P *et al.* Differential expression of stem cell markers in lichen planopilaris and alopecia areata. *Br J Dermatol* 2011; 165: 1149–1151.
17. Sellheyer K. Stem cell markers can help identify adnexal tumor differentiation when evaluated in the context of morphology: methodology matters. *J Cutan Pathol* 2011; 38: 460–474.
18. Gross TL, Ihrke PJ, Walder EJ, *et al. Follicular tumours.* In: *Skin Diseases of the Dog and Cat: Clinical and Histopathologic Diagnosis*, 2nd edition. Oxford: Blackwell Publishing Ltd, 2005; 604–640.
19. Abbas O, Mahalingam M. Epidermal stem cells: practical perspectives and potential uses. *Br J Dermatol* 2009; 161: 228–236.
20. Lyle S, Christofidou-Solomidou M, Liu Y *et al.* The C8/144B monoclonal antibody recognizes cytokeratin 15 and defines the location of human hair follicle stem cells. *J Cell Sci* 1998; 111: 3179–3188.
21. Kloepper JE, Tiede S, Brinckmann J *et al.* Immunophenotyping of the human bulge region: the quest to define useful *in situ* markers for human epithelial hair follicle stem cells and their niche. *Exp Dermatol* 2008; 17: 592–609.
22. Jih DM, Lyle S, Elenitsas R *et al.* Cytokeratin 15 expression in trichoepitheliomas and a subset of basal cell carcinomas suggests they originate from hair follicle stem cells. *J Cutan Pathol* 1999; 26: 113–118.

23. Schirren CG, Rutten A, Kaudewitz P *et al.* Trichoblastoma and basal cell carcinoma are neoplasms with follicular differentiation sharing the same profile of cytokeratin intermediate filaments. *Am J Dermatopathol* 1997; 19: 341–350.
24. Kanitakis J, Bourchany D, Faure M *et al.* Expression of the hair stem cell-specific keratin 15 in pilar tumors of the skin. *Eur J Dermatol* 1999; 9: 363–365.
25. Yamamoto O, Asahi M. Cytokeratin expression in trichoblastic fibroma (small nodular type trichoblastoma), trichoepithelioma and basal cell carcinoma. *Br J Dermatol* 1999; 140: 8–16.
26. Kanoh M, Amoh Y, Sato Y *et al.* Expression of the hair stem cell-specific marker nestin in epidermal and follicular tumors. *Eur J Dermatol* 2008; 18: 518–523.
27. Weedon D. Tumors of cutaneous appendages. In: *Weedon's Skin Pathology*, 3rd edition. London: Churchill Livingstone Elsevier, 2010; 767.
28. Abbas O, Richards JE, Yaar R *et al.* Stem cell markers (cytokeratin 15, cytokeratin 19 and p63) in *in situ* and invasive cutaneous epithelial lesions. *Mod Pathol* 2011; 24: 90–97.

Supporting Information

Additional Supporting Information may be found in the online version of this article:

Table S1. Clinical data and results of the immunohistochemical investigation on different tumours of follicular and epidermal origin.

To cite this article, please use DOI: 10.1111/j.1365-3164.2012.01116.x

6.4

Epithelial-to-mesenchymal transition: immunohistochemical investigation of related molecules in canine cutaneous epithelial tumours

Laura Bongiovanni*, Alessandra D'Andrea*, Mariarita Romanucci*, Daniela Malatesta*, Melissa Candolini*, Leonardo D. Salda*, Luca Mechelli†, Monica Sforna† and Chiara Brachelente†

*Department of Comparative Biomedical Sciences, Faculty of Veterinary Medicine, University of Teramo, Teramo, Italy
†Department of Biopathological Sciences and Hygiene of Animal and Alimentary Productions, Faculty of Veterinary Medicine, University of Perugia, Perugia, Italy

Correspondence: Laura Bongiovanni, Department of Comparative Biomedical Sciences, Faculty of Veterinary Medicine, University of Teramo, 64100 Teramo, Italy. E-mail: lbongiovanni@unite.it

Background – Epithelial-to-mesenchymal transition (EMT) is a multistep process, important in tumour invasion and metastasis, characterized by loss of epithelial markers, redistribution of β-catenin and gain of mesenchymal markers.

Hyposthesis/Objectives – Our aim was to investigate the immunohistochemical aberrant expression of cytokeratin, vimentin, survivin and heat shock protein 72 (Hsp72) in canine cutaneous epithelial tumours, to understand the association of expression of these molecules with features of malignancy and their role in the EMT phenotype.

Methods – Ten canine squamous cell carcinomas (SCCs; one with lymph node metastasis), 30 canine hair follicle tumours (six pilomatricomas, eight infundibular keratinizing acanthomas, six trichoepitheliomas and 10 trichoblastomas) and five normal skin samples were investigated by immunohistochemistry using specific anti-vimentin, -cytokeratin, -survivin and -Hsp72 antibodies. A semi-quantitative method was used to analyse the results, as follows: 0 to <5%; ≥5 to <10%; ≥10 to <25%; and ≥25% of positive cells. Immunofluorescence was performed to investigate survivin–vimentin and survivin–Hsp72 colocalization in selected SCCs.

Results – In malignant hair follicle tumours and SCCs, a reduced intensity of cytokeratin and increased survivin and Hsp72 expression were observed. In SCCs, loss of cytokeratin expression and vimentin immunolabelling, suggestive of the EMT phenotype, were evident in <5% of neoplastic cells in the front of tumour invasion. In the same areas, strong nuclear survivin and cytoplasmic Hsp72 staining was evident, often colocalizing. Only a few neoplastic cells in the front of tumour invasion showed vimentin–survivin colocalization.

Conclusions and clinical importance – A possible simultaneous involvement of survivin and Hsp72 in tumour invasion and the multistep process of EMT of cutaneous epithelial tumours of dogs is suggested.

Introduction

In order to grow, infiltrate and invade, epithelial tumour cells need to acquire new properties, allowing them to survive without cell-to-cell contact, to pass through basal membranes, to interact with stromal cells and molecules and, finally, to gain access to the vessels for metastatic dissemination. All these cellular proprieties have recently been grouped under the name of epithelial-to-mesenchymal transition (EMT).[1] The process of EMT is believed to be one of the key steps towards metastatic dissemination.[2] Epithelial-to-mesenchymal transition is characterized by diminished epithelial characteristics and increased mesenchymal attributes[3] induced by several pathways, such as transforming growth factor-β (TGF-β)[4] and Wnt[5] pathways, using the transcription factors Snail, Slug and Twist.[6] The exact phenotypic changes associated with EMT are difficult to define. The exact contribution of EMT to the metastatic cascade is still a subject of debate,[7,8] although the expression of EMT markers in circulating tumour cells has been demonstrated.[9] It has been suggested that many intermediate phenotypes, ranging from epithelial to mesenchymal differentiation, are likely to coexist in a tumour population.[10] The EMT phenotype has been associated with several features, as follows: increased invasive ability; improved resistance to apoptotic signals; and augmented ability to promote angiogenesis.[3] Cells undergoing EMT are characterized by weakness of cell-to-cell adhesion, which favours the ability to degrade the matrix and modify the cell cytoskeleton, facilitating cell motility.[3] During EMT, many cytokeratins are downregulated, whereas vimentin is upregulated.[3] Vimentin can be upregulated by central EMT transcription factors, such as Snail[11] and Twist,[12] as

Accepted 29 June 2012
Sources of Funding: This study was self-funded.
Conflict of Interest: No conflicts of interest have been declared.

well as the β-catenin pathway,[13] showing a functional role in both epithelial and mesenchymal cell migration.[14–16] Vimentin expression by epithelial neoplastic cells has been considered a hallmark of the EMT phenotype, as a marker of mesenchymal differentiation and as a useful marker of carcinomas with a more aggressive behaviour in several types of human cancers.[17–19]

Activation of the Wnt/β-catenin pathway has been related to the EMT process.[6] As a consequence of adherens junction reorganization, β-catenin can accumulate in the cytoplasm and translocate into the nucleus, where it activates the expression of EMT target genes, such as vimentin, or EMT regulators, such as Snail and Twist.[6,13,20] In canine cutaneous squamous cell carcinomas (SCCs), we have recently found an altered subcellular β-catenin distribution[21] and co-expression with vimentin in SCCs with a more aggressive behaviour.[22] These findings suggest that EMT molecular modifications might take place in a subset of neoplastic cells in these canine skin neoplasms.

Based on these previous results and on knowledge of the functions and properties of survivin and heat shock proteins (HSPs),[23,24] we hypothesized a possible association of these molecules with tumour-associated EMT, because several links are evident between their roles in neoplastic cells and the EMT phenotype.

Survivin is a member of the inhibitor of apoptosis (IAP) protein family. It has low or undetectable expression in most adult tissues and is upregulated in the majority of cancers, suggesting that it is one of the most specific cancer proteins identified to date. It plays a fundamental role in cell proliferation and survival, with anti-apoptotic functions.[25] Survivin has been implicated in several aspects of tumour malignancy. In skin tumours, its expression can correlate with tumour severity, metastases, neoangiogenesis and decreased patient survival and it has been inversely correlated with sensitivity to cytotoxic agents used in anticancer therapy.[23] Upregulation of survivin has been demonstrated in both human[23,26–28] and canine[28] cutaneous SCCs.

The HSPs are a wide group of highly conserved molecules that act as molecular chaperones and play an important role in the cellular maintenance of homeostasis, in both physiological conditions and during stress.[29] Altered expression of HSPs has been reported in several human[30] and canine[24] tumours, because they are involved in tumour proliferation, impaired apoptosis, tumour-associated angiogenesis, invasion and metastasis.[29] Several HSPs have been demonstrated to exert anti-apoptotic roles,[31] particularly Hsp72, the expression of which has been observed in canine cutaneous SCC;[32,33] however, their exact role in EMT is still poorly understood. Heat shock protein 72 has recently been implicated in EMT and seems to act by protecting cells from TGFβ-induced EMT in different types of cellular processes, through an interaction with the Smad proteins.[34–36]

The aims of the present study were to perform a comparative immunohistochemical evaluation of the pattern and levels of expression of cytokeratin, vimentin, survivin and Hsp72 in canine cutaneous epithelial tumours, in order to understand the association of expression of these molecules with features of malignancy and to discuss their possible role in the EMT phenotype.

Materials and methods

Tumour samples

In this retrospective study, 40 samples of canine cutaneous epithelial tumours (10 canine SCCs, including one SCC lymph node metastasis, and 30 canine hair follicle tumours) and five normal skin samples were selected from the database of the Departments of Comparative Biomedical Sciences, University of Teramo, Italy, and Biopathological Sciences and Hygiene of Animal and Alimentary Productions, University of Perugia, Italy. Table 1 summarizes the tumour location and signalment of affected animals. Tissue samples were unrelated to those used in previous studies by the authors.[28,32,33]

Histological examination

All specimens were fixed in 10% neutral buffered formalin, embedded in paraffin, sectioned at 4–5 μm, stained with haematoxylin and eosin and examined by light microscopy. Tumours were classified according to the World Health Organization[37] criteria for canine

Table 1. Tumour location and signalment of affected animals

Case	Sex	Age (years)	Location	Dog breed
Squamous cell carcinomas				
1	M	7	Digit	Schnauzer
2	NF	6	Abdomen	Dogo Argentino
3	—	11	Eyelid	Newfoundland dog
4	NM	5	Scrotum	American bulldog
5	M	10	Prepuce	Pitbull
6	M	11	Lip	Pitbull
7	NF	9	Digit	Rottweiler
8	F	15	Footpad	Schnauzer
9	NF	13	Neck	Poodle
10*	NF	3	Abdomen	Mixed breed
Pilomatrichomas				
11	F	8	Chest	German shepherd dog
12	M	10	Back	Shih tzu
13	F	5	Shoulder	Yorkshire terrier
14	—	12	—	Poodle
15	M	—	—	Poodle
16	M	10	Tail	Mixed breed
Infundibular keratinizing acanthomas				
17	F	4	Neck	Yorkshire terrier
18	M	—	Tail	Yorkshire terrier
19	F	4	Tail	Mixed breed
20	M	6	Tail	Rottweiler
21	M	9	Thigh	German shepherd dog
22	NM	6	Head	Mixed breed
23	M	8	Scapula	German shepherd dog
24	F	8	Elbow	German shepherd dog
Trichoepitheliomas				
25	NM	13	Back	German shepherd dog
26	M	3	Shoulder	Giant schnauzer
27	F	8	Back	German shepherd dog
28	M	8	Interscapular	Pitbull
29	F	8	Tail	Setter
30	M	11	Flank	Mixed breed
Trichoblastomas				
31	M	12	Prescapular area	Mixed breed
32	F	9	Lateral face	Setter
33	F	8	Head	German shepherd dog
34	M	11	Chest	Mixed breed
35	F	10	Perianal area	Shih tzu
36	M	3	Tarsus	Mixed breed
37	M	5	Thigh	Mixed breed
38	M	3	Neck	Mixed breed
39	M	11	Neck	—
40	F	9	Lateral face	Setter

Abbreviations: F, female; M, male; NF, neutered female; and NM, neutered male.
*Metastatic.

cutaneous neoplasms and according to the classification of Gross *et al.*[38] by two pathologists (L.B. and C.B.) in an independent way. Squamous cell carcinomas were subclassified into well, moderately and poorly differentiated. For each sample, the degree of invasiveness into the surrounding tissue and the degree of inflammatory reaction were evaluated as additional features.

Immunohistochemistry

Deparaffinized and rehydrated tissue sections were immunostained by the streptavidin–biotin peroxidase complex method using commercially available antibodies, including the following: full-length survivin (rabbit polyclonal, diluted 0.7 μg/mL; Novus Biologicals, Littleton, CO, USA), vimentin (mouse monoclonal, V-9, diluted 1:200; DakoCytomation, Ely, UK), pancytokeratin (mouse monoclonal, AE1/AE3, diluted 1:50; Dako, Glostrub, Denmark) and Hsp72 (mouse monoclonal, C92 F3A-5, diluted 1:100; StressGen, Kampenhout, Belgium). Endogenous peroxidases were blocked with 3% hydrogen peroxide in absolute methanol for 45 min. Antigen retrieval was undertaken by heat-treating sections in citrate buffer at pH 6 in a pressure cooker for 20 min for survivin and in a microwave oven (3 × 5 min) for vimentin, pancytokeratin and Hsp72. To reduce non-specific binding, slides were incubated in 5% bovine milk (Bio-Rad, Deeside, UK) in Tris-buffered saline for 15 min at room temperature. Overnight incubation with primary antibodies was performed in a humidified chamber at 4°C. Slides were treated with secondary biotinylated goat anti-mouse + rabbit antibodies (Biospa, Milan, Italy), and detected with streptavidin-peroxidase (Kit Vectstain ELITE ABC; Vector Laboratories, Burlingame, CA, USA), incubated at room temperature for 30 min. The reaction was visualized with 3-3′-diaminobenzidine (D5905; Sigma-Aldrich, St Louis, MO, USA) solution, which was applied for 5 min, and finally lightly counterstained with Mayer's haematoxylin (Merk, Darmstadt, Germany) for 2 min. Samples of canine cutaneous SCC were used as positive controls. A negative control was performed in all instances by incubating tissue sections with an antibody directed against an unrelated antigen (mouse anti-human desmin monoclonal antibody; Dako) dissolved in Tris-buffered saline instead of the primary antibody.

Quantification of immunolabelling

Immunolabelling was classified based on the subcellular localization (cytoplasmic/nuclear) and the percentage of positive cells found on analysis of 10 high-power fields (×40 magnification; semi-quantitative method), as follows: 0 to <5%; ≥5 to <10%; ≥10 to <25%; and ≥25% of positive cells. Cytokeratin and vimentin expression was also evaluated as positive (+), negative (–) or with a reduced intensity of expression (–/+).

Immunofluorescence

Immunofluorescence was also used to investigate the colocalization of survivin–vimentin and survivin–Hsp72 expression in four selected canine infiltrative SCC samples and one SCC lymph node metastasis. Tissue samples were treated as described for the immunohistochemical procedure. A mixture of primary antibodies against survivin–vimentin (diluted 0.5 μg/mL and 1:100, respectively) and survivin–Hsp72 (diluted 0.5 μg/mL and 1:50, respectively) was applied overnight at 4°C. The first secondary antibody, biotinylated goat anti-rabbit (Vector Laboratories), diluted 1:200, was applied and incubated for 30 min at room temperature, and slides were then incubated with fluorescein-conjugated avidin (Vector Laboratories) diluted 1:100 in sodium bicarbonate buffer 0.1 mol/L, NaCl 0.15 mol/L (pH 8.2–8.5) for 10 min at room temperature. A blocking step was performed by incubating slides for 15 min with avidin and then biotin, at room temperature. The second secondary antibody, biotinylated goat anti-mouse (Vector Laboratories), diluted 1:200, was applied and incubated for 30 min at room temperature, and slides were then incubated with Texas Red-conjugated avidin (Vector Laboratories) diluted 1:100 in sodium bicarbonate buffer 0.1 mol/L, NaCl 0.15 mol/L (pH 8.2–8.5) for 10 min at room temperature. Nuclei were counterstained with 4′,6-diamidino-2-phenylindole (DAPI) (Vector Laboratories).

Results

Histological examination

Histologically, the 40 canine cutaneous tumour samples were identified as 10 canine SCCs, all with an infiltrative growth, of which seven were well differentiated, three poorly differentiated and one was associated with lymph node metastasis; four benign and two malignant pilomatricomas; eight infundibular keratinizing acanthomas; three benign and three malignant trichoepitheliomas; and 10 trichoblastomas.

Immunohistochemical evaluation

Normal skin (skin of control dogs, as well as epidermis and hair follicles adjacent to the neoplastic tissue).
In normal epidermis, all keratinocytes were negative for vimentin and positive for pancytokeratin. Vimentin immunostaining was noted in scattered cells, compatible with melanocytes and epidermal dendritic cells.

Weak Hsp72 cytoplasmic immunolabelling was observed in all layers of the epidermis, except the stratum corneum. Scattered survivin-positive nuclei were found in the basal cell layer.

In normal hair follicles, vimentin was negative in epithelial cells, while positive cells were observed in the dermal papilla. Diffuse cytokeratin staining was observed, excluding the matrix cells and dermal papilla. The Hsp72 staining was diffuse in the cytoplasm of the outer root sheath, with scattered positive nuclei in the basal cell layer.

Survivin-positive nuclei were present in the basal cell layer of the outer root sheath and matrix cells.

Benign hair follicle tumours.
All immunohistochemical results are shown in Table 2.

Neoplastic cells were positive for cytokeratin, although cells with matrical differentiation (pilomatricomas and trichoepitheliomas) were negative.

Vimentin was not expressed, other than in scattered cells representing melanocytes and epidermal dendritic cells accompanying the tumour growth. In three of 10 cases of trichoblastomas, small clusters of spindle-shaped cells (so-called 'follicular papillary mesenchymal bodies', similar to abortive dermal papillae)[38] accompanying the tumour were vimentin positive (Figure 1a).

Cytoplasmic survivin was present in all the cases evaluated with no significant differences among tumour types. However, survivin marked the highest number of positive cells in trichoblastomas (Figure 2a), where in most of the cases (seven of 10) the number of positive nuclei was >25%. Benign pilomatrichomas showed moderate (≥10 to <25%) to high (>25%) nuclear expression (Figure 2b). Two of three trichoepitheliomas had survivin immunolabelling, and the survivin-positive nuclei were mostly present among neoplastic cells with matrical differentiation (Figure 2c). In infundibular keratinizing acanthomas the expression of nuclear survivin ranged between 0 to <5 and ≥5 to <10%, mostly present in cells with basal cell morphology (Figure 2d).

The Hsp72 staining showed the highest number of positive cells in trichoblastomas, where in most of the cases both cytoplasmic and nuclear staining were evident

Table 2. Immunohistochemical results for hair follicle tumours

	Cytokeratin	Vimentin	Nuclear survivin (%)	Cytoplasmic Hsp72 (%)	Nuclear Hsp72 (%)
Pilomatricomas					
11	MC−	−	≥25	≥25	≥25
12	MC−; DC+	−	≥10 to <25	≥5 to <10	≥10 to <25
13	MC−	−	≥10 to <25	0 to <5	0 to <5
14	MC−; DC+	−	≥25	—	—
15*	I −/+	−	≥25	0 to <5	—
16*	I −/+	−	≥25	0 to <5	0 to <5
Infundibular keratinizing acanthomas					
17	+	−	≥5 to <10	≥10 to <25	≥5 to <10
18	+	−	0 to <5	≥10 to <25	≥5 to <10
19	+	−	≥5 to <10	—	—
20	+	−	0 to <5	>25	≥10 to <25
21	+	−	0 to <5	≥25	0 to <5
22	+	−	≥5 to <10	≥25	0 to <5
23	+	−	0 to <5	0 to <5	—
24	+	−	≥5 to <10	0 to <5	—
Trichoepitheliomas					
25	+; MC−	−	≥5 to <10	≥10 to <25	≥10 to <25
26	+	−	≥10 to <25	≥25	≥25
27	+	−	—	≥25	≥25
28*	+	−	≥10 to <25	≥25	≥25
29*	I −/+	−	≥10 to <25	0 to <5	0 to <5
30*	+	−	≥5 to <10	≥25	≥10 to <25
Trichoblastomas					
31	+	−	≥25	≥10 to <25	≥5 to <10
32	+	−	≥25	≥10 to <25	>25
33	+	−	≥25	≥10 to <25	≥10 to <25
34	+	−	≥5 to <10	0 to <5	0 to <5
35	+	−; DP+	≥5 to <10	≥5 to <10	0 to <5
36	+	−	≥25	≥25	≥25
37	+	−; DP+	≥25	≥25	≥25
38	+	−; DP+	≥10 to <25	≥25	≥25
39	+	−	≥25	≥25	≥25
40	+	−	≥25	≥25	≥25

Abbreviations and symbols: +, positive; −, negative; −/+, reduced intensity of expression; DC, differentiated cells; DP, abortive dermal papillae; Hsp72, heat shock protein 72; I, infiltrative areas; MC, matrical cells.
*Malignant.

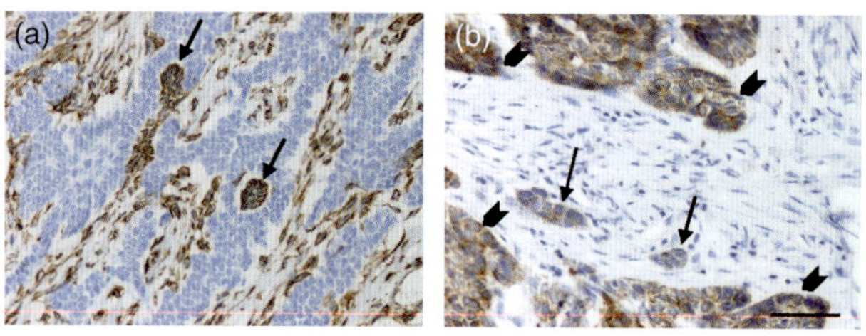

Figure 1. Immunohistochemical evaluation of trichoblastoma. Mayer's haematoxylin counterstain. (a) Benign trichoblastoma with vimentin immunohistochemistry showing negative neoplastic cords surrounded by positive connective tissue. There is intense immunolabelling in small clusters of spindle-shaped cells accompanying the tumour (so-called 'follicular papillary mesenchymal bodies'; arrows). (b) Malignant trichoblastoma with cytokeratin immunohistochemistry showing neoplastic cords with high cytokeratin expression (arrowheads) and small clusters of neoplastic cells showing a reduction of immunostaining (arrows). Scale bar represents 50 μm.

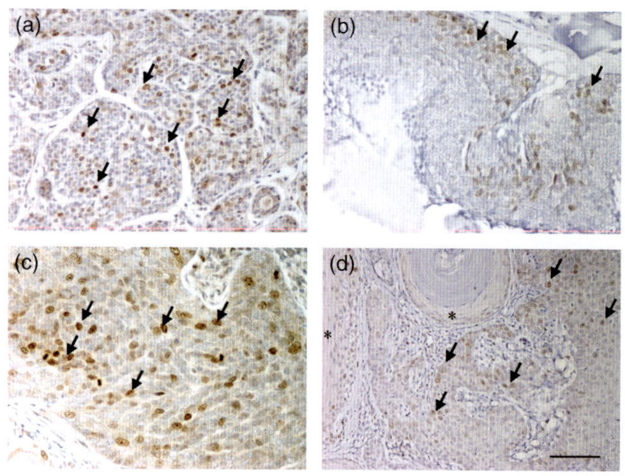

Figure 2. Survivin immunohistochemical evaluation in hair follicle tumours. Mayer's haematoxylin counterstain. (a) Trichoblastoma showing numerous positive nuclei in neoplastic cords (arrows). (b) Pilomatrichoma with positive nuclei evident in the external areas of the wall of the cystic structure (arrows). (c) Trichoepithelioma with numerous survivin-positive nuclei (arrows) present among neoplastic cells with matrical differentiation. (d) Infundibular keratinizing acanthoma with survivin-positive nuclei in the neoplastic cords among cells with basal morphology, but absent in the areas of squamous differentiation (*). Scale bar represents 50 μm in (a), (b) and (c) and 100 μm in (d).

(Figure 3a). Nuclear immunolabelling was less frequent. Follicular papillary mesenchymal bodies were negative.

In benign pilomatrichomas, limited or absent immunostaining was observed among tumour cells with matrical differentiation, while intense cytoplasmic immunostaining was evident in cells detaching from

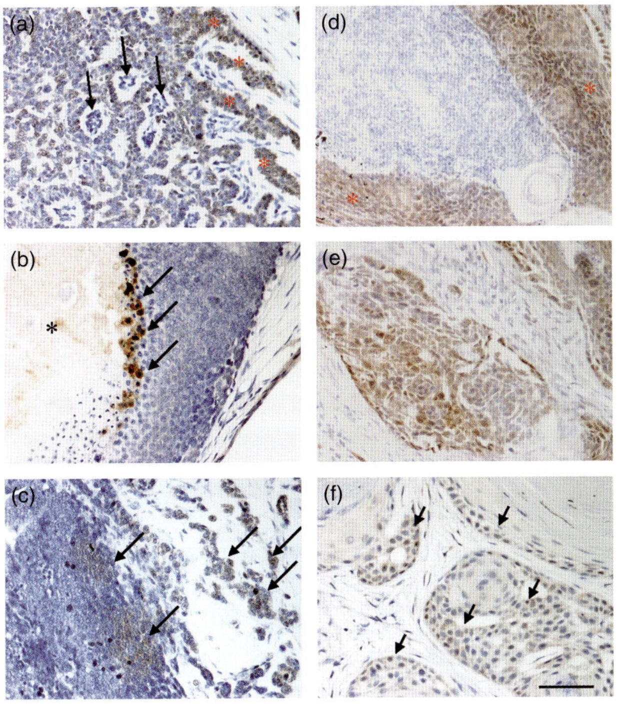

Figure 3. Heat shock protein 72 (Hsp72) immunohistochemical evaluation in hair follicle tumours. Mayer's haematoxylin counterstain. (a) Trichoblastoma. The cytoplasmic immunostaining is more intense in the external part of the tumour mass (*). Negative 'follicular papillary mesenchymal bodies' (arrows). (b) Benign pilomatrichoma. There is an absence of immunolabelling among tumour cells with matrical differentiation, but intense cytoplasmic immunostaining in cells detaching from the wall of the cystic structures into the lumen (arrows) where they become 'ghost cells' (*). (c) Malignant pilomatrichoma with a low number of positive neoplastic cells (arrows) in the external portion of the cystic structures. (d) Benign trichoepithelioma showing cytoplasmic and nuclear immunolabelling in cells with matrical differentiation (*). (e) Malignant trichoepithelioma with diffuse cytoplasmic and nuclear immunolabelling. (f) Infundibular keratinizing acanthoma. There is cytoplasmic immunostaining among neoplastic basal cells of neoplastic cords (arrows). Scale bar represents 100 μm in (a) and 50 μm in (b)–(f).

the wall of the cystic structures into the lumen where they become 'ghost cells' (Figure 3b). Benign trichoepitheliomas had an unpredictable number of positive cells, varying from case to case based on the predominant type of follicular differentiation (Figure 3d). Nuclear immunolabelling was more numerous in cells with basal and matrical differentiation, while cytoplasmic staining was evident in areas with squamous differentiation. Most of the infundibular keratinizing acanthoma cases showed cytoplasmic staining mainly within cords of neoplastic basal cells (Figure 3f). In the same areas, positive nuclei were evident in five of eight cases.

Squamous cell carcinomas.
Cytokeratin immunolabelling intensity was decreased in 0 to <25% of neoplastic cells (Figure 4a) while loss of cytokeratin expression was evident only in a very low number of cells (<5%) which were often single, infiltrative neoplastic cells, detaching from the front of tumour invasion.

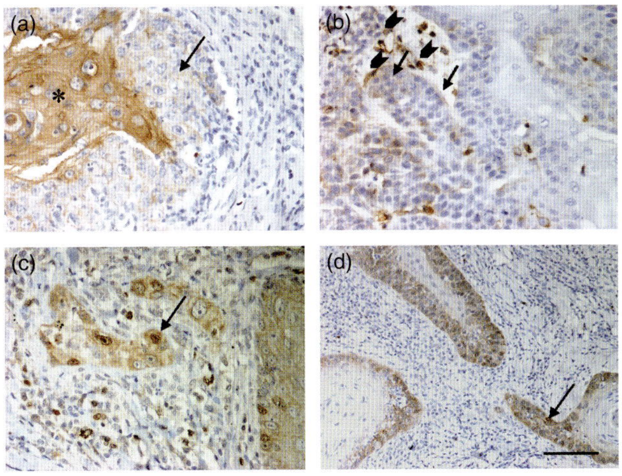

Figure 4. Immunohistochemical evaluation of squamous cell carcinoma. Mayer's haematoxylin counterstain. (a) Cytokeratin immunohistochemistry. There are areas with squamous differentiation with intense cytoplasmic immunolabelling (*) and areas of reduction and loss of immunolabelling (arrow). (b) Vimentin immunohistochemistry. There is focal acquisition of vimentin expression at the front of tumour invasion (arrows), with positive surrounding connective tissue and endothelial cells (arrowheads). (c) Survivin immunohistochemistry showing nuclear survivin expression in small clusters of neoplastic cells (arrow). (d) Heat shock protein 72 immunohistochemistry. There is intense cytoplasmic immunolabelling at the front of tumour invasion where scattered positive nuclei were also found (arrow). Scale bar represents 50 μm in (a), (b) and (c) and 100 μm in (d).

Acquisition of vimentin immunolabelling was evident in only a very low number (<5%) of neoplastic cells observed at the front of tumour invasion (Figure 4b).

Cytoplasmic survivin expression was observed in six of 10 cases, as well as in the lymph node metastasis, often (four of six cases) with a high expression (>25% of tumour cells).

Survivin nuclear immunolabelling was observed in neoplastic cells showing a basal cell morphology at the front of tumour invasion and in small clusters of infiltrative neoplastic cells (Figure 4c). In these areas, expression of survivin reached the highest levels (eight of 10 of the cases showed >10% expression, of which four of eight showed >25%; Table 3).

Cytoplasmic Hsp72 immunolabelling was found in all the cases examined and was intense in the infiltrative portions of the neoplastic mass. Seven of 10 cases showed >10% of positive cells (Figure 4d and Table 3).

Nuclear immunolabelling was absent in most of the cases analysed. In only three cases, nuclear staining was present in the external portion of tumour cords and nests (Figure 4d, arrow).

Malignant hair follicle tumours.
Immunohistochemical results are shown in Table 2.

In malignant trichoepitheliomas, reduced intensity of cytokeratin expression was observed in a low number of cells in the infiltrative areas of the neoplastic mass (Figure 1b). In malignant pilomatricomas, as for their benign counterparts, cytokeratin expression was negative.

In malignant hair follicle tumours, vimentin was not expressed other than in scattered cells representing

Table 3. Immunohistochemical results for squamous cell carcinomas

SCC	Cytokeratin loss (%)	Vimentin (%)	Survivin (%)	Hsp72 (%)
1	—	—	C ≥25 N ≥10 to <25	C ≥5 to <10
2	0 to <5 I	0 to <5 I	C ≥25 N, I ≥10 to <25	C ≥10 to <25
3	≥10 to <25 S	≥25 S	N ≥25 S	C ≥10 to <25 S
4	0 to <5 FTI	0 to <5 FTI	N ≥25 FTI	C ≥25 N ≥10 to <25
5	≥5 to <10 FTI	0 to <5 FTI	C ≥10 to <25 N ≥5 to <10	C ≥25 N 0 to <5
6	0 FTI; 0 to <5 V	–	C, N ≥25	C 0 to <5 FTI
7	≥5 to <10 FTI	0 to <5 FTI	N ≥10 to <25	C ≥25 N 0 to <5
8	0 to <5 FTI	0 to <5 FTI	N 0 to <5	C ≥25
9	≥5 to <10 FTI	0	N ≥25	C ≥25
10	0 to <5 FTI	0 to <5 FTI	C ≥25 N, FTI ≥10 to <25	C, FTI ≥5 to <10
10*	≥25 FTI	0 to <5 FTI	C ≥10 to <25 N ≥25	C, FTI ≥5 to <10

Abbreviations: C, cytoplasmic; FTI, front of tumour invasion (comprising single/small clusters of infiltrating cells); Hsp72, heat shock protein 72; I, infiltrative areas; N, nuclear; S, spindle cells; SCC, squamous cell carcinoma; and V, infiltrating cells around vessels.
*Lymph node metastasis of case 10.

melanocytes and epidermal dendritic cells accompanying the tumour growth.

Cytoplasmic survivin was observed in all the cases evaluated. No significant differences in nuclear survivin expression were observed between benign and malignant trichoepitheliomas and pilomatricomas.

In the two cases of malignant pilomatrichoma, a low number (0–5%) of Hsp72-positive neoplastic cells were observed, mainly in the external portion of the cystic structures in infiltrative areas, and as small clusters of cells invading the surrounding connective tissue (Figure 3c). Malignant trichoepitheliomas had an unpredictable number of positive cells, varying from case to case based on the predominant type of follicular differentiation (Figure 3e).

Immunofluorescence evaluation

Survivin–Hsp72 colocalization was observed in several (0–10%) neoplastic cells (Figure 5b). As far as survivin–vimentin double immunolabelling was concerned, different patterns were observed. Survivin–vimentin colocalization was present in only a few (0–5%) neoplastic cells at the front of tumour invasion (Figure 5a, arrows); survivin-positive, vimentin-negative cells and vimentin-positive, survivin-negative cells (Figure 5a, arrowheads) were also present. In the lymph node metastasis the expression patterns of the molecules were similar to those observed in the primary neoplastic tissue.

Discussion

In the present study, we showed that in canine cutaneous SCCs the expression of vimentin, survivin and Hsp72 is induced and that there is focal loss of expression of pancytokeratin. Furthermore, we demonstrated an induction of survivin expression associated with focal acquisition of vimentin and intense Hsp72 cytoplasmic expression. In addition, Hsp72 and survivin expression in normal hair follicles and in hair follicle tumours suggests a potential role of these molecules in hair follicle growth and carcinogenesis.

The immunohistochemical staining for vimentin and cytokeratin was evaluated as a simple and rapid approach in order to identify the EMT phenotype. Unlike SCCs, the complexity of cell differentiation of hair follicle tumours makes the EMT process difficult to evaluate by this method. Despite its limitations, vimentin is considered a hallmark of the EMT phenotype and a useful marker of carcinomas with a more aggressive behaviour.[17,19] The use of immunohistochemical evaluation of vimentin in canine skin neoplasms showed several limitations, as follows: (i) vimentin-positive inflammatory cells often accompany and infiltrate neoplastic masses; (ii) there is a tight interconnection between tumour cells and surrounding positive connective tissue; and (iii) neoplastic cells undergoing EMT may change their morphology to become spindle shaped and phenotypically indistinguishable from fibroblasts.[6] These limitations caused difficulty when interpreting the results. In general, the margins of the cords and nests of neoplastic tissue were evaluated in order to detect the presence or absence of vimentin and cytokeratin immunostaining, because it was very difficult to evaluate single infiltrative cells or very small clusters of tumour cells, especially for vimentin. The immunofluorescence was performed in four SCC selected cases without or with minimal inflammatory infiltrate.

Epithelial-to-mesenchymal transformation within malignant tumours, characterized by loss of cytokeratin and variable vimentin expression, was evident in a small subpopulation of tumour cells along the front of tumour invasion. These changes coincided with high nuclear survivin and cytoplasmic Hsp72 expression, as demonstrated by double-labelling immunofluorescence. These findings are in accordance with previous studies.[39] Indeed, EMT takes place at the periphery of the tumour where cells are exposed to cytokines and an extracellular environment that promotes EMT.[40] Interestingly, the induction of EMT

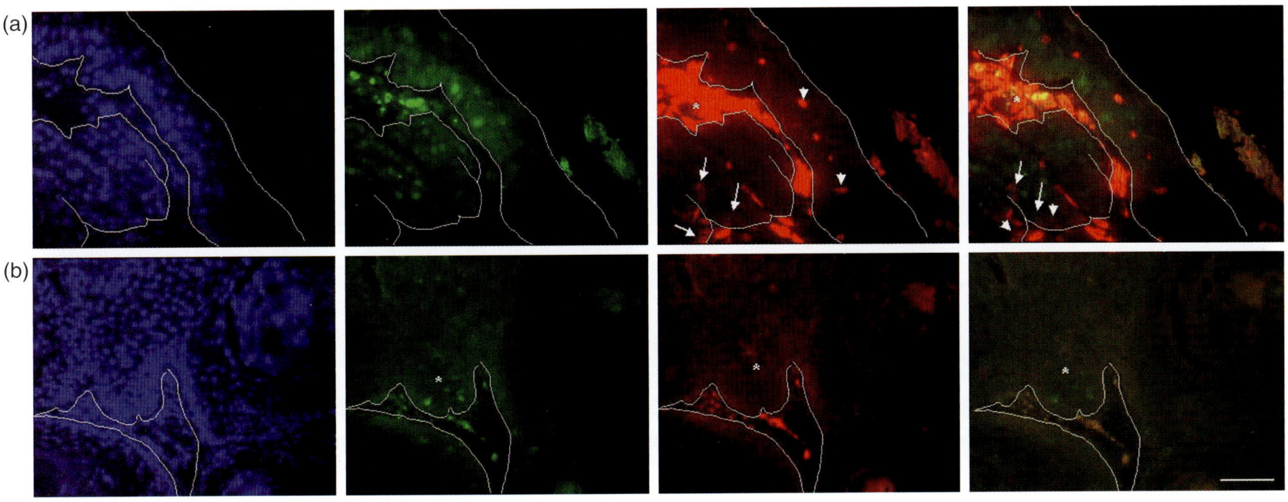

Figure 5. Immunofluorescence in squamous cell carcinomas. First column, shows blue nuclei with DAPI counterstain. Second column shows survivin stained green. Note several positive nuclei and a diffuse cytoplasmic immunolabelling in neoplastic cords. Third column shows vimentin stained red (a) with a low number of neoplastic cells present at the front of tumour invasion showing immunolabelling (arrows). There are positive cells among the neoplastic cells compatible with melanocytes and epidermal dendritic cells (arrowheads). Third column also shows Hsp72 stained red (b) with intense cytoplasmic staining of cells at the front of tumour invasion (*). Fourth column shows the merged image (orange). (a) Presence of vimentin-positive and survivin-negative cells (arrowheads) and vimentin-positive and survivin-positive cells (arrows) at the front of tumour invasion. (b) Presence of numerous Hsp72 and survivin double-immunolabelled cells (*). Scale bar represents 100 μm.

also regulates the interaction of a tumour cell with the microenvironment, including the immune cells, which produce immunosuppressive cytokines and impair tumour surveillance mechanisms.[41]

Furthermore, the evaluation of EMT in cancer is complicated by the fact that at the secondary site the metastatic cells undergo a reverse process, named mesenchymal-to-epithelial transition. This process leads neoplastic cells to reproduce a neoplastic tissue similar to the primary tumour.[42] Although a single case of SCC lymph node metastasis was examined, our results showed a pattern of molecular expression very similar to the primary tumour, in accordance with this theory.

The low metastatic potential of hair follicle tumours[38] could explain the data observed herein, characterized by a rarely complete lack of cytokeratin immunostaining and no vimentin expression. However, few cases were evaluated and a larger number of cases, with no or mild inflammatory infiltrate should be examined to study the EMT process further.

In general, in canine malignant epithelial tumours, loss or reduction of cytokeratin immunostaining appears to be more frequent than the acquisition of vimentin expression. These data confirm that the EMT process is a multi-step process and that few cells eventually acquire the ability to leave the primary tumour and invade.

Nuclear survivin-positive cells were more numerous than the number of cells showing loss of cytokeratin expression and acquisition of vimentin immunolabelling. These results are in agreement with the wide role that survivin plays in neoplastic transformation as well as in the early phases of carcinogenesis, in accordance with its anti-apoptotic and cell-cycle regulatory functions.[23] Recently, a link between survivin and the EMT process has been investigated in hepatocellular carcinoma cells.[43] A lack of survivin expression seemed to be able to induce vimentin expression and enhance cancer metastasis.[43] In order to investigate the simultaneous expression of survivin and vimentin we performed a double immunofluorescence labelling. Beside double-immunolabelled cells, there were cells showing only vimentin expression. Although survivin functions seem to contribute to the EMT process, Tai *et al.*[43] in accordance with our results, showed an opposite role and further studies are needed to understand better the exact role of survivin in this process.

As far as Hsp72 expression is concerned, data obtained are similar to previous reports.[32,33] Heat shock protein 72 is strongly upregulated in cancers,[44] but its significance for tumour induction and growth is poorly understood. Its upregulation may reflect a biological stress condition of tumour cells,[45,46] as well as the increased cell proliferation rate[45] in accordance with its role in the control of cell growth.[47] The present study produced preliminary results that suggest an involvement of Hsp72 in the acquisition of the EMT phenotype by the epithelial cancer cells. However, further studies are necessary to clarify the involvement of Hsp72, and HSPs in general, in pathological tumour-associated EMT processes. In particular, it should be clarified whether the involvement of Hsp72 is to promote this process, as indicated by its anti-apoptotic functions,[31] or to counteract it as suggested by recent studies conducted on pathological EMT.[34–36,48] Nevertheless, previous studies have been conducted on pathological but not tumour-associated EMT where Hsp72 might also play a different role.

Furthermore, data obtained from immunofluorescence evaluation of the survivin–Hsp72 potential colocalization suggest that these molecules could be activated in the same subset of tumour cells mostly present at the periphery of the tumour.

The expression of survivin and Hsp72 in normal hair follicles and their upregulation in hair follicle tumours suggest a potential role of these molecules in the pathogenesis of these canine neoplasms. In particular, a role of survivin could be hypothesized in matrix cells as well as in tumours with matrical differentiation, such as trichoepithelioma and pilomatrichoma. In these neoplasms, Hsp72 seems to be intensively produced in stressed cells which become 'ghost cells'. Furthermore, both survivin and Hsp72 showed the highest level of expression in trichoblastomas, according to their expression in the basal cells of the outer root sheath in normal hair follicles, from which this tumour is thought to originate.[38]

Data presented herein suggest that in canine cutaneous malignant epithelial tumours, neoplastic cells might undergo EMT and that the acquisition of the EMT phenotype is a multistep process involving a restricted number of cells. Furthermore, our results suggest that in addition to the well-known contribution in neoplastic transformation, there is a possible simultaneous involvement of survivin and Hsp72 in tumour invasion and the EMT process of cutaneous epithelial tumours of dogs.

References

1. De Wever O, Pauwels P, De Craene B *et al.* Molecular and pathological signatures of epithelial–mesenchymal transitions at the cancer invasion front. *Histochem Cell Biol* 2008; 130: 481–494.
2. Yang J, Weinberg RA. Epithelial-mesenchymal transition: at the crossroads of development and tumor metastasis. *Dev Cell* 2008; 14: 818–829.
3. Bonnomet A, Brysse A, Tachsidis A *et al.* Epithelial-to-mesenchymal transitions and circulating tumor cells. *J Mammary Gland Biol Neoplasia* 2010; 15: 261–273.
4. Zavadil J, Böttinger EP. TGF-β and epithelial-to-mesenchymal transitions. *Oncogene* 2005; 24: 5764–5774.
5. Kim K, Lu Z, Hay ED. Direct evidence for a role of beta-catenin/LEF-1 signaling pathway in induction of EMT. *Cell Biol Int* 2002; 26: 463–476.
6. Micalizzi DS, Farabaugh SM, Ford HL. Epithelial-mesenchymal transition in cancer: parallels between normal development and tumor progression. *J Mammary Gland Biol Neoplasia* 2010; 15: 117–134.
7. Thompson EW, Newgreen DF, Tarin D. Carcinoma invasion and metastasis: a role for epithelial-mesenchymal transition? *Cancer Res* 2005; 65: 5991–5995.
8. Garber K. Epithelial-to-mesenchymal transition is important to metastasis, but questions remain. *J Natl Cancer Inst* 2008; 100: 232–239.
9. Bonnomet A, Syne L, Brysse A *et al.* A dynamic in vivo model of epithelial-to-mesenchymal transitions in circulating tumor cells and metastases of breast cancer. *Oncogene* 2012; 31: 3741–3753.
10. Klymkowsky MW, Savagner P. Epithelial-mesenchymal transition: a cancer researcher's conceptual friend and foe. *Am J Pathol* 2009; 174: 1588–1593.
11. Cano A, Pérez-Moreno MA, Rodrigo I *et al.* The transcription factor Snail controls epithelial-mesenchymal transitions by repressing E-cadherin expression. *Nat Cell Biol* 2000; 2: 76–83.
12. Yang J, Mani SA, Donaher JL *et al.* Twist, a master regulator of morphogenesis, plays an essential role in tumor metastasis. *Cell* 2004; 117: 927–939.
13. Gilles C, Polette M, Mestdagt M *et al.* Transactivation of vimentin by β-catenin in human breast cancer cells. *Cancer Res* 2003; 63: 2658–2664.
14. Eckes B, Dogic D, Colucci-Guyon E *et al.* Impaired mechanical stability, migration and contractile capacity in vimentin-deficient fibroblasts. *J Cell Sci* 1998; 111: 1897–1907.
15. Gilles C, Polette M, Zahm JM *et al.* Vimentin contributes to human mammary epithelial cell migration. *J Cell Sci* 1999; 112: 4615–4625.
16. Eckes B, Colucci-Guyon E, Smola H *et al.* Impaired wound healing in embryonic and adult mice lacking vimentin. *J Cell Sci* 2000; 113: 2455–2462.
17. Handra-Luca A, Hong SM, Walter K *et al.* Tumour epithelial vimentin expression and outcome of pancreatic ductal adenocarcinomas. *Br J Cancer* 2011; 104: 1296–1302.
18. Luo WR, Chen XY, Li SY *et al.* Neoplastic spindle cells in nasopharyngeal carcinoma show features of epithelial–mesenchymal transition. *Histopathology* 2012; 61: 113–122.
19. Kim SH, Kim JM, Shin MH *et al.* Correlation of epithelial-mesenchymal transition markers with clinicopathologic parameters in adenocarcinomas and squamous cell carcinoma of the lung. *Histol Histopathol* 2012; 27: 581–591.
20. Brembeck FH, Rosário M, Birchmeier W. Balancing cell adhesion and Wnt signaling, the key role of β-catenin. *Curr Opin Genet Dev* 2006; 16: 51–59.
21. Bongiovanni L, Malatesta D, Brachelente C *et al.* β-Catenin in canine skin: immunohistochemical pattern of expression in normal skin and cutaneous epithelial tumours. *J Comp Pathol* 2011; 145: 138–147.
22. Bongiovanni L, Di Antonio M, Romanucci M *et al.* Tumour epithelial vimentin expression in canine cutaneous squamous cell carcinoma. *J Comp Pathol* 2012; 146: 86 (abstract).
23. Bongiovanni L, Müller EJ, Della Salda L. Survivin in skin pathologies. *Exp Dermatol* 2011; 20: 457–463.
24. Romanucci M, Bastow T, Della Salda L. Heat shock proteins in animal neoplasms and human tumours - a comparison. *Cell Stress Chaperones* 2008; 13: 253–262.
25. Altieri DC. New wirings in the survivin networks. *Oncogene* 2008; 27: 6276–6284.
26. Grossman D, McNiff JM, Li F *et al.* Expression of the apoptosis inhibitor, survivin, in nonmelanoma skin cancer and gene targeting in a keratinocyte cell line. *Lab Invest* 1999; 79: 1121–1126.
27. Lo Muzio L, Staibano S, Pannone G *et al.* Expression of the apoptosis inhibitor survivin in aggressive squamous cell carcinoma. *Exp Mol Pathol* 2001; 70: 249–254.
28. Bongiovanni L, Colombi I, Fortunato C *et al.* Survivin expression in canine epidermis and in canine and human cutaneous squamous cell carcinomas. *Vet Dermatol* 2009; 20: 369–376.
29. Calderwood SK, Khaleque MA, Sawyer DB *et al.* Heat shock proteins in cancer: chaperones of tumorigenesis. *Trends Biochem Sci* 2006; 31: 164–172.
30. Ciocca DR, Calderwood SK. Heat shock proteins in cancer: diagnostic, prognostic, predictive, and treatment implications. *Cell Stress Chaperones* 2005; 10: 86–103.
31. Arya R, Mallik M, Lakhotia SC. Heat shock genes – integrating cell survival and death. *J Biosci* 2007; 32: 595–610.
32. Romanucci M, Bongiovanni L, Marruchella G *et al.* Heat shock proteins expression in canine intracutaneous cornifying epithelioma and squamous cell carcinoma. *Vet Dermatol* 2005; 16: 108–116.
33. Bongiovanni L, Romanucci M, Fant P *et al.* Apoptosis and anti-apoptotic heat shock proteins in canine cutaneous infundibular keratinizing acanthomas and squamous cell carcinomas. *Vet Dermatol* 2008; 19: 271–279.
34. Banh A, Deschamps PA, Vijayan MM *et al.* The role of Hsp70 and Hsp90 in TGF-β-induced epithelial-to-mesenchymal transition in rat lens epithelial explants. *Mol Vis* 2007; 13: 2248–2262.
35. Li Y, Kang X, Wang Q. HSP70 decreases receptor-dependent phosphorylation of Smad2 and blocks TGF-β-induced epithelial-mesenchymal transition. *J Genet Genomics* 2011; 38: 111–116.
36. Zhou Y, Mao H, Li S *et al.* HSP72 inhibits Smad3 activation and nuclear translocation in renal epithelial-to-mesenchymal transition. *J Am Soc Nephrol* 2010; 21: 598–609.
37. Goldschmidt MH, Dunstan RW, Stannard AA *et al.* *Histological Classification of Epithelial and Melanocytic Tumors of the Skin of Domestic Animals.* Washington, DC: World Health Organization,

International Histological Classification of Tumors of Domestic Animals, Armed Forces Institute of Pathology, American Registry of Pathology, 1998; 20–22.

38. Gross TL, Ihrke PJ, Walder EJ *et al.* Epidermal tumors and follicular tumours. In: *Skin Diseases of the Dog and Cat.* 2nd edn. Oxford: Blackwell Publishing Ltd, 2005: 562–640.
39. Brabletz T, Jung A, Reu S *et al.* Variable β-catenin expression in colorectal cancers indicates tumor progression driven by the tumor environment. *Proc Natl Acad Sci USA* 2001; 98: 10356–10361.
40. Brabletz T, Hlubek F, Spaderna S *et al.* Invasion and metastasis in colorectal cancer: epithelial-mesenchymal transition, mesenchymal-epithelial transition, stem cells and β-catenin. *Cells Tissues Organs* 2005; 179: 56–65.
41. Kudo-Saito C, Shirako H, Takeuchi T *et al.* Cancer metastasis is accelerated through immunosuppression during Snail-induced EMT of cancer cells. *Cancer Cell* 2009; 15: 195–206.
42. Kalluri R, Weinberg RA. The basics of epithelial-mesenchymal transition. *J Clin Invest* 2009; 119: 1420–1428.
43. Tai CJ, Chin-Sheng H, Kuo LJ *et al.* Survivin-mediated cancer cell migration through GRP78 and epithelial-mesenchymal transition (EMT) marker expression in Mahlavu cells. *Ann Surg Oncol* 2012; 19: 336–343.
44. Sherman M. Major heat shock protein Hsp72 controls oncogene-induced senescence. *Ann N Y Acad Sci* 2010; 1197: 152–157.
45. Kaur J, Srivastava A, Rahlan R. Expression of 70-kDa heat shock protein in oral lesions: marker of biological stress or pathogenicity. *Oral Oncol* 1998; 34: 496–501.
46. Jolly C, Morimoto RI. Role of the heat shock response and molecular chaperones in oncogenesis and cell death. *J Natl Cancer Inst* 2000; 92: 1564–1572.
47. Helmbrecht K, Zeise E, Reinsing L. Chaperones in cell cycle regulation and mitogenic signal transduction: a review. *Cell Prolif* 2000; 33: 341–365.
48. Mao H, Li Z, Zhou Y *et al.* HSP72 attenuates renal tubular cell apoptosis and interstitial fibrosis in obstructive nephropathy. *Am J Physiol Renal Physiol* 2008; 295: F202–F214.

To cite this article, please use DOI: 10.1111/j.1365-3164.2012.01106.x

6.5

Canine inflamed nonepitheliotropic cutaneous T-cell lymphoma: a diagnostic conundrum

Peter F. Moore, Verena K. Affolter and Stefan M. Keller

Department of Pathology, Microbiology and Immunology, University of California, Davis, CA 95616, USA

Correspondence: Peter F. Moore, Department of Pathology, Microbiology and Immunology, 4206 VM3A, University of California, Davis, 1 Shields Avenue, CA 95616, USA. E-mail: pfmoore@ucdavis.edu

Background – Cutaneous T-cell lymphoma (CTCL) in dogs is a heterogeneous disease complex, which consists of nonepitheliotropic (NE) and epitheliotropic forms. These lymphomas are readily recognized by the presence of dominant populations of cytologically atypical lymphocytes.

Objective – The objective of this study was to introduce the key features of inflamed NE-CTCL, which is easily confused with reactive, inflammatory histiocytic disease.

Animals – Twenty-four dogs (mean age 7.5 years) presented with inflamed NE-CTCL. Lesions presented as nodules, plaques or masses. An initial diagnosis of cutaneous reactive histiocytosis (11 dogs) or histiocytic neoplasia (three dogs) was made by primary pathologists.

Methods – Lesions were assessed by histology and immunohistochemistry to detect canine leukocyte antigens. Lesional genomic DNA was extracted and gene rearrangement analysis of the T-cell receptor γ locus was assessed.

Results – The cutaneous lesions consisted of pleocellular infiltration of the dermis with variable extension into the subcutis. The lesions often surrounded vessels and adnexae. Epitheliotropism was minimal or lacking. Small lymphocytes, plasma cells and intermediate to large, cytologically atypical lymphocytes were scattered between prominent histiocytic infiltrates. Atypical lymphocytes often had marked variation in the intensity of CD3 expression. Molecular clonality analysis of the T-cell receptor γ locus revealed clonal expansion of T cells in 22 of 23 dogs tested.

Conclusion – The recognition of inflamed NE-CTCL and its differentiation from cutaneous reactive histiocytosis depends on careful assessment of lymphocyte morphology and immunostaining patterns. Confirmation of the diagnosis is best accomplished by T-cell antigen receptor gene rearrangement analysis.

Introduction

Cutaneous T-cell lymphoma (CTCL) is a heterogeneous group of disorders, with a variety of clinical presentations and morphological features in both humans and dogs. Epitheliotropic CTCL, also known as mycosis fungoides (MF), accounts for the majority of cases of CTCL, and is readily recognized by virtue of the prominent epitheliotropism of the T-cell infiltrates for epidermis and adnexal structures.[1–4] Nonepitheliotropic CTCL (NE-CTCL) is an uncommon but well-recognized entity in dogs.[2,5–7] The World Health Organization (WHO) classification of tumours of haematopoietic and lymphoid tissues considers most NE-CTCL as peripheral T-cell lymphomas (PTCL), unspecified.[8] However, the extreme heterogeneity of diseases included in this classification is becoming increasingly recognized.[9,10] In time, a number of specific lymphoma entities will be extracted from the PTCL unspecified category. For example, an indolent form of NE-CTCL was recently described in dogs.[5] Also, primary cutaneous $\gamma\delta$ T-cell lymphoma and two other provisional CTCL entities have been added to the WHO lymphoma classification for humans.[9,11]

In dogs, NE-CTCL are readily recognized when they occur as relatively homogeneous dermal infiltrates of large, cytologically atypical lymphocytes with clear CD3 expression revealed by immunohistochemistry.[2] However, diagnosis of NE-CTCL is more difficult when the dermal infiltrate is heterogeneous with respect to cell lineage, or if CD3 expression by neoplastic T cells is diminished or absent. The hierarchy of pan-T-cell antigen loss in human PTCL is well documented.[10,12] The goal of the present study was to present the morphological, immunohistochemical and molecular characteristics of canine NE-CTCL in which the neoplastic T cells are associated with a dominant pleocellular inflammatory response.

Accepted 13 July 2012

Sources of Funding: Centre for Companion Animal Health and Leukocyte Antigen Biology Laboratory, University of California, Davis, CA, USA.

Conflict of Interest: No conflicts of interest have been declared.

Materials and methods

Canine patients

Four dogs were presented to the Veterinary Medical Teaching Hospital of the University of California at Davis for evaluation and treatment of their lesions. The remaining 20 dogs were patients at private veterinary hospitals, and the original surgical biopsy specimens from skin were submitted to private pathology laboratories (IDEXX Laboratories, USA; ANTECH Diagnostics, USA; or VDx Veterinary Diagnostics, Davis, CA, USA). These latter cases were submitted for second opinions regarding the original diagnosis and/or for molecular diagnostic investigation to confirm suspected lymphoma. Surgical biopsy specimens of skin lesions were obtained from 24 canine patients. Multiple accessions were received for five dogs, and multiple skin sites were sampled from all but four dogs. Specimens consisted of formalin-fixed tissue samples, paraffin blocks or unstained slides. All specimens were obtained with the informed consent of the pet owners. Dogs had not received chemotherapy for their lesions prior to initial surgical biopsy sampling.

Statistical methods

Accurate survival data were obtained for 19 of 24 dogs with inflamed NE-CTCL. The Kaplan–Meier survival curve and median survival time were estimated using the survfit function in R version 2.15.0 (R Development Core Team 2012; R: a language and environment for statistical computing; R Foundation for Statistical Computing, Vienna, Austria).

Tissue handling and immunohistochemistry

The tissues were collected over an 8 year period from 2004 until the present. Tissues were fixed in 10% neutral buffered formalin. Formalin-fixed tissue was embedded in paraffin, and 5-μm-thick sections were stained with haematoxylin and eosin (H&E). For immunohistochemistry, sections were stained by a streptavidin–horseradish peroxidase method according to the manufacturer's instructions (Zymed, South San Francisco, CA, USA) using previously described methods.[13] Monoclonal antibodies (MAb) or polyclonal antibodies specific for canine leukocyte antigens were applied to sections as diluted tissue culture supernatants. Negative controls consisted of substitution of specific MAb with isotype-matched irrelevant MAb (FE1.7B12, mouse IgG1, specific for feline CD4) or omission of the primary antibody.

Antibodies

Antibodies specific for canine leukocyte antigens included MAb specific for CD3 (CD3-12, rat IgG1, AbD Serotec, Kidlington, UK), CD79a (HM57, mouse IgG1, AbD Serotec, Kidlington, UK), CD18 (CA16.3C10, mouse IgG1), CD11d (CA18.3C6, mouse IgG1) and CD45 (CA12.10C12, mouse IgG1). Polyclonal antibodies specific for conserved epitopes on human CD20 (rabbit IgG; Lab Vision, Freemont, CA, USA) and human granzyme B (rabbit IgG; Spring Bioscience, Pleasanton, CA, USA) were used in some instances.

Lymphocyte antigen receptor gene rearrangement analysis

Genomic DNA was extracted from two (25-μm-thick) unmounted sections of formalin-fixed, paraffin-embedded lesional tissue using the manufacturer's recommended protocol (DNeasy tissue kit; Qiagen, Valencia, CA, USA). Extracted genomic DNA was quantified spectrophotometrically using an Ultraspec 2100 pro spectrophotometer (Amersham Pharmacia Biotech, Uppsala, Sweden). All PCRs were performed on GeneAmp PCR system 2700 thermocycler or a Veriti thermocycler (Applied Biosystems, Foster City, CA, USA). Two primer sets were used to assess T-cell receptor γ locus (TRG) rearrangements. All dogs (except dog 5) were analysed with a simplex PCR primer set as previously described.[14,15] Thirteen dogs (dogs 11–22 and dog 24) were analysed with a multiplex PCR primer set that detects all rearranged variable and joining genes.[16] The PCR products were size separated by conventional polyacrylamide gel electrophoresis as previously described, or by capillary electrophoresis using an eGene HDA-GT12 capillary electrophoresis analyser (renamed QIAxcel; Qiagen). All PCRs were run in duplicate or triplicate. Duplicate or triplicate PCRs were used to assist distinction between true clonal samples and pseudoclonal samples. A sample was regarded as clonal if one or two sharp bands of the appropriate and same size were present in duplicate or triplicate samples run in adjacent lanes (conventional electrophoresis) or if clonal peaks were at least twice the height of the polyclonal background (capillary electrophoresis). If the bands differed in size in duplicate/triplicate samples, the sample was considered pseudoclonal.

Results

Clinical summary

Twenty-four dogs, 14 males and 10 females, with a mean age of 7.5 years (range 2–15 years) were included in this study. No breed predilection was observed. Demographic details are summarized in Table 1. Lesions presented as nonpruritic nodules, plaques or masses up to 4 cm in maximal dimension; some lesions were associated with alopecia, ulceration and crust formation. Lesions occurred throughout the skin. Frequently affected sites included the face (lips, nasal planum, eyelids), lower extremities (paws, interdigital folds), neck and trunk (Table 1 and Figure 1).

Clinical follow-up

Treatments and clinical outcome are listed in Table 1. Owing to progression of the lesions, 11 dogs were euthanized and two died within 1–24 months. The median survival time was 9 months as determined by the Kaplan–Meier method (based on 19 dogs; Figure 2). A broad range of treatments were administered to the dogs with inflamed NE-CTCL (Table 1) and, as such, limits the value of the survival data in this retrospective study. Seven dogs are currently alive. Six of these are free of lesions (5 months to 3 years). The remaining dog (dog 22) was treated with Lomustine (CCNU) and developed new lesions within 2 months, and currently receives palliative treatment only. Clinical follow-up was not available for four dogs, and the date of euthanasia was not available for dog 11.

Histological features of inflamed NE-CTCL

Three main topographic patterns of skin infiltration were observed (Figure 3). Pattern A consisted of a lichenoid infiltrate located immediately beneath the epidermis. Pattern B consisted of a prominent perivascular and periadnexal infiltrate located in the mid to deep dermis. Pattern C consisted of an infiltrate localized to the septal and lobular panniculus, with minimal encroachment on the deep dermis. Often, combinations of these basic patterns were present, and in advanced lesions the infiltrates merged to create diffuse effacement of the dermis and panniculus with extension into the adjacent musculature. Partial or complete ulceration of the epidermis was a frequent accompaniment (eight dogs). Infiltration of epithelial structures (epidermis or adnexae) was minimal (dog 8; small epidermal clusters) or nonexistent.

The cellular infiltrates were diverse. Prominent histiocytic infiltrates were consistently observed. Histiocytes did not manifest cytological atypia, and radiated from perivascular locations to coalesce in the deep dermis and

Table 1. Signalment, lesion topography, treatment, response to treatment, follow-up and outcome for dogs with inflamed nonepitheliotropic cutaneous T-cell lymphoma

Dog no.	Breed	Sex	Age (years)	Location	Treatment	Response*	Follow-up	Outcome
1	Bernese mountain dog	MC	6	Digit, mandible, carpus	CCNU, amputation of digit	PD	Lymphadenomegaly after 5 months	Euthanasia – 9 months
2	Standard poodle	MC	7	Muzzle, medial canthus	Radiation, prednisone	CR	—	Alive – 36 months
3	Siberian husky	MC	7	Nasal planum, eyelid	Surgery, prednisone	CR	Weaned off prednisolone after 9 months	Alive – 13 months
4	Beagle	FS	15	Lip margins, conjunctiva, third eyelid	Retinoids, dexamethasone	PR; later PD	Developed pulmonary infiltrates	Euthanasia – 3 months
5	Boxer	F	11	Above eye	Surgery, palliative treatment	PD	—	Euthanasia – 5 months
6	Rottweiler	M	8	Multiple skin sites, not specified	Doxycycline, prednisone, vincristine	PD	—	Euthanasia – 6 months
7	Pit bull terrier	MC	10	Chin, leg, neck	Antibiotics, CCNU	PD	—	Euthanasia – 9 months
8	Shetland sheepdog	MC	6	Dorsal and ventral trunk	n.a.	n.a.	—	n.a.
9	Yorkshire terrier	F	3	Dorsum, adjacent to vulva	Cefalexin, prednisone	PD	—	Euthanasia – 1 month
10	Beagle	FS	12.5	Ventral abdomen, tongue, neck, thorax	Antibiotics, doxycycline, metronidazole, prednisone	PD	—	Euthanasia – 4.5 months
11	French mastiff	M	3	Eyelid, lip	No information	n.a.	Developed seizures	Euthanasia – time (?)
12	Border collie	MC	3	Generalized	n.a.	n.a.	—	n.a.
13	Bulldog	FS	4	Widespread, interdigital	Repeated surgical excision at 6 weeks	PD	—	Euthanasia – 9 months
14	Bassett hound	MC	11	Dorsal neck	Vitamin C, intravenous infusions	PD	Prescapular lymph node; secondary leukaemia	Died – 24 months
15	Bernese mountain dog	MC	8	Lateral thorax	CCNU, cytoxan, vincristin, diphenhydramine famitidine	PR; later PD	—	Euthanasia – 20 months
16	Poodle	FS	10	Scapula, more nonspecified locations	Adriamycin	PR; later PD	—	Died – 10 months
17	Labrador retriever	MC	4	Caudal and ventral abdomen	Cefpodoxime proxetil, metronidazole, hydroxyzine	PD	—	Euthanasia – 1 month
18	Boxer	MC	10	Lower thigh, paw	Surgery only	CR	—	Alive – 12 months
19	German shepherd	M	8	Perianal mass	Chemotherapy (protocol unknown)	CR	—	Alive – 7 months
20	Schnauzer mix	FS	5	Dorsal lumbar	Two surgeries, CCNU, chlorambucil, denosyl	CR	—	Alive – 8 months
21	Shetland sheepdog	F	10	Ventral jaw	Surgery only	CR	—	Alive – 5 months
22	Boxer	F	9	Leg	CCNU; palliative treatment currently	PD	—	Alive – 2 months
23	Mixed breed	FS	8	n.a.	n.a.	n.a.	—	n.a.
24	Golden retriever	MC	2	Chest, back, flank	Asparaginase, prednisone	PD	—	n.a.

Abbreviations: CCNU, lomustine; F, female; FS, female spayed; M, male; MC, male castrated; and n.a., not available.

*Response evaluation in solid tumours: CR, complete response; PR, partial response; SD, stable disease; and PD, progressive disease.

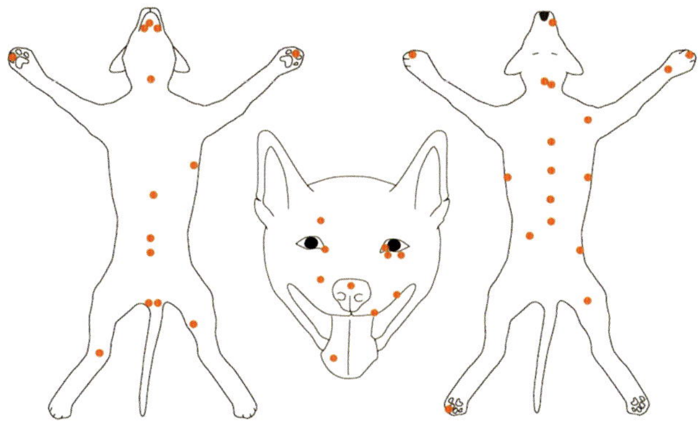

Figure 1. Skin sites (when specified) associated with inflamed non-epitheliotropic cutaneous T-cell lymphoma.

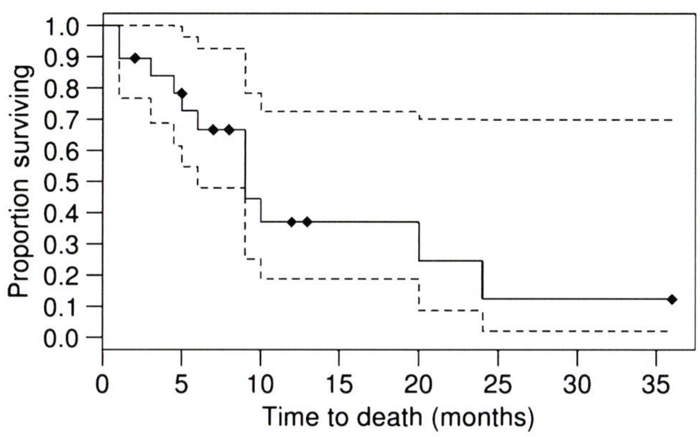

Figure 2. Kaplan–Meier survival curve with 95% upper and lower confidence intervals (dashed lines). The filled diamonds indicate dogs that are still alive.

subcutis (Figure 4). Lymphocytic infiltrates consisted of small, uniformly sized lymphocytes and a variable proportion of intermediate to large lymphocytes, which were intimately associated with the prominent histiocytic expansion (Figures 5 and 6). The intermediate to large lymphocytes often had large vesicular or hyperchromatic nuclei, prominent nucleoli, a high nuclear-to-cytoplasmic ratio and, in some regions, formed clusters of similar cells (Figure 6). Mitotic figures (10–40 per 10 ×400 fields) were also observed in the latter cell population. Small foci of plasma cells and neutrophils were encountered in the majority of lesions (14 dogs). A prominent eosinophil infiltrate was observed in the lesions from seven dogs. Eosinophils were either diffusely scattered, formed intense aggregates, or both, and sometimes contained embedded Splendore-Hoeppli-like material, which appeared to be deposited on collagen fibres (Figure 7).

The topographic pattern of the infiltrate (especially patterns B and C) and the prominent histiocytic infiltrate in inflamed NE-CTCL closely mimicked cutaneous reactive histiocytosis. In fact, 11 dogs were referred with an initial diagnosis of cutaneous histiocytosis and three dogs had an initial diagnosis of histiocytic neoplasia (histiocytic sarcoma or histiocytoma). The distinction of reactive histiocytosis from inflamed NE-CTCL was clearly challenging without further diagnostic investigation, which utilized immunohistochemistry and T-cell antigen receptor gene rearrangement analysis.

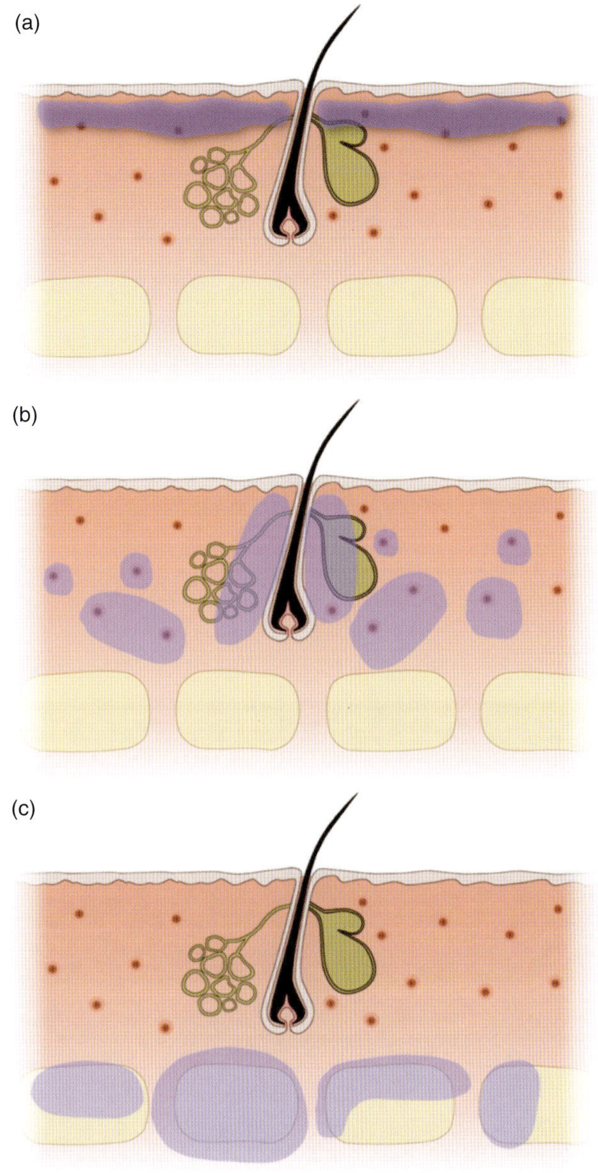

Figure 3. (a) Topographical pattern A, characterized by lichenoid infiltrates beneath the dermal–epidermal junction. (b) Topographical pattern B, characterized by periadnexal and perivascular infiltrates in the mid to deep dermis. (c) Topographical pattern C, characterized by infiltration of the lobular and septal panniculus.

Immunophenotypic features of inflamed NE-CTCL

Histiocytic infiltrates expressed abundant CD18 and CD45 (Figure 8). Small lymphocytes were mostly T cells with uniform strong expression of CD3. Large, cytologically atypical lymphocytes were T cells; most commonly, there was a marked variation in the intensity of CD3 expression in these cells from strong to almost negative (Figure 9). In other instances, CD3 expression was uniform and strong in both small and large, atypical T cells. Large, atypical T cells commonly expressed CD18, CD45 and, less commonly, CD11d. A sizable subpopulation of large, atypical T cells expressed granzyme B in the five dogs in which this stain was conducted. Expression of CD20 and CD79a was limited to minor populations of small lymphocytes in the lesions.

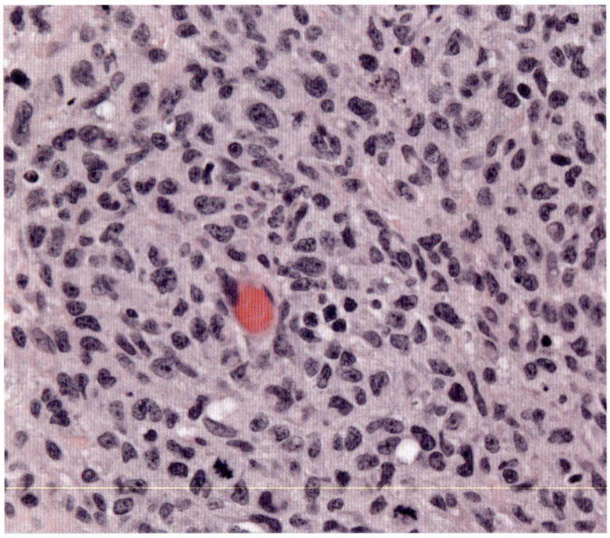

Figure 4. Skin from dog 1; inflamed nonepitheliotropic cutaneous T-cell lymphoma. Perivascular histiocytic infiltrate radiates from the central vessel. H&E stain.

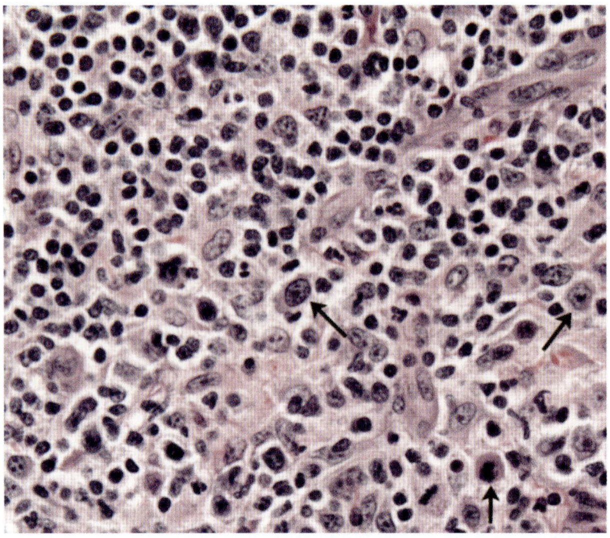

Figure 5. Skin from dog 18; inflamed nonepitheliotropic cutaneous T-cell lymphoma. Dermal infiltrate rich in cytologically normal, small lymphocytes also contains large, cytologically atypical lymphocytes (angled arrows); mitotic figures are evident in these latter cells (vertical arrow). H&E stain.

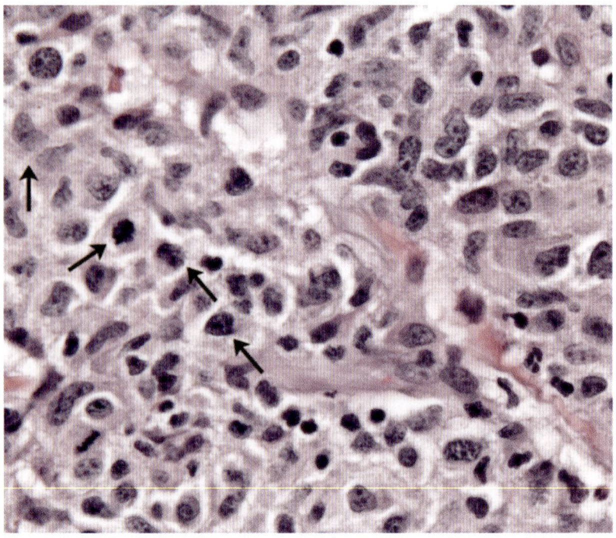

Figure 6. Skin from dog 1; inflamed nonepitheliotropic cutaneous T-cell lymphoma. Dermal infiltrate contains mainly large, cytologically atypical lymphocytes (angled arrows) and abundant histiocytes (vertical arrows). H&E stain.

T-Cell antigen receptor gene rearrangement analysis in inflamed NE-CTCL

Molecular clonality determination was performed in 23 dogs by amplifying the CDR3 region of the TRG locus in genomic DNA extracted from paraffin blocks. The simplex PCR primer set was used in all 23 dogs available for testing. Clonal T-cell populations were detected in 18 of 23 dogs (78%). In most instances, the clonal T-cell population was evident within a noticeable polyclonal background. Two dogs had a pseudoclonal result (dogs 11 and 21); two dogs (dogs 18 and 24) had a polyclonal result, and the DNA from another dog failed to amplify (dog 13). The multiplex PCR primer set was more recently developed.[16] Thirteen dogs were assessed with this primer set. Clonal T-cell populations were detected in 11 of 13 dogs (85%); two dogs (dogs 12 and 24) had a polyclonal result. Four dogs that did not have clonal results with the simplex PCR primers exhibited clonal T-cell populations with the multiplex PCR primers. If the results for both primer sets were pooled, clonal T-cell populations were detected in 22 of 23 dogs (96%).

Discussion

Canine inflamed NE-CTCL targets the skin. The frequently affected sites included face (lips, nasal planum and eyelids), lower extremities (paws and interdigital folds), neck and trunk. Lesions presented as nonpruritic nodules, plaques or masses, which were frequently ulcerated and crusted. An initial diagnosis of cutaneous reactive histiocytosis (11 dogs) or histiocytic neoplasia (three dogs) was made by primary pathologists. The clinical course was quite variable and covered a range of 1–36 months. However, inflamed NE-CTCL behaved most like a high-grade PTCL in the majority of dogs, with a median survival of only 9 months.

The difficulty in distinguishing cutaneous reactive histiocytosis from inflamed NE-CTCL was evident in the submissions to our laboratory. This is probably because cutaneous reactive histiocytosis lesions present with a merged histological pattern B plus C lesion topography. The identification of clusters of cytologically atypical, large lymphocytes in the lesions was an important feature, which raised concern for lymphoma. These clusters of cytologically atypical cells are most often lacking in cutaneous reactive histiocytosis. However, the diagnosis of inflamed NE-CTCL was most indicated by examination of CD3 immunostains and by T-cell receptor gene rearrangement analysis. Marked variation in the density of CD3 expression by large, atypical T cells was an important feature, which fortunately was commonly observed. The T cells often showed evidence of almost complete loss of CD3 expression. One of the key immunophenotypic features for diagnosis of T-cell lymphoma is hierarchical

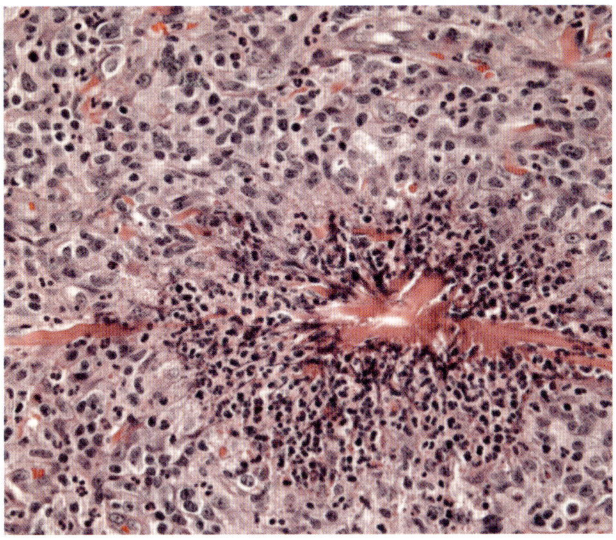

Figure 7. Skin from dog 21; inflamed nonepitheliotropic cutaneous T-cell lymphoma. Histiocytic and lymphocytic dermal infiltrate surrounds a focus of eosinophils gathered around a collagen fibre with deposits of Splendore-Hoeppli-like material. H&E stain.

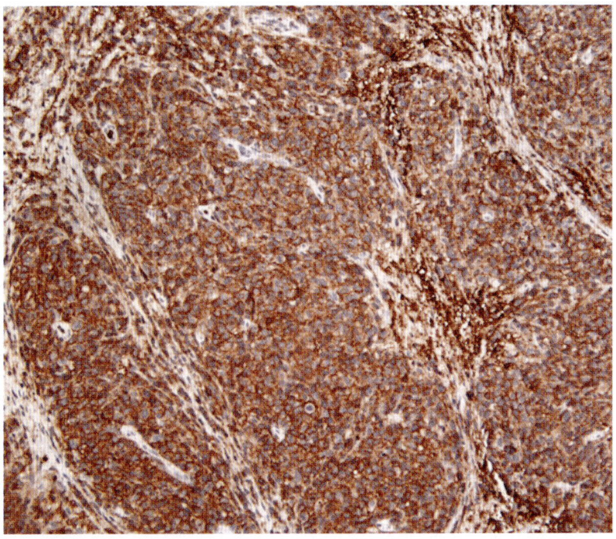

Figure 8. Skin from dog 1; inflamed nonepitheliotropic cutaneous T-cell lymphoma. Perivascular histiocytes express abundant CD18. Immunoperoxidase method with Vector Red substrate and Gill's haematoxylin counterstain.

loss of antigens expressed by all normal T cells. In human PTCL, antigen loss, in decreasing order of frequency, occurs with CD7, CD5, CD3 and CD2.[10,12,17] In the dog, only CD3 is assessable in formalin-fixed tissue, which is commonly available for diagnosis.

The T-cell antigen receptor gene rearrangement analysis, using the TRG locus, confirmed clonal T-cell populations in 96% of dogs purported to have inflamed NE-CTCL. This is a very high success rate for T-cell antigen receptor gene rearrangement utilizing a single locus, and is likely to be due to the unique structure of the canine TRG locus.[18,19] In a previous study of canine epitheliotropic CTCL, clonal T-cell populations were detected in the lesions of 80% of dogs; in that study, only the simplex TRG primer set was available. The multiplex TRG primer set was developed after the structure of the canine TRG locus was discovered.[16,18] The multiplex TRG primer set amplifies all rearranged variable (V) and joining (J) genes in the canine TRG locus. The structure of the canine TRG is unique, comprising eight tandem cassettes with up to three V genes, two J genes and a single constant (C) gene each. Seven TRG cassettes per allele can rearrange independently; this makes the canine TRG locus very sensitive for the detection of clonal T-cell expansions in lymphoproliferative diseases. In a study of a group of canine T-cell lymphomas, an average of 4.6 rearrangements was found per lymphoma. These data indicate that canine T cells rearrange multiple TRG cassettes per allele.[20] In the present study, the multiplex TRG primer set detected clonal T-cell populations in four of five dogs in which the simplex TRG primer set failed to detect clonality. These results further validate the superiority of the multiplex canine TRG primer set for clonality determination.

Failure to detect clonality in the neoplastic T-cell infiltrate occurred in one dog with morphological and immunophenotypic evidence of inflamed NE-CTCL. A likely explanation may involve the substantial polyclonal T-cell background infiltrate, which is commonly encountered in lesions of this type. The sensitivity of TRG amplification within a lesion is influenced by the frequency of the neoplastic clone in the population of infiltrating cells and by the complexity of the associated polyclonal repertoire. The neoplastic clone needs to occur at a frequency of about 5–10% for detection to occur.[21,22] Also, minor clonal populations are at greater risk of going undetected if they involve frequently rearranged Vγ and Jγ segments, which will be lost amidst the polyclonal repertoire.[22]

The demonstration of clonal T-cell populations in inflamed NE-CTCL by T-cell receptor gene rearrangement

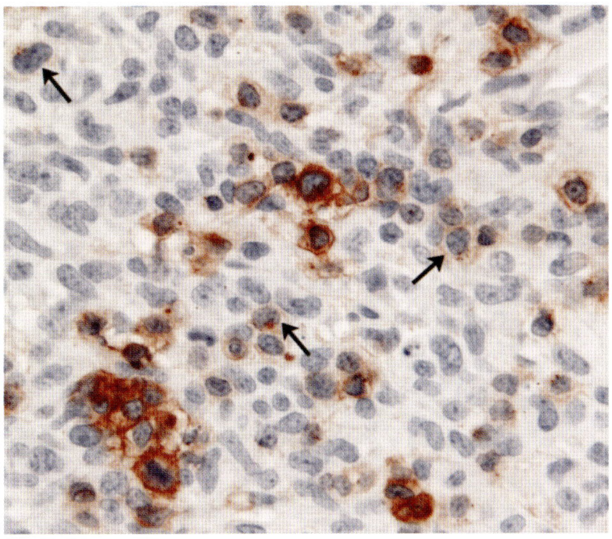

Figure 9. Skin from dog 1; inflamed nonepitheliotropic cutaneous T-cell lymphoma. Marked variation in the intensity of CD3 expression by large, cytologically atypical T cells. T cells show very weak CD3 expression (angled arrows). Immunoperoxidase method with aminoethyl carbazole substrate and Gill's haematoxylin counterstain.

analysis was critical to establishing the diagnosis. An important question arises; is it possible to demonstrate clonal T-cell populations in reactive inflammatory lesions? Investigation of cutaneous lymphoproliferative disease in humans has revealed a low incidence of clonal T-cell expansion in reactive inflammatory disease.[19] In that study, the authors urged caution in the interpretation of PCR clonality data, and recommended integration of clinical data and the results of morphological and immunohistochemical analyses. We also believe in the importance of integrative diagnostics. We have conducted limited molecular clonality analyses (with simplex and multiplex TRG primer sets) on known cases of cutaneous reactive histiocytosis (four dogs); the results so far indicate polyclonal T-cell expansion. We intend to continue this investigation in the future. It is also imperative to determine clinical outcomes in the inflamed NE-CTCL case series. For the majority of cases (13 dogs), clinical follow-up confirmed that the lesions progressed as expected for high-grade T-cell lymphoma; these dogs died or were euthanized with a median survival time of 9 months. Seven dogs are still alive (1–36 months after diagnosis). This marked heterogeneity in clinical behaviour is a feature of inflamed NE-CTCL, and may in some part be due to the intense host inflammatory response to the lymphoma.

A significant inflammatory component in cutaneous lymphoma of humans has been noted in both B- and T-cell lymphomas, although uncommonly.[23–26] Two variants of human MF, namely granulomatous MF and granulomatous slack skin, have a prominent histiocytic component, which can mimic sarcoidosis, granuloma annulare or granulomatous dermatitis.[23,25,26] In humans, NE-CTCL can also have a prominent histiocytic infiltration, which has led to misdiagnosis of granulomatous dermatitis.[26] T-cell antigen receptor gene rearrangement analysis was invaluable for obtaining the correct diagnosis in these instances. Clonal T-cell expansion can occur rarely in cutaneous inflammatory lymphoproliferative diseases.[19] One solution to this potential pitfall is to conduct dual TRG clonality assessment (i.e. to conduct the analysis on two separate sites), which largely excludes false-positive results.[23] Systematic application of this approach has not been conducted in veterinary medicine due to cost constraints. However, in some instances dual TRG clonality assessment may be warranted and should be considered if clinical data are not in agreement with the results of molecular analyses.

In conclusion, the recognition of inflamed NE-CTCL and its differentiation from reactive cutaneous histiocytosis depends on careful assessment of clinical disease progression, lymphocyte morphology and immunostaining patterns. Clusters of cytologically atypical lymphocytes with highly variable CD3 expression, especially partial to almost complete loss of expression, are important features. Confirmation of the diagnosis is best accomplished by T-cell antigen receptor gene rearrangement analysis. Application of these procedures, which are now more widely available, should enable increased recognition of inflamed NE-CTCL and ensure that appropriate treatment is selected earlier in the clinical course. It is anticipated that some improvement in survival time will result.

Acknowledgements

The authors thank the numerous clinicians and pathologists who submitted case material for this study. We also thank Rick Hayes for assistance with artwork, Chris Barker for statistical assistance and Kristy Harman for able technical assistance.

References

1. Moore PF, Affolter VK, Graham PS *et al.* Canine epitheliotropic cutaneous T-cell lymphoma: an investigation of T-cell receptor immunophenotype, lesion topography and molecular clonality. *Vet Dermatol* 2009; 20: 569–576.
2. Moore PF, Olivry T. Cutaneous lymphomas in companion animals. *Clin Dermatol* 1994; 12: 499–505.
3. Moore PF, Olivry T, Naydan DK. Canine cutaneous epitheliotropic lymphoma (mycosis fungoides) is a proliferative disorder of CD8+ T cells. *Am J Pathol* 1994; 144: 421–429.
4. Ralfkiaer E, Cerroni L, Sander CA *et al.* Mycosis fungoides. In: Swerdlow SH, Campo E, Harris NL *et al.*, eds. *WHO Classification of Tumors of the Haematopoietic and Lymphoid Tissues.* 4th edn. Lyon: International Agency for Research on Cancer (IARC), 2008; 296–298.
5. Affolter VK, Gross TL, Moore PF. Indolent cutaneous T-cell lymphoma presenting as cutaneous lymphocytosis in dogs. *Vet Dermatol* 2009; 20: 577–585.
6. Day MJ. Immunophenotypic characterization of cutaneous lymphoid neoplasia in the dog and cat. *J Comp Pathol* 1995; 112: 79–96.
7. Valli VE, Jacobs RM, Parodi AL, *et al.* eds. *World Health Organization International Histological Classification of Tumors of Domestic Animals.* vol. VIII (2nd edn.). Washington, DC: Armed Forces Institute of Pathology, 2002; 43.
8. Swerdlow SH, Campo E, Harris NL, *et al.* eds. *WHO Classification of Tumors of the Haematopoietic and Lymphoid Tissues,* 4th edn. Lyon: International Agency for Research on Cancer (IARC), 2008; 12. (abstract)
9. Agostinelli C, Piccaluga PP, Went P *et al.* Peripheral T cell lymphoma, not otherwise specified: the stuff of genes, dreams and therapies. *J Clin Pathol* 2008; 61: 1160–1167.
10. Rodriguez-Abreu D, Filho VB, Zucca E. Peripheral T-cell lymphomas, unspecified (or not otherwise specified): a review. *Hematol Oncol* 2008; 26: 8–20.
11. Gaulard P, Berti E, Willemze R, *et al.* Primary cutaneous peripheral T-cell lymphomas, rare subtypes. In: Swerdlow SH, Campo E, Harris NL, *et al.* eds. *WHO Classification of Tumors of the Haematopoietic and Lymphoid Tissues.* 4th edn. Lyon: International Agency for Research on Cancer (IARC), 2008; 302–305.
12. Knowles DM. Immunophenotypic and antigen receptor gene rearrangement analysis in T cell neoplasia. *Am J Pathol* 1989; 134: 761–785.
13. Affolter VK, Moore PF. Localized and disseminated histiocytic sarcoma of dendritic cell origin in dogs. *Vet Pathol* 2002; 39: 74–83.
14. Valli VE, Vernau W, de Lorimier LP *et al.* Canine indolent nodular lymphoma. *Vet Pathol* 2006; 43: 241–256.
15. Vernau W, Moore PF. An immunophenotypic study of canine leukemias and preliminary assessment of clonality by polymerase chain reaction. *Vet Immunol Immunopathol* 1999; 69: 145–164.
16. Keller SM, Moore PF. A novel clonality assay for the assessment of canine T cell proliferations. *Vet Immunol Immunopathol* 2012; 145: 410–419.
17. Picker LJ, Weiss LM, Medeiros LJ *et al.* Immunophenotypic criteria for the diagnosis of non-Hodgkin's lymphoma. *Am J Pathol* 1987; 128: 181–201.
18. Massari S, Bellahcene F, Vaccarelli G *et al.* The deduced structure of the T cell receptor gamma locus in *Canis lupus familiaris.* *Mol Immunol* 2009; 46: 2728–2736.

19. Sandberg Y, Heule F, Lam K *et al.* Molecular immunoglobulin/T-cell receptor clonality analysis in cutaneous lymphoproliferations. Experience with the BIOMED-2 standardized polymerase chain reaction protocol. *Haematologica* 2003; 88: 659–670.
20. Keller SM, Moore PF. Rearrangement patterns of the canine TCRγ locus in a distinct group of T cell lymphomas. *Vet Immunol Immunopathol* 2012; 145: 350–361.
21. Hsiao PF, Hsiao CH, Lin YC *et al.* Histopathologic-molecular correlation in early mycosis fungoides using T-cell receptor γ gene rearrangement by polymerase chain reaction with laser capture microdissection. *J Formos Med Assoc* 2007; 106: 265–272.
22. van Dongen JJ, Langerak AW, Bruggemann M *et al.* Design and standardization of PCR primers and protocols for detection of clonal immunoglobulin and T-cell receptor gene recombinations in suspect lymphoproliferations: report of the BIOMED-2 Concerted Action BMH4-CT98-3936. *Leukemia* 2003; 17: 2257–2317.
23. Dabiri S, Morales A, Ma L *et al.* The frequency of dual TCR-PCR clonality in granulomatous disorders. *J Cutan Pathol* 2011; 38: 704–709.
24. Li S, Griffin CA, Mann RB *et al.* Primary cutaneous T-cell-rich B-cell lymphoma: clinically distinct from its nodal counterpart? *Mod Pathol* 2001; 14: 10–13.
25. Pfaltz K, Kerl K, Palmedo G *et al.* Clonality in sarcoidosis, granuloma annulare, and granulomatous mycosis fungoides. *Am J Dermatopathol* 2011; 33: 659–662.
26. Scarabello A, Leinweber B, Ardigo M *et al.* Cutaneous lymphomas with prominent granulomatous reaction: a potential pitfall in the histopathologic diagnosis of cutaneous T- and B-cell lymphomas. *Am J Surg Pathol* 2002; 26: 1259–1268.

Part 7

Equine Dermatology

To cite this article, please use DOI: 10.1111/j.1365-3164.2012.01080.x

7.1

Comparison of hair follicle histology between horses with pituitary pars intermedia dysfunction and excessive hair growth and normal aged horses

Marie Innerå*[,1], Annette D. Petersen*, Danielle R. Desjardins†[,2], Barbara A. Steficek†, Edmund J. Rosser Jr* and Harold C. Schott II‡

*Department of Small Animal Clinical Sciences, †Diagnostic Center for Population and Animal Health and ‡Department of Large Animal Clinical Sciences, College of Veterinary Medicine, Michigan State University, East Lansing, MI 48824, USA

Correspondence: Annette D. Petersen, Department of Small Animal Clinical Sciences, Veterinary Medical Center, 736 Wilson Road, Room D208, Michigan State University, East Lansing, MI 48824, USA. E-mail: petersen@cvm.msu.edu

Background – Pituitary pars intermedia dysfunction (PPID) in older equids is commonly recognized by a long hair coat that fails to shed.

Objective – The aim of this study was to compare hair follicle stages in PPID-affected horses with excessively long hair coats with the stages of normal aged horses (controls) and to compare hair follicle stages in PPID-affected horses after 6 months of treatment with pergolide mesylate with those of control horses.

Animals – Eight PPID-affected horses and four normal, age-matched, control horses.

Methods – Skin biopsies were collected from the neck and rump of PPID-affected and control horses. A diagnosis of PPID was established based on hair coat changes and supportive overnight dexamethasone suppression test results. Skin biopsies were repeated after 6 months of treatment with pergolide. The number of hair follicles in anagen (A) or telogen (T) was counted for each skin biopsy using transverse sections.

Results – Pretreatment biopsies had a greater percentage of A follicles (neck 96%, rump 95%) and a lower percentage of T follicles (neck 4%, rump 5%) in PPID-affected horses than in control horses (A, neck 15%, rump 25%; and T, neck 85%, rump 75%). After treatment with pergolide, all PPID-affected horses had improved shedding, and the percentages of A follicles (neck 69%, rump 70%) and T follicles (neck 31%, rump 30%) were not different from untreated control horses (A, neck 68%, rump 82%; and T, neck 32%, rump 18%).

Conclusions – These findings document that excessive hair growth (hypertrichosis) in PPID-affected horses is due to persistence of hair follicles in A. Furthermore, treatment with pergolide improved shedding and reduced the percentage of A follicles in PPID-affected horses.

Introduction

Pituitary pars intermedia dysfunction (PPID), also known as equine Cushing's disease, is the most common endocrinopathy of equids.[1,2] This disease increases in prevalence with age and may affect 15–20% of equids over 15 years of age.[3] Furthermore, a recent report documented clinical findings consistent with PPID in nearly 40% of equids over 30 years of age.[4]

Several clinical signs are observed in PPID-affected equids; a pathognomonic sign in over 80% of cases is a long and often curly hair coat that fails to shed.[1] Hair coat changes with PPID typically progress over several years. Initial changes include delayed shedding and persistence of long hairs under the jaw, along the jugular grooves and ventral neck, and on the palmar and plantar aspects of the limbs. End-stage PPID-affected equids have a generalized, long and shaggy hair coat that fails to shed regardless of season or climate. Other dermatological problems may include excessive or decreased sweating and recurrent pyoderma, notably dermatophilosis.[1,2] Non-dermatological clinical signs can include lethargy, muscle wasting, regional fat deposits, polyuria and polydipsia, recurrent infections and chronic laminitis.[1,2]

The excessively long hair coat of PPID-affected horses has been described to be caused by hair follicle arrest in

Accepted 28 May 2012

Sources of Funding: American College of Veterinary Dermatology Resident Research Award.

Conflict of Interest: Harold Schott is a consultant for Boehringer-Ingelheim Vetmedica, Inc., and skin samples examined in this study were collected from a cohort of horses enrolled in an open field trial for Prascend[TM].

An abstract with preliminary data on this study has been published: *Vet Dermatol* 2011; 22: 300.

[1]Marie Innerå's present address is Finnsnes Dyreklinikk AS, PB 228, 9305 Finnsnes, Norway.

[2]Danielle Desjardin's present address is Phoenix Central Laboratory, 4338 Harbour Pointe, Boulevard SW Mukilteo, WA 98275, USA.

anagen (A) or telogen (T);[5,6] however, no data have been presented to support these opposing claims. An equine dermatology textbook stated: 'To the authors' knowledge, no studies have been published concerning the hair follicle stages from horses with PPID'.[7] In our experience, trichograms from horses with PPID reveal hairs in A; furthermore, these hairs are difficult to epilate. Consequently, we hypothesize that excessive hair growth in PPID-affected horses is due to a persistence of hair follicles in the A stage.

The treatment of choice for PPID-affected equids is pergolide mesylate.[8–11] Pergolide is a dopamine agonist that activates dopamine type 2 receptors on pars intermedia melanotrophs, leading to decreased production of pro-opiomelanocortin and pro-opiomelanocortin-derived peptides responsible for the varied clinical signs of PPID. A recent open field trial of pergolide (Prascend™ 1 mg tablets; Boehringer-Ingelheim Vetmedica, Inc., St Joseph, MO, USA) reported improvement in hair coat in 99 of 111 (89%) PPID-affected equids after 6 months of treatment.[12] We hypothesize that the percentages of A and T stages of hair follicles will be similar in PPID-affected horses post-treatment and normal aged horses.

Materials and methods

All procedures performed were approved by the Animal Care and Use Committee of Michigan State University and included owner consent.

Animals

The affected horses were eight horses with PPID, five mares and three geldings, ranging from 20 to 29 years of age (mean 24 years). The group included two Morgan horses, two quarter horses, one Arabian and three mixed breed horses. The eight PPID-affected horses were either client owned (n = 5) or had been donated (n = 3) to Michigan State University and were enrolled in an open field trial to assess the efficacy of pergolide mesylate (Prascend™ 1 mg tablets; Boehringer-Ingelheim Vetmedica, Inc.) for the control of clinical signs of PPID.

The diagnosis of PPID was confirmed by clinical signs (characteristic excessively long hair coats) and overnight dexamethasone suppression test (ODST) results (failure of endogenous cortisol to suppress below 1 μg/dL 19 h after intramuscular administration of 40 μg/kg dexamethasone).[13] Normal controls were four horses, three mares and one gelding, ranging in age from 21 to 29 years (mean 25 years). The group included two standardbred horses, one quarter horse and one thoroughbred. The aged control horses were reported to have had normal hair coat sheds the previous spring, normal winter hair coats at the study start, and normal ODST results (nonsupportive of PPID). These horses were all donated animals with similar husbandry to the donated PPID-affected horses. During the 6 month treatment period, all 12 horses were housed at pasture, with supplemental hay feeding until pasture grass was available (either at Michigan State University or at the home pasture). All horses had spent their entire lives in the northern hemisphere.

Sample collection

The hair coat was clipped from a 5 cm × 5 cm area of skin on the left side of the neck and a site overlying the left gluteal region. Skin biopsy sites were infiltrated subcutaneously with 1 mL of lidocaine HCl (APP Pharmaceuticals LCC, Schaumburg, IL, USA), and two 8 mm skin punch biopsy samples (Acu-Punch® Acuderm Inc., Fort Lauderdale, FL, USA) were obtained, one from each site. Samples were fixed in 10% neutral buffered formalin and stored at room temperature until all samples were collected. Specimens were embedded in paraffin and sectioned in a routine longitudinal (vertical) fashion. In addition, biopsies were also sectioned in a transverse (horizontal) plane parallel to the surface of the epidermis, at the level of, or slightly below, entry of the sebaceous duct in the mid-dermis ('Swiss cheese' cut).[14] The correct level was approximated to reflect the normal sebaceous gland dermal anatomical placement within the upper one-third of the dermis. Five-micrometre-thick sections were mounted on slides and stained with haematoxylin and eosin. Additional deeper or more superficial sections of the paraffin blocks were made as needed to achieve cross-sectioning at the level of the follicular infundibulum–isthmus junction. Slides were randomly numbered to blind the investigators during histological examination.

Clinical evaluation

For the open field trial, hair coat changes were scored on a 0–3 scoring system, as follows: 0 = normal, no unusual hair growth; 1 = regional hair coat changes, long hair growth restricted to discrete areas (lower jaw, jugular area, and palmar or plantar aspects of limbs); 2 = generalized hair coat changes (slightly to moderately long hair coat that fails to shed out as in previous years); and 3 = severe hair coat changes (severely long and/or curly hair coat over the entire body that fails to shed). All eight PPID-affected horses were enrolled between 1 November and 31 January and had a hair coat score of '3' when pretreatment skin biopsy samples were collected. The four control horses had a hair coat score of '0', and skin biopsy samples were collected during the same time period.

Pergolide treatment

The PPID-affected horses were treated with pergolide (2 μg/kg, orally, once daily). They were re-evaluated by clinical examination and an ODST after 3 and 6 months of treatment. If ODST results remained supportive of PPID after 3 months of treatment, the dose of pergolide was increased to 4 μg/kg, orally, once daily. At the 6 month evaluation (between 1 May and 31 July), a second set of skin biopsy samples from the neck and rump were collected from sites adjacent to the original skin biopsy sites. These biopsy samples were processed as previously described.

Histological examination

Longitudinal (vertical) sections were initially evaluated at low- (×4) and high-power magnification (×20 and ×40) to assess general histological features, including inflammation. Transverse sections were subsequently evaluated under low-power magnification (×4) independently by two investigators (M.I. and A.D.P.). Using a standard light microscope equipped with a 1 mm^2 optical grid reticule, the number of hair follicles within the same grid area was counted by each investigator, and the growth stage (A or T) was classified for each hair follicle. Criteria previously described for morphological evaluation of human scalp[14] and canine hair follicles[15] were used to classify equine hair follicle growth stages. Anagen follicles were characterized by a hair shaft surrounded by a well-defined inner root sheath, presence of trichohyaline granules in the inner root sheath, and absence of tricholemmal keratinization (Figure 1). Telogen follicles were characterized by absence of a well-defined inner root sheath, tricholemmal keratinization, and volumetric reduction of the outer root sheath (Figure 2). As catagen follicles are difficult to identify on transverse sections and are typically few in number, when suspected they were counted as T, because catagen represents a transition to T.[14,15]

Statistical analysis

Results are reported as means ± SEM. Agreement (interclass correlation) of hair follicle categorization between the two investigators was good (>90% for all biopsy samples). Thus, mean percentages of the two investigators' observations of A and T follicles for each biopsy were analysed by a split-plot ANOVA using grouping factors of disease status (PPID or normal) and growth stage (A or T) and a repeat factor of site (neck or rump). ANOVA was performed with a commercial software package (SAS version 9.1; SAS Institute, Cary,

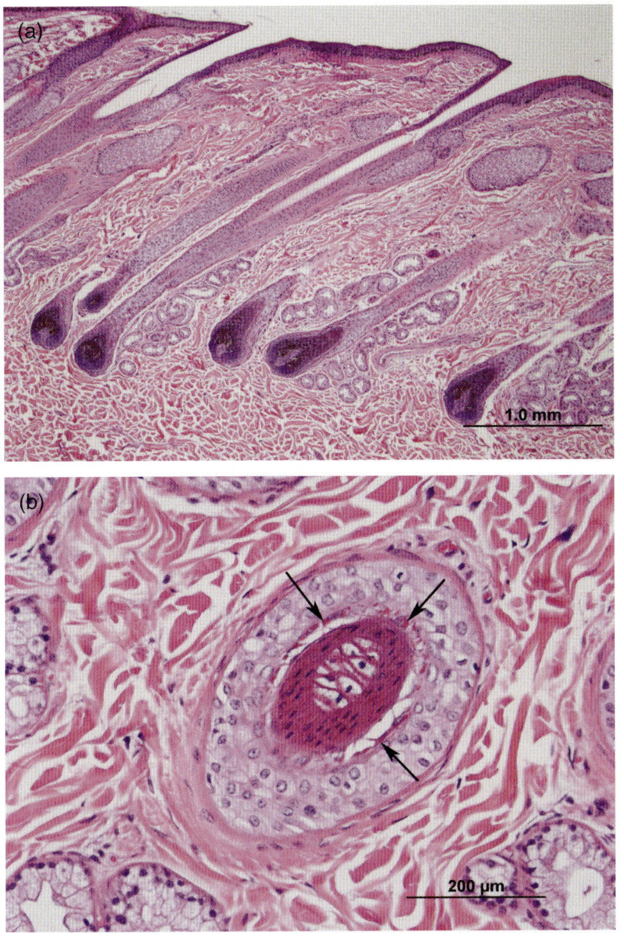

Figure 1. (a) Low-power photomicrograph of a haematoxylin and eosin stained longitudinal section of a skin biopsy collected from a horse with pituitary pars intermedia dysfunction showing hair follicles primarily in anagen. (b) A high-power photomicrograph of the same biopsy in transverse section showing an anagen hair follicle with a well-defined inner root sheath, presence of trichohyaline granules in the inner root sheath, and absence of tricholemmal keratinization. The arrows point to the trichohyaline granules in the inner root sheath.

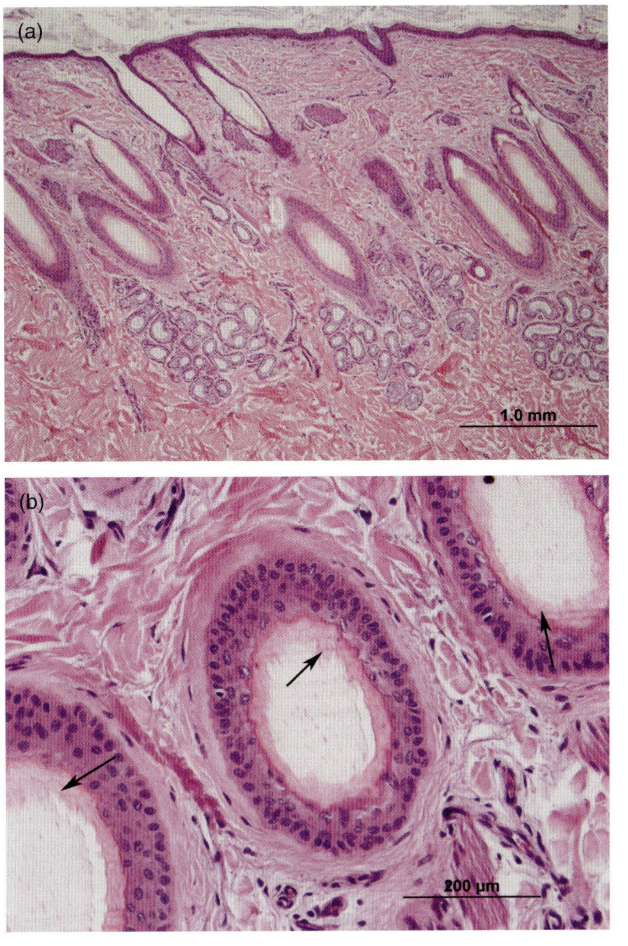

Figure 2. (a) Low-power photomicrograph of a haematoxylin and eosin stained longitudinal section of a skin biopsy collected from a normal aged horse showing hair follicles primarily in telogen. (b) A high-power photomicrograph of the same biopsy in transverse section showing a telogen hair follicle characterized by absence of a well-defined inner root sheath, tricholemmal keratinization and volumetric reduction of the outer root sheath. The arrows point to the tricholemmal keratinization.

NC, USA). When significant *F* ratios were detected, using a *P* value of <0.05, multiple comparisons were performed with the Bonferroni correction for least significant differences.

Results

Longitudinal (vertical) skin biopsy sections were evaluated at all levels, including epidermis, dermis, pilosebaceous units and hypodermis. These sections contained between eight and 24 hair follicles for examination, with no evidence of follicular structural abnormalities, inflammation or fibrosis being seen in either PPID-affected or normal aged horse skin at either time point. For transverse (horizontal) sections of neck and rump biopsy samples from both PPID-affected horses and control horses, there were no significant differences in the number of hair follicles counted within the grid area by investigators 1 and 2 at either time point (Table 1). Using the combined counts of both investigators, PPID-affected horses had a greater percentage of A follicles (neck 96%, rump 95%) and a lower percentage of T follicles (neck 4%, rump 5%) than control horses (A, neck 15%, rump 25%; and T, neck 85%, rump 75%) prior to pergolide treatment (Table 2).

After 3 months of treatment with pergolide, clinical improvement in PPID-affected horses was largely limited to improved attitude, decreased sweating, and decreased polyuria and polydipsia. Median hair coat score in PPID-affected horses had decreased to 2.5 (range 2–3), and ODST results remained supportive of PPID in all horses. Consequently, the dose of pergolide was increased to 4 μg/kg, orally, once daily in all horses. After 6 months of pergolide treatment, improved shedding was apparent in all eight treated horses, and median hair coat score had decreased to 1 (range 0–2). Furthermore, ODST results were normal (no longer supportive of PPID) in four of eight horses. There was no significant difference in median hair coat scores for horses with normal ODST results (0.5; range 0–1) when compared with horses with abnormal ODST results (2; range 0–2); however, statistical power (0.2) was low owing to the small sample size. The four control horses remained healthy during the study period, and ODST results at the time when the second biopsy specimens were collected remained normal.

Table 1. Number (mean ± SEM) of hair follicles counted by investigators 1 and 2 in skin biopsy samples collected from the neck and rump of eight horses with pituitary pars intermedia dysfunction (PPID) and four aged normal horses at two time points ('pre' and 'post')

	Investigator 1	Investigator 2
PPID-affected horses (*n* = 8)		
Neck, pre	71 ± 10	70 ± 10
Rump, pre	57 ± 7	56 ± 7
Neck, post	59 ± 7	60 ± 7
Rump, post	53 ± 7	53 ± 7
Control horses (*n* = 4)		
Neck, pre	69 ± 9	67 ± 8
Rump, pre	55 ± 12	57 ± 12
Neck, post	78 ± 16	77 ± 16
Rump, post	66 ± 5	64 ± 4

There were no significant differences between hair follicle counts at either site or time point by either investigator.

Table 2. Percentage of anagen and telogen hair follicles in skin biopsy samples collected from the neck and rump of eight horses with PPID and four aged normal horses

	Percentage anagen (mean ± SEM)	Percentage telogen (mean ± SEM)
Pretreatment (autumn and winter)		
PPID-affected horses (*n* = 8)		
Neck	$96 \pm 3^{a,1}$	$4 \pm 3^{b,1}$
Rump	$95 \pm 3^{a,1}$	$5 \pm 3^{b,1}$
Control horses (*n* = 4)		
Neck	$15 \pm 12^{a,2}$	$85 \pm 18^{b,2}$
Rump	$25 \pm 22^{a,2}$	$75 \pm 20^{b,2}$
Post-treatment (spring and summer)		
PPID-affected horses (*n* = 8)		
Neck	69 ± 10^{a}	31 ± 9^{b}
Rump	70 ± 11^{a}	30 ± 11^{b}
Control horses (*n* = 4)		
Neck	68 ± 20^{a}	32 ± 19^{b}
Rump	82 ± 15^{a}	18 ± 15^{b}

Pretreatment samples were collected in autumn and winter months, and post-treatment samples (only PPID-affected horses were treated with pergolide mesylate) were collected in spring and summer months. For each time period, different letter superscripts within a row indicate significant differences ($P < 0.05$) between hair follicle stages, and different number superscripts within a column indicate significant differences ($P < 0.05$) between PPID-affected and control horses.

Using the combined counts of both investigators, there were no significant differences in percentages of A and T follicles between all eight PPID-affected horses treated for 6 months with pergolide and control horses (Table 2). However, as is evident from the large SEM values, there was substantial variability in hair follicle stages in PPID-affected horses after the treatment period. Furthermore, although not a significant difference (again, sample size was small), the four PPID-affected horses with abnormal ODST results after 6 months of treatment tended to have a higher percentage of A follicles (neck 83%, rump 92%) compared with the four PPID-affected horses with normal ODST results after 6 months (neck 58%, rump 54%). Finally, considerable variability in hair follicle stages was found in the normal aged horses at both biopsy times.

Discussion

This study demonstrated that the excessively long hair coat in horses with advanced PPID is a consequence of persistence of hair follicles in the A stage. As limited information exists on hair follicle morphology in PPID, horses with obvious hair coat changes consistent with advanced disease were selected for this study to characterize hair follicle histology. Furthermore, based on the findings of Headington[14] and Credille *et al.*,[15] skin biopsy samples were sectioned in a transverse (horizontal) plane to increase the number of hair follicles available for histological examination. By using this method, PPID-affected horses with markedly long hair coats were found to have a higher percentage of A follicles and a lower percentage of T follicles when compared with aged control horses, supporting the hypothesis that the excessively long hair coat of PPID-affected horses is due to persistence of hair follicles in the A stage of hair growth. Next, treatment with pergolide mesylate improved hair coat shedding and reduced the number of A follicles in PPID-affected horses to values similar to those of normal aged horses. Although not a statistically significant finding, it is of interest that there was a tendency for a greater reduction in the percentage of A follicles in the four PPID-affected horses that had normal ODST results after 6 months of treatment in comparison to the four PPID-affected horses with persistently abnormal ODST results.

Hirsutism is the term commonly used to describe the essentially pathognomonic long and shaggy hair coat characteristic of equids with advanced PPID.[1,2] Use of this term appears to have been introduced in an early case report by Eriksson *et al.* [16] in 1956, and it subsequently became firmly ingrained in the equine veterinary literature. By definition, hirsutism refers to excessive growth of coarse and pigmented terminal hairs in women in androgen-dependent areas of the body where hair is not typically present (e.g. beard or chest).[17] Hirsutism is commonly associated with polycystic ovary syndrome in women, but it can also accompany Cushing's disease and pituitary tumours. The association of hirsutism with Cushing's disease and the common description of PPID in horses as equine Cushing's disease probably resulted in the accepted use of this term to describe the abnormal hair coat of PPID-affected equids.

The pathogenesis of the hair coat changes in PPID-affected equids remains poorly understood and contrasts sharply with alopecia observed in dogs with pituitary-dependent hyperadrenocorticism.[5,6] An early suggestion was that both increased sweating and excessive hair growth could be a consequence of pressure exerted on the hypothalamic thermoregulatory centre due to an enlarged pituitary gland.[18] Other explanations have included effects of excess androgenic steroids (testosterone) produced by the adrenal gland[19] (again, probably due to comparison of PPID with Cushing's disease in people) or excess α-melanocyte-stimulating hormone produced by the pars intermedia.[20] To our knowledge, no data exist to support these purported mechanisms. However, because excessive hair growth with PPID in horses is similar in both sexes, as well as in castrated males, excess androgenic steroid effects would seem an unlikely cause of persistent hair growth.

In contrast to androgen-induced hair growth in women, the term hypertrichosis is used to describe excessive hair growth on any part of the body, beyond accepted limits for a particular age, race or sex.[21] Hypertrichosis may be generalized or localized and can be a consequence of congenital disorders or a marker of systemic disease. In agreement with more recent pathology[6,22] and equine dermatology textbooks,[7] we support use of the term hypertrichosis as being more appropriate than hirsutism to describe the nearly pathognomonic hair coat pattern of PPID-affected equids.

Compared with many disorders accompanied by alopecia, acquired hypertrichosis, especially in a generalized form, is uncommon.[21,23] In humans, hypertrichosis has been observed with autoimmune hepatitis, porphyria, hypothyroidism, malabsorption syndromes, juvenile dermatomyositis and acrodynia.[21,23] Development of hypertrichosis has also been associated with central nervous system trauma and diseases, including encephalitis, multiple sclerosis, schizophrenia and anorexia nervosa.[23] Furthermore, hypertrichosis can be an adverse effect of medications, notably with use of ciclosporin in both humans and animals.[23,24] In equids, with the exception of spontaneous hypertrichosis in the Bashkir curly breed,[25] PPID is the only recognized cause of naturally occurring hypertrichosis and has been documented to be the most accurate diagnostic indicator for PPID.[26]

Considerable variability in hair follicle stages was found at both time points in this study. Owing to the design of the open field drug trial, each skin biopsy sampling period lasted 3 months, with a 6 month interval between sampling periods. Potential seasonal effects were unavoidable and may have contributed to the variability observed. Skin biopsy samples from both PPID-affected and control horses were initially obtained during late autumn and winter months in a temperate area of the northern hemisphere (latitude 43°N, longitude 84°W). Although there has been limited investigation of the equine hair growth cycle, horses in this region typically shed the winter hair coat from March to May. As a consequence, the majority of hair follicles would have been expected to be in T during the late autumn and winter months, as was found in the control horses. Thus, we considered these months to be an ideal time of year to collect biopsy samples to compare hair follicle stages between untreated PPID-affected and normal horses. Another factor that may have contributed to the variability observed was that several breeds of horses were included in this study. Little is known about breed variations in horses, and this could potentially affect both hair density and shedding pattern; therefore, breed variation should be another area of further investigation.

It was not surprising that there was little improvement in hair coat in PPID-affected horses after only 3 months of pergolide treatment, because this re-evaluation occurred in late winter to early spring (February–April). The fact that the cohort of PPID-affected horses studied had advanced disease was supported by their marked hair coat changes at the start of the study and persistently abnormal ODST results after 3 months of treatment with 2 μg/kg of pergolide daily. After the dosage was increased to 4 μg/kg daily and the time of year progressed to May–July, improved shedding was observed in all PPID-affected horses, and ODST results were normal in 50% of the cohort. Consequently, collection of skin biopsy samples at this time point was considered ideal for comparison of treated PPID-affected horses with control horses. Clearly, it would also have been useful to have studied a group of hypertrichotic PPID-affected horses that did not receive pergolide treatment. Nevertheless, our data provide initial support that pergolide treatment produces a 'normalization' of the hair growth cycle in PPID-affected horses. Ideally, in future investigations the sampling periods would be more tightly controlled and could also include more frequent sampling times throughout the year.

For this study, skin biopsy specimens were obtained from the lateral neck and the gluteal region of the rump, areas that were convenient to sample. Given that all PPID-affected horses had marked, generalized hypertrichosis, we considered these appropriate regions to sample, and the similar findings in both locations suggest that persistence of the hair follicle in A may be a common feature of all areas of the body manifesting hypertrichosis. In the future, it would be of interest to compare skin biopsy results collected from multiple sites from horses in the earlier stages of PPID with regional hypertrichosis under the lower jaw, along the ventral neck, and the palmar and plantar aspects of the limbs. Further investigations could also apply techniques used to identify canine hair follicle stages in greater detail to explore whether or not canine criteria apply to the equine hair cycle and to elucidate further the cause of equine hypertrichosis.[27]

In conclusion, the results of this study demonstrate that the excessively long and curly hair coat that is essentially pathognomonic for PPID in equids is due to persistence of hair follicles in anagen. Treatment with pergolide appeared to reduce the number of anagen follicles in PPID- affected horses to values similar to those of normal aged horses. Further investigation is needed to elucidate the mechanism(s) underlying development of hypertrichosis in PPID-affected horses.

Acknowledgements

The authors thank Sue Wismer, Lauren Groppi and Julie Rapson for technical assistance, Ingeborg Langohr for assistance with photomicrographs, and Joe Hauptman for assistance with statistical analysis.

References

1. Schott HC. Pituitary pars intermedia dysfunction: equine Cushing's disease. *Vet Clin North Am Equine Pract* 2002; 18: 237–270.
2. McFarlane D. Equine pituitary pars intermedia dysfunction. *Vet Clin North Am Equine Pract* 2011; 27: 93–113.
3. McGowan TW, Pinchbeck GL, Phillips C *et al.* A survey of aged horses in Queensland, Australia. Part 2: clinical signs and owner

perceptions of health and welfare. *Aust Vet J* 2010; 88: 465–471.
4. Ireland JL, Clegg PD, McGowan CM *et al.* A cross-sectional study of geriatric horses in the United Kingdom. Part 2: health care and disease. *Equine Vet J* 2011; 43: 37–44.
5. Corke MJ. The pathogenesis of cutaneous signs in endocrine disease. *Equine Vet Educ* 1992; 4: 127–130.
6. Capen CC. Endocrine glands. In: Maxie MG, ed. *Jubb, Kennedy, and Palmer's Pathology of Domestic Animals.* 5th edn, volume 3. Philadelphia: Elsevier, 2007; 325–428.
7. Scott DW, Miller WH. *Equine Dermatology.* 2nd edn. Philadelphia: Elsevier, 2011; 360–377.
8. Beech J. Treatment of hypophyseal adenomas. *Compend Cont Educ Pract Vet* 1994; 16: 921–923.
9. Donaldson MT, LaMonte BH, Morresey P *et al.* Treatment with pergolide or cyproheptadine of pituitary pars intermedia dysfunction (equine Cushing's disease). *J Vet Intern Med* 2002; 16: 742–746.
10. Perkins GA, Lamb S, Erb HN *et al.* Plasma adrenocorticotropin (ACTH) concentrations and clinical response in horses treated for equine Cushing's disease with cyproheptadine or pergolide. *Equine Vet J* 2002; 34: 679–685.
11. Schott HC, Graves EA, Refsal KR *et al.* Diagnosis and treatment of pituitary pars intermedia dysfunction (classical Cushing's disease) and metabolic syndrome (peripheral Cushing's syndrome) in horses. In: Hillier A, Foster A, Kwochka KW, eds. *Advances in Veterinary Dermatology.* volume 5. Oxford: Blackwell Publishing Ltd, 2005; 159–169.
12. Freedom of Information Summary – NADA 141-331 – Prascend tablets for the control of clinical signs associated with pituitary pars intermedia dysfunction (equine Cushing's disease) in horses. Available at: http://www.fda.gov/downloads/AnimalVeterinary/Products/ApprovedAnimalDrugProducts/FOIADrugSummaries/UCM280354.pdf. Accessed April 12, 2012.
13. Dybdal NO, Hargreaves KM, Madigan JE *et al.* Diagnostic testing for pituitary pars intermedia dysfunction in horses. *J Am Vet Med Assoc* 1994; 204: 627–632.
14. Headington JT. Transverse microscopic anatomy of the human scalp. A basis for a morphometric approach to disorders of the hair follicle. *Arch Dermatol* 1984; 120: 449–456.
15. Credille KM, Slater MR, Moriello KA *et al.* The effects of thyroid hormones on the skin of beagle dogs. *J Vet Intern Med* 2001; 15: 539–546.
16. Eriksson K, Dyrendahl S, Grimfelt D. A case of hirsutism in connection with hypophyseal tumour in a horse. *Nord Vet* 1956; 8: 807–814.
17. Somani N, Harrison S, Bergfeld WF. The clinical evaluation of hirsutism. *Dermatol Ther* 2008; 21: 376–391.
18. Capen CC. The endocrine glands. In: Jubb KVF, Kennedy PC, Palmer N, eds. *Pathology of Domestic Animals.* volume 3, 3rd edn. Orlando: Academic Press Inc, 1985; 237–303.
19. Holscher MA, Linnabary RL, Netsky MG *et al.* Adenoma of the pars intermedia and hirsutism in a pony. *Vet Med Small Anim Clin* 1978; 73: 1197–2000.
20. van der Kolk JH, Kalsbeek HC, van Garderen F *et al.* Equine pituitary neoplasia: a clinical report of 21 cases. *Vet Rec* 1993; 133: 594–597.
21. Trüeb RM. Causes and management of hypertrichosis. *Am J Clin Dermatol* 2002; 3: 617–627.
22. Hargis AM, Ginn PE. The integument. In: Zachary JF, McGavin MD, eds. *Pathologic Basis of Veterinary Disease.* 5th edn, Philadelphia: Elsevier, 2012; 927–1084.
23. Paus R, Olsen EA, Messenger AG. Hair growth disorders. In: Wolff K, Goldsmith LA, Katz SI *et al.*, eds. *Fitzpatrick's Dermatology in General Medicin.* 7th edn. New York, NY: McGraw-Hill Medical, 2008; 753–777.
24. Radowicz SN, Power HT. Long-term use of cyclosporine in the treatment of canine atopic dermatitis. *Vet Dermatol* 2005; 16: 81–86.
25. Scott DW. Skin of the neck, mane and tail of the curly horse. *Equine Vet Educ* 2004; 16: 201–206.
26. Frank N, Andrews FM, Sommardahl CS *et al.* Evaluation of the combined dexamethasone suppression/thyrotropin-releasing hormone stimulation test for detection of pars intermedia pituitary adenomas in horses. *J Vet Intern Med* 2006; 20: 987–993.
27. Müntener T, Doherr MG, Guscetti F *et al.* The canine hair cycle – a guide for the assessment of morphological and immunohistochemical criteria. *Vet Dermatol* 2011; 22: 383–395.

To cite this article, please use DOI: 10.1111/j.1365-3164.2012.01108.x

7.2

Equine sarcoidosis: clinical signs, diagnosis, treatment and outcome of 22 cases

Marianne M. Sloet van Oldruitenborgh-Oosterbaan* and Guy C. M. Grinwist†

*Departments of Equine Sciences and †Pathobiology, Faculty of Veterinary Medicine, Utrecht University, Yalelaan 114, 3584 CM Utrecht, The Netherlands

Correspondence: Marianne Sloet van Oldruitenborgh-Oosterbaan, Department of Equine Sciences, Faculty of Veterinary Medicine, Utrecht University, Yalelaan 114, 3584 CM Utrecht, The Netherlands. E-mail: m.sloet@uu.nl

Background – Equine sarcoidosis may present as a generalized or localized exfoliative dermatitis and/or as a granulomatous inflammation of multiple organs.

Objectives – To report the clinical signs, diagnosis, treatment and outcome for 22 horses with histologically confirmed sarcoidosis.

Animals – Twenty-two horses of different breeds, between 3 and 17 years of age.

Methods – Diagnosis was based on clinical signs and histopathological findings.

Results – The following three forms of equine sarcoidosis were identified: generalized (13.6%), partially generalized (18.2%) and localized (68.2%). High-dose systemic corticosteroids were used as the initial treatment in all three forms, followed by lower doses for a variable number of weeks. No local treatment was prescribed. Case outcome was variable; one of three cases of generalized sarcoidosis was euthanized immediately and the remaining two were euthanized after 2–3 months of unsuccessful treatment; all four cases of partially generalized sarcoidosis deteriorated despite treatment and were euthanized after 3.5–12 months; two cases with localized disease showed no response or insufficient response to treatment and were euthanized; four cases recovered fully with or without treatment, and one showed partial recovery without treatment; and eight cases improved whilst receiving prednisolone but required continuous low doses to maintain remission.

Conclusions and clinical importance – Recognition of the different forms of sarcoidosis based on history, clinical appearance and histopathology assisted in making an informed choice between treatment and euthanasia and prevented unnecessary local treatment. Equine sarcoidosis should be included in the differential diagnosis of a localized exfoliative dermatitis of unknown origin.

Introduction

Equine sarcoidosis (ES) has also been referred to as 'equine idiopathic granulomatous disease', 'equine generalized granulomatous disease', 'equine systemic granulomatous disease', 'equine histiocytic disease' and 'equine histiocytic dermatitis'.[1–4]

Equine sarcoidosis is a rare disease complex that initially may present as an exfoliative dermatitis or as a nodular form characterized by granulomatous inflammation of multiple organs.[3–6] Both forms have similar outcomes; horses with exfoliative dermatitis frequently develop nodules, and horses with the nodular form will usually develop exfoliative dermatitis.[4,5] Sarcoidosis can also be categorized into the following three clinical presentations based on disease extension: 'generalized', 'partially generalized' and 'localized'. Peripheral lymphadenopathy may be present in the generalized and partially generalized presentations.[3–5,7] The localized presentation tends to remain localized, without the development of systemic clinical signs.[8] The onset of sarcoidosis may be insidious or rapid.[2,4]

The skin lesions are variable but mostly characterized by focal, multifocal or generalized scaling and crusting, with varying degrees of alopecia.[2–4] Lesions are often well demarcated.[3]

In the generalized form, nodules may be found in order of decreasing frequency in the lungs, lymph nodes, liver, gastrointestinal tract, spleen, kidneys, bones and central nervous system.[2–4] There may be serious skin involvement or no skin involvement.[9] Most horses with generalized sarcoidosis develop a wasting syndrome characterized by one or more of the following clinical signs: exercise intolerance, increased respiratory rate at rest, mild dyspnoea, poor appetite, weight loss, ventral oedema, and persistent or fluctuating low-grade fever.[2,4]

No age or sex predilections have been recognized,[2–5] although Spiegel *et al.*[10] noted a predisposition for thoroughbreds and geldings. This was also described by

Accepted 13 July 2012
Sources of Funding: This study was self-funded.
Conflict of Interest: No conflicts of interest have been declared.

Loewenstein *et al.*[11] There is no documented seasonality.[4,10] In contrast to human sarcoidosis, pruritus is rarely encountered in ES.[3–6,10,12,13] There is no proven aetiology or causative agent, although many triggering factors have been suggested.[2–4] In humans, it is believed that sarcoidosis may be an aberrant reaction to an infectious agent or an antigen, and this may also be true in the horse.[2,7,14] Spiegel *et al.*[10] could not identify any infectious aetiological agent, and these authors concluded that ES is unlikely to have a microbial aetiology. White *et al.*[15] reported a failure in detecting DNA from equine herpesvirus 1 and 2 in paraffin-embedded skin of eight cases of ES, but these authors did not discount equine herpesvirus 1 or 2 as a cause in some cases. A putative causative role for *Mycobacterium* spp. has been proposed for human sarcoidosis, and was suggested in a single equine case.[16]

Most authors suggest that glucocorticoids are the therapy of choice.[2,4,17] In addition to glucocorticoids, dietary ω3/ω6 fatty acids for at least 3–12 weeks (dosage depending on manufacturer) and pentoxifylline [10 mg/kg twice daily orally (p.o.)] may be used as adjunctive therapy, but the benefits have not been established.[4] Dietary changes may be helpful, given that diseases similar or identical to ES have been caused by hairy vetch (*Vicia villosa*), and those horses responded to dietary changes.[3,18]

The prognosis for generalized sarcoidosis is poor,[1,5,6,12] although some authors describe that weight gain may occur during glucocorticoid therapy and that euthanasia may not be required.[19] Spontaneous resolution has also been reported.[2,4]

The aim of the present study was to report the clinical signs, diagnosis, treatment and outcomes for 22 horses with confirmed equine sarcoidosis seen between 2002 and 2011.

Materials and methods

The Animal Ethics Committee of Utrecht University concluded that this study did not require its approval because it was a patient-based study.

Horses

Twenty-two cases of ES were seen between 2002 and 2011. Twenty animals were referred to the Utrecht University clinic, and two were cases seen at the Utrecht University outpatient clinic. Information collected included the following: age, breed, sex, onset of clinical signs, distribution and type of skin lesions, diagnostic investigations, treatment and response to treatment.

Diagnosis

All horses were tentatively diagnosed with sarcoidosis (Figures 1,3,5,7 and 9) based on the characteristic of skin lesions (exfoliation, crusting alopecia, increased local skin temperature, subcutaneous oedema and/or nodule formation) and/or systemic signs (e.g. fever, weight loss, lymphadenopathy). The tentative diagnosis was confirmed by histological examination of skin biopsies (Figures 2,4,6,8 and 10) and/or other tissue biopsies (e.g. Tru-Cut needle biopsy) by a board-certified veterinary pathologist (G.C.M.G.). Patients were included in the study when the biopsies revealed a multifocal to diffuse lympho-granulomatous dermatitis with multinucleated giant cells.

Clinical presentations of sarcoidosis based on extent of lesions

Horses with 'generalized sarcoidosis' showed cutaneous signs and/or (sub)cutaneous nodules all over the body, had no pruritus and

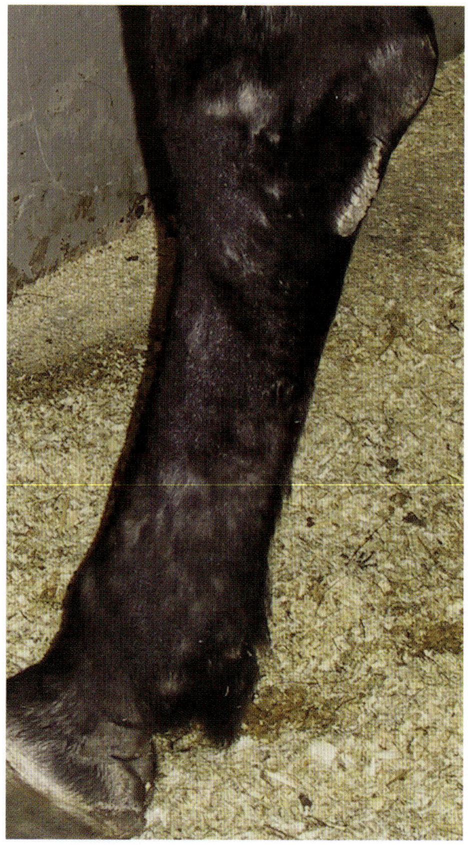

Figure 1. Localized sarcoidosis: 13-year-old standardbred gelding (case 1) with crusting, scaling and hair loss on the right hindlimb.

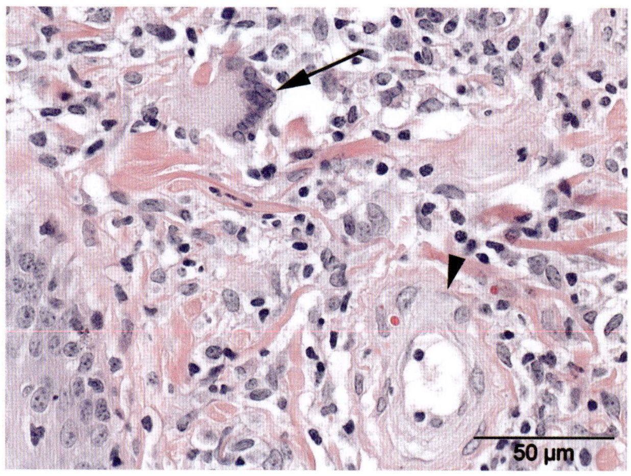

Figure 2. Skin biopsy of case 1 (shown in Figure 1) revealed marked lymphohistiocytic dermatitis with multinucleated giant cells (arrow). Vessels in the superficial and mid dermis show swelling of the vessel wall and occasional extravasation of erythrocytes (arrowhead). Haematoxylin and eosin stain.

showed one or more of the following signs: persistent low-grade fever, exercise intolerance, pain when touched, mild respiratory distress, weight loss and/or peripheral lymphadenopathy.

Horses with 'partially generalized sarcoidosis' showed exfoliative dermatitis on one or two pigmented or nonpigmented limb(s) and/or (sub)cutaneous nodular lesions on a limited body region (e.g. a forelimb and the chest or a hindlimb and the thigh, etc.).

Horses with 'localized sarcoidosis' had localized area(s) of nonpruritic exfoliative dermatitis, often showed oedema of the lower limb,

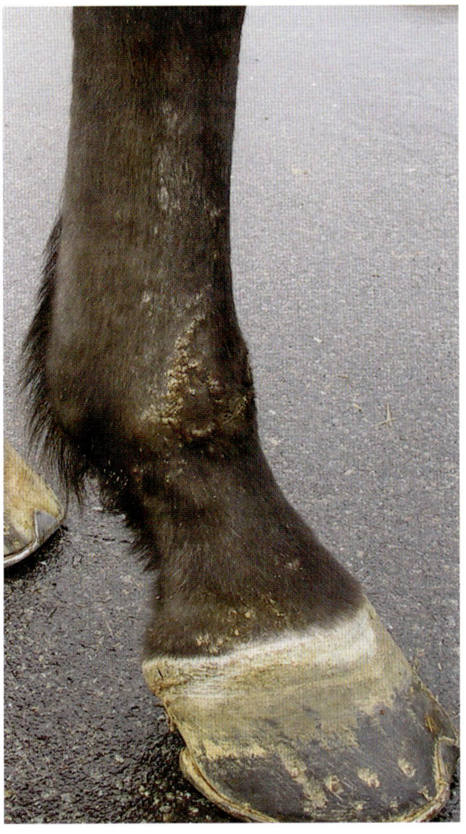

Figure 3. Localized sarcoidosis: 8-year-old Dutch warmblood mare (case 4) with crusting, scaling and alopecia of the right forelimb.

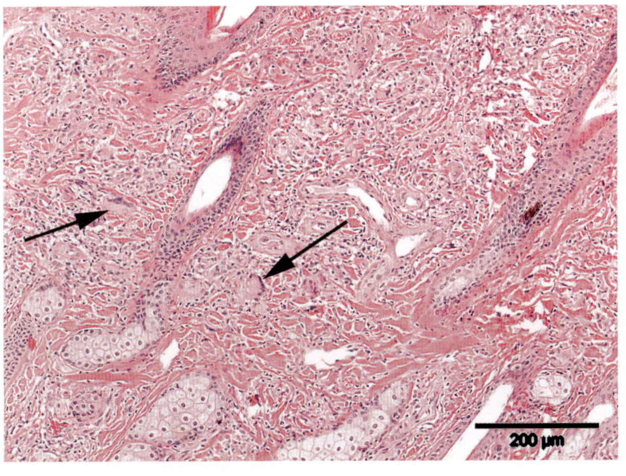

Figure 4. Skin biopsy of case 4 (shown in Figure 3) with a marked lymphohistiocytic infiltrate in the dermis. Several scattered multinucleated giant cells are indicated by arrows. Haematoxylin and eosin stain.

sometimes were painful to the touch and, in severe cases, lameness was seen. Lesions occurred on one or two pigmented or nonpigmented lower limb(s), extending not further than the elbow or the knee, or occurred elsewhere on the body, limited to one area maximally 20 cm × 20 cm.

Follow-up

All owners and/or their private veterinarians were contacted by telephone at least once, and often several times, for follow-up.

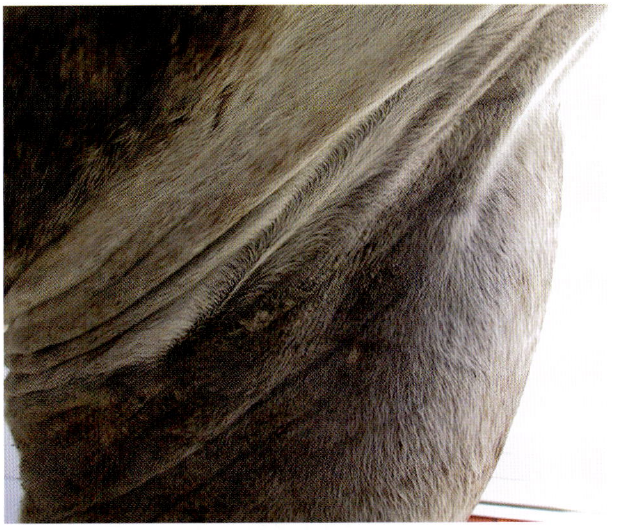

Figure 5. Partially generalized sarcoidosis: 12-year-old Dutch warmblood mare (case 10) with exfoliative dermatitis on the left forelimb and some subcutaneous nodules on the chest.

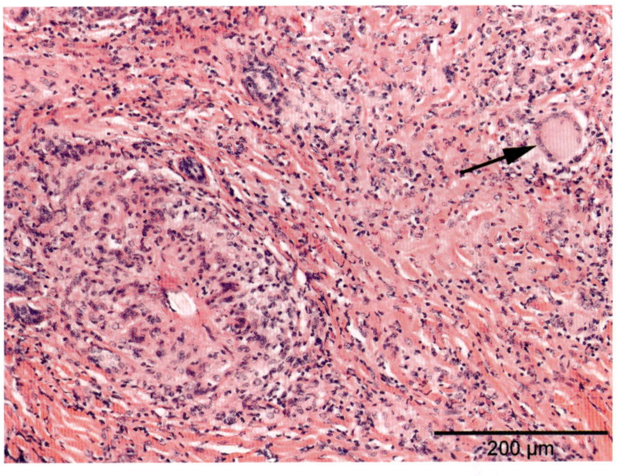

Figure 6. Skin biopsy of case 10 (shown in Figure 5) with a marked histiocytic and neutrophilic infiltrate. At the left side of the picture is a pyogranulomatous focus with a centrally located hair fragment. Note the multinucleated giant cell (arrow). Haematoxylin and eosin stain.

Data analysis

Data analysis was descriptive.

Results

Twenty-two horses were included in the study, six geldings (27%) and 16 (73%) mares. The mean age at the time of diagnosis was 10 ± 4.6 years (range 3–17 years). Case signalment, breed, clinical presentation, form, treatment and outcomes are summarized in Table 1.

Most of the horses received an initial high dose of systemic glucocorticosteroids [prednisolone at 1.0–2.0 mg/kg p.o. once daily or dexamethasone at 0.04–0.08 mg/kg intramuscularly once daily (n = 2)] for 7–14 days, followed by a lower dose of prednisolone (0.20–1.0 mg/kg p.o. once daily) for several weeks or longer. All glucocorticosteroid therapy was administered between

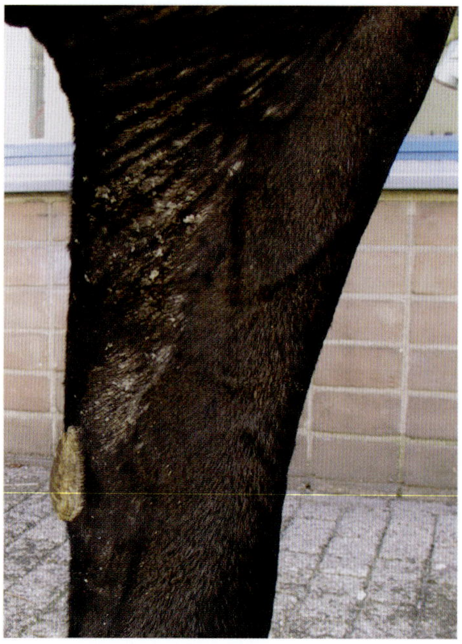

Figure 7. Partially generalized sarcoidosis: 4-year-old Friesian mare (case 11) with exfoliative dermatitis of the left forelimb and also some lesions on the head and neck and enlarged retropharyngeal lymph nodes.

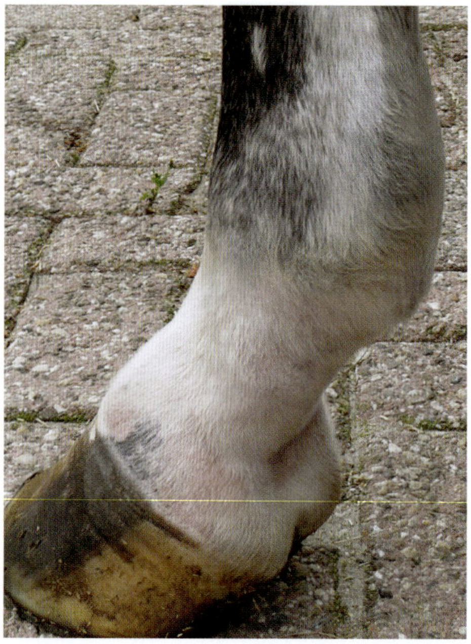

Figure 9. Localized sarcoidosis: 6-year-old Dutch warmblood mare (case 20) with some crusting, scaling and hair loss on the left forelimb.

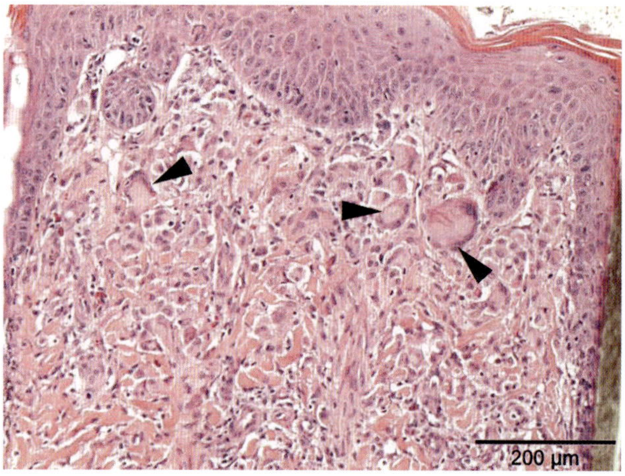

Figure 8. Skin biopsy of case 11 (shown in Figure 7), showing haired skin with moderate epidermal hyperplasia and several multinucleated giant cells (arrowheads). Haematoxylin and eosin stain.

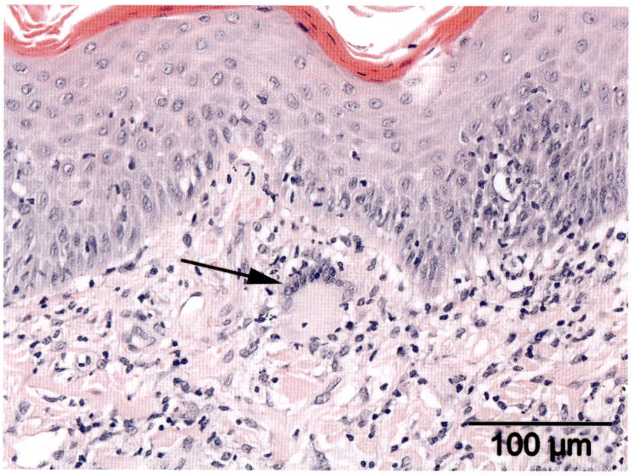

Figure 10. Skin biopsy of case 20 (shown in Figure 9) with moderate epidermal hyperplasia and a mixed lymphohistiocytic and neutrophilic inflammatory infiltrate with a multinucleated giant cell (arrow). Haematoxylin and eosin stain.

07.00 and 09.00 h to support the endogenous day–night rhythm of cortisone. Topical treatments were not prescribed because the skin was painful and fragile, given that most horses had already been treated at home with one or more topical therapies with no success.

'Generalized sarcoidosis' occurred in three horses (13.6%) and presented with generalized exfoliative dermatitis and/or generalized (sub)cutaneous nodules. Lesions started as nodules in two horses and as exfoliative dermatitis in another horse. Two of these three horses have been described earlier in detail by Reijerkerk *et al.*[6] One of three horses was euthanized immediately, and the remaining two were euthanized after 2–3 months of unsuccessful treatment.

'Partially generalized sarcoidosis' was diagnosed in four horses (18.2%). In two horses, skin lesions started with nodules and in the other two cases lesions were localized (one on a limb and one on the chest). All four cases deteriorated despite treatment and were euthanized after 14 weeks to 12 months.

'Localized sarcoidosis' occurred in 15 horses (68.2%). In two of the localized cases with lesions on the lower limb, the histological examination of the biopsies also showed some vasculitis. One horse with a localized affected area on the body (right flank 5 cm × 5 cm) improved after receiving prednisolone. Following cessation of therapy, the lesion waxed and waned but the owner did not consider this to be problematic. The outcome of the 14 horses with lesions on the lower limbs was: two cases showed no improvement or insufficient improvement on treatment and were euthanized; four

Table 1. Number, sex, age, breed, clinical problem, form of sarcoidosis, treatment and outcome of 22 cases with equine sarcoidosis

Case no.	Sex	Age (years)	Breed	Clinical problem	Form	Treatment and outcome
1	Gelding	13	Standardbred	ED right hind, mainly lower limb	Localized	Insufficient response to prednisolone, deteriorated, lesions extended over the body, weight loss, and was euthanized after 8 months
2	Gelding	17	KWPN	ED right hind lower limb, some lesions neck and under abdomen	Partially generalized	After 8 months was slaughtered because the owner did not want continuous treatment
3	Mare	11	Trakener	Generalized sarcoidosis, with whole body ED	Generalized	Owner decided on immediate euthanasia; pathology also showed enlarged pulmonary lymph nodes
4	Mare	8	KWPN	ED right fore lower limb	Localized	Improved with prednisolone but was not completely 'cured' and thus was slaughtered 2 months later
5	Gelding	6	KWPN	ED left hind lower limb	Localized	Improved without therapy and remained in remission
6	Mare	3	KWPN	ED right hind lower limb	Localized	Some permanent alopecia and scaling but has remained stable for 7 years on prednisolone 0.5 mg/kg/day orally
7	Mare	12	Pony	ED right hindlimb	Localized	After 2 years, spontaneous regression
8	Mare	3	Friesian	ED localized area, right chest 5 cm × 5 cm	Localized	Improved after a 4 week course of prednisolone but was still lesional
9	Gelding	11	KWPN	ED left hind lower limb	Localized	Acceptable response to prednisolone and cod-fish-oil ointment, but lesions did not resolve and after 3.5 years was slaughtered for sarcoidosis and ataxia
10	Mare	12	KWPN	ED left forelimb and nodules on chest	Partially generalized	First improved with dexadreson and prednisolone, but deteriorated after 3.5 months and was slaughtered
11	Mare	4	Friesian	ED face, chest and left forelimb localized areas and few nodules	Partially generalized	Owner did not want to continue treatment; nodules became generalized everywhere and horse was euthanized within 6 months
12	Gelding	10	KWPN	ED left hind lower limb	Localized	Improved with prednisolone, and cured completely 6 months later after a 'home remedy'
13	Gelding	16	Arabian	ED right fore lower limb; incidentally, a lesion elsewhere	Localized	Stable with 0.2 mg/kg/day prednisolone
14	Mare	9	KWPN	ED right forelimb	Localized	Almost normal with 0.3 mg/kg/day prednisolone
15	Mare	7	KWPN	Generalized sarcoidosis; started with nodular form	Generalized	Improved with prednisolone, but owner refused continuous treatment; horse deteriorated, developed generalized lesions and was euthanized
16	Mare	17	German warmblood	ED right fore lower limb	Localized	0.5–1 mg/kg/day prednisolone; lesions are acceptable to owner, but treatment cannot be discontinued
17	Mare	16	KWPN	ED right fore lower limb	Localized	Prednisone 1.2 mg/kg/day, decreased to 0.3 mg/kg/day; horse has some lesions but owner is satisfied
18	Mare	4	KWPN	ED right hind lower limb	Localized	After foaling, horse was slightly better but still lesional; owner declines treatment
19	Mare	16	KWPN	Subdermal nodules on some areas of the body	Partially generalized	Prednisolone for 6 months, nodules resolved but if discontinued horse relapsed; was euthanized due to injury
20	Mare	6	KWPN	ED left fore lower limb (histology also vasculitis)	Localized	Pregnant and was not treated; lesions resolved without treatment
21	Mare	9	KWPN	Generalized sarcoidosis, both ED and nodules	Generalized	Pregnant, treated only with prednisolone; mare died and necropsy revealed extensive pulmonary sarcoidosis
22	Mare	9	Arabian	ED both hind lower limbs (histology also vasculitis)	Localized	Improved with dexadreson 0.05 mg/kg/day for 6 days and then treated with prednisolone 1.2 mg/kg/day; horse relapses when dose is decreased

Unless indicated differently, dosages of prednisolone and dexamethasone were as described in the text. Abbreviations: ED, exfoliative dermatitis; KWPN, Dutch warmblood.

cases showed full recovery with or without treatment; one showed partial recovery without treatment; and seven cases improved after receiving prednisolone but required continuous low doses to maintain the improvement.

Discussion

The assumption that ES may occur more frequently in geldings was not supported in the present case series; only 27% were geldings, and the sex difference in the overall patient load in the University Equine Clinic is about equal. Furthermore, the finding in the present study that 73% of the cases were mares was similar to the findings in humans, where women have a higher rate of sarcoidosis than men.[14]

Although sarcoidosis has been described to occur as early as 3 months of age,[3,11] all of the horses in this case series were older than 3 years of age at the time of diagnosis. This age distribution is also found in several other equine studies[5,9,10,12,16,19,20] and is consistent with the occurrence in humans, where the disease is also very rare in children.[14]

Treatment in this case series was similar to other reports. The treatment of choice was glucocorticosteroid therapy either intravenously or intramuscularly (dexamethasone) or p.o. (prednisolone).[2–5] Fatty acids or pentoxifylline as mentioned by Scott and Miller[4] were not used in horses in this case series but may be useful if efficacy can be demonstrated. Tumour necrosis factor-α inhibitors have been shown to be beneficial in refractory human sarcoidosis cases,[14] and these substances could also be considered in the future for use in horses.

The outcome for the generalized and partially generalized forms in the horses reported here was disappointing and concurs with some earlier studies;[9,12,16,20] however, others have reported a more favourable outcome.[10,19] The prognosis of the localized form is good with respect to the fact that it is not life threatening, but guarded given that localized skin lesions are viewed as problematic by the owners. This is consistent with the findings of a previous report of nine cases of localized sarcoidosis.[8] In that study, two of nine horses (four geldings and five mares, 5–20 years of age) with localized sarcoidosis showed a full recovery and seven showed only some improvement in clinical signs. These results are comparable with the results of the localized sarcoidosis cases in the present study. However, in the present study two horses were euthanized because the skin lesions did not resolve and the owners did not want a horse that required continuous treatment. One horse was euthanized within 2 months and the other after 3 months. One other horse was euthanized after 3.5 years, but mainly for a reason not related to sarcoidosis. In some of the equine patients with localized sarcoidosis, concurrent vasculitis was found. It is possible that vasculitis and ES may share a common underlying immune-mediated mechanism.

Although the number of cases in this series is small and includes two cases from a previous study, this is still the largest collection of cases of sarcoidosis to date. The increase in case numbers may be due to either earlier recognition of the disease and its clinical subsets and/or a real increase in prevalence. Loewenstein *et al.*[11] presented six cases collected over four continents, and most other published studies described only one or two cases. More sarcoidosis cases will undoubtedly be collected as a result of increased recognition of the importance of equine skin diseases in general and as a result of earlier diagnosis of equine sarcoidosis.

Based upon this case series of 22 horses, the following conclusions were drawn: (i) the prognosis of 'generalized' and 'partially generalized' ES is poor; (ii) the prognosis of 'localized' ES is good with respect to survival but guarded for the localized skin problem, because only 26.7% recovered fully with or without treatment and 53% needed continuous low maintenance doses of prednisolone (0.2–0.5 mg/kg/day); (iii) recognition of the different forms of sarcoidosis based on history, clinical signs and histopathology assisted owners in making an informed choice between treatment and euthanasia and prevented unnecessary topical treatment strategies; and (iv) localized ES should always be considered in the differential diagnosis of a localized exfoliative dermatitis of unknown origin.

Acknowledgements

The authors thank the referring veterinarians and owners for giving us access to the patients and for providing follow-up information.

References

1. Heath SE, Bell RJ, Clark EG *et al.* Idiopathic granulomatous disease involving the skin in a horse. *J Am Vet Med Assoc* 1990; 197: 1033–1036.
2. Stannard AA. Systemic granulomatous disease. *Vet Dermatol* 2000; 11: 170–172.
3. Knottenbelt DC. Sarcoidosis (generalized granulomatous disease). In: Knottenbelt DC, ed. *Pascoe's Principles and Practice of Equine Dermatology.* 2nd edn. Edinburgh: Saunders Elsevier, 2009; 280–281.
4. Scott DW, Miller WH. Sarcoidosis. In: *Equine Dermatology*, 2nd edn. Missouri: Elsevier Saunders, 2011: 453–455.
5. Sloet van Oldruitenborgh-Oosterbaan MM, Koeman JP. Recognition and therapy of sarcoidosis, in *Proceedings. 45th Annu Congr Br Equine Vet Assoc* 2006: 184–185.
6. Reijerkerk EPR, Veldhuis Kroeze EJB, Sloet van Oldruitenborgh-Oosterbaan MM. Generalized sarcoidosis in two horses. *Tijdschr Diergeneeskd* 2008; 133: 654–661.
7. Fadok VA. An overview of equine dermatoses characterized by scaling and crusting. *Vet Clin N Am: Equine Pract* 1995; 11: 43–51.
8. Sloet van Oldruitenborgh-Oosterbaan MM, Koeman JP. Equine sarcoidosis: a systemic disease or a localised dermatosis? in *Proceedings. 41th Annu Congr Br Equine Vet Assoc* 2002: 210–211.
9. Peters M, Graf G, Pohlenz J. Idiopathic systemic granulomatous disease with encephalitis in a horse. *J Vet Med Assoc* 2003; 50: 108–112.
10. Spiegel IB, White SD, Foley JE *et al.* A retrospective study of cutaneous equine sarcoidosis and its potential infectious aetiological agents. *Vet Dermatol* 2006; 17: 51–62.
11. Loewenstein C, Bettenay SV, Mueller RS. A retrospective study of equine sarcoidosis. *Vet Dermatol* 2004; 15(Suppl 1): 67 (Abstract).
12. Hansmann F, Venner M, Hewicker-Trautwein M *et al.* Sarkoidose bei einer Warmblutstute. *Tierarztl Prax Grosstiere* 2007; 5: 363–368.

13. Goldberg A, Lang A, Mekori YA. Prolonged generalized pruritus associated with selective elevation of IgA as the presenting symptoms of sarcoidosis. *Ann Allergy Asthma Immunol* 1995; 74: 387–389.
14. Haimovic A, Sanchez M, Judson MA *et al.* Sarcoidosis: a comprehensive review and update for the dermatologist. Part 1: cutaneous disease. *J Am Acad Dermatol* 2012; 66: 699, e1–18.
15. White SD, Foley JE, Spiegel IB *et al.* Lack of detectable equine Herpesviruses 1 and 2 in paraffin-embedded specimens of equine sarcoidosis. *J Vet Intern Med* 2009; 23: 623–625.
16. Oliveira-Filho JP, Monteiro LN, Delfiol DJZ *et al. Mycobacterium* DNA detection in liver and skin of a horse with generalized sarcoidosis. *J Vet Diagn Invest* 2012; 24: 596–600.
17. Schlipf JW Jr. Dermatological conditions associated with crusts and scales: sarcoidosis. In: Robinson NE, ed. *Current Therapy in Equine Medicine*, 4th edn. Philadelphia: W.B. Saunders, 1997; 384.
18. Woods LW, Johnson B, Hietala SK *et al.* Systemic granulomatous disease in a horse grazing pasture containing vetch (*Vicia* sp.). *J Vet Diagn Invest* 1992; 4: 356–360.
19. Rose JF, Littlewood JD, Smith K *et al.* A series of four cases of generalized granulomatous disease in the horse. In: Kwochka KW, Willemse T, von Tscharner C, eds. *Advances in Veterinary Dermatology, volume 3.* Oxford: Butterworth Heinemann, 1998; 562–563.
20. Axon JE, Robinson P, Lucas J. Generalised granulomatous disease in a horse. *Aust Vet J* 2004; 82: 48–51.

Part 8

Workshop Reports

Co-editors:
Dr Karen L. Campbell, University of Illinois, Illinois, USA
Dr Kinga Gortel, Lake Country Veterinary Specialist Hospital, Lake Country, BC, Canada

8.1

Nonpruritic hair loss

R. Cerundolo[1] (Chairperson), J.R. Rest[2] (Secretary)

[1]Dick White Referrals, Veterinary Specialist Centre, Station Farm, London Road, Six Mile Bottom, Suffolk, CB8 0UH, UK
[2]Focus Veterinary Histopathology International, The Heath Science and Technology Park, PO Box 13, Runcorn, WA7 4QF, UK

Monika Welle (*Switzerland*) opened the workshop by explaining that because many forms of alopecia in dogs are associated with hair cycle arrest, it is important to understand the hair cycle. Recently, two new stages have been characterized in dogs – exogen (shedding) and kenogen (hairless resting stage). The hair cycle consists of the phases anagen, catagen, telogen and exogen (shedding) with a resting kenogen (hairless telogen) phase.

In order to progress to anagen, stem cells from the bulge (an anatomical feature in mice but not in dogs or humans) grow down to form the inner root sheath and hair shaft. The precise stimulus is unknown. Later in anagen, the hair grows upwards. It then regresses in catagen and the lower part undergoes apoptosis producing a telogen follicle. The telogen resting phase hair is firmly attached to hair follicle and it is not pushed out. Exogen, or shedding, is an enzymatic process between the hair and root sheath and can occur at any time during the following cycle.

Kenogen follicles are hairless resting follicles (called hairless telogen by Dunstan) that need stimulation to enter anagen. Normally, 15–20% of follicles are in this phase and when activated enable dogs to grow more hair at colder times of year. The numbers of hair follicles in kenogen may be increased three to four times in clinical alopecia when stimuli to make hair downgrowth are missing.

The hair cycle is governed by epithelial and dermal tissues with systemic modifiers. Various mediators are involved in the hair cycle.

Canine recurrent flank alopecia (CRFA) (S. Vandenabeele)

Sophie Vandenabeele (*Belgium*) discussed CRFA in dogs. The typical presentation is a bilaterally symmetrical flank alopecia. However, not all cases are on the flanks or seasonal or symmetrical.

Clinical syndromes:

1 Typical: bulldogs and boxers have a clear breed predilection with symptoms developing from 8 months to 11 years. The lesions are classical bilaterally symmetrical areas of alopecia. Some also have a little alopecia on the dorsal muzzle. There is hyperpigmentation in some breeds but not the Dalmatian. Some dogs also have the dorsum affected, and other breeds, such as the great dane, show only hypotrichosis.

2 Atypical presentations include alopecia that is predominantly facial: on the bridge of the nose and periocular regions. Breeds developing this form include golden and Labrador retrievers. The hair may regrow and the dogs do not have concurrent hypothyroidism. Some have multifocal lesions and involvement of dorsal facial and pinnal folds.

3 Atypical presentations also occur in some bulldogs and boxers. In these dogs areas of alopecia develop inflammation with crusts and pigmentation. An interface dermatitis is found on histopathology.

4 An atypical presentation is also found in Rhodesian ridgeback dogs. These dogs exhibit a change in coat colour and not alopecia. The change occurs annually. Histopathology shows hyperkeratosis and malformed follicles.

The pathogenesis involves the photoperiod and the disease is usually seen at latitudes from 35 degrees upwards. The photoperiod may act directly or indirectly via prolactin secretion. There may be decreased endogenous melatonin production in genetically predisposed animals.

Shoulder (normal-haired) and flank (hairless) biopsies were transplanted to nude (athymic) mice from two classically affected 3-year-old dogs, a boxer and a mixed breed. After 30 days there was hair regrowth on both the affected and nonaffected skin biopsies. Both donor dogs stayed alopecic for a further 50 days. These results indicate that the pathogenesis of CRFA is mediated by systemic factors. A systemically induced alopecia can explain the diversity of clinical presentations of this disease.

Stefanie Kobrich (*Germany*) commented that Rhodesian ridgeback dogs have hair that looks different and asked if this is the same syndrome.

Sophie Vandenabeele replied that it is.

Monika Welle added that affected dogue de Bordeaux and cane corso dogs appear mucinotic.

Sophie Vandenabeele stated that she has not biopsied these breeds.

Jan Declercq (*Belgium*) added that he saw a Yorkshire terrier with texture and colour change that progressed to alopecia later in the season.

Ann Hargis (*USA*) stated that histologically there is a mix of growing and nongrowing hair types.

Sophie Vandenabeele agreed that both types are seen.

Sherry Myers (*Canada*) asked if the growth is in one implanted site.

Sophie Vandenabeele clarified that the transplanted biopsies taken from the shoulder area of the dogs regrew hair but not those taken from the flank.

Valerie Fadok (*USA*) commented that the disease is common in pitbulls in the USA and that melatonin is used regularly as a treatment. She asked if melatonin affects hair regrowth.

Sophie Vandenabeele answered that melatonin has only recently become available in Belgium. One group had reported that their experience is that regrowth is faster.

Valerie Fadok added that Ed Rosser (*USA*) believes that if the timing of the hair loss cycle is established, starting treatment with melatonin before the hair falls out results in less alopecia.

Rosario Cerundolo recommended starting treatment with melatonin 2 months before hair loss is expected to develop.

Dominique Heripret (*France*) recommended starting melatonin treatment in December.

Rosario Cerundolo added that he uses melatonin starting daily in November/December and continuing until spring as the majority of the dogs who had a previous episode would start to show alopecia again in the spring.

Geoff Orbell (*New Zealand*) added that he has seen the condition in Australia.

Rangson Saliuploy (*Thailand*) commented that he does not see it on the Equator.

Alopecia in silver Labrador retrievers (V. Fadok and C. Vitale)

Valerie Fadok and **Carlo Vitale** (*USA*) posted requests for cases on the VetDerm and International Society for Veterinary Dermatopathology (ISVD) listservs. Responses from 33 veterinarians included information on 45 dogs. Affected European dogs were imported from the USA. Age at presentation was 12 weeks to 2 years.

Of the 45 silver Labrador retrievers, 2 were reported to have normal coats, while 43 had alopecia and a brittle coat affecting the trunk, with the head and lower limbs being spared. Thirty-two percent of the dogs had developed pyoderma at least once, 20% had hyperpigmentation, 20% had follicular cysts and 20% had comedones. Many dogs had other associated diseases including atopic dermatitis, food allergy and also congenital abnormalities such as absence of one kidney or ocular dystrophies. Nearly all dogs had microscopic examination of hairs that revealed mild to moderate clumping of melanin within the hair shaft. A small number had large melanin clumps that distorted the hair shafts. The coat changes were similar to those in other breeds of dogs with colour dilution alopecia. For most dogs, treatment focused on controlling the ancillary diseases such as pyoderma.

The silver coat colour is not recognized by the American Kennel Club (AKC), with only black, yellow and chocolate colours being considered as expressing the breed standard. The origin of silver Labradors is in dispute. They may derive by crossing Weimaraners with chocolate Labradors. Weimaraners are homozygous recessive at the *D* locus. Breeding a Weimaraner (homozygous *d/d*) with a chocolate Labrador (heterozygous *D/d*) would result in a subset of *d/d* puppies being homozygous recessive and thus exhibiting diluted coat colour. Alternatively, the silver modifier may have arisen spontaneously in Labradors and may not even be associated with the *D* locus. The silver modifier in black Labradors results in a charcoal colour, in yellow Labradors as a champagne colour, and in chocolate Labradors as the silver colour. Some breeders claim the AKC has performed DNA tests to verify that these dogs are purebred Labradors. However, the AKC DNA testing is only for assigning or proving parentage and not for assessing purity of the breed.

Fifteen dogs have been biopsied. Histopathology evaluations by Sherry Myers shows common findings of mild-to-moderate clumping of pigment within the hair shafts, the follicular lumen, the follicular walls and the hair bulbs. The melanin clumping does not appear to be as marked as that seen in classic colour dilution alopecia. In some dogs, however, the aggregates were observed to cause a bulge in the hair shaft. Some hairs were miniaturized and atrophic, with secondary hairs more severely affected than primary hairs. Melanophages below the hair follicles were common. In nearly all dogs, the lower segments of the hair follicle were wavy or curved, as is seen in hair follicle dysplasia.

At this time there is debate whether the disease in silver Labradors is a true colour dilution alopecia or if it should be called 'follicular dysplasia of the dilute Labrador colour'.

Monika Welle reported that she had seen this in two dogs, possibly imported to Switzerland.

Ann Hargis commented that the histopathology is similar to colour dilution alopecia with hairs and epidermis affected. The irises are colour dilute. She asked whether anyone knew if the ocular pathology of affected dogs had been evaluated.

Rosario Cerundolo mentioned that a similar condition has been reported in Munsterlanders.[1]

Stephanie Kobrich reported that two young Labradors, not silver but similar in appearance, had parents from

USA. These dogs had 'rough hair' at 4–6 months. The owner was pleased to have a different greyish colour.

Tyler Udenberg (*USA*) remarked that as a Canadian dog judge he sees abnormal coat coloured dogs.

Monika Welle commented that in her opinion this disease has to be a dysplasia. Melanocytic dysplasia can only occur in anagen because melanin is only picked up by anagen hairs.

Description and characterization of a hair coat disorder in schipperkes (E.R. May)

Elizabeth May (*USA*) reported on a hair coat disorder she has studied in schipperkes. The clinical sign in affected schipperkes is that the black coat has hair that lightens, turns red and becomes brittle. Friction areas develop alopecia. The head and legs remain normal, similar to other plush-coated dogs. In her local area the condition is known as 'red coat disorder' of schipperkes. There is regrowth of hair at biopsy sites. It is speculated that Pomeranians were introduced into the breed to 'improve' the hair coat.

To determine if this disease is similar to alopecia X in Pomeranians, three normal-coated (1 male, 1 female, 1 neutered male) and 10 affected (2 male, 2 female, 3 neutered male, 3 spayed female) schipperkes were evaluated. Complete blood count (CBC), serum chemistry panel, urinalysis (UA), urine cortisol:creatinine ratio (UCCR), total thyroxine (TT_4), free thyroxine by equilibrium dialysis (fT_4ed), thyroid stimulating hormone (TSH), and pre- and post-ACTH stimulation cortisol and sex hormone analysis were done for all dogs. Complete blood count, serum chemistry panel and UA results did not reveal abnormalities consistent with an endocrine disorder. Total thyroxine, fT_4ed and TSH concentrations were within normal limits for all dogs. The UCCR results were increased in 1/3 healthy and 4/10 affected dogs; post-ACTH cortisol concentrations were within normal limits for all dogs; androstenedione concentrations pre- and post-ACTH were elevated in 2/3 healthy and 5/10 affected dogs; pre- and post-ACTH oestradiol concentrations were increased in 3/3 healthy and 5/10 affected dogs; pre- and post-ACTH progesterone concentrations were increased in 2/3 healthy and 3/10 affected dogs; pre- and post-ACTH 17-hydroxyprogesterone concentrations were increased in 2/10 affected dogs; aldosterone concentrations were within normal limits for all dogs.

Similar to the disease in Pomeranians, there were no significant differences regarding any of the tests performed between normal and affected dogs. Skin biopsies showed an atrophic pattern in affected dogs.

Geoff Orbell asked if the affected dogs have responded to any treatment and if they progress to have alopecia.

Elizabeth May replied that they have not responded to treatment. The use of mitotane has been discussed but not yet tried. The dogs do progress to develop areas of alopecia.

Jan Declercq stated that hair colour lightens in sable and black Pomeranians before the dogs become alopecic.

Elizabeth May commented that she has only seen the condition in black schipperkes.

Treatment of alopecia X with progesterone (L.A. Frank)

Linda Frank (*USA*) asserted that while older studies with growth hormone injections have resulted in hair regrowth, the studies were poorly done and the use of growth hormone was associated with adverse side effects. She has completed a more recent study to determine if the administration of progesterone is safe and effective in inducing endogenous growth hormone to a level that results in hair growth in Pomeranians with alopecia X.

Progesterone side effects may include endometrial hyperplasia and mammary nodules, so only neutered dogs were recruited. Entry criteria included exclusion of hyperadrenocorticism and hypothyroidism. Methylprogesterone acetate was injected subcutaneously every 4 weeks for a total of four injections. Two males and three females received 5 mg/kg and one male and two females received 10 mg/kg methylprogesterone acetate. Dogs were monitored monthly and serum was saved for insulin-like growth factor-1 (IGF-1) analysis.

On the lower dose, one dog died of disease considered to be unrelated to treatment. Two of the four remaining dogs had partial hair regrowth. On the higher dose, one dog had partial hair regrowth and one dog had complete hair regrowth 2 months after completion of the study. The IGF-1 concentrations were low and remained unchanged throughout the study. They were proportional to body weight.

This study showed the effects of progesterone to be similar to other studies of therapies for dogs with alopecia X, with approximately 40% of affected dogs exhibiting hair regrowth. Hair regrowth always occurs at approximately the same time after treatment has started.

Rosario Cerundolo asked whether different formulations of progesterone such as proligestone make a difference in the efficacy.

Linda Frank replied that the mechanism seems to be the same.

Dominique Heripret stated that he treats with a testosterone inhibitor, which gives the same pattern of regrowth that he previously achieved with growth hormone, and that hair follicles have both sex and growth hormone receptors.

Rosario Cerundolo reported that one injection of deslorelin (Suprelorin, Virbac), commonly used for chemical castration, also induces hair regrowth and lasts 6 months. Deslorelin is a gonadotropin-releasing hormone (GnRH) agonist.

Joan Rest summarized the workshop.

Monika Welle described the new exogen and kenogen stages in the hair follicle. Exogen (shedding) is an active process. Kenogen is the pool of inactive follicles that can be stimulated to change the rate of growth.

Sophie Vandenabeele discussed her group's work on a *short-hair type* alopecia, recurrent (seasonal, flank) alopecia. She described the various clinical presentations including a facial type, demonstrating that it is not always recurrent, seasonal or flank in distribution. Experimental grafting work of skin biopsies from affected dogs showed that hair could regrow in the new host, indicating that neither hair follicle nor perifollicular connective tissue failure was the cause of the alopecia. A systemic factor is involved. Pigmentation of skin does not follow the alopecia.

Valerie Fadok introduced a *colour-related disease* of silver Labrador retrievers. The source of this colour-modifying gene appears to be the USA, with European dogs traced back to importation. The disease progresses from noninflammatory to inflammatory. It is likely a dysplasia.

Elizabeth May introduced an alopecia in schipperke dogs that appears similar to that in other breeds with plush coats such as the Pomeranian. Melanocytes are sensitive cells so loss of pigment precedes alopecia. She explored endocrine aspects concluding that there were no endocrine abnormalities.

Linda Frank presented her latest study on alopecia X, revisiting early work when it was reported as a *growth hormone-responsive* disease. To explore the mechanism of action, she used two doses of progesterone, which is linked to production of IGF-1. Her achievement of 40% regrowth in some dogs is consistent with Tony Stannard's comment that 'any kick' could induce temporary hair growth in these dogs. It is also compatible with Monika Welle's group's finding of approximately 35% of hairless kenogen follicles.[2] These hairless follicles are ready to progress to anagen. Regrowth lasts as long as there are kenogen follicles to stimulate. Search for the ideal treatment continues but will probably not be found until the hair cycle is fully understood.

References

1. von Bomhard W, Mauldin EA, Schmutz SM, Leeb T, Casal ML. Black hair follicular dysplasia in Large Münsterländer dogs: clinical, histological and ultrastructural features. *Vet Dermatol* 2006; 17: 182–188.
2. Muntener T, Schuepbach-Refula G, Frank L, Rufenacht S, Welle MM. Canine noninflammatory alopecia: a comprehensive evaluation of common and distinguishing histological characteristics. *Vet Dermatol* 2012; 23: 206–221.

8.2

Dietary management of skin disease: elimination diets and dietary approach to canine allergic disease

D.N. Carlotti[1] (Chairperson), R.G. Harvey[2] (Secretary)

[1]Aquivet Clinique Vétérinaire, Avenue de la Forêt, Parc d'Activités Mermoz Eysines, France
[2]The Veterinary Centre, 207 Daventry Road, Coventry, UK

Didier Carlotti (*France*) gave a brief introduction to the session and acknowledged the help of the session's sponsors, Proctor and Gamble Pet Care (IAMS). He announced the two topics: the first would be the dietary management of skin disease with emphasis on food allergy and choosing an elimination diet, and the second would address the dietary management of canine allergic disease. There were 34 delegates in the session. Hilary Jackson was identified as the first speaker.

Hilary Jackson (*UK*) acknowledged that a substantial portion of her presentation was work performed by a former PhD student, Rebecca Ricci, who is currently undertaking a nutrition residency in Europe, and that the work was in press.[1] Their study looked at the presence of antigens in pet food and compared 12 commercially produced kibble diets. The diets were of European origin, both novel protein and a hydrolysed soya-based diet. The declared protein sources were rabbit, horse, fish, deer and duck. The fats, when declared by the manufacturer, were of fish and animal origin.

The first part of the study used standardised microscopic techniques to look for mammalian, fish and poultry bone fragments (identification microscopy) within a preparation made from a ground portion of the food treated with tetrachloroethylene. The results were graded positive or negative. The second study utilized polymerase chain reaction (PCR) techniques to look for DNA of mammalian, avian or piscine origin in samples of the food.

Unexpected contamination with bone fragments was found in 10 of the 12 diets; for example, a fish-based diet contained mammalian bone fragments. The PCR confirmed the results in some cases, whereas in other cases there were discordant results between microscopy and PCR. The only fish-based diet tested was free of contamination using PCR, and the hydrolysed soya-based diet was also found to be free of contamination.

Ed Rosser (*USA*) enquired as to whether the diets were veterinary exclusive ('prescription only') or commercially available.

Hilary Jackson confirmed that many of the diets were veterinary exclusive.

The Chairman then introduced Ralf Mueller, who presented his personal approach to the process of conducting an elimination diet study.

Ralf Mueller (*Germany*) was happy to announce, in the light of the first speaker's presentation, that his preference to use home-cooked diets for the diagnosis of food allergy makes complete sense. He emphasized that home-cooked diets are used for the diagnosis of food allergy in adult dogs. The diets he subsequently uses for maintenance are essentially whatever can be tolerated by the patient. He said that he had not researched cross-reactivity between ingredients. He advocated feeding the diagnostic diet for 8 weeks and trying to find a novel protein and carbohydrate combination. For example, if the animal was fed ruminant-based food he might advocate poultry and millet. If it was fed a fish-based diet, he would advocate rabbit (or hare, or kangaroo) and sweet potato or pumpkin. If the dog was fed soya-based food then he avoids soya hydrolysates. If the dog had a very varied diet, or refused to eat home-cooked food, then he advocates an appropriate commercially produced selected-protein diet or a hydrolysed protein diet. However, he avoids the commercial chicken hydrolysates in dogs fed poultry, and avoids soya hydrolysate if the dog was fed soya. Otherwise, provided that there was no such protein cross-match, he was happy to use hydrolysates.

In growing dogs, particularly rapidly growing dogs, Ralf Mueller stated that he avoids simple home-cooked diets and hydrolysed diets, preferring to use a commercially produced restricted-protein diet. If he must use home-cooked diets he takes great care to optimize nutrient balance with appropriate supplements, making use of an internet-based diet-balancing tool, whose company would send out an appropriate mineral balance mix (http://www.ernaehrung.vetmed.uni-muenchen.de/service/ernaehrungsberatung/eb_hunde/index.html).

Ralf Mueller also advocates an 8-week duration for restrictive diet trials in cats. He advises the owner to feed a protein-only diet. In his experience, cats refuse to eat potatoes or rice, and a protein-only diet usually results in better compliance. A problem arises if the clients of the cats are strict vegetarians who refuse to have raw meat in the house, and for those cases a commercial novel-protein or hydrolysed diet might be necessary. Cats frequently have been fed foods with very varied protein content, making a novel protein difficult to identify.

Ralf Mueller reported that he has started to use patch testing in dogs exposed to a very varied diet or in cases where the owner was sceptical of food allergy. He used both cooked and raw samples of feed placed onto the skin. The relevant foods are ground, aliquoted and frozen until needed. He has found a good correlation with a negative cutaneous patch reaction and suitability for the diet. For example, a negative reaction to potato meant it could be used in the diet. He said that a positive reaction was regarded as meaningless for allergen selection, being possibly false-positive or even perhaps irritant. He described this technique as useful to convince sceptical owners that a diet trial is necessary, and in identifying suitable food trial ingredients in dogs fed very varied diets.

In response to a question from the Chairman, Ralf Muller described how he had also back-tested proven food-allergic dogs against a commercial food enzyme-linked immunosorbent assay (ELISA). The likelihood ratio (a statistical technique that is less dependent on the prevalence of the disease in a population) of the results from this study of 23 dogs suggested that ELISA assay for food allergy was not reliable.

Hilary Jackson asked which ELISA was used.

Ralf Mueller replied that he used the Avacta test.

Michael Stephan (*USA*) asked what the value of patch testing would be if the dog was intolerant, rather than allergic.

Ralf Mueller pointed out that he did not know if the dogs were simply intolerant rather than allergic – they just reliably responded to challenge. Commenting further on patch testing, he pointed out that it was a very time-consuming procedure, taking about 45 minutes to prepare and apply the patches to the dog. The dogs are allowed to return home after the patches are affixed.

Ed Rosser said that in his hands patch testing was a 3-day procedure and that he preferred the dogs to be hospitalized.

Ralf Mueller said that during an in-house study of these 32 dogs they read 132 reactions at 24, 48 and 72 hours. Only one reaction was only positive at 72 hours. Only six were positive only at 24 hours, and that four of these were subsequently judged to be false-positive. All the other reactions were positive at both 24 and 48, or 48 hours only, or 48 and 72 hours, so he now reads these food patch tests at 48 hours.

Ed Rosser, commenting on Ralf Mueller's 8-week diagnostic protocol, said that he still recommended that food trials be continued for 12 weeks. He could recall dogs, and still sees dogs, that showed no improvement at all at 8 weeks, only to respond by 12 weeks.

Didier Carlotti asked what percentages of dogs do not respond at all at 8 weeks but will by 12 weeks.

Ed Rosser replied that not many, maybe 5% at most.

Ralf Mueller said that he had not had a single dog with demonstrated food allergy that had failed to show some improvement by 8 weeks, over a 2-year period when in practice in Melbourne.

Ed Rosser further added that he had always advocated home-cooked food and would continue to do so, particularly in the light of Hilary's presentation.

Michael Stephan asked Ralf Mueller if he had ever used pork as it is very rarely included in commercial dog foods.

Ralf Mueller replied that he did use cooked pork if the dog had been fed a fish-based diet. However, in Germany, porcine by-products are present in meat-based dog diets and, therefore, pork was unsuitable for these dogs.

Ed Rosser reminded members of the audience from the USA that the palatability enhancer in heartworm medication was pork. He expressed interest in the assumption by many dermatologists that food allergy was IgE mediated. For example, he said, in all other IgE-mediated diseases, if the allergen was removed from the environment, it only takes 5–7 days for remission to be obtained, not 8 or 12 weeks.

Ralf Mueller said he agrees that food allergies may not be IgE-mediated. He had published a study investigating serum IgE concentrations before and after challenging dogs with proven food allergy, and had found no difference in IgE concentrations.[2] He thought maybe IgE production is a bystander phenomenon, except perhaps in dogs with urticaria, which is very rare. Maybe IgE titres are just a marker for immunological disturbance.

Didier Carlotti commented that there have been publications that state that cross-reactivity exists between lamb and beef. Bovine IgG has been identified as a major cross-reactive vertebrate meat allergen in beef, lamb, venison and milk.[3] A study based on 10 dogs with identified food allergy has shown that bovine IgG is a major allergen in cow's milk and that it can be a source of cross-reactivity with beef and probably with lamb because of the high homology with ovine immunoglobulins (similarly as for meat allergy in humans). Also it was shown that phosphoglucomutase is an important allergen involved in allergic reaction to lamb and beef.[4]

Ralf Mueller commented that he has seen some poly-sensitised animals (which reacted to six or seven allergens) but that those are the exception. Most react to only one or two allergens. The prevalence or relevance of cross-reactivity is not known. He had seen lamb and beef cross-reactions, and also dogs known to be allergic to beef that could tolerate lamb.

Catherine Milley (*Canada*) questioned if Ralf Mueller had ever used a vegetarian diet.

Ralf Mueller replied that a vegetarian diet is useful in dogs that have been fed so many types of food that it is hard to identify a novel protein, or in dogs living in vegan households. The problems are two-fold: it is hard to stop dogs losing weight on an all-vegetarian diet, and flatulence is also a problem.

Ed Rosser said that beans must be soaked for at least 24–48 hours and then the water should be changed. He said that cross-reactivity is mostly molecularly based and not a clinical problem.

The Chairman then introduced Phil Roudebush, who would discuss aspects of food cross-reactivity.

Phil Roudebush (*USA*) commented that he had been involved in clinical diet trials for over 25 years. He said that adverse reactions to foods can occur alone, but more often they reflect a multifaceted, complex disease of allergic dermatitis in which food allergy is only a part. He reminded the audience that food-induced hypersensitivity and non-flea-induced allergy (e.g. atopy) cannot be differentiated clinically in either dogs or cats.[5] He presented data from 330 food-allergic dogs reported in published studies over the past 45 years. The most recent data were from research abstracts at this World Congress. The four most common ingredients causing adverse reactions in dogs were beef, dairy products, chicken and wheat, which accounted for 78% of all reported adverse reactions. The top three ingredients (beef, dairy and wheat allergens) account for around two-thirds (66%) of all reported reactions in which the allergen had been identified. In cats there is a paucity of data. He could only identify trials involving 56 cases in cats where challenge studies were reported, and the major allergens were beef, dairy and fish. Interestingly, there are very few dairy ingredients in commercial pet foods. Most dairy products are fed by owners in addition to the pet food.

The chemical nature of the allergens had been identified in some cases, at least in dogs:

- chicken – chicken serum albumin
- beef – bovine serum albumin
- milk and beef – bovine IgG
- lamb – ovine IgG
- beef and lamb – muscle phosphoglucomutase (may cross-react in all mammalian tissue)
- soya – glycoproteins of 50 and 75 kDa.

Phil Roudebush stated that chicken serum albumin was easily broken down by hydrolysis so that he had no problem, in principle, with chicken hydrolysates. Further, commercial chicken-based dog foods contain chicken by-products (e.g. viscera, feet), which might not contain chicken albumin. Likewise, challenging with chicken breast may not expose the animal to the relevant allergen.

Phil Roudebush noted that phosphoglucomutase is present in nearly all mammalian cells, where it helps to regulate glucose metabolism. This allergen might account for some of the beef and lamb cross-reactions that have been recorded.

In humans, cross-reactivity is seen between cow's milk and other milks, between chicken and eggs, between fish and different fish, and between domestic poultry and wild fowl. Tropomyosin is highly conserved across insects and swimming invertebrates such as squid and may be highly sensitizing. Cross-reactions across vegetable oils are very rare as they contain virtually no protein. Cross-reactions between vegetables and legumes are also virtually nonexistent. Very few such cross-reaction studies have been performed in dogs. It has been demonstrated, albeit in a very small number of dogs, that those allergic to beef could tolerate milk.

Phil Roudebush then discussed studies of various diets that have been advocated as suitable for screening dogs and cats for food allergy. In a study published in *Veterinary Dermatology* in 1992, he looked at 150 home-cooked diet recipes recommended by 116 veterinarians with an interest in dermatology (members of the American Academy of Veterinary Dermatology and American College of Veterinary Dermatology).[6] Only 10% of diets advocated for initial investigation were nutritionally adequate. Much more concerning, however, is that between 50% (canine) and 65% (feline) of diets advocated for long-term management of food-allergic animals were nutritionally deficient. Only 16 of the more than 60 commercial diets advocated as suitable for the diagnosis of food allergy have been subject to published studies into efficacy. Collectively, these studies indicate 65–85% efficacy in diagnosis of adverse food reactions. Addressing this figure, he again pointed out that most of the dogs in these studies would have had chronic, complex disease, and that some probably did not even have adverse food reactions.[7–10]

With regard to the hydrolysed protein diets, there have been 13 studies into four diets, with similar efficacy to the nonhydrolysed diets.

Phil Roudebush emphasized the importance of getting the owner to keep a diet diary. The diary often contains important information that the owners fail to report in the clinic. It must record details of all food offered, the clinical signs observed, faecal output, etc. He reported one dog with an apparent beer-related reaction.

Ed Rosser commented that chicken serum albumin was a major allergenic component in chicken. He wondered if chicken serum albumin was present in diets containing chicken by-products.

Phil Roudebush replied that it was. There may also be other allergens present.

Ed Rosser stated that with regard to the hydrolysed chicken-based diets, the best hydrolysis leaves around 1% original protein. If so, that was 1% too much.

Phil Roudebush said that was true, and additionally we should recognize the difference between ingredients versus allergens. The chicken serum albumin was eliminated but there may be other allergens present within these hydrolysed products that we have yet to recognize.

An unidentified delegate asked why no one recommended the use of two, or even three, hypoallergenic diets in order to increase the chance of diagnosis?

Didier Carlotti replied that the answer is time and money.

Phil Roudebush stated that he routinely recommends a 60-day trial with one commercial novel protein or hydrolysed diet and, if there is no response, he follows it with another commercial 'hypoallergenic' diet trial. Occasionally, he uncovers food allergy in this second stage.

The Chairman then opened the second part of the workshop, dedicated to diets and essential fatty acids (EFAs) in the management of allergic skin disease. He introduced Nina Glos as the first speaker.

Nina Glos (*Germany*) described enrolling 42 atopic dogs into a multicentre, randomized, placebo-controlled, 8-week study with CADESI clinical scoring and pruritus assessment (using a visual analogue scale) every 4 weeks.[11] Three commercially available veterinary 'dermatologic' diets were used – Diet A: Hill's Prescription Diet Salmon and Rice (Hill's Pet Nutrition); Diet B: Eukanuba Dermatosis FP (Procter & Gamble Pet Care); Diet C: Royal Canin Canine Hypoallergenic (Royal Canin) – and one over-the-counter placebo diet.

Eukanuba Dermatosis FP was the only diet that was associated with both a decrease in CADESI (47%) and pruritus scores (14%), whereas Hill's Salmon and Rice was associated with a 28% reduction in pruritus score alone.

The diets contained different combinations and ratios of *n*-6 and *n*-3 EFAs, with the lowest ratio (2.7:1) in the Eukanuba Dermatosis FP. What is unknown is the relevance of *n*-3, *n*-6 or *n*-6/*n*-3 ratio to these results, for as **Ralf Mueller** commented, this was an early study.

Phil Roudebush made a general point about oil supplementation: oils are 97–98% absorbed whatever the source. This high bioavailability suggests that the source of oil, be it *n*-3 or *n*-6, is irrelevant – the way in which it is metabolized physiologically is important.

Ralf Mueller said that we do not know what the ideal dose of these oils should be, what type of EFA might be best and whether it is best when given as a component of the diet or as a supplement or topically. He advocated, personally, *n*-3 (or a combination of *n*-3 and *n*-6) EFAs, at a dose of 50–100 mg/kg/day. He had no particular favourite product, tending to use what the owner felt most comfortable using. Not forgetting that supplementing EFAs at this dose adds to the daily calorie load, a commensurate reduction in food calories might be necessary. He also highlighted a recent blinded study that he had completed, citing work reported from France (Didier Pin), using a topical EFA preparation (Dermoscent® Essential 6 Spot-On Skin Care for Dogs, Dermoscent). Application resulted in an 18–30% reduction in CADESI score, although the strong odour (herbal scent) was undesirable to some clients. A Virbac topical product (Allerderm®) was also useful, and not as fragrant.

Ed Rosser pointed out that although the application of topical *n*-6 EFA (Dermoscent Essential 6 Spot-On Skin Care for Dogs) to the skin of dogs with recalcitrant sebaceous adenitis is helpful, the mechanism of action is not known – does it result in barrier enhancement or is it absorbed and exerting an anti-inflammatory effect?

The Chairman then introduced Hilary Jackson again, to talk further about EFAs.

Hilary Jackson thanked Phil Roudebush for providing some current information regarding EFAs in diet. Summarizing the *n*-3 and *n*-6 cascade, she wondered if *n*-9 EFAs might be important in the anti-inflammatory cascade, although we know little about them in the context of skin disease. She reminded delegates that arachidonic acid is essential for cats, which are obligate carnivores. Hilary Jackson also reminded delegates that 6–12 weeks are required for orally provided EFAs to be incorporated into cell membranes, and that this ought to be the minimum period for which clinicians should supplement these oils before making a decision about efficacy. She pointed out that all commercial diets are more than adequately supplemented with oils, vis-á-vis normal dietary requirements. Neither Δ^5- nor Δ^6-desaturase are present in the epidermis, so unless necessary EFAs are present in the diet they will not reach the skin. She referred to **Ed Rosser's** point as to whether, for example, topically applied EFAs might be incorporated into ceramides. Given that there is no epidermal capability to metabolize topically applied linoleic acid, she doubted that they could be incorporated into ceramides. There is some evidence that orally administered EFAs (Karen Campbell's work) can decrease the concentrations of circulating and intracellular inflammatory molecules.[12,13] There was also a Nordic study demonstrating that oral supplementation with EFAs could significantly reduce steroid requirement in atopic dogs.[14] She reviewed some of the European EFA supplements and commented that if she wants an *n*-3 supplement she is currently using Yumega Plus® (Medic Animal, UK). If she wishes to address a perceived skin barrier defect she looks to an *n*-6 supplement.

Phil Roudebush pointed out that extensive EFA data were available in his presentation in the otitis symposium yesterday. Furthermore, the EFA data relating to most commercial diets available in the USA and Canada are available on the Mark Morris Institute website (www.markmorrisinstitute.org) and that they are reviewed and updated annually.

The Chairman then introduced Didier Pin to discuss barrier enhancement in atopic dogs.

Didier Pin (*France*) described his ultrastructural and lipid study into the benefits of using an *n*-3 and *n*-6 lipid supplement in atopic dogs. His results were based on using Megaderm® (Virbac SA, France), a commercially prepared mixture of *n*-6 and *n*-3 EFAs, for 8 weeks plus a 1-week washout.

The stratum corneum lipids originate from lamellar bodies within the differentiating corneocytes. Enzymatic action results in this lipid organizing into intercellular lipid lamellae (free lipid). In addition there is some protein-bound lipid that is included within the lipid envelope of the corneocyte.

The stratum corneum free lipids (cholesterol, fatty acids and ceramides) had similar concentrations in both normal controls and atopic dogs. However, the protein-bound lipid portion was different: atopic dogs had significantly decreased concentrations of protein-bound fatty acids and ceramides. If we look at fatty acids, for example: in healthy dogs the fatty acids are evenly distributed throughout the successive layers of the stratum corneum, whereas in atopic dogs they are barely detectable and are heterogeneously distributed.

Didier Pin's research group had previously shown, through ultrastructural studies of the stratum corneum, that in healthy dogs the corneocytes are long and flat and coalesce closely.[15] This is particularly true in the deeper part of the stratum corneum, the stratum compactum. In atopic dogs the corneocytes of the stratum corneum are properly shaped but do not coalesce as closely, and the intercellular spaces are wide and empty – this can be termed stratum disjunctum. Furthermore, a closer view shows that the intercellular spaces between squames in the normal dogs are filled with well-organized intercellular lipid lamellae. In contrast, the intercellular spaces in the atopic dogs are wide and empty and contain small, distorted lipid lamellae.

After 8 weeks of oral supplementation, the protein-bound lipid concentrations in atopic dogs returned towards normal and the concentration of free lipid (which was not abnormal before the study) increased. Ultrastructural studies of the deeper stratum corneum compactum demonstrated that in normal dogs the well-organized lamellae occupied 90% of the intercellular spaces. In atopic dogs the pre-treatment value was 26% and after treatment this had increased to 59%, still well below normal.

In conclusion, Didier Pin's research group observed an improvement in the concentration of protein-bound ceramides, and this may be responsible for observation of an increase in lamellar lipids in the stratum corneum compactum. The failure to restore the defects to normal may reflect an imperfect mix of oils, or a too short period of supplementation.

Didier Carlotti asked if this dietary approach to restoring the skin barrier was clinically relevant at the level of Megaderm prescribed in this study.

Didier Pin answered that he did indeed use EFA with this aim in atopic dogs but that he was unsure of the clinical relevance. Perhaps the barrier improvement, while significant enough to be measured, was too little to be assessed as providing clinical improvement.

Ed Rosser observed that the lamellar improvement did in fact double, and particularly since it was so deep in the stratum corneum, it must have some clinical relevance.

The Chairman closed the workshop by thanking the speakers for their excellent contributions.

References

1. Ricci R, Granato A, Palagiano C *et al.* Detection of food antigens in dog foods used as elimination diets. In: *Abstract Proceeding* 15th Congress of the European Society of Veterinary and Comparative Nutrition, Zaragoza, Spain, September 14–16, 2011.
2. Zimmer A, Bexley J, Halliwell RE *et al.* Food allergen-specific serum IgG and IgE before and after elimination diets in allergic dogs. *Vet Immunol Immunopathol* 2011; 44: 442–447.
3. Ayuso R, Lehrer SB, Lopez M *et al.* Identification of bovine IgG as a major cross-reactive vertebrate meat allergen. *Allergy* 2000; 55: 348–354.
4. Martín A, Sierra MP, González JL, Arévalo MA. Identification of allergens responsible for canine cutaneous adverse food reactions to lamb, beef and cow's milk. *Vet Dermatol* 2004; 15: 349–356.
5. Jackson HA, Murphy KM, Tater KC *et al.* The pattern of allergen hypersensitivity (dietary or environmental) of dogs with non-seasonal atopic dermatitis cannot be differentiated on the basis of historical or clinical information: a prospective evaluation 2003-2005 [abstract]. In: *Proceedings 20th N Am Vet Dermatol Forum* 2005; 96.
6. Roudebush P, Crowell CS. Results of a hypoallergenic diet survey of veterinarians in North America with a nutritional evaluation of homemade diet prescriptions. *Vet Dermatol* 1992; 3: 23–28.
7. Roudebush P, Guilford WG, Jackson HA. Adverse reactions to food. In: Hand MS, Thatcher CD, Remillard RL *et al.*, eds. *Small Animal Clinical Nutrition,* 5th edn. Topeka, KS: Mark Morris Institute, 2010; 609–635.
8. Fritsch DA, Roudebush P, Allen TM *et al.* Effect of two therapeutic diets in dogs with chronic nonseasonal pruritic dermatitis. *Intern J Appl Res Vet Med* 2010; 8: 146–154.
9. Loeffler A, Lloyd DH, Bond R *et al.* Dietary trials with a commercial chicken hydrolysate diet in 63 pruritic dogs. *Vet Rec* 2004; 154: 519–522.
10. Loeffler A, Soares-Magalhaes R, Bond R *et al.* A retrospective analysis of case series using home-prepared and chicken hydrolysate diets in the diagnosis of adverse food reactions in 181 pruritic dogs. *Vet Dermatol* 2006; 17: 273–279.
11. Glos K, Linek M, Loewenstein C *et al.* The efficacy of commercially available veterinary diets recommended for dogs with atopic dermatitis. *Vet Dermatol* 2008; 19: 280–287.
12. Byrne KP, Campbell KL, Whiteley HF, Schaeffer DJ. The effects of dietary n-3 vs n-6 fatty acids on canine skin after intradermal injection of interleukin-8. *Vet Dermatol* 2000; 11: 123–132.
13. Campbell KL, Laflamme D. Effects of four diets with varying omega 6:omega 3 ratios on the health and appearance of the skin and hair coat in normal dogs. *Vet Dermatol* 2000; 11(S1): 18.
14. Sævik, BK, Bergvall, K, Holm, BR *et al.* A randomized, controlled study to evaluate the steroid sparing effect of essential fatty acid supplementation in the treatment of canine atopic dermatitis: *Vet Dermatol* 2004; 15: 137–145.
15. Piekutowska A, Pin D, Rème CA *et al.* Effects of a topically applied preparation of epidermal lipids on the stratum corneum barrier of atopic dogs. *Comp Pathol* 2008; 138: 197–203.

Secretary's Note: Philip Roudebush has requested that anyone interested in accessing the large number of papers on diets and diet trials that he cited can find these citations in:

Roudebush P, Guilford WG, Jackson HA. Adverse reactions to food. In: Hand MS, Thatcher CD, Remillard RL *et al.*, eds. *Small Animal Clinical Nutrition*, 5th edn. Topeka, KS: Mark Morris Institute, 2010; 609–635.

8.3

Fun with lasers

M. Boord[1] (Chairperson), C.S. Nett-Mettler[2] (Secretary)

[1]Animal Dermatology Clinic of San Diego, California, USA
[2]vetderm.ch – Dermatologie und Allergologie für Tiere, c/o ESK – Ennetsee Klinik fuer Kleintiere, Huenenberg, Switzerland

Mona Boord (*USA*) welcomed the audience to the workshop. She noted that she has used a CO_2 laser since 1999 and finds that it allows her to perform procedures that could not be done with traditional surgery. She introduced three speakers (George Peavy, David Duclos and Claudia Nett) who would be presenting four different talks during the session on the use of lasers in medicine and surgery. The goal of the session was to help participants gain knowledge about the use of lasers in veterinary dermatology and help participants in deciding whether a laser would fit into their practice setting.

Claudia Nett-Mettler served as the secretary for this workshop.

Mona Boord also thanked Peter Vitruk (*USA*), a co-founder of Aesculight, who made it possible for the first speaker, George Peavy, to attend today. George Peavy is a Diplomate of the American Board of Veterinary Practitioners. He is a Project Scientist, Director of Comparative Medicine Programs, and Manager of the Military Photomedicine Program at the Beckman Laser Institute and Medical Clinic, College of Medicine at the University of California, Irvine. He is a leader in the field of laser biomedical research for veterinary and human applications.

Light, tissue and magic: a peek behind the curtain (G.M. Peavy)

George Peavy (*USA*) introduced how laser light interacts with tissue, to help the audience to understand some of the newer technologies currently under investigation that would be presented later in the session, and also to help members of the audience for whom lasers and laser tissue interactions are new concepts.

There are many types of different lasers, each named after the laser media comprising the laser. Different lasers emit light of different wavelengths. The wavelength is specific for the energy state of the laser media. Eximer lasers, which are excited dimer lasers, produce light in the ultraviolet spectrum.

Types of lasers:

- argon, krypton and KTP laser (blue-green light)
- dye and diode laser (577–780 nm wavelength)
- helium neon (the old standard of red laser pointers before diode lasers entered the market)
- gold vapour, ruby laser (red region)
- Nd:YAG, holmium and near infrared diode lasers (910–2100 nm wavelength)
- erbium:YAG (mid-infrared region)
- CO_2 (far infrared region).

Laser selection for a procedure is dependent upon the wavelength of the laser and optical properties of the target tissue. There are a variety of ways that light can interact with tissue. In the following, the basic laser tissue mechanisms are described.

Laser light and interaction with tissue

1 *Reflection.* Light can be completely reflected from tissue – that is why teeth are white: white light is composed of all the wavelengths in the visible spectrum, and all are reflected from the enamel surface.

2 *Transmission.* Light can be transmitted through the tissue (like light going through a glass with clear water in it). Putting a flashlight on one's palm will result in some wavelengths being reflected; the blue and green light is absorbed by chromophores in the tissues of the hand, while the red light is transmitted through the palm and out the other side.

3 *Scattering of light.* Light can be scattered in the tissue. If some milk is added to a glass with clear water, the water becomes cloudy and soon it is impossible to see through because the milk fat molecules dispersed in the water scatter the light.

4 *Absorption of light – photothermal reaction.* Light is absorbed by chromophores in the tissue and transformed into thermal energy, causing a photothermal reaction, with changes to the tissue. This property of light is used to cut or ablate tissue.

5 *Photodisruption – photomechanical action.* High-energy short-duration pulses result in rapid heating and cooling of the tissue generating a shockwave. This is called a photomechanical action, a property that is used in laser lithotripsy.

6 *Photochemistry.* A chemical agent in the tissue is illuminated with a light, which the chemical absorbs. This energy stimulates a chemical reaction, which may be used to selectively destroy a target tissue such as cancer.

7 *Fluorescence emission.* Molecules in the tissue absorb photons of one wavelength, utilize some of that energy, and then release the excess energy in the form of another photon in a lower energy state (and therefore of a different wavelength).

Choosing the correct laser

There are four things that influence the outcome of applying a laser to tissue. Only three of those will be discussed here. These three things are important whether you are cutting or ablating tissue or whether you are using laser as a source of energy for a diagnostic application.

1 *Wavelength selection.* The wavelength needs to be selected so that the target tissue most efficiently absorbs it. There are a variety of chromophores in the body that will absorb light:

- Melanin/haemoglobin. These chromophores absorb light in the blue and green but not in the red wavelengths. This is why haemoglobin is red: it absorbs the green, blue, orange and yellow light but not red light.
- Water. Water is a chromophore that absorbs infrared light (it does not absorb in the visible spectrum – which is why it appears transparent). Lasers in the mid- and far-infrared spectrum will cut with more efficiency than a laser that is absorbed by melanin or haemoglobin, because soft tissues contain more water than either haemoglobin or melanin.

2 *Photothermal reactions.* When tissue is heated but does not reach 60°C, the tissue is only warmed up. If the heating is continued and reaches 60–65°C, denaturation of proteins occurs and tissue will no longer be viable. At 100°C, water goes through a phase change and vaporizes, which results in increased pressure within the tissue. Once the pressure exceeds the strength of confinement in the tissue, explosive vaporization occurs. If the heating continues for too long, all the oxygen, nitrogen and hydrogen elements are released, resulting in carbonization of the tissue.

3 *Beam intensity (watts/cm^2).* Beam intensity (power density, irradiance) describes the rate at which photons are being delivered by the laser beam per unit area of tissue; this determines how efficient the laser exposure is going to be. A 10 W laser being put into a spot diameter of 2 mm will allow the delivery of approximately 320 W/cm^2. This intensity results only in warming of the tissue. Vaporization does not necessarily require a higher power laser, instead the laser can be focused or adjusted into a smaller spot size. Using a 0.2 mm focal spot, the same laser at 10 W will be delivering 32 000 W/cm^2. Changes of the spot diameter by a factor of two will change the intensity (e.g. the number of photons per unit area) by a factor of four. When using a CO_2 laser, it is very important to have a power density of 4500–5000 W/cm^2 in order to get good and efficient ablation. A 10 W laser beam delivered in a 0.8 mm focal spot delivers 2000 W/cm^2, a setting that will allow cutting, but with reduced efficiency, resulting in thermal injury. By switching to a 0.4 mm focal spot diameter, the intensity will increase to 10 000 W/cm^2.

4 *Time domain of beam delivery.* The longer it takes to cut or ablate tissue, the more time is allowed for heat to diffuse to the surrounding tissue, resulting in collateral thermal injury. Using higher power settings speeds cutting and ablating, thus resulting in less collateral thermal injury to surrounding tissue. Some lasers have a superpulse mode that delivers an ablation threshold level of energy in an individual pulse that is less than the thermal relaxation time of the tissue. Consequently the ablation is accomplished before there is enough time for heat diffusion into the surrounding tissue to cause thermal injury. The amount of thermal injury is thus *both* wavelength and time dependent

George Peavy explained that in his opinion there are two advantages of using a CO_2 laser instead of traditional surgical techniques:

a Simultaneous haemostasis when excising tissue.

b Tissue can be removed with high precision moving between the focused and defocused regions of the beam, enabling the user to ablate cell layer by cell layer and remove tissue without damaging any sensitive structures.

5 *Selective photothermolysis.* This uses a technique where the target tissue, which is to be eliminated, has one optical property and the surrounding normal tissue has different optical properties. If using a laser that is absorbed by the target tissue but transmitted by the normal surrounding tissue, the target tissue is destroyed while sparing the surrounding tissue as it passes through. Examples for the use of selective photothermolysis are angiomatosis, distichiasis (individual pigmented hairs can be removed), and cyclophotocoagulation for treating glaucoma.

6 *Photodynamic therapy.* This is a process where an individual is administered a photochemical drug that localizes in cancer tissue. The area is then illuminated with a laser that produces a wavelength that excites that chemical agent (i.e. photochemical interaction) and produces singlet oxygen that destroys the tissue where the photochemical agent is localized. One typical clinical application is actinic keratosis in cats.

Mona Boord introduced David Duclos, the next speaker, as someone who is interested in CO_2 lasers and has used them since 1992.

CO_2 laser use in dermatology (D. Duclos)

David Duclos (*USA*) explained that when he first started to use a CO_2 laser, his main goal was to find out whether there were areas where a laser would do a better job than a surgical knife. His talk would concentrate on indications for CO_2 laser therapy – such as when lasers are the best or only option. Currently, David Duclos prefers using the laser for most standard operations and rarely uses a surgical knife.

David Duclos prefers the Aesculight CO_2 laser. It is the only self-calibrating laser with calibration at the tip. This means that the rate of delivered energy is measured right at the tip of the laser; if set to 2 W, 2 W will be delivered from the tip of the laser.

He uses general anaesthesia in most cases; local anaesthesia is only used for single lesions.

Examples of procedures amenable to CO_2 laser therapy were discussed, as follows.

Nodular sebaceous hyperplasia (multiple) and sebaceous gland tumours ('senile warts')

1 Cosmetic use of laser to ablate nodular glands causing neither pain nor pruritus. Therefore, animals rarely lick at the laser surgery sites.

2 No sutures needed, much shorter surgery time.

3 Laser settings:

a Typically uses the 0.8 mm tip or the paint brush tip.

b Power: starts at high power at 20 W and reduces to super pulse and 5 W at the base of the tumour.

4 Without a laser, those nodular growths would not be removed, as they are mainly a cosmetic problem. Using laser surgery to remove them generates new income and helps to pay for the laser.

Apocrine gland tumours and apocrine cysts

1 Mainly in cats affecting the ears, face and chin.

2 Laser is used for ablation of all cystic tissue.

3 Easiest if lesions are not yet large clusters, obstructing the ear canal.

4 No sutures needed, heals within 2–3 weeks.

Viral lesions

1 These include papilloma viral warts, pigmented viral plaques, Bowen's disease/bowenoid in situ carcinoma.

2 Laser can be used as a good alternative to imiquimod or other topical therapies especially in Bowen's disease where it is often difficult to treat all lesions topically.

3 Procedure for treating Bowen's disease/bowenoid carcinoma in situ:

a Obtain biopsy whenever possible to establish a diagnosis prior to laser ablation.

b Disadvantage of the laser: evaporates the tissue, nothing to submit for histopathology.

c Repeated treatment may be necessary in many of the larger tumours and especially in Bowen's disease.

d Settings for Bowen's disease/bowenoid carcinoma in situ:

i Start with the paintbrush tip, and then switch to a smaller spot size tip 0.8 mm.

ii 10 W at continuous wave until lesion is mostly ablated, and then reduce settings to super pulse at about 2 W. The lesion is completely ablated once the pigment is completely gone.

iii To cut tissue increase power to 25 W with 0.4 mm tip, which cuts like a knife with no collateral damage. Use of laser to cut with lower power density increases collateral damage and delays healing.

4 Canine pigmented viral plaques:

a Primarily seen in schnauzers, caused by papilloma virus.

b These lesions are mainly treated for cosmetic reasons: owners dislike their appearance but they do not cause pain or pruritus. There are some literature statements that they could potentially progress into carcinomas.

c Lesions are associated with hyperpigmentation; need to continue ablation until pigment is no longer seen.

d Settings:

i Since the CO_2 laser is best absorbed by water and these lesions consist of mainly melanin and collagen, it takes a lot of energy to ablate them with the CO_2 laser.

ii Paintbrush tip at 20 W and continuous wave. Takes much more time compared to, e.g., sebaceous gland tumours due to the little amount of water in these plaques. At the base of the lesion, the power is reduced to 2 W at super pulse.

5 Viral papilloma:

a Laser as an adjunctive if needed.

b Administer systemic interferon subcutaneously for 1 month, 3 times weekly.

c If there is not complete resolution with interferon therapy, CO_2 laser can be used as an adjunctive therapy.

d If viral papillomas are only treated with laser, they will regrow approximately three to five times. This rarely occurs when interferon is used prior to laser therapy.

e For single papilloma virus lesions, laser can be used with local anaesthesia.

Lentigo simplex

1 Hyperpigmented macules in cats mainly seen on the mucocutaneous junctions of the nose, eyes and lips.

2 Laser can be used to ablate those, even though they are only cosmetic.

3 Settings: continuous wave at 20 W with paintbrush tip; after reaching normal, nonpigmented skin, reduce power to 2–5 W at super pulse setting.

Squamous cell carcinoma, actinic keratosis

1 For surgical excisions, extremely small spot sizes should be used to prevent collateral thermal injury. In such cases, David Duclos suggests using a very small spot size of 0.2 mm and setting the power high (25 W). At this setting the CO_2 laser will cut like a knife and not cause collateral damage. If a larger spot size at a lower power is used, damaged collateral tissue will likely slough at the incision site.

2 These are treatable with laser ablation but may need multiple surgeries. Will need deeper ablation of the neoplastic tissue than with other tumour types.

3 Some are too large for surgery; for these cases laser ablation may serve as a palliative treatment.

Spindle cell tumours

Usually not treatable with laser surgery because of the depth of the lesions.

Plasma cell pododermatitis

1 Only affects footpads resulting in swollen, soft and spongy footpads, primarily seen in cats. Usually only the large central pad is affected.

2 David Duclos uses laser surgery, but only if medical therapy fails. Some can be successfully treated with laser; some will return and require multiple surgeries.

3 Settings:

a Small spot size 0.2 mm at high power of 25 W continuous wave to cut and peel away the affected tissue.

b Sutures are necessary after this procedure.

c Pain medication is used after treatment. One may also need to bandage for several days.

Miscellaneous tumours amenable to laser surgery

1 Examples in this category include fibromas, naevi, mixed epitheliomas, plasma cell tumours, follicular tumours, gingival tumours and follicular cysts.

2 The laser is used in these cases for either ablation if the lesions are more superficial or as a cutting knife if they are deeper (e.g. trichoblastoma and other follicular tumours). For follicular cysts, make a very small incision and peel the lesion out through the incision.

3 Gingival hyperplasia and masses:

- **a** If no response to azithromycin, the laser can be used.
- **b** Since the laser can burn enamel, the teeth should be protected from the laser energy with a metal spatula positioned underneath the gingiva.

Mona Boord then introduced Claudia Nett-Mettler as the final speaker and secretary of this workshop.

Diode laser use in the dermatological practice (C.S. Nett-Mettler)

Claudia S. Nett-Mettler (*Switzerland*) explained that the diode laser can be used for many procedures as previously shown with the CO_2 laser. She uses a class IV diode laser with an energy range of 10–15 W. The spot sizes are 0.2 and 0.4 mm, and in addition there is a therapy hand-piece.

She uses the diode laser primarily for the removal of skin masses, eyelid tumours, and ear polyps. She also uses it as a 'laser shower' for aural haematomas and to accelerate wound healing. As a therapy laser, the diode laser is also commonly used by surgeons to accelerate wound healing, by physiotherapists to alleviate chronic pain of muscles and joints, and by acupuncturists.

Claudia Nett-Mettler uses local anaesthesia and cold packs or ice cubes to laser small tumours in sedated dogs. Cold anaesthetic sprays should not be used with lasers because they are highly flammable. For the same reason oxygen masks should not be used for anaesthesia in laser patients, and tracheal tubes should be tight fitting to avoid oxygen leakage.

If aural haematomas do not respond to medical therapy or if an owner is reluctant to have his/her dog undergo surgery, Claudia Nett-Mettler uses the diode laser to first create a small hole at the tip of the pinna to allow the bloody exudate to drain. This hole should be created large enough to prevent it from closing for at least 7–10 days. To help heal the separated cartilage, the 0.2 mm flexible hand-piece is introduced into the cavity to scarify the tissue within the cavity thus accelerating the healing process. The power is set to 2 W. Claudia Nett-Mettler remarked that with the diode laser it is difficult to visualize how deeply the laser is penetrating into tissues. Since the diode laser is a near-infrared laser at 680–910 nm it reaches far deeper into the tissue than a CO_2 laser thus creating more collateral damage.

Because the diode laser has a flexible fibre, it can be used in conjunction with a video-otoscope to treat glandular hyperplasia and polyps originating from the lateral ear canal walls. Care has to be taken over how long and how much energy is applied to such lesions in order to prevent collateral thermal injury to the ear canals. The laser fibre is small and flexible enough to be introduced into the working channel of the video-otoscope.

Laser shower/laser radiation

The diode laser can also be used as a laser shower. This application of laser radiation is used to treat painful conditions of soft tissue, muscles and joints. It is also used to reduce exuberant granulation tissue formation and to accelerate wound healing. The effects of laser radiation on tissue include the reduction of inflammation, pain and oedema formation. It accelerates wound healing by increasing mitochondrial ATP production, improving microcirculation, promoting peripheral nerve regeneration and reducing the number of micro-organisms.

For laser radiation, the energy is set at 1.5–5 W (depending on the tissue type) and the therapy hand-piece is used to provide a defocused laser beam. The hand-piece is slowly moved over the affected area without touching the tissue (non-touch technique) for a total of 3–5 minutes. Laser therapy is usually repeated every 2–3 days for five to seven treatments. Claudia Nett-Mettler has successfully used laser radiation therapy for chronic wounds in a snake and for thrombovascular necrosis of the pinnae in multiple dogs. Unfortunately no controlled studies have been published. However, Claudia Nett-Mettler successfully treated a Magyar vizsla with severe bilateral thrombovascular necrosis of the pinnae, which was previously on various topical and systemic medication including corticosteroids. After six sessions, the dog could be weaned off all medication, and after seven treatments there were no active lesions. The dog has not relapsed in over 1.5 years.

New frontiers in structural and functional optical diagnostics (G.M. Peavy)

George Peavy introduced his second talk by saying that Mona Boord had asked him to give a preview of future uses of medical lasers including new frontiers in structural and functional optical diagnostics. There are multi-day conferences presented on photonics and biophotonics and the different kinds of technologies being developed that use light as a source of energy. He decided to focus on a few technologies that have applications in the field of dermatology and hoped these would be of interest to the audience.

Optical coherence tomography (OCT)

This is a photonic version of ultrasound. It uses reflection that occurs at the interface of tissues with different refractive indices. If you have two different tissues with slightly different optical properties, there is a change in refractive index, and some light will reflect back. Differences in the reflected light compared to the entering light are detected and used to generate a tissue image. Ophthalmology is one area where there are clinically available OCT units, in human clinical practice. They are primarily used for mapping retinas and provide a very high quality image.

For an example of what these images are like he showed an OCT unit image of the palm of a hand. Epidermal folds of the epidermis, the dermis and apocrine sweat glands can be seen. The technique produces images of tissues to a depth of 2 cm and can be used to plot changes in the skin much as ultrasound devices are used to look into the abdominal cavity.

Multiphoton microscopy (MPM)

Multiphoton microscopy is a technology that induces and detects natural tissue fluorescence. In standard fluorescence microscopy an optical lens is used to look at tissue planes. There is a light source and molecules within the tissue that are labelled using a fluorescent marker. The marker may be a fluorescent dye or it may be a fluorescence-tagged antibody, and the light source elicits a fluorescent response. Fluorescence is seen at the level of the focal point of the lens and there is fluorescence below and above it adding background noise. This makes fluorescence microscopy difficult. There is a trade-off between resolution and clarity.

Multiphoton microscopy (MPM) takes advantage of a phenomenon whereby some chemical structures, if they absorb two photons of the same wavelength at exactly the same time, combine the energy of both photons into a single photon and then release that single photon. This is called frequency doubling. Collagen does this without any loss of energy. An 800 nm incident beam is used and collagen combines two of these photons at the same time and releases a 400 nm wavelength photon, which is in the green region. In order to get a two-photon event, the laser beam, which is monochromatic at 800 nm, must be focused into a very small spot. By increasing the population of photons in a very small area, the chance that a two-photon event will occur is increased.

A benefit of multiphoton microscopy is that the fluorescence is generated right at the focal point, and not above or below it. The lens objective can be used to change the focal length and thereby scan through the thickness of the tissue being examined; the fluorescence emission is from natural chemical agents in the tissue, and the fluorescence is generated right at the focal point of the lens. Collagens yield a second harmonic generation, and a variety of chemical agents also provide two-photon fluorescence. Examples of these include riboflavin, NADH, folic acid, cholecalciferol, retinol, pyridoxine and elastin, all of which will fluoresce in the 450–600 nm range.

The synovium is an area in which George Peavy has been involved in research using two-photon microscopy to study joint disease. The intima is the lining of the joint capsule and is about two to three cell layers thick. Below it is the subintima, which is composed of collagen, next is a layer of adipocytes and below that are blood vessels. These are the primary structures that make up synovium. When visualized using two-photon microscopy, the blue material is all collagen. Green fluorescence is produced by chemicals that are inside the individual cells. The individual cells have a fluorescence shadow enabling visualization of both the outside of the cell and inside the nucleus. Red blood cells can be seen within blood vessels, and adipocytes may be found encased in collagen. The adipocytes have nuclear material and a blank space that is occupied by lipid, which does not fluoresce. A typical multiphoton image is about 250 μm square; when these are collected successively and tiled together a larger image is produced that demonstrates the intima, collagen, subintima, blood vessels and adipocytes.

With regard to joint cartilage, similar to individual planar images that can be scanned, a stack of these planar images of joint cartilage, which are 100 μm deep, can be put together to form a three-dimensional image. An example image was shown of joint cartilage. The blue represented collagen and the red represented elastin not previously thought to be found in cartilage.

There is also a clinical MPM imaging unit for dermatology. It is not licensed by the FDA in the USA. There is a prototype unit being made by a startup company in Germany. These can be purchased from the company for approximately US$700 000. Veterinarians in Germany may be able to make arrangements with the company (JenLab) to use one of the units. The name of the unit is MPTflex. Images can be obtained to a depth of 200 μm (100 μm is about the thickness of a human hair). Images taken of the skin surface, the keratin layer, 20, 40 and 60 μm down into tissue were presented. Collagen appears blue. Fat cannot be imaged using standard MPM. To study fat, MPM can be combined with a coherent anti-Stokes Raman scattering (CARS). This involves taking two photons from a pump laser into tissue that stimulates vibration in C_2H bonds and releases a 600 nm photon.This allows visualization of adipocytes and/or lipid-containing structures such as sebaceous glands. A picture of skin histology was shown that included sebaceous glands and a hair follicle imaged by MPM plus CARS imaging technology on an *ex vivo* skin sample. The tissue structures can be visualized without a biopsy sample being taken.

Diffuse optical spectroscopy

This is a functional imaging technology in which lasers are used to detect and quantify physiological changes in tissue. As light enters tissue it scatters and some of it is absorbed, attenuating the light. The intensity of the beam coming back out of the tissue is dependent upon the number of scatters and absorbers in the tissue. Diffuse optical spectroscopy directs laser light into the tissue and then detects the reflected light coming back out of the tissue after interaction with the tissue constituents. The light molecules detected can be used to determine the amount of oxyhaemoglobin, deoxyhaemoglobin, water, lipid and cytochrome *c* oxidase in the tissue. There are a variety of applications in trauma and critical care, for example in detection of impending haemorrhagic shock, evaluating response to blood replacement and a variety of other things that can improve patient management.

Spatial frequency domain imaging

This is mapping or plotting tissue oxygenation and haemoglobin content in each pixel of an image of the tissue. An example was shown of skin flaps on a pig. One flap had normal circulation and one had compromised circulation (a vessel was ligated). This technology is being developed to assess wounds such as burns in humans. One of the challenges in the treatment of burns is being able to predict where within the burn the tissue will not survive. The standard way of doing this is looking and watching over a few days until the eschar forms and tissue begins to slough; however, waiting this long increases the risk of infection within the tissue. There is real interest in being able to determine what is nonviable tissue and debriding it early to minimize the risk of secondary infections. An image of a burn wound was shown. The degree of oedema could be visualized, and areas with poor oxygenation could be detected and then debrided.

Laser speckle contrast imaging

This uses a laser beam directed through a lens into tissue and depicts the reflections coming back through digital photography. Where there is motion inside the tissue, such as capillaries with red blood cells, there is a loss of speckle imaging. By taking a series of speckle images and subtracting from each one the places where the speckle disappears, a flow map can be developed. The disappearance of speckles can be translated into a flow map of how fast in a tissue the blood cells are flowing through the vessel. A large camera system that can capture whole body images can map people with larger areas of burns to better predict tissue viability and follow the healing of burns. Speckle imaging can also be used to monitor a pulse laser treatment of a birthmark. Light green translates into normal circulation going through a portwine stain while dark-blue areas are sites where treatment with the laser is creating thermolysis and blanching. Speckle imaging can therefore be used as a method of monitoring the response intraoperatively to know when an area has been adequately treated.

Mona Boord invited the audience to ask questions to the three speakers.

G. Ghibaudo (*Italy*) asked whether it would be possible to use the CO_2 laser for both surgery and low-light laser therapy (LLLT) treatment of patients and how one knows when laser surgery has reached its end-point.

George Peavy replied that not everybody believes in therapeutic laser therapy (LLLT), but if one does, the CO_2 laser cannot be used for this purpose. CO_2 laser beams cannot reach deep into the tissue because water is such a good absorber of infrared light. For therapeutic purposes it is necessary to choose a near infrared laser at 680–910 nm that achieves deeper penetration of the tissue.

The next question was how to know what laser to use and when to stop when using the laser in the ear canal.

Mona Boord responded that there are various types of lasers. The diode lasers are contact lasers, whereas the CO_2 laser is a noncontact laser. A CO_2 laser has a little back suction through the tip that allows the surgeon to see into the ear canal when using short pulses of energy. With a diode laser there is deeper penetration of the tissue causing more tissue damage that will only become apparent after a few days. She thus suggested that in order to minimize the collateral tissue damage in an ear canal it is best to use a snare to remove the bulk of the mass prior to using the laser surgery to ablate the base.

Ralf Mueller (*Germany*) commented he has found it difficult to use a CO_2 laser for feline ear polyps as the base of the lesion is usually too deep to visualize.

Mona Boord agreed and said she does not use a CO_2 laser in ear polyps unless the base tears. She first grasps the mass as far towards the base as possible and applies tension in a twisting motion. If needed a second step, CO_2 laser can be used to ablate the base of the stump while avoiding creating too much heat in the ear canal to minimize collateral thermal tissue damage.

Mona Boord commented that laser surgery has a steep learning curve. The laser cuts slower than a knife and if the surgeon stays too long in one spot a lot of peripheral tissue damage can be caused.

Ursula Mayer (*Germany*) made a comment that, in her clinical experience, animals are rarely painful after laser surgery and it has been theorized that this is because the laser seals nerve endings, but that she had never seen any scientific evidence to prove this and that in humans this is not the case. She asked whether lasers truly are nerve-sealing or whether the decrease in pain is because lasers cause less damage to the tissue compared to conventional surgery.

George Peavy answered that laser wounds in humans are, by self-experience, painful. In the early 1980s, a study that was never published used CO_2 laser surgery in horses for digital neurectomy and scanning electron microscopy images of excised nerves demonstrated melting and sealing of the nerves.

Mona Boord made a comment that prior to utilizing laser surgery, she used electrocauterization to perform rhinectomy and generally the patients exhibited signs of severe pain after the surgery, but that when she started to use laser surgery for this procedure the pain was much less obvious.

Ursula Mayer further queried whether the reduced pain could be due to the fact that with laser surgery less tissue damage is created and that this fact would result in reduced pain regardless of whether or not the nerve endings were sealed.

Mona Boord answered that in addition to nerve endings being sealed there is also sealing of lymphatic and vascular structures. This reduces the perfusion in the wounded tissue and minimizes the 'inflammatory shower'.

George Peavy commented that more thermal damage is caused by using low-power settings compared to high-power settings, and this may lead to increased pain compared to standard surgical techniques. However, he believes that an appropriate laser used correctly can result in a less painful procedure. Caution is warranted because if not used correctly lasers can cause large problems.

Mona Boord thanked the speakers and audience for their attendance before she closed the session.

8.4

Allergen-specific immunotherapy

A. Hillier[1] (Chairperson), J.S. Pendergraft[2] (Secretary)

[1]The Ohio State University, Columbus, Ohio, USA
[2]Colorado State University, Fort Collins, Colorado, USA

Andrew Hillier (*USA*) thanked Heska for sponsoring the workshop and introduced himself as Chairperson. He introduced Jennifer Pendergraft as Secretary for the session. He noted that the content of the workshop was intended to be specific, and not a general discussion of the basics of allergen-specific immunotherapy. Three discussion topics for the workshop and their contributors were introduced: rush immunotherapy by Abby Foust, sublingual immunotherapy in a canine model of atopic dermatitis by Rosanna Marsella followed by early experiences in the use of sublingual immunotherapy in canine patients by Valarie Fadok, and lastly, how to utilize allergen cross-reactivity for the formulation of immunotherapy by Ken Lee. Andrew Hillier observed that it has become clear that sublingual immunotherapy was a hot topic at this congress, and he was pleased to include it in the workshop. Abby Foust was introduced as a University of Florida-trained dermatologist practising for nearly 5 years at MedVet, a multispecialty practice in Columbus, Ohio.

Rush immunotherapy (A. Foust)

Abby Foust (*USA*) noted that rush immunotherapy is the technique of advancing an allergic patient to a maintenance dose of extract over a short period of time. At MedVet this is performed within 6–8 hours. Abby Foust emphasized that there are few articles in the veterinary literature on rush immunotherapy, with the exception of Ralf Mueller and Sonya Bettenay's article in the *American Journal of Veterinary Research* 2001 that described approximately 30 patients,[1] and the report of several cats by Trimmer *et al.* in an article in *Veterinary Dermatology* in 2005.[2] There appears to be more information regarding rush immunotherapy for desensitization of feline asthma patients.

Abby Foust has been performing rush immunotherapy since January 2008. She admitted that initially she was reluctant to try it. However, after observing the technique of her colleague who has been successfully performing rush immunotherapy for many years, she adopted the protocol. Their practice completes approximately 32 rush immunotherapy procedures annually. Upon review of their records, 93% of their rush immunotherapy patients were dogs, and only 7% were cats. As a small animal-only specialty practice, they do not have experience in rush immunotherapy for large animals. Although Abby Foust does test for Hymenoptera venom, she has no experience in rush immunotherapy for these cases. All antigens used at MedVet are aqueous.

Patients are brought to the dermatology service between 8.00 and 9.00 a.m. The clients are asked to read and sign a drop-off form and a consent form prior to admission. For the first 30 minutes, the patients are allowed to acclimate to the environment, consisting of a small room, 2.4 × 3 m. A baseline erythema and pruritus score is established. The patient is supervised throughout the day by a designated veterinary technician, who also prepares the immunotherapy solution. The patient is confined by a barrier in the room, but at least three veterinary technicians and two veterinarians in an adjoining room may also readily view the patient throughout the day. When the designated technician must leave the room for a break or a meal, another technician replaces her during that time, ensuring the patient is monitored continuously.

The rush protocol begins after the 30-minute acclimation period. A three-vial system is used. An injection is administered every 30 minutes until the 13 injection series is completed. The protocol lasts for 6.5 hours and the patients are discharged between 4.00 and 5.00 p.m. The concentration of the allergens is unique: instead of a typical 200 PNU/mL concentration in Vial 1, a 2000 PNU/mL solution in Vial 2, and a 20 000 PNU/mL solution in Vial 3, the concentrations are all twice these standard solutions. The first injection from Vial 1 (400 PNU/mL) is a volume of 0.1 mL, followed by 0.2, 0.4 and 0.8 mL given sequentially 30 minutes apart. The protocol similarly proceeds with Vial 2 (4000 PNU/mL) injected at a volume of 0.1 mL, followed by 0.2, 0.4 and 0.8 mL given sequentially 30 minutes apart. Vial 3 (40 000 PNU/mL) is then injected at a volume of 0.1 mL, followed by 0.2, 0.3, 0.4 and 0.5 mL given sequentially 30 minutes apart. The maintenance dose is a total of 20 000 PNU of allergen (0.5 mL of 40 000 PNU/mL solution). Abby Foust explained that the concentrations chosen are for the convenience of the client; a full 1.0 mL injection as maintenance can be cumbersome for the clients compared to a volume of 0.5 mL.

An intravenous catheter is not placed for the rush protocol, nor is the patient premedicated with antihistamines or corticosteroids. Antihistamines and corticosteroids are continued as previously dosed in patients receiving them on a maintenance basis at the time of rush immunotherapy. Review of the cases showed that 73% of patients experienced no adverse events, and she pointed out this is very similar to the percentage reported by Mueller and

Bettenay in their aforementioned manuscript. Adverse events are typically witnessed 5–10 minutes after an injection. If there is uncertainty regarding an adverse event or if there is only a mild change, such as an escalation in pruritus from 3/10 to 4/10, a subcutaneous injection of the identical concentration and volume is repeated at the next time point to see if the event is repeatable. Abby Foust reported that she and her colleagues at MedVet tend to be very cautious in their approach to adverse events, and attribute probable significance to even mild adverse reactions.

The most common adverse events are increased pruritus and erythema. The patient is thoroughly assessed for erythema including the interdigital spaces and the groin and axillae. Erythema is most often observed on the muzzle, face and, in particular, the concave surfaces of the pinnae. Urticaria is a relatively rare event, as only one patient of the last 26 receiving rush immunotherapy developed urticaria. One canine patient was observed to have ptyalism. Abby Foust remarked that she debated whether or not this should be mentioned in her presentation, as this dog was previously reported to have ptyalism at other veterinary visits and this was presumed to be a stress response and unrelated to rush immunotherapy.

The most common reason for offering rush immunotherapy is convenience for the client. Examples provided included clients with phobias of needles, elderly or disabled owners, or families leaving town for an extended period of time. Rush immunotherapy may reduce stress and confusion for the clients under these circumstances. She commented that one of the best features of rush immunotherapy is ensuring compliance, as a traditional induction period provides ample opportunity for missteps. It was also suggested that rush immunotherapy is a good option for patients with fluctuating pruritus. Because induction is completed in one day, natural day-by-day fluctuations in pruritus prompted by events such as cutting the grass or a hike outdoors do not interfere with the client's or practitioner's interpretations of adverse events. It was additionally noted that seasonally pruritic patients approaching their offending season are offered rush immunotherapy to reduce such confusion as well. Abby Foust has not noted a more rapid clinical response with rush immunotherapy although she admitted that she did not review records in search of this information.

Few patients are excluded from rush immunotherapy. Size is not a factor for exclusion as the protocol has been successfully employed in cats and very small dogs. Number and intensity of positive reactions on intradermal tests are also not factors for exclusion. Patients are primarily excluded for unacceptable behaviour; patients demonstrating incessant barking, separation anxiety or aggression are not offered rush immunotherapy – for the comfort and safety of the veterinary staff.

Abby Foust mentioned that Mueller and Bettenay have experience with alum-precipitated extracts in rush immunotherapy, and that they are preparing a case series of approximately 20 dogs to report their experiences.

Abby Foust offered to entertain questions from the attendees.

Ilan Skorinsky (*Israel*) enquired about the fees for rush immunotherapy and asked how immunotherapy is continued after the rush protocol.

Abby Foust stated that the cost is approximately $100, and that injections are continued every 14 days at 0.5 mL of the 40 000 PNU/mL solution if the patient completed the rush immunotherapy protocol.

Andrew Hillier highlighted Abby Foust's previous observation that there was not noticeable reduced time to improvement with rush immunotherapy relative to a traditional induction protocol. He commented that further dose adjustments in his traditionally induced patients are often required, and asked if rush immunotherapy patients were more stable in this regard after a rush immunotherapy induction.

Abby Foust remarked that there is increased confidence in maintenance dosing after rush immunotherapy. She has had occasional patients that have required a dose reduction after maintenance dosing was initially established. Further, if the patient is stable on the maintenance dose 4–6 weeks later but with no clinical improvement, she will try to slowly increase the maintenance dose.

Craig Griffin (*USA*) asked if she routinely stops the induction at the dose at which the reaction occurred, and if that dose is maintained thereafter every 14 days. He additionally asked if any effort was made to increase the dose.

Abby Foust stated that it depends on the response of the patient. If there is no clinical improvement over time, she attempts a slow dose increase. If the patient is improving then she maintains that lower concentration/lower volume dose.

Craig Griffin asked what is done if the patient reacts during Vial 1 (400 PNU/mL) during induction.

Abby Foust responded that she would continue that low dose as her maintenance dose initially and then observe for clinical benefit over time. She would slowly increase the dose if there was no clinical benefit.

Andrew Hillier asked for clarification if the concentration and volume that induced the reaction during induction was given once again to confirm a reaction prior to stopping the induction and confirming a maintenance dose.

Abby Foust confirmed that she uses that strategy.

Craig Griffin asked for clarification if the maintenance dose was the last dose that did not cause a reaction during the induction or if the maintenance dose was the last dose that induced a side effect.

Abby Foust stated that it depended on the severity of the reaction observed. They often do use the last dose that did not elicit a reaction as a maintenance dose. She emphasized that some patients on a low concentration of immunotherapy do not tolerate higher concentrations, but still respond very well to immunotherapy with a low concentration maintenance dose.

Regina Wagner (*Austria*) asked if after a reaction has been confirmed, whether the same dose and concentration is again repeated 6 hours later, or if the patient is then sent home.

Abby Foust responded that they are comfortable sending the patient home within an hour of that last injection. She reiterated that the majority of the patients do not have adverse events during induction and are maintained on a full dose of 20 000 PNU (0.5 ml of 40 000 PNU/mL).

Sam Sadeghi (*Canada*) asked whether intradermal testing or serum testing was utilized as the basis of allergen selection.

Abby Foust responded that intradermal testing is most frequently used because she sees patients that are not doing as well on immunotherapy based on a serum test. Many of her patients are referred because immunotherapy, based on serum testing, has failed.

Sam Sadeghi observed that some dermatologists use both methods to increase accuracy of testing and asked for comments based on her experience.

Abby Foust commented that if a patient is presenting for intradermal testing and has had a previous serum test, she will note the results of the serum test, and compare the results to her intradermal test findings. She will consider the history and seasonality of the patient to select from antigens deemed positive on the tests. For new patients, she will perform intradermal testing alone as a matter of personal preference.

Andrew Hillier remarked that the rapidity of the observations mentioned (5–10 minutes) was intriguing, as he has noted possible late-phase reactions to immunotherapy. He calculated that most patients would be discharged 30 minutes after the last injection in the aforementioned protocol and asked for confirmation of this, because he would be inclined to keep them longer afterwards for observation.

Abby Foust noted that the patient is typically discharged 30–60 minutes (at 4.30–5.00 p.m.) after the last injection, and she confirmed that rarely are reactions seen after approximately 15 minutes following an injection.

Therese Demanuelle (*USA*) asked if brachycephalic breeds were considered a risk factor for rush immunotherapy.

Abby Foust answered that they have not seen adverse events in these breeds.

Therese Demanuelle asked the attendees if anyone had experience with rush immunotherapy in horses.

None of the attendees offered any experience with rush immunotherapy in horses.

Abby Foust commented that Ralf Mueller may have experience with horses, and confirmed that he was not present to offer his opinion.

Andrew Hillier asked what percentage of immunotherapy patients receive rush immunotherapy induction at MedVet.

Abby Foust acknowledged that she had not looked at that statistic within her practice.

Andrew Hillier thanked Abby Foust for her participation and introduced Rosanna Marsella, Professor and head of the dermatology service at the University of Florida.

Investigations of the effects of sublingual immunotherapy on clinical signs and immunological parameters using a canine model of atopic dermatitis: a prospective, double-blinded, randomized, controlled study (R. Marsella)

Rosanna Marsella (*USA*) reported that sublingual immunotherapy (SLIT) has been used in the treatment of human atopic disease for many years, particularly for allergic rhinitis and less so for atopic dermatitis. Some clients do not like the idea of using needles on their pets for administration of subcutaneous immunotherapy (SCIT). For these reasons, Rosanna Marsella developed an interest in exploring SLIT as a possible treatment for canine atopic dermatitis, and aimed to evaluate this treatment in her canine model of atopic dermatitis.

She reported on a prospective, randomized, controlled study aimed to evaluate clinical and immunological effects of one year of SLIT. Eighteen atopic beagle dogs, epicutaneously sensitized to *Dermatophagoides farinae*, timothy grass and ragweed were randomly divided into control (n = 6, vehicle) and active (n = 12, three allergens) groups. Allergen challenge and scoring of clinical signs during challenge was done before and at the end of SLIT. The SLIT preparation was composed of a mixture of *D. farinae*, timothy and ragweed allergens provided by Nelco laboratories, administered sublingually once daily with a purpose-designed metered bottle to ensure volume consistency. The dose was three pumps once daily for the first month, then six pumps once daily for the second month, then eight pumps once daily in months 3–12. The total duration of the study was 12 months.

Clinical signs (without challenge) were scored after 1, 2, 3, 4, 8 and 12 months during SLIT, and then 2 months after stopping SLIT. Blood was drawn at baseline, 4, 8 and 12 months of SLIT and 2 months after stopping for allergen-specific IgE, interleukin-10 (IL-10), and transforming growth factor β (TGF-β). For clinical scores, ANOVA showed a significant effect of time (end < beginning). One dog in each group worsened at the end of study. Improvements were as follows: in the controls 0 >80%, 1/6 61–80%, 2/6 41–60%; 2/6 21–40%, 0 <20%; in the active group 0 >80%, 1/12 61–80%, 7/12 41–60%, 2/12 21–40%, 0 <20%. Overall the percentage of dogs that improved >40% was 50% in the control and 66% in the active group. For allergen-specific IgE a significant effect of time ($P < 0.05$) was found for *D. farinae* (end < beginning), ragweed (end > beginning). For TGF-β, significant effects of group (active > control) and time (end > beginning) were found for ragweed. For IL-10 a significant effect of group (active > control) and time (end > beginning) was found for ragweed. Also for IL-10, a significant effect of time (end > beginning) and group × time interaction were found for timothy grass.

Rosanna Marsella remarked that she was impressed with the ease of sublingual dosing, and SLIT was very well tolerated by the beagles. She further commented that in hindsight, this may not have been frequent enough dosing to observe maximal benefit, given our current knowledge of SLIT. She concluded that SLIT shows much promise as a treatment in a clinical setting, and acknowledged that her experience with SLIT is presently limited to the beagle model of atopic dermatitis. It was reiterated that there were some dogs in the active group that noticeably improved, and she additionally proposed that small study numbers may have hampered the ability to appreciate more dramatic changes in the active group.

Rosanna Marsella offered to entertain questions from the attendees.

Klaus Loft (*USA*) requested comment about the onset of the study relative to pollen season for timothy and ragweed.

Rosanna Marsella explained that although the study started and ended in the fall, the beagles were kept strictly indoors in a climate-controlled environment with controlled exposures to allergen. Personnel entering the environment were entirely gowned per Institutional Animal Care and Use Committee Guidelines, eliminating exposure to outside allergens. She further commented that because the potentially confounding factors of diet and environment were entirely controlled in her study, the variability of CADESI-03 scores within groups demonstrated individual variability in disease severity.

Cecelia Friberg (*USA*) asked for the ages of the beagles.

Rosanna Marsella replied that they were 6 and 7 years of age.

Andrew Hillier asked whether the individuals who responded well to SLIT continued to have mild disease.

Rosanna Marsella confirmed that two individuals continue to do very well. Given their level of improvement, these two will be adopted out of her programme because they are no longer of investigative value.

Andrew Hillier was curious if she had challenged these individuals after the study.

Rosanna Marsella replied that upon allergen challenge they did develop clinical signs of atopic dermatitis. However, the flares were of dramatically diminished intensity. They had mild signs of atopic dermatitis in between challenges.

Andrew Hillier asked what period of time has now passed since their last SLIT treatment.

Rosanna Marsella stated that the SLIT was discontinued in the fall of 2011. The beagles were challenged again throughout the winter of 2011–12, and in the spring of 2012. She had recent blood samples, therefore cytokine profiles could again be assessed in these individuals, but she has not evaluated the cytokine levels at this time.

Craig Griffin asked if she had attempted other methods of immunotherapy in the beagles.

Rosanna Marsella responded that other methods such as SCIT had not been attempted with these individuals. At the commencement of the study, she did not have enough dogs to form additional groups, and acknowledged that a SCIT group would have been ideal as well as a second placebo group. Given these limitations, she prioritized the study groups in order to answer the question of whether or not SLIT was well tolerated, and if it could lead to clinical improvement. If given sufficient resources and new beagles, she would perform a more comprehensive study to assess and compare both SLIT and SCIT. She commented that in her experience, patients that do not have house dust mite allergy tend to respond to SCIT better, and she would be interested in studying beagles sensitized to grass and weeds only. She suspects that the response to immunotherapy in general may be more rewarding in that subpopulation.

Craig Griffin asked for comment about the efficacy of anti-inflammatory drugs used in the beagle model. He expressed concern that the model may represent a high allergen challenge, and therefore it may be more difficult to elicit a therapeutic response compared to a clinical population. He was curious if the beagles responded to corticosteroids or ciclosporin.

Rosanna Marsella replied that corticosteroids work well in her model. Prednisone is used as a rescue drug protocol for individuals that have severe clinical signs necessitating removal from a study. Ciclosporin does not work as well in the model. She agreed that some individuals in the study colony have very severe clinical signs and that it can be a challenging model to assess potential efficacy of treatments. Further, if a treatment is helpful in the model, then she finds it is quite likely to be successful in the clinical population. She agreed that if a treatment is not working well in her model, it does not necessarily mean that a clinical population will not respond. Rosanna Marsella emphasized that although her model may present inherent challenges with regard to treatment response, the benefit of the beagle model is the ability to control confounding factors.

Andrew Hillier recalled that Rosanna Marsella had stated in retrospect that she would have liked to dose the SLIT more than once daily and asked for comment.

Rosanna Marsella affirmed this statement. After speaking to people receiving SLIT and other investigators, she thinks that twice to three times daily treatment would be a better protocol for assessing efficacy. Three times daily treatment may be more difficult with regard to compliance, but she suspects perhaps even twice-daily dosing may increase efficacy. She admitted that she is not sure how increasing the SLIT frequency would affect the cost of immunotherapy in practice, as a greater amount of allergen is delivered in general via the sublingual route relative to the subcutaneous route.

Andrew Hillier observed that Mary Morris was in attendance, and that she had previously mentioned in a different forum that antigen is present on dendritic cells for up to 48 hours after exposure. However, given dosing of SLIT in humans is twice daily, he asked for comment regarding this apparent discrepancy.

Mary Morris (*USA*) confirmed that frequent dosing is important in humans, and ideally SLIT is administered three times daily, as a better response is achieved than twice daily. She mentioned that there is at least one study demonstrating that only approximately 5% of the antigen is needed if given three times daily versus once daily.

Gila Zur (*Israel*) asked if there are any oral side effects of SLIT.

Rosanna Marsella reminded the attendees that she was blinded during the study. A technician checked the beagles daily to note any increase in behaviours associated with pruritus such as rubbing of the face. There were some reports of increased overall pruritus, but not necessarily oral effects. There were no reports of urticaria or facial angioedema. She suggested that perhaps the oral sensations that humans experience may occur in the beagles, but it is unlikely that this could be detected by investigators. Some individuals in the SLIT group did require a more gradual escalation in antigen volume (number of metered pumps) in the induction phase, in particular, the beagles with more severe manifestations. However, all beagles in the active study group did eventually achieve the final volume eight pumps of the SLIT once daily.

Ken Lee (*USA*) requested clarification about the vehicle used in the SLIT and control groups.

Rosanna Marsella replied that only glycerin was used.

Andrew Hiller thanked Rosanna Marsella for her participation and mentioned that a poster detailing her study was available for review at the congress. He introduced Valerie Fadok, noting that she has some early experiences in the use of SLIT in canine patients.

Early experiences in sublingual immunotherapy (V. Fadok)

Valerie Fadok (*USA*) participated in a clinical study with Doug DeBoer and Mary Morris evaluating the efficacy of SLIT in canine patients. The protocol involved delivering two pumps of the vaccine sublingually twice daily with a purpose-designed metered bottle. There were two vials: Vial A and Vial B, lasting approximately 5 months. Then a maintenance dose of two pumps twice daily was administered from Vial C.

Valerie Fadok described her first patient treated with SLIT, 'Patty', a mature female spectacled bear at the Houston Zoo. Patty had a several year history of partly seasonal, partly perennial facial pruritus. The pruritus and resultant hypotrichosis prompted the zoo to take her off exhibit from March to October. She explained that every 24 months Patty is placed under general anaesthesia for comprehensive diagnostic, maintenance and preventive medical care. Intradermal skin testing was opportunistically performed during one of Patty's medical care sessions. Testing revealed numerous positive reactions to regional pollens as well as house dust mites. Valerie Fadok commented that she would typically recommend SCIT, but the Houston Zoo has a policy that noxious stimuli are not permitted for the animals in their charge, unless they are trained and rewarded to accept the procedure. Patty had not been trained to accept injections, and the zoo did not want to compromise the positive working relationship that Patty maintained with her keeper. For this reason SLIT was offered. After evaluating primary literature about SLIT, she decided to quadruple the dose of 20 000 PNU/mL antigen delivered in her standard subcutaneous formulations for the sublingual solution. A three-vial startup set was created. Following the suggestion of the Houston Zoo, the solution was mixed in honey prior to administration, and Patty enthusiastically accepted this method of delivery, reliably consuming the entire dose. This solution was initially given every 72 hours, and Valerie Fadok suggested that in retrospect she would have recommended more frequent dosing. In the second year of immunotherapy, Patty improved significantly and she was once again displayed year round. To date, approximately 4 years later, she continues to be clinically normal, with minimal pruritus, and is on display at the Houston Zoo. Patty's SLIT is delivered every 14 days to maintain her response.

This experience gave her faith in the benefits of SLIT, particularly for patients that do not tolerate subcutaneous administration. Valerie Fadok's practice has approximately 32 canine patients and three feline patients receiving SLIT, many of which have only very recently commenced therapy. Selection criteria for SLIT include: clinical failure of SCIT, preference of the client not to administer subcutaneous injections, or lack of patient cooperation in receiving subcutaneous injections. Valerie Fadok acknowledged that some patients fail to respond to SCIT even with perfect compliance. However, many clinical failures of SCIT in her practice apparently stem from lack of client compliance. In her experience, some clients are uncomfortable giving injections, but are reluctant to admit it, because they desire to do what is best for their pet. Upon offering SLIT in cases of clinical failure, clients often subsequently confess their dislike of administering injections and lack of previous compliance.

Valerie Fadok then wished to discuss the clinical progress of two dogs she had been treating with SLIT for approximately 6 months. 'Sasha' is a female mixed breed dog abandoned in the parking lot of her clinic at approximately 4 months of age. Sasha was severely pruritic and emaciated, and Valerie Fadok agreed to foster Sasha and provide medical care. Sasha's initial treatment plan involved treatment for possible sarcoptic mange and treatment of bacterial pyoderma with bathing. An elimination diet trial was immediately instituted. After 6 weeks of the trial it was determined that she had cutaneous adverse food reaction to chicken. Sasha's pruritus was reduced by approximately 40%. However, oral glucocorticoids were required to control the remaining severe pruritus. In order to avoid lifelong corticosteroid administration in such a young dog, Valerie Fadok opted to institute immunotherapy. An intradermal test and serum allergy test were both performed. SLIT was instituted using the Allergychoices vaccine (Allergychoices, Inc.) with Doug DeBoer's protocol. Sasha's initial CADESI score was approximately 40. At a 3-month reassessment, her score was 15, and by 6 months she was skin lesion-free. At the onset of immunotherapy she was treating Sasha with a combination of antihistamines and pentoxifylline to avoid use of glucocorticoids; this combination did not appear to be effective in reducing pruritus. Valerie Fadok found Sasha's subsequent clinical response to SLIT to be remarkably noticeable; Sasha's pinnal alopecia resolved, and her quality of life dramatically improved. The dog's initial pruritus score assessed on a visual analog scale was approximately 80 mm and was reduced to 10 mm in 6 months. Valerie Fadok reiterated that she lived with Sasha so she could assess her progress well. At present she is only slightly more pruritic than a normal dog, and is lesion-free. Valerie Fadok displayed for the attendees of the workshop pictures of Sasha's progress throughout her treatment.

'Rocky' is a 7-year-old neutered male Scottish terrier with atopic dermatitis and recurrent bacterial pyoderma, first presenting in 2007. A serum allergy test and intradermal test were performed at that time, and SCIT was initiated shortly thereafter. The client was compliant with the administration of subcutaneous injections. Rocky failed immunotherapy after 1 year of administration, and he also failed treatment with ciclosporin (Atopica®, Novartis Animal Health). He had recurrent methicillin-resistant staphylococcal infections, requiring treatment with amikacin and rifampin. Prednisolone and trimeprazine + prednisolone (Temaril P®, Pfizer Animal Health) failed to control pruritus; only triamcinolone provided relief. Approximately 4 months ago, Rocky presented with pruritus and alopecia. He was receiving twice weekly oral triamcinolone to control his atopic dermatitis. SLIT was instituted. Retesting was not performed given the abundance of positive results of the aforementioned allergy tests. Rocky responded rapidly to SLIT. He was asymptomatic with regard to his CADESI score at his recheck 3 months later, with dramatic hair regrowth. His pruritus score also remarkably improved during that time. In light of his dramatic improvement, triamcinolone was successfully discontinued 6 weeks after instituting SLIT. Rocky continues to be well at this time. Valerie Fadok feels it is inappropriate to suggest that SLIT will work for all dogs. However, based on the data and experiences she is aware of, SLIT is as effective as, if not more effective than SCIT. It appears to elicit a more rapid response, and it does work in some dogs that have failed SCIT. She offers clients the option of SLIT or SCIT. She finds that most clients are very happy to have the option to forego giving injections, and that they are very willing to comply with twice-daily dosing of SLIT. She finds that administration of SLIT, per her personal experience with treating Sasha, is quite easy. Valerie Fadok is of the opinion that SLIT is going to allow more dogs to experience the benefit of immunotherapy via increased compliance and ease of administration for the client and the patient. She is awaiting with interest studies that compare the efficacy of SLIT and SCIT. She lastly assured the attendees that her next atopic West Highland white terrier patient will be receiving oral immunotherapy. She asked the attendees if they have had experience in SLIT, either commercial or formulated in-house. Approximately 10 attendees raised their hands in response.

Klaus Loft remarked that he has been using SLIT since May 2012. After practising in the US Midwest as well as Europe, he finds that the most intense client needle phobia is observed on the East Coast of the USA, where he currently practises. In the midwestern USA, the cost of SCIT was a greater limiting factor. Thus far, he likes SLIT and finds it to be particularly useful in the treatment of service dogs.

Alison Diesel (*USA*) commented that she was part of Doug DeBoer's initial study of Allergychoices SLIT. She concurs that some dogs failing SCIT may still respond to SLIT, and she feels fortunate to have SLIT as another option for treating atopic patients. She also allows clients to choose between SCIT and SLIT. Some clients prefer the intermittent injections, and others prefer the twice daily sublingual route. She remarked that if one route does not work, fortunately the other route is available to try as another option. Alison Diesel has also treated some patients that have failed SLIT but responded to SCIT as well.

Karri Beck (*Canada*) remarked that she has had a few dogs experience anaphylactic reactions to SCIT, and asked if SLIT may be a reasonable option for such patients. She also asked Valerie Fadok if she would recommend premedicating such patients prior to administration of SLIT. She also mentioned that SLIT is not commercially available in Canada.

Valerie Fadok responded that based on some discussions earlier in the meeting, patients with severe reactions to SCIT were safely treated with SLIT with no adverse reactions. She suggested that Karri Beck contact

Dawn Logas, as she has practical experience with formulating SLIT.

Andrew Hillier asked Mary Morris to comment about the incidence of anaphylactic reactions with SLIT in humans.

Mary Morris responded that in her clinic they have treated approximately 125 000 patients since 1970 with no reported anaphylactic reactions.

Valerie Fadok shared that she had undergone rush immunotherapy. Her allergist had quipped that he was going to try to kill her, and she ultimately felt that sentiment to be true, although clearly he did not succeed.

Cecilia Friberg concurred with Alison Diesel's comments, and was also a participant in Doug DeBoer's study. She has observed patients respond as dramatically as Rocky. She emphasized that the clients must commit to the twice-daily dosing to optimize results.

Valerie Fadok added that SLIT has the added convenience of not requiring refrigeration, which is particularly helpful for travelling patients and clients.

Craig Griffin asked Valerie Fadok if the patients failing SCIT that respond to SLIT used formulations based on the original allergy test. He also asked if the allergen source/company used for SLIT differed from that used for the SCIT.

Valerie Fadok responded that Rocky was not re-tested because he had so many positive results with the initial tests, she did not think that re-testing would be a valuable use of time or resources. She has always used Greer aqueous allergens for subcutaneous injection. During the study, she did not know the source of the sublingual allergens; she just knows they were formulated according to the Allergychoices protocol, and now she is ordering the solutions from HESKA.

Craig Griffin asked if the allergens included for Rocky were the same in the subcutaneous formulation as in the sublingual formulation.

Valerie Fadok confirmed that the allergens were the same.

Craig Griffin questioned if Sasha has been re-challenged with chicken now that she is doing so well with immunotherapy.

Valerie Fadok observed that Sasha accessed a bag of Science Diet and she did have a flare, but it was not as severe as the food challenges she performed with Sasha prior to the SLIT. She thinks that the immunotherapy may be helping her cutaneous adverse food reaction as well, likely via the allergy threshold concept.

Regina Wagner questioned the attendees if anyone had experienced a SLIT failure that subsequently responded to SCIT.

Valerie Fadok commented that Alison Diesel had, but she has personally not been performing SLIT long enough to make this observation.

Alison Diesel confirmed that during the pilot study in which she had participated, some dogs failing SLIT responded to SCIT.

Lisa Reiter (*USA*) asked the attendees to comment about their experiences using SLIT in cats.

Valerie Fadok replied that she has treated one cat for 6 months with SLIT. The cat is owned by an elderly person whose arthritis limited her ability to give injections. She has been communicating with the client weekly, and the client and the primary veterinarian have been impressed with the response. She recently initiated SLIT in another cat with a history of SCIT failure, but insufficient time has passed to judge efficacy.

Jill Abraham (*USA*) shared that she recently initiated SLIT in a cat with a history of rabies vaccine-associated fibrosarcoma, circumventing trepidation regarding injections; this scenario is another potential indication for SLIT in cats.

Andrew Hillier thanked Valerie Fadok for sharing her experiences, and introduced Ken Lee from Greer.

How to utilize allergen cross-reactivity for formulation of immunotherapy (K. Lee)

Ken Lee (*USA*) stated that allergen cross-reactivity is a practical and important concept in formulating immunotherapy for canine patients. Principles of rational allergen selection and cross-reactivity in human immunotherapy may be valuable in creating canine immunotherapy solutions; however, the possibility of species-specific differences must be considered as well. Ken Lee has investigated allergen cross-reactivity in dogs and his goal was to present a brief overview of translatable concepts for formulating immunotherapy as well as to present his canine cross-reactivity results. He observed that the immunotherapy successes described in the previous presentations may be in part due to evaluation of allergen cross-reactivity and appropriate allergen selection by the clinician.

Ken Lee introduced three concepts in formulating immunotherapy: enzymatic degradation of allergens, optimizing dose amount of each constituent, and allergen cross-reactivity. Protease-producing allergens must be recognized to avoid degradation of other allergens in solution. He acknowledged that some veterinary dermatologists are not concerned about proteases, and are of the opinion that they do not appear to affect their clinical results. He has noticed that many veterinary dermatologists as a general rule recommend immunotherapy solutions consisting of 12 allergens or less, and he additionally noted that practitioners he conversed with from the UK suggested that the maximum number should be eight allergens. In contrast, upon discussing the subject with other veterinary dermatologists, Ken Lee discovered that some place no limit on the number of allergens in their solutions. He reiterated the concept that limiting the allergen numbers may optimize the therapeutic doses of the included constituents, increasing the likelihood of a desired immunological response. Knowledge of allergen cross-reactivity allows one to include relevant antigens with a lower number of constituents.

Cross-reactivity occurs within pollen groups, even at the taxonomic rank of family (Table 1). The grasses have well-recognized cross-reactivity within the subfamily Pooideae, with the exception of the unique antigens of Bermuda grass (*Cynodon dactylon*). Ken Lee stated that if the patient has reactions to multiple grasses, then including Bermuda grass allergen in the formulation as well as another grass of the subfamily Pooideae, likely provides sufficient antigen representation. Weeds also have a recognized cross-reactivity within the taxonomic rank of family, including Chenopodiaceae (goosefoot), Asteraceae (aster) and Amaranthaceae (amaranth). Trees are more diverse with a greater number of families, with fewer members within families, and thus are more complex in cross-reactivity. Relevant families include Aceraceae (maple), Betulaceae (birch), Cupressaceae (cyprus), Fagaceae (beech), Juglandaceae (walnut), Olacaceae (olive and ash), and Salicaceae (willow).

Ken Lee pointed out that although much is known with regard to allergen cross-reactivity in humans, less is known about canine cross-reactive allergens. However, it appears that species-specific differences are present. For example, it has been demonstrated that the major *D. farinae* allergens in humans (Der f 1 and 2) differ from that of dogs (Der f 15).

Ken Lee reported that he investigated canine allergen cross-reactivity via ELISA inhibition studies utilizing serum samples from 50 dogs. The 50 canine serum samples evaluated were selected because they contained IgE recognizing all allergens investigated. Solid-phase ELISA tests were developed with grass, weed and tree antigens. Cross-inhibition studies were performed. For example, Bermuda antigen was placed in a solid phase, and a liquid phase of another grass antigen admixed with canine serum was added to the solid phase. If the canine IgE recognizing Bermuda also recognized the liquid phase antigen, the liquid phase allergen rather than the solid-phase Bermuda would be bound, and the optical density of the ELISA signal would be attenuated. Every allergen investigated was tested in the solid phase with all other antigens in the liquid phase (Figure 1).

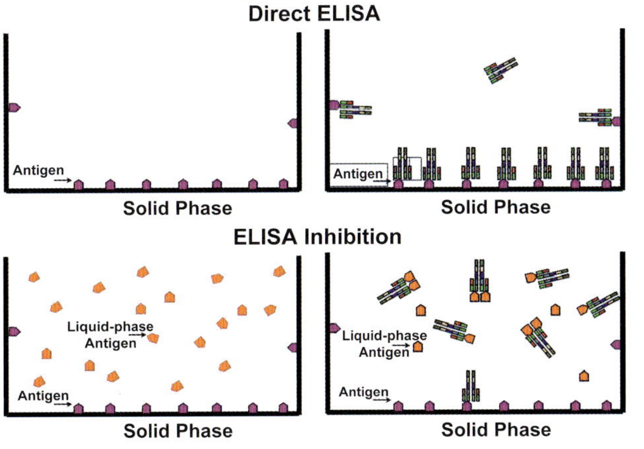

Figure 1. Cross-inhibition studies performed using the solid-phase ELISA test.

The results of these assays with the solid Bermuda phase suggest that at a concentration of 10 ng/mL, other grass antigens will inhibit IgE binding to Bermuda by 50%, indicating cross-reactivity. Ken Lee emphasized that the concentration of weed antigen required for 50% inhibition of Bermuda solid phase with weeds in the liquid phase is only approximately two to five times greater as required for the grasses in some individual samples, and greater in others. This indicates that there can be a substantial degree of cross-reactivity but there are differences in individual dogs. He also discovered that ash and oak can have substantial cross-reactivity with Bermuda, requiring approximately five to six times more antigen than the grasses for 50% inhibition.

In general when weeds were examined in the solid phase and liquid phase, the results were similar to grasses in both liquid and solid phase, but there was greater divergence in cross-reactivity upon comparing individual weed species, where 50% inhibition was only achieved at very high concentrations of allergen tested at liquid phase. Grasses did appear to cross-react with

Table 1. Cross-reacting pollen groups

	Family	Genera
Grasses	Pooideae	*Poa* (bluegrass), *Dactylis* (orchard), *Festuca* (fescue), *Lolium* (perennial rye), *Agrostis* (redtop), *Anthoxanthum* (vernal), *Phleum* (timothy)
Weeds	Chenopodiaceae	*Atriplex* (saltbrush), *Chenopodium* (lamb's quarter), *Salsola* (Russian thistle), *Kochia* (firebush)
	Asteraceae	*Artemisia* (sage, mugwort), *Ambrosia* (ragweeds), *Xanthium* (cocklebur)
	Amaranthaceae	*Amaranthus* (careless weed/pigweed), *Acnida* (water hemp)
Trees	Aceraceae	*Acer* (maples, boxelder)
	Betulaceae	*Alnus* (alder), *Betula* (birch), *Corylus* (hazelnut)
	Cupressaceae	*Cupressus* (cypress), *Juniperus* (juniper, cedar), *Taxodium* (bald cypress)
	Fagaceae	*Quercus* (oaks), *Fagus* (beech)
	Juglandaceae	*Carya* (hickory, pecan), *Juglans* (walnut)
	Olacaceae	*Olea* (olive), *Fraxinus* (ash), *Ligustrum* (privet)
	Salicaceae	*Populus* (cottonwood, poplar), *Salix* (willows)

weeds to some extent. When oak was utilized in the solid phase it was found that some individual serum samples displayed significant cross-reactivity. To summarize, Ken Lee remarked that, based on his data, a considerable degree of allergen cross-reactivity occurs in dogs, and it may be more extensive than what is observed in humans. Based on new research in this area, it appears that some of the target antigens may be carbohydrates rather than proteins. That said, regardless of the target antigen involved, the findings with regard to cross-reactivity do parallel those of the groupings defined for humans, and he assured the attendees that following those groupings in canine patients is appropriate. In conclusion he thanked those who performed the ELISA experiments.

Andrew Hillier thanked Ken Lee for his presentation and asked for clarification about Bermuda as an outlier in regard of reduced cross-reactivity compared to other grasses.

Ken Lee confirmed that Bermuda is still an outlier overall, but not in all individuals; in some there is significant cross-reactivity with other grasses. Regardless, it does appear that Bermuda has a unique antigen.

Andrew Hillier asked the attendees if they use principles of cross-reactivity to formulate immunotherapy. Approximately 20 attendees raised their hands in response.

Regina Wagner asked if these data had been published, so they may be cited.

Ken Lee stated they have not been published yet, and explained that there are much more extensive data than were presented at the workshop, and he aims to have the study published.

Stacy Johnson (*USA*) asked Ken Lee and the attendees if they are using concepts of allergen cross-reactivity to choose regional allergens for intradermal testing.

Ken Lee suggested that the cross-reactivity may allow one to reduce the number of allergens tested, and acknowledged that his experience is limited to use of the *in vitro* serum allergy testing.

Andrew Hillier asked the attendees if anyone had considered their intradermal test results and decided to pare down the number of allergens tested. He suggested that in his experience he could likely exclude many of the grasses he tests for, given the redundancy.

Klaus Loft replied that he presently works at two locations: Boston and Maine. In Maine he tests with a seven grass mix as well as Bermuda and Johnson, whereas in Boston he tests with 13 grass allergens individually. Although he has not formally gathered data, his clinical impression is that when using mixes to desensitize patients he has difficulty in controlling patients with seasonal signs, particularly relating to the grass pollens.

Andrew Hillier thanked the presenters and attendees for their participation.

References

1. Mueller RS, Bettenay SV. Evaluation of the safety of an abbreviated course of injections of allergen extracts (rush immunotherapy) for the treatment of atopic dermatitis. *Am J Vet Res* 2001; 62: 307–310.
2. Trimmer AM, Boord MJ, Rosenkrantz WS. Rush allergen specific immunotherapy protocol in feline atopic dermatitis: a pilot study of four cats. *Vet Dermatol* 2005; 16: 324–329.

8.5

Pododermatitis: canine interdigital follicular cysts and feline plasma cell pododermatitis

R. Muse[1] (Chairperson), B.E. Wildermuth[2] (Secretary)

[1]Animal Dermatology Clinic, Tustin, California, USA
[2]Tierdermatologie Dr. Wildermuth, Wiesbaden, Hessen, Germany

Rusty Muse (*USA*) welcomed the participants to the workshop and presented a brief overview of pododermatitis. He then explained that the workshop would focus on two specific diseases that are both interesting and frustrating to treat: canine interdigital cysts and feline plasma cell pododermatitis. During the first half of the workshop, the aetiology, diagnosis and carbon dioxide (CO_2) laser ablation of canine interdigital cysts would be presented by David Duclos, followed by the medical management of this disease by John Angus. For the second half of the workshop, Brett Wildermuth would present an overview of feline plasma cell pododermatitis, followed by a clinical case presented by Sarah Bartlett.

Interdigital cysts (D. Duclos)

David Duclos (*USA*) began his presentation by stating that he prefers to call this disease interdigital follicular cysts rather than interdigital cysts, as the lesions originate in the hair follicle. He first explained that his initial thought was to use the laser to sterilize these lesions because they were described in the literature as strictly bacterial lesions. While ablating these lesions, he found that the dorsal interdigital draining tracts originated from dilated cystic hair follicles located deeper in the ventral interdigital space.

He then discussed the pathogenesis of this disease. It is proposed that friction on the ventral surface of the interdigital space causes thickening of the skin, secondarily plugging the follicular infundibulum. The hair follicle continues to produce keratin and dilates, forming a cyst. Hair growth in the follicle is inhibited, resulting in alopecia. Some dogs form follicular cysts but remain asymptomatic, while in others the follicular cyst ruptures, dissects through the tissue dorsally and perforates the skin of the interdigital space resulting in a chronic draining tract with secondary bacterial infection. These cysts do not rupture ventrally due to the constant friction pushing on the hyperplastic epidermis.

David Duclos then showed numerous videos and photos detailing the surgical ablation of follicular cysts using the CO_2 laser. Prior to the surgical procedure, he recommends administering an appropriate antibiotic to reduce the size of infected lesions as much as possible. He feels that the use of glucocorticoids is acceptable, but he prefers not to as these lesions are a form of deep pyoderma.

The first video showed a 5-year-old male Alaskan malamute with follicular cysts between the fourth and fifth digits of both forepaws. There were draining tracts dorsally, with a corresponding thickening of the skin on the ventral interdigital spaces with numerous comedones and alopecia. David Duclos explained that to assist with the diagnosis of interdigital follicular cysts, this thickened ventral interdigital skin could be squeezed to exude keratin from the many small cysts that have formed. This should not be performed on a dog while it is awake, however, as it is painful.

To perform the ablation, David Duclos uses a CO_2 laser with a wide tip, set in continuous mode at 25 W power. He places a metal probe in the draining tract of the dorsal interdigital space to act as a landmark for the ventral approach with the laser. He begins by ablating the upper layer of the epidermis on the ventral interdigital skin of the affected area. The laser easily vaporizes the soft tissue of the dermis, making the keratin of the cysts stand out. The tissue is squeezed after each layer of ablation, exuding keratin to guide the next layer of laser ablation. Additionally, the metal probe may be manipulated to help guide the direction of ablation towards the main fistula that has perforated to the dorsal surface. The previous steps are repeated until all the follicular cysts have been vaporized leaving only normal tissue dorsally. Occasionally grape-cluster-like pyogranulomatous lesions are encountered while ablating through the tissue; these bleed easily and are best excised rather than ablated.

Some cysts are so deep that one may need to laser almost through to the other side, though typically the dorsal interdigital skin can remain intact. In general it is recommended to ablate these lesions with a wide margin to vaporize additional hair follicles that would otherwise be the source of future lesions.

David Duclos also informed the audience that the surgeon must naturally be familiar with the vasculature of the paw prior to attempting this surgery. The laser is very precise and will cauterize small blood vessels of less than 1 mm, and in most cases large blood vessels can be visualized and avoided, but a tourniquet is necessary in case a larger blood vessel is damaged.

As this is not a sterile surgery and there is a large amount of tension on the paw when the dogs walk, David Duclos leaves the lesions open to heal by second intention. The paw is bandaged postoperatively with bandage changes performed twice weekly during weeks 1 and 2, then weekly for 1 month. In approximately 4 weeks most dogs will have healed completely.

In summary, follicular interdigital cysts present as recurrent draining tract lesions most commonly on the forepaws of younger dogs with or without obvious conformational abnormalities. The lesions begin ventrally as a follicular cyst, and progress to form a draining tract dorsally. Laser ablation of the cysts is an effective long-term solution with a success rate of approximately 70%.[1]

Medical therapy of interdigital furunculosis (J.C. Angus)

John Angus (*USA*) began his presentation by reiterating that this disease was initially thought by many veterinary dermatologists to be only bacterial and/or allergic in origin prior to David Duclos' report published in 2008,[1] and today he sees that it is often misdiagnosed in general practice as a foxtail foreign body. He noted that affected dogs tend to be large breed, short-coated dogs, with Labradors, retrievers and English bulldogs apparently over-represented. Additionally, it is not uncommon for dogs to have both interdigital follicular cysts and allergic dermatitis with secondary bacterial interdigital furunculosis.

John Angus's diagnostic approach for these cases includes obtaining a sample for cytological evaluation from the affected area(s) as well as performing a deep skin scraping to rule out demodicosis. It is important to evaluate the dorsal and ventral aspects of both paws, as bilateral disease in different stages of severity is common. It is unknown how valuable cytological samples from the dorsal draining tract lesions are, as they may not represent what is present in deeper tissue where the follicular cyst originates. An intact follicular cyst is not typically infected with bacteria and is not a lesion responsive to antibiotic therapy; however, once the cyst ruptures secondary bacterial infection may occur, and a partial clinical response to antibiotics can be seen. If there is evidence of cystic rupture with secondary bacterial infection, such as a purulent discharge with intracellular bacteria on cytological examination, antimicrobial therapy is indicated. The cephalosporin antibiotics are a good first choice, and if there is a lack of response then bacterial culture and susceptibility testing can be helpful. John Angus reported that rifampin is an effective reserve antibiotic for these cases as it has anti-inflammatory properties and methicillin-resistant staphylococci are often susceptible to it. Biopsy performed on the ventral interdigital tissue from which the lesion originates can confirm the diagnosis of an interdigital follicular cyst. Finally, when clinical signs of allergic disease are present a diet trial and specific allergy testing may also be indicated.

John Angus explained that the main goal of treating this disease is to open occluded hair follicles to prevent the formation of large cysts. Pets with early clinical signs of alopecia, ventral interdigital hyperplasia, and small comedone formation are good candidates for preventive therapy. Once a large cyst has formed and the pet is symptomatic, surgical intervention is most likely necessary. Benzoyl peroxide, known for its follicular flushing action, is widely available in shampoos, wipes and gels, thus making it a good candidate for treatment of this disease. John Angus has been using Douxo Chlorhexidine 3% PS pads (Sogeval, USA) to clean the interdigital spaces as a potential preventive therapy. Additionally for early lesions and as preventive therapy, he recommends applying either Essential 6® spot-on (Dermoscent, France), Duoxo Seborrhea Spot-on (Sogeval, USA) or ALLERDERM® Spot-on Skin Lipid Complex (Virbac Animal Health, USA) to the affected ventral interdigital tissue once weekly. In 3 to 6 months this can slowly improve the state of the skin. Finally, whirlpool soaks and astringent solutions could potentially be beneficial in combination with comedolytic agents, though the response is expected to be variable.

The second goal of therapy emphasized by John Angus is to reduce the inflammatory component of this disease. He recommends avoiding glucocorticoids as they are comedogenic and deep pyoderma may also be present. Instead, he recommends pentoxifylline since it has mild anti-inflammatory properties via suppression of tumour necrosis factor α (TNF-α), which is likely released in large amounts from the plentiful macrophages in these chronic lesions. He postulates that peripheral blood flow to the diseased areas may be improved, facilitating healing and enhancing antibiotic penetration into these lesions. John Angus finds nonsteroidal anti-inflammatory drugs helpful to decrease lameness, and dietary therapy with omega-3 fatty acids may also help. He recommends either Prescription Diet® j/d® Canine Mobility (Hill's Pet Nutrition, Inc., USA), or Skin Support (Royal Canin, USA). Finally, he does not believe oral vitamin A supplementation is effective for interdigital follicular cysts and recommends against synthetic retinoids due to their expense and risk of side effects. Topical retinoids, however, may be of benefit.

Amanda Booth (*Canada*) asked if John Angus was applying the spot-on lipid products between the toes ventrally, to which he replied yes, and that he demonstrates the application for the owner.

Kallahalli Umesh (*India*) asked if John Angus had used tacrolimus in these cases, to which he replied not, but that it may be beneficial.

Otto Fischer (*Austria*) added that he uses tacrolimus with a good response.

Jan Declercq (*Belgium*) emphasized that he refers to the disease as conformational pododermatitis, and several factors are contributory: conformation, high body weight, short feet and narrow interdigital spaces. He stated that the body reacts to anatomical deformation with callus and cyst formation, which can result in rupture and secondary foreign body inflammation. He also reiterated that pets could have concurrent allergic skin disease with secondary bacterial furunculosis as a cause for relapses.

John Angus agreed he too finds the term conformational pododermatitis useful as well.

David Duclos added that he was very careful to exclude pets with allergic disease from his previous study. He had followed many of the dogs for 10 years afterwards and they did not develop allergic symptoms and most did not have recurrences of cysts.

Feline plasma cell pododermatitis (B.E. Wildermuth)

Brett Wildermuth (*Germany*) introduced his overview of feline plasma cell pododermatitis (PCP) as a lead into Sarah Bartlett's case presentation, which was to follow.

He reported that there is no apparent breed or sex predisposition and the disease can affect cats as young as 6 months of age and as old as 12.5 years.[2,3] Disease duration prior to consultation may vary from months to years,[4] and the cats are often presented with pain or lameness[2,3,5] or occasionally paw pad haemorrhage.[6]

Dermatological findings in mildly affected cats may include: asymptomatic swelling, softening, and erythematous to violaceous discoloration of one or more metacarpal, metatarsal or digital paw pads. Additionally, as the paw pad is stretched the striations of the paw pad may become more prominent, white and scaly. Advanced clinical signs may include severe swelling and discoloration of the paw pads, ulceration with secondary haemorrhagic and/or purulent crusts, or prolapse of the deep paw tissue outward.

Concurrent diseases are occasionally present, including plasma cell stomatitis, plasmacytic infiltrates in the liver, kidney and lung, feline immunodeficiency virus (FIV), feline leukaemia, glomerulonephritis, renal and/or hepatic amyloidosis, as well as nasal swelling and upper respiratory infection.[2,4,5,7–10] Clinical pathological changes reported in the literature include hypergammaglobulinaemia, thrombocytopenia, leukocytosis, lymphopenia and normochromic anemia.[4,6,11]

While the clinical presentation is relatively characteristic, biopsy is necessary to definitively diagnose PCP. Histopathological patterns of the disease may include: a perivascular or diffuse to nodular plasmacytic dermatitis with or without lymphocytic aggregates; a neutrophilic infiltrate; granulomatous inflammation or leukocytoclastic vasculitis.[2,8,12]

Brett Wildermuth reiterated that the aetiology of the disease is still unknown. It is most commonly stated that an immune-mediated pathogenesis is likely,[13] while other references describe the disease as inflammatory[14] or as a reaction pattern with multiple aetiologies.[2,10]

It is unlikely that bacteria, fungi or *Leishmania* cause plasma cell pododermatitis based on previous studies,[4,15] but the association with viral disease is more interesting, in particular with FIV. In the literature more than half of the cats with plasma cell pododermatitis that were tested for FIV were positive[2–5] with evidence of FIV in lesional skin in two studies.[2,16] An association of upper respiratory viral infection with PCP has been reported, but infrequently, and attempts to find either herpes or calicivirus in lesional tissue have been negative.[10,15]

Brett Wildermuth reported that traditional scalpel excision of the affected paw pad is reported to be curative for PCP,[2,5] and more recently a case was successfully treated with cryotherapy.[17] Traditionally, medical therapy with glucocorticoids has been reported to be effective,[13] and more recently medical therapy with doxycycline as well.[3,4] Ciclosporin has been mentioned in textbooks as an option;[14,18] however, studies showing its efficacy have not yet been reported. Placebo-controlled studies proving the efficacy of various therapies for PCP are unfortunately lacking, most likely due to the rarity of the disease. In addition, spontaneous resolution and seasonal improvement have been reported.[5,8,11,19]

Brett Wildermuth closed his presentation by stating that many questions still remain about this disease. Is plasma cell pododermatitis simply an autoimmune disease? Is there perhaps a genetic predisposition that we are not yet aware of? What is different structurally or immunologically so that the footpads are targeted? Is this disease only a reaction pattern and if so what role might viruses play as so many cats are FIV positive?

Complicated plasma cell pododermatitis in a domestic medium-hair cat (S. Bartlett)

Sarah Bartlett (*USA*) presented a case of plasma cell pododermatitis in a 5-year-old domestic medium-hair cat with a 1-year history of swollen, ulcerated and haemorrhagic metacarpal paw pads. The cat had previously responded to treatment with injectable methylprednisolone along with short courses of antibiotics, but this therapy was no longer effective. Doxycycline at 5.5 mg/kg twice daily was also ineffective, and the cat had developed lameness on the right forepaw, was lethargic and had lost weight.

At presentation, the cat had significant swelling of the metacarpal paw pads of both forepaws, with purple discoloration and tightly adherent honey-coloured crusts. A few of the digital pads were also slightly swollen. On the dorsal right forepaw there was a large area of alopecia and cellulitis with multiple draining tracts and serosanguinous discharge. The dorsal left forepaw had a single fistulous tract with peripheral erythema and swelling.

Cytological examination of the exudate from the dorsal aspects of both forepaws showed numerous neutrophils, macrophages and both coccoid and rod-shaped bacteria. Biopsies were taken for histopathological evaluation of the dorsal paw lesions and revealed a pyogranulomatous dermatitis and panniculitis. A methicillin-resistant *Staphylococcus sciuri* was cultured from the dorsal paw, while fungal and mycobacterial cultures were negative. The cat tested negative for feline leukaemia virus and FIV, and a toxoplasmosis antibody titre was negative.

The diagnosis was ultimately plasma cell pododermatitis with a secondary deep pyoderma, and the question is: How did this happen? It is common to see ulceration and infection on the paw pad, but in this case the deep pyoderma seems to have dissected its way dorsally through the paw in a fashion similar to that described with rupture of canine interdigital follicular cysts.

The cat was initially treated with enrofloxacin alone, and after 2 weeks there was a marked decrease in the swelling of the dorsal paws and the draining tracts had healed. Since there had been a poor response to both doxycycline and methylprednisolone prior to presentation, ciclosporin (Atopica®, Novartis) was initiated at 5.3 mg/kg once daily.

By day 45 of treatment, the dorsal surfaces of the paws were normal and the metacarpal pads were much less swollen. However, more digital pads of the rear paws were involved and, therefore, doxycycline was reintroduced at 7 mg/kg twice daily. Over the next 4 months enrofloxacin and doxycycline were discontinued separately. At the 6-month recheck examination, the cat was receiving only ciclosporin. The left front paw pad was nearly normal, and the right front paw pad had only mild swelling. This was considered a successful therapeutic outcome, and as of the time of this presentation the cat was still well controlled with ciclosporin 5.5 mg/kg orally once daily.

Following the feline portion of the workshop, there were no further questions.

Rusty Muse thanked all participants and the workshop was ended.

References

1. Duclos DD, Hargis AM, Hanley PW. Pathogenesis of canine interdigital palmar and plantar comedones and follicular cysts, and their response to laser surgery. *Vet Dermatol* 2008; 19: 134–141.
2. Gauguere E, Prelaud P, Degorce-Rubiales F *et al.* Feline plasma cell pododermatitis: a retrospective study of 26 cases. *Vet Dermatol* 2004; 15(Suppl. 1): 20–40.
3. Bettenay SV, Mueller RS, Dow K, Friend S. Prospective study on the treatment of feline plasmacytic pododermatitis with doxycycline. *Vet Rec* 2003; 152: 564–566.
4. Scarampella F, Ordeix L. Doxycycline therapy in 10 cases of feline plasma cell pododermatitis: clinical, haematological and serological evaluations. *Vet Dermatol* 2004; 15(Suppl. 1): 20–40.
5. Pereira PD, Faustino AMR. Feline plasma cell pododermatitis: a study of 8 cases. *Vet Dermatol* 2003; 14: 333–337.
6. Taylor JE, Schmeitzel LP. Plasma cell pododermatitis with chronic footpad hemorrhage in two cats. *JAVMA* 1990; 197: 375–377.
7. Scott DW. Feline dermatology 1900–1978: a monograph. *J Am Anim Hosp Assoc* 1980; 16: 417.
8. Scott, DW. Feline dermatology 1979-1982: introspective retrospections. *J Am Anim Hosp Assoc* 1984; 20: 537–564.
9. Scott, DW. Secret sits 1983-1985. *J Am Anim Hosp Assoc* 1987; 23: 255.
10. Declercq J, De Man M. Swelling of the nose in three cats with plasmacytic pododermatitis. *Vlaams Diergeneeskundig Tijdschrift* 2002; 71: 277–281.
11. Gruffydd-Jones TJ, Orr CM, Lucke VM. Foot pad swelling and ulceration in cats: a report. *J Small Anim Pract* 1980; 21: 381–389.
12. Gross TL, Ihrke PJ, Walder EJ *et al.* Plasma cell pododermatitis. In: Gross TL, Ihrke PJ, Walder EJ, eds. *Skin Diseases of the Dog and Cat. Clinical and Histopathologic Diagnosis*, 2nd edn. Oxford, UK: Blackwell Publishing Ltd, 2005; 363–364.
13. Scott DW, Miller WH, Griffin CE. Feline plasma cell pododermatitis. In: Scott DW, Miller WH, Griffin CE, eds. Muller & Kirk's Small Animal Dermatology, 6th edn. Philadelphia, PA: WB Saunders, 2001; 1129–1130.
14. Griffin CE. Ciclosporin use in dermatology. In: Bonagura JD, Twedt DC, eds. *Kirk's Current Veterinary Therapy XIV*. St Louis, MO: Saunders; 386–388.
15. Bettenay SV, Lappin MR, Mueller RS. An immunohistochemical and PCR reaction evaluation of feline plasmacytic pododermatitis. *Vet Pathol* 2007; 44: 80–83.
16. Simon M, Horvath, C, Pauley D. Plasma cell pododermatitis in feline immunodeficiency virus-infected cats. *Veterinary Pathol* 1993; 30: 477.
17. Gruchouskei L, de Marco Viott A, Santana R *et al.* Pododermatite plasmocitaria felina. *Arch Vet Sci* 2012; 17: 32–36.
18. Hnilica KA. Hypersensitivity disorders. In: Hnilica KA, ed. *Small Animal Dermatology: A Color Atlas and Therapeutic Guide.* St Louis, MO: Elsevier Saunders, 2011; 175–226.
19. Drolet R, Bernard J. Plasma cell pododermatitis in a cat. *Can Vet J* 1984; 25: 448–449.

8.6

Hot topics in zoonosis

J.S. Weese[1] (Chairperson), C.C. Pye[1] (Secretary)

[1]Ontario Veterinary College, University of Guelph, Ontario, Canada

Scott Weese (*Canada*) introduced himself as the chairperson of the workshop and encouraged questions and further discussion at the end. He stated that 'zoonotic 'diseases' is a broad category and so the workshop would focus on resistant staphylococci and the most important questions relating to staphylococcal zoonoses: namely, how to disseminate information more widely regarding current guidelines for management, including what is being done in veterinary hospitals; how to improve patient care; and how to reduce anxiety. He introduced the secretary and the different speakers and their topics for the workshop.

Overview of zoonotic methicillin-resistant staphylococci (S. Weese)

Scott Weese began by reviewing the different groups of staphylococci, each with different clinical relevance and zoonotic disease potential. There has been an evolution in our identification of staphylococci from *Staphylococcus aureus* to *S. aureus* versus *S. intermedius* and more recently recognition of *S. pseudintermedius*, *S. aureus* and *S. schleiferi* coagulans as the main coagulase-positive staphylococcal pathogens in dogs and cats. Coagulase-negative staphylococci are common and, even when methicillin resistant (MR), are much less of a concern. One of the major issues with zoonotic organisms is discussing them with clients; unfortunately the internet can provide misleading information regarding infection with MR staphylococci. Methicillin-resistant *S aureus* (MRSA) is a major issue in human medicine, although dogs and cats can also be infected and involved in transmission. Other species of staphylococci include resistant *S. schleiferi* and methicillin-resistant *S. pseudintermedius* (MRSP). *S. pseudintermedius* is the canine *Staphylococcus* species and consequently is more concerning from an animal health standpoint.

MRSA is widely publicized because of its scope of disease morbidity and mortality in the human population. There are various reports of MRSA transmission from animals to people and most companion animal data are focused on this transmission and not any other underlying cause of disease. Transmission from animals may be a true risk but may also be overestimated due to a reporting bias. While evidence of concurrent colonization of MRSA by humans and pets is relatively common, evidence implicating pets as causes of disease in humans is still rather weak.

Workers in the veterinary field are at increased risk of exposure to MR staphylococci; even with a small percentage of a veterinary clinic's caseload carrying MRSA, that percentage is multiplied by the large number of patients, the worker's hygiene status, infection control practices and risk of inoculation associated with handling animals. Studies show variable results but the general consensus is that veterinarians are a higher risk group than the average population for carrying MRSA. No evidence indicates that veterinarians should be routinely tested or treated for MR staphylococcal carriage, but veterinarians (and their physicians) should understand the occupational risk and increased likelihood that a veterinarian is a MRSA carrier.

There are reports of *S. pseudintermedius* infections in humans but here we need to consider the relative risk. Most dogs carry *S. pseudintermedius*, and 60% of the human population has contact with dogs regularly. Thus a large proportion of the population is touching *S. pseudintermedius* every day but there are just single case reports of infection in humans. This implies that *S. pseudintermedius* is not very capable of causing infection in people. However, *S. pseudintermedius* can cause severe infections such as meningitis, so while rare, the risk must not be dismissed. The same applies for MRSP, which is no more virulent than methicillin-susceptible S. *pseudintermedius* (MSSP). Since MSSP infections are rare in people, MRSP infections should be of equally limited frequency.

In terms of relative risk, MRSA is the primary concern in humans, with MRSP of secondary importance. *S. schleiferi schleiferi* appears to be a human bacterium that might be crossing from human to animal or in both directions. *S. schleiferi coagulans* is probably associated more with dogs but there is debate about how different the two subspecies are. There is a close degree of contact between humans and animals, and with these resistant bacteria becoming more common the likelihood of transmission is increasing. Therapy and other service animals are brought into long-term care facilities with high-risk patients. MRSA is known to be capable of moving readily from humans to animals and back in these types of populations. There is a range of concerns from low risk for typical owners and their families to high risk for certain individuals (e.g. young, old or immunocompromised individuals); the latter can comprise 20–40% of the total population. Veterinary personnel may be included in the high-risk groups. A study undertaken in Ontario, Canada, with physician offices showed that 64% of households had one or more pets and 37% of non-pet-owning households also had frequent contact with animals so there is a large population that has contact with animals. When these figures are multiplied by the number of high-risk individuals, it is evident that attention must be paid to the increasing prevalence of MRSP and MRSA in animals.

Transmission of methicillin-resistant *Staphylococcus* (L. Frank)

Linda Frank (*USA*) stated that the two main staphylococcal species are *S. pseudintermedius* and *S. aureus,* as not much is known about *S. schleiferi*. Looking at *S. pseudintermedius* in the human literature, there are uncommon case reports where the bacterium seems to be more of an opportunistic organism whereby infection is usually associated with immunosuppression or dog bites. Almost always the person has had contact with a dog or another pet. In a study by Mahoudeau *et al.*,[1] looking at thousands of coagulase-positive staphylococci cultured from hospital patients, only two were *S. pseudintermedius* and both people had animal contact. A case report of a MRSP human sinus infection identified the organism as the same as that being carried by the dog in the house, based on pulse-field gel electrophoresis.[2] There was another report of MRSP type 71, the main European strain, in a person with recurrent sinusitis who had contact with a number of animals including a dog with health issues, cats and horses.[3] It has been shown that people are more likely to be infected with the organism they are colonized with; therefore, whether *S. pseudintermedius* can colonize people needs to be studied. Guardabassi *et al.* looked at dogs with deep pyoderma due to a susceptible staphylococcus.[4] In 7 of 13 dog owners, *S. pseudintermedius* was isolated from their nares. Six had the same organism as their pet, confirmed by pulsed-field gel electrophoresis. Colonization, however, appeared to be short lived as five of these owners who were re-tested 2 months later had negative cultures. Linda Frank did a similar study looking at whether there was a risk of genes being transferred from the dog *Staphylococcus* to the owner *Staphylococcus*.[5] Dogs were selected if they had recurrent pyodermas or pyodermas while on antibiotics, as these cases were more likely to be methicillin resistant. Of 25 dog and owner pairs, 15 dogs had MRSP and two of the owners cultured positive from their nares with the same pulse-field gel electrophoresis. Two dogs had methicillin-resistant *S. schleiferi schleiferi*, and one of those owners had methicillin-susceptible *S. schleiferi coagulans*. These organisms were most likely unrelated as the resistance patterns were not the same between the two bacteria. One dog had a resistant *S. schleiferi coagulans* and the owner was not affected. All owners had coagulase-negative staphylococci cultured from their nares, indicating that this is a common finding and probably not pathogenic. Many times owners will call dermatologists and veterinarians panicking that they have MRSA, but upon discussion the bacterium is identified as coagulase negative. Coagulase-negative bacteria may be pathogens but this is uncommon. The coagulase-negative bacteria in the study had different susceptibility patterns and different SCC*mec* (staphylococcal cassette chromosomal *mec*) types than the MRSP, so genes were not being shared. One owner in the study, whose pet did not have a MR staphylococcus, did have a MR coagulase-negative staphylococcus with the same antibiogram often seen with MRSP (solely susceptible to chloramphenicol). This owner was a veterinary hospital employee so may have acquired resistance from the workplace. Engeline van Duijkeren *et al.* took 45 nasal swabs from humans in 20 households.[6] Two were MRSP positive and both were from the same household where the resident cat had cystitis. The same group performed another study where owners were cultured monthly for 6 months.[7] On first sampling three owners were MRSP positive and all three had pets with MRSP. Two of these owners had repeat cultures performed, which were negative, highlighting the fact that owners only cultured positive when their dog had an active infection. Also, two individuals from the same household cultured positive on the last sampling, when their dog had an active infection. To summarize, MRSP infections in humans are relatively uncommon and often associated with pet contact. MRSP infrequently colonizes owners and if colonization does occur, it appears to be temporary. As the pets clear the infection, their owners are no longer carriers of the organism. Results from a limited number of studies show that the methicillin-resistance gene is not being transferred from pets to their owners.

Staphylococcus aureus is the bacterium people are most concerned about. A number of case reports document people with recurrent infections where the pet is thought to be the source of these recurrent infections. Once the pet was treated for carriage, infection in the humans was cleared. It is hypothesized that this may be a reverse zoonosis, where the pets are acquiring the organism from the owner and then re-infecting them. One case report of a diabetic individual with concurrent renal insufficiency, and another individual in the same house with recurrent MRSA infections, found that the dog was carrying MRSA in the nares.[8] The isolates in this household had the same pulsed-field gel electrophoresis pattern. This organism was resistant to mupirocin so topical vancomycin was used on lesions and the nares of the dog to resolve the infection. Boost *et al.* looked at colonization of owners and their pets in Hong Kong.[9] Twenty-four percent of humans had *S. aureus*, which is similar to the 20–40% previously noted. However, of those, only 0.5% had MRSA. A fraction (8.8%) of dogs living with these people were also colonized with *S. aureus*, and 0.7% were colonized by MRSA. This study showed that owner colonization was rarely associated with canine colonization as only 10% of owners with nasal colonization had colonized dogs. Dogs of healthcare workers were more likely to be colonized, and dogs that stayed in the bedroom were also more likely to be colonized. Six of 17 dog/owner pairs had the same organism based on pulsed-field gel electrophoresis, and only one pair was co-colonized with MRSA. Faires *et al.* looked at 22 households with MRSA in a pet.[10] Six of these households had MRSA colonization in a person and 20% of people were colonized. Comparing this with the previously reported 20% of people colonized with susceptible *S. aureus,* there is an increase in colonization with MRSA with a pet in the household. Eight households had infected individuals and only one of these households had a pet with

MRSA colonization. In that same household one of three people and both dogs were colonized with MRSA. Loeffler *et al.* looked at 120 owners with MRSA in a pet and of these 9 people cultured MRSA positive (7.5%).[11] This value is higher than the normal population rate. The percentage of the population with positive cultures varies depending on region; in Hong Kong it was 0.5% and in Britain it is closer to 1.5%. When owners of pets with susceptible *S. aureus* were cultured, no owners carried MRSA and 20% carried susceptible *S. aureus*. When there is a pet in the household with MRSA, there are often more people carrying the MRSA. Dan Morris *et al.* surveyed humans infected with MRSA and cultured pets to determine whether the pets were carriers of MRSA.[12] One hundred dogs and cats were screened from 66 households with people with MRSA. Eleven-and-a-half percent of pets from nine households were MRSA positive but only six of the households had concordant human and animal strains. With an increased delay between obtaining the human and pet cultures there was a decreased chance of isolating the organism, indicating that carriage was brief.

To summarize, interspecies transmission of *S. aureus* is possible but there appears to be a higher population of people colonized with MRSA when pets have MRSA, compared to the general population. The number of pets with MRSA has been increasing. The current literature is missing longitudinal studies with *S. aureus* to follow the incidence of infection in people and pets. There is no standardization of sampling methodology and, therefore, it is difficult to compare studies.

Heather Peikes (*USA*) asked where Linda Frank would recommend sampling for carriage.

Linda Frank replied that she would swab four sites: nose, mouth and skin on one swab and then swab the perianal region separately to prevent bacterial overgrowth.

Scott Weese commented that he typically recommends swabbing the nose and rectum, but that the pharynx might be a bigger reservoir than assumed in the past; therefore, obtaining nose, mouth and rectal swabs might be more sensitive. He explained his concern with culturing the skin for carriage – in an MRSA household an MRSA-positive skin sample could represent the owner having just touched the dog. He also mentioned that if skin was to be cultured, he would recommend using a different swab than the one used for other body sites. He stated that different groups may have different colonization patterns and sampling of 'both ends' seems to be particularly important for dogs like hospital therapy dogs where colonization is predominantly gastrointestinal (GI). There are a lot of nasal-negative and rectal-positive cultures as the dogs may be licking surfaces and hands.

Heather Peikes asked Scott Weese to confirm that he would do a nasal swab separately.

Scott Weese replied that he can perform cultures in his lab for a few dollars whereas screening through a diagnostic lab may cost US$80 to US$100 per sample. In this case pooling the samples may be warranted. He noted that prior to sampling one must ask the questions 'when do we screen and why do we screen?'.

Linda Frank commented that when she submitted four regions on one swab there was bacterial overgrowth even using staphylococcal selection media. She recommended sampling the perianal region on a separate swab. In an 'ideal world', three swabs would be taken.

Scott Weese explained that research was needed to look at separate sites and standardization of sampling procedures. He remarked that nasal swabs are variable in quality between dogs. If a diagnostic lab is using nonselective culture media, there may be decreased ability to find MRSA or MRSP versus a selective culture through surveillance screening.

David Lloyd (*UK*) remarked that the purpose for screening should first be identified. He considered that *S. aureus* was less likely to be carried for a long period of time on a dog unless the dog was infected. Sampling a dog once is inconclusive, as with one sample colonization cannot be confirmed. He pointed out that within the room the participants were exchanging staphylococci and some would continue to be carriers for short periods of time. He noted that Linda Frank had quoted the study performed in the UK that showed that owners of pets with MRSA infection were more likely to have MRSA nasal carriage than owners of pets with MSSA infection.[11] A parallel study using the same group of animals had shown there was also a significant relationship between human hospital visits and pet MRSA infections, and that isolates were nearly always hospital isolates.[13] The implication was that the MRSA originate from hospitals, are carried by the owner and then transferred to susceptible pets.

Scott Weese noted that the big question is whether there is an indication to screen. He remarked that there continue to be situations where a human is infected with MRSA and the cat is deemed the reservoir of infection when screening of the cat has not been performed.

Christine Prost (*UK*) asked how many samples should be taken to determine whether an animal is colonized and at what interval.

David Lloyd responded that there are many different definitions of 'colonization' in the literature. Sommerville-Millar and Noble state that if less than 25% of samplings are positive then this is carriage.[14] If 25–75% are positive it is transient carriage, and if sampling is positive more than 75% of the time then this is colonization. This means that a minimum of four samples is required.

Once infectious, always infectious. So what about persistence of MRS? (D. Lloyd)

David Lloyd remarked that because staphylococci are ubiquitous, dogs and other animals in our clinics can carry bacteria from all sorts of sources. Dogs can transfer staphylococci to people, other animals and the environment where staphylococci can survive. Endogenous staphylococci are being transferred around the animal all the time. Staphylococci found on the skin have likely been transferred from a mucosal site such as the mouth or perianal region. The staphylococcal flora in dogs consists of both coagulase-positive and coagulase-negative species and is first acquired from the dam when the dog is born or shortly afterwards.[15] In humans transmission occurs from around the breasts during suckling. Coagulase-positive staphylococci are acquired from an individual's parents, and typically one or two dominant strains become prominent. Throughout the life of the dog, a variety of strains will be transiently carried and may even have short-term colonization, but will then be lost leaving the dominant strains.[16] Fusidic acid has been used previously to remove populations of *S. intermedius* from mucosal sites. The population decreases and cannot be detected in many regions on the skin for a short time but will return several weeks later.[17] Therefore, fusidic acid could be used to decolonize an animal but the process is not well understood.

S. pseudintermedius adheres better than *S. aureus* to dog's skin, so *S. pseudintermedius* is likely to persist better in dogs and other animals than *S. aureus*. Loeffler *et al.* looked at dogs and cats, both healthy and those visiting veterinary clinics, in the London region.[18] This study showed that healthy dogs and cats in the community tended to have lower percentages of MRSA carriage than those in veterinary clinics, but these differences were not significant. Data from the USA by Gingrich *et al.* showed that 0.5% of both dogs and cats carried MRSA.[19] Couto *et al.* in Lisbon showed carriage rates of 1.4% in cats and 0.7% in dogs,[20] whereas in Belgium, Vanderhaeghen *et al.* showed rates of 1.1% in dogs.[21] Carriage of MRSA in animals occurs at low levels but appears to be higher in animals that visit veterinary clinics. When Loeffler *et al.* were studying MRSA carriage in London,[22] one dog in a rescue facility was found to have a MRSA wound infection, and 7.8% of the other dogs were found to be carrying MRSA. All isolates had the same lineage and resistance pattern. All of the carrier dogs lived in shared kennels but their 16 kennel partners sampled negative on two occasions. This supports the concept that MRSA transfer between healthy dogs does not readily occur. The kennels in the facility were cleaned and disinfected twice daily and following antimicrobial treatment of the infected dog, MRSA carriage resolved in all of the dogs. There was no MRSA transfer from dog to dog so transfer was likely by kennel staff. Floras *et al.* showed that there was a similar loss of MRSA over time after an outbreak in a breeding kennel.[23] Without a constant source of exposure to MRSA, dogs are likely to lose their MRSA colonization. Patel *et al.* studied both feral and domestic cats in veterinary practices.[24] *S. aureus, S. pseudintermedius* and coagulase-negative staphylococci were all isolated. In domestic cats 91% of the isolates were susceptible to all of the antimicrobials tested. Only 81% of the feral cat isolates were susceptible, indicating that the feral cats carried more resistance. This demonstrated that even without therapy, cats can harbour resistant staphylococci.

Coagulase-negative staphylococci also carry resistance genes, which can be transferred to other bacteria. It is believed that MRSA acquired its capacity for methicillin resistance from a coagulase-negative *Staphylococcus*. This highlights the fact that unnecessary use of antimicrobials may promote resistance not only in pathogens but also in nonpathogens, with unexpected long-term consequences. Rota *et al.* looked at the misuse of antimicrobials and selection of MRSP in two breeding kennels over a 2-year period.[25] In both kennels, antimicrobials, including third-generation cephalosporins, fluoroquinolones and macrolides, had commonly been given without supervision. In kennel A, in which antibiotic use had been dramatically reduced, there were few infections, whereas in kennel B, which had not reduced antimicrobial use, MRSP infections continued to be a problem. He commented that he recommends clients ask their veterinarian why an antibiotic is being prescribed and whether it is necessary. Beck *et al.* looked at prevalence of methicillin-resistant *S. pseudintermedius* on skin and carriage sites after treatment of methicillin-resistant or methicillin-susceptible staphylococcal pyoderma.[26] In this study, skin, nasal and rectal swabs were cultured at referral and again after resolution of the pyoderma. Initially MRSP from the skin was cultured in 40.5% of cases, MRSA in 1.7% and MR *S. schleiferi coagulans* in 2.9%. Samples from carriage sites, nose and rectum, showed MRSP in 34.1% of cases, MRSA in 6.4% of cases and MR S. *schleiferi coagulans* in 4%. After clinical cure, of the 42 cases initially diagnosed with MRSP pyoderma, MRSP was cultured from the skin in 45.2% of cases and from carriage sites in 47%. Of the 60 without MRSP pyoderma initially, MRSP was found on the skin in 28.3% of cases and from carriage sites in 26.7%. This study proves that MRSP can be acquired by animals during the treatment period. With antibiotic treatment, susceptible flora is reduced so if these animals come into contact with other animals or people with MRSP, they are more likely to acquire the MR bacteria.

Veterinary clinics are a major area where transmission can occur and stringent cleaning protocols should be followed. Infected animals should enter the hospital via a different route and be handled separately. Cleaning and disinfection should occur between patients. Laarhoven *et al.* took dogs with a recent MRSP infection (index dogs) and sampled those dogs, owners and other contact animals once a month for 6 months.[7] Samples were obtained from the nose, perineum and infection sites of the affected dogs, as well as contact animals and from the nares of owners. Index dogs were positive for long periods of time, with two dogs being positive every month. In 5 of the 12 households, index cases were intermittently MRSP positive. This highlights the need for repeated samples to determine colonization versus carriage and also shows that long-term carriage of MRSP is possible. Four households had positive cultures from the environment but negative cultures from humans and animals, indicating that MRSP can survive well in the environment. MRSP isolates are generally similar within households, but in two households in this study genetically distinct isolates were found. If factors that promote colonization by one isolate are present then other isolates may also be able to colonize the susceptible hosts. Humans were rarely positive and never more than once, exhibiting rapid loss of nasal carriage.

In summary, dogs have dominant staphylococcal strains but transiently acquire others during their life. Coagulase-negative staphylococci commonly acquire methicillin resistance and can serve as a reservoir of resistance. Carriage of MRSA by pets is low but probably increased by exposure to veterinary clinics; fortunately carriage of MRSA by dogs tends to be lost in hygienic environments. Antimicrobial misuse can promote MRSP persistence in healthy dogs, and MRSP can be acquired during periods of antimicrobial treatment. MRSP can persist for long periods after a clinical cure, and MRSA can survive for 6 to 9 months or longer in a hospital. Environmental contamination may also persist in the absence of carrier animals and people.

Valerie Fadok (*USA*) asked David Lloyd what he advises owners to do in a household with a dog with MRSP pyoderma to limit environmental contamination when the dog is being bathed.

David Lloyd commented that topical therapy can be used, such as bathing with an antibacterial shampoo to reduce shedding of the bacteria. He remarked that owners should be informed that the animal will carry the bacteria on mucosal sites and so contact with these sites should be minimized. Surfaces in the house should be disinfected once or twice a day, and if the animal has an exudative lesion the animal should be restricted to a certain part of the house that can easily be disinfected. Contact with other animals should be reduced so the affected animal should be kept on a leash. When the infection has resolved, cleaning should continue to reduce contamination. He commented that he asks owners to follow these recommendations but cautions that it is unlikely to be 100% effective.

Recommendations for management (V. Fadok)

Valerie Fadok mentioned that at her clinic in Houston, numerous referral cases of pyoderma are treated, many of which are atopic dogs or dogs with demodicosis with a secondary pyoderma. Many of these animals have been treated for over a year with serial or continual antibiotics without being cultured. An indication that an animal may have an MR infection is a poor response to antibiotic therapy. With these cases cytology is performed to confirm a bacterial pyoderma. Most pyodermas are due to staphylococci, so a culture and susceptibility testing is performed with no oral antimicrobial treatment until the culture results are obtained. While waiting for the culture results, aggressive topical therapy can be instituted. Once the culture results are returned, the dog is often clinically improved and owners are willing to continue the topical treatment following a discussion of the limited options for oral antibiotics.

Typical resistance patterns of MR staphylococci show susceptibility to only rifampin and amikacin. Both of these antibiotics have the potential to cause serious adverse effects, such as kidney damage with amikacin use, and liver damage with rifampin use. Topical therapy is the least expensive option when the cost of monitoring is included (e.g. renal monitoring with amikacin). In a small unpublished study performed in Houston, 10 owners were asked to bathe their dog with pyoderma with either 3% or 4% chlorhexidine daily. A contact time of 10 minutes was requested. A scoring system looking at erythema, crusting, odour and pruritus was used to determine improvement. At a 2-week recheck all dogs were at least 50% improved in score and some had almost complete resolution. By 4 weeks all dogs had resolved with no active lesions and hair regrowth. One outlier remained pruritic but was noted to be atopic. After they have bathed their animals on a daily basis, asking owners to bathe their pets once or twice weekly is typically well received for maintenance to help prevent recurrence of infection.

In Houston (Texas), the Douxo® chlorhexidine regimen has also been used for the initial therapy. This regimen includes shampooing two or three times per week and using the spray in between. This regimen provides similar results to daily chlorhexidine bathes but is more expensive. There are many topical products that can be used, such as bleach rinses or the Douxo® gel spray, but the most important factor is identifying the pyoderma early. If a pyoderma develops focally on the abdominal skin and is identified, the owners can treat aggressively locally and prevent the spread to the rest of the body. Zymox® spray (PKB Animal Health) is available and efficacious but it may be more difficult to use due to the small size of the spray. Vetericyn VF® (Innovacyn, Inc.) is an oxygenated chlorine spray, used a minimum of twice daily in treating bacterial pyodermas. This product is available as a water spray and hydrogel; the hydrogel is best for glabrous skin. Nisin wipes are dairy wipes containing an antibiotic used to reduce staphylococcal mastitis. These wipes can be used twice daily on glabrous areas and may be beneficial if frequent bathing is not an option. Some clinics may offer owners a bathing protocol within the clinic for a set fee. This would ensure animals receive at least five baths on a weekly basis. Staphage Lysate® (Delmont Laboratories, Inc.) immunotherapy and topical barrier repair products may be used to help minimize the use of antibiotics. Staphage Lysate® may be useful for dogs with staphylococcal hypersensitivity and dogs with recurrent pyoderma. Valerie Fadok commented that she is an advocate of barrier repair and feels that there is a reduced frequency of pyoderma when barrier repair is used. One such product she has had good results with is Allerderm spot on® (Virbac).

If there is a recurrence of pyoderma in an animal that had a previous MR staphylococcal infection, a culture should always be taken. On reculture, some infections are still caused by MR strains yet some will be susceptible. Topical therapy can then be reinstituted while awaiting results.

It is very important to counsel clients, as many will ask if the infection is contagious. Making use of handouts is recommended, including those from Scott Weese's 'worms and germs' blog.[27] An MRSP handout can be provided but it is recommended to distribute an MRSA handout only if MRSA is cultured, due to anxiety surrounding this particular organism. By explaining that infection with MR staphylococci is of greatest public health concern for young children, the elderly and immunocompromised individuals, people will often volunteer whether they or family members are within one of these high-risk groups and then precautions can be discussed. For example if there is an elderly mother on chemotherapy it is best to recommend that she does not touch the dog while it has an infection and that the dog is bathed in the clinic.

Discussing common-sense hygiene at home, such as hand washing after touching the dog and using a separate tub to bathe the dog, is important in MR infection cases. Owners may not need to wear gloves as they will have their hands submerged in products such as chlorhexidine and therefore should not become colonized. After use, the tub should be bleached. In Valerie Fadok's clinic in Houston, there are alcohol sanitizers in every exam room, tables are wiped and floors washed between patients. Keyboards and door handles are wiped at least once a day and bleach sprays are used on exam tables. Test cultures of the treatment area are taken but are often not positive for staphylococci. In the medical and surgical wards, if there are MRSP-positive patients, signs are posted requiring personal protective equipment to be worn (disposable booties, gowns and gloves). Often the medical and surgical departments will consult with dermatology prior to procedures to check whether the animal has a pyoderma that would prevent surgery from occurring. Another hygiene measure worth undertaking is to mop floors and wipe chairs and other items in the waiting area with bleach twice daily.

Linda Frank commented that at her clinic they recommend bathing every other day. Chlorhexidine gluconate 2% solution poured into a spray bottle can be used twice daily between bathing. She has noted the occasional contact reaction so clients should be instructed to call if the animal's skin condition appears to worsen.

Christine Prost asked whether the dogs are shaved for this treatment regimen.

Linda Frank stated that she does not shave the animal; she recommends that owners move the hair to apply spray to the skin.

Heather Peikes asked what to use if the animal had a contact reaction.

Linda Frank mentioned that only very few had this type of reaction to chlorhexidine. An alternative would be the use of nisin wipes on hairless areas or shaved areas; however, these wipes do not have activity against yeast or *Pseudomonas*.

Helen Power (*USA*) asked how clipper blades were being handled in clinics after being used on a patient with an MR infection. She commented that she disposed of the blades after use.

Valerie Fadok remarked that she soaks the blades in chlorhexidine for several hours and then scrubs them.

Helen Power stated that she would not want her dog clipped with these same clipper blades and that she has a dedicated clipper for MR cases.

Scott Weese highlighted the key point that MRSP is no more virulent than MSSP and can be killed with disinfectants. He mentioned that the blades can be soaked in accelerated hydrogen peroxide.

Helen Power was concerned that the technicians in the hospital would still be handling the blade.

Scott Weese replied that whatever is the most practical and cost-effective route of disinfecting blades should be followed.

Helen Power asked where the blades should be cleaned in a small hospital, where often a treatment area is shared by several veterinarians, to minimize exposure to other dogs.

David Lloyd commented that clipping causes damage to the skin so the organism is actually being inoculated through the stratum corneum and hair follicles are being disrupted. Clipping should only be performed to shorten the hair so the skin is untouched. He noted that as 70% alcohol kills staphylococci, the blades could be soaked in alcohol to kill the bacteria.

Helen Power commented that discussion had revolved around how persistent staphylococci are in households and asked whether this soaking would be sufficient to kill the microbes.

David Lloyd replied that these concerns with environmental contamination are regarding typical ambient conditions, not situations where the bacteria are exposed to 70% alcohol or high concentrations of chlorhexidine.

Maron Calderwood (*USA*) introduced herself as a diagnostic pathologist. She stated that she recommends practitioners send an aseptic tissue biopsy for tissue culture. She asked whether she should continue to do this.

Linda Frank commented that it would depend on the type of infection present. If a deep pyoderma is present then tissue should be collected aseptically. If it is a superficial pyoderma then she does not recommend aseptic preparation of the skin.

Scott Weese recommended talking to clients about basic infection control including avoiding biohazardous sites such as the dog's nose and perianal region and any lesions. He recommended routine hand washing and identifying high-risk areas such as food bowls. In rare instances a dog can be sent away to another house, not a veterinary clinic, for a few weeks, where the dog should be able to decolonize itself.

Heather Peikes asked about recommendations for the use of accelerated hydrogen peroxide.

Scott Weese commented that the product is new to the USA but has been in Canada for a while and is becoming the standard of care in human hospitals for environmental disinfection. He noted that accelerated hydrogen peroxide is his standard for disinfection of the environment because it has a broad spectrum, a short kill time, works in the presence of organic debris and the breakdown product is water. It does not appear to be corrosive like other disinfectants such as Virkon® (DuPont). Accelerated hydrogen peroxide is more expensive than other disinfectants but has a label claim for *Trichophyton*, poliovirus, parvovirus and clostridial spores. This spectrum of activity is unique to this product. Brand names include Accel®, Virox® and Peroxigard® (all manufactured by Sonosite, Inc.) and are the same product licensed through different companies. He mentioned that Virox® will send you links to different sites containing information about these products if requested via the website or by phone. There is also a shampoo containing accelerated hydrogen peroxide, although the only data currently available concern efficacy in the environment. Unpublished work at the Ontario Veterinary College showed that at the concentration used, there should be no cytotoxic effect on the skin. Whether accelerated hydrogen peroxide is more efficacious on skin than chlorhexidine is unknown. It is useful for any equipment as a mid-level disinfectant after removal of organic debris.

Helen Power asked whether clipper blades could be disinfected using accelerated hydrogen peroxide.

Scott Weese replied that soaking the blades for a few minutes, cleaning debris and then soaking for a further 30 seconds is recommended. This short contact time combined with rinsing should prevent damaging the metal. He commented that there are also wipes containing accelerated hydrogen peroxide available for use on keyboards, etc. Human data suggest that laundering within households will wash off the majority of microbes and the dryer will subsequently kill most microbes.

Scott Weese asked if there was anything else participants would like to see on information sheets for clients, such as pet bathing recommendations for animals with MR infections. He asked participants to contact him if they had any ideas for other information sheets. He concluded the workshop by thanking the speakers and the participants for coming.

References

1. Mahoudeau I, Delabranche X, Prevost G *et al.* Frequency of isolation of *Staphylococcus intermedius* from humans. *J Clin Microbiol* 1997; 35: 2153–2154.
2. Kempker R, Mangalat D, Kongphet-Tran T *et al.* Beware of the pet dog: a case of *Staphylococcus intermedius* infection. *Am J Med Sci* 2009; 338: 425–427.
3. Stegmann R, Burnens A, Maranta CA *et al.* Human infection associated with methicillin-resistant *Staphylococcus pseudintermedius* ST71. *J Antimicrob Chemoth* 2010; 65: 2047–2048.
4. Guardabassi L, Leober ME, Jacobson A. Transmission of multiple antimicrobial-resistant *Staphylococcus intermedius* between dogs affected by deep pyoderma and their owners. *Vet Microbiol* 2004; 98: 23–27.
5. Frank L, Kania SA, Kirzeder EM *et al.* Risk of colonization or gene transfer to owners of dogs with methicillin-resistant *Staphylococcus pseudintermedius*. *Vet Dermatol* 2009; 20: 496–501.
6. Van Duijkeren E, Kamphuis M, van der Mije IC. Transmission of methicillin-resistant Staphylococcus pseudintermedius between infected dogs and cats and contact pets, humans and the environment in households and veterinary clinics. *Vet Microbiol* 2011; 150: 338–343.
7. Laarhoven LM, de Heus P, van Luijn J *et al.* Longitudinal study on methicillin-resistant *Staphylococcus pseudintermedius* in households. *PLoS One* 2011; 6: 1–6.
8. Manian FA. Asymptomatic nasal carriage of mupirocin-resistant, methicillin-resistant *Staphylococcus aureus* (MRSA) in a pet dog associated with MRSA infection in household contacts. *Clin Infect Dis* 2003; 36: e26–e28.
9. Boost MV, O'Donoghue MM, James A. Prevalence of S. *aureus* carriage among dogs and owners. *Epidemiol Infect* 2008; 136: 953–964.
10. Faires M, Tater K, Weese JS. An investigation of methicillin-resistant *Staphylococcus aureus* colonization in people and pets in the same household with an infected person or infected pet. *J Am Med Vet Assoc* 2009; 235: 540.
11. Loeffler A, Pfeiffer DU, Lloyd DH *et al.* Methicillin-resistant *Staphylococcus aureus* carriage in UK veterinary staff and owners of infected pets: new risk groups. *J Hosp Infect* 2010; 74: 282–288.
12. Morris DO, Lautenbach E, Zaoutis T *et al.* Potential for pet animals to harbour methicillin-resistant *Staphylococcus aureus* when residing with human MRSA patients. *Zoonoses Public Hlth* 2012; 59: 286–293.
13. Soares Magalhaes RJ, Loeffler A, Lindsay J *et al.* Risk factors for methicillin-resistant Staphylococcus aureus (MRSA) infection in dogs and cats: a case-control study. *Vet Res* 2010; 41: 55.
14. Somerville-Millar DA, Noble WC. Resident and transient bacteria of the skin. *J Cutan Pathol* 1974; 1: 260–264.
15. Saijonmaa-Koulumies L, Lloyd DH. Colonisation of neonatal puppies by Staphylococcus intermedius. *Vet Dermatol* 2002; 13: 123–130.
16. Saijonmaa-Koulumies L, Myllys V, Lloyd DH. Diversity and stability of the Staphylococcus intermedius flora in three bitches and their puppies. *Epidemiol Infect* 2003; 131: 931–937.
17. Saijonmaa-Koulumies L, Parsons E, Lloyd DH. Elimination of Staphylococcus intermedius in healthy dogs by topical treatment with fusidic acid. *J Small Anim Pract* 1998; 39: 341–347.
18. Loeffler A, Pfeiffer DU, Lindsay JA *et al.* Prevalence of and risk factors for MRSA carriage in companion animals: a survey of dogs, cats and horses. *Epidemiol Infect* 2010; 14: 1–10.
19. Gingrich EN, Kurt T, Hyatt DR *et al.* Prevalence of methicillin-resistant staphylococci in northern Colorado shelter animals. *J Vet Diagn Invest* 2011; 23: 947–950.
20. Couto N, Pomba C, Moodley A *et al.* Prevalence of meticillin-resistant staphylococci among dogs and cats at a veterinary teaching hospital in Portugal. *Vet Rec* 2011; 169: 72.
21. Vanderhaeghen W, Van de Velde E, Crombe F *et al.* Screening for methicillin-resistant staphylococci in dogs admitted to a veterinary teaching hospital. *Res Vet Sci* 2011; 93: 133–136.
22. Loeffler A, Pfeiffer DU, Lindsay JA *et al.* Lack of transmission of methicillin-resistant *Staphylococcus aureus* (MRSA) between

apparently healthy dogs in a rescue kennel. *Vet Microbiol* 2010; 141: 178–181.

23. Floras A, Lawn K, Slavic D *et al.* Sequence type 398 meticillin-resistant *Staphylococcus aureus* infection and colonisation in dogs. *Vet Rec* 2010; 166: 826–827.
24. Patel A, Lloyd DH, Lamport AL. Antibiotic resistance amongst feline staphylococci in south-eastern England. *Vet Dermatol* 1999; 10: 257–262.
25. Rota A, Milani C, Corro M *et al.* Misuse of antimicrobials and selection of methicillin-resistant *S. pseudintermedius* strains in breeding kennels: genetic characterization of bacteria after a two-year interval. *Reprod Domest Anim* 2012; doi: 10.1111/j.1439-0531.2012.02012.x [Epub ahead of print].
26. Beck KM, Waisglass SE, Dick HLN *et al.* Prevalence of meticillin-resistant *S. pseudintermedius* (MRSP) from skin and carriage sites of dogs after treatment of their meticillin-resistant or meticillin-sensitive staphylococcal pyoderma. *Vet Dermatol* 2012; 23: 369-e67.
27. Weese JS, Anderson M. Worms and Germs Blog. URL: http://www.wormsandgermsblog.com/articles/diseases/test-subcategory/. Accessed 30 July 2012.

8.7

Responsible use of antimicrobials

D.H. Lloyd[1] (Chairperson), J.D. Littlewood[2] (Secretary)

[1]Royal Veterinary College, University of London, UK
[2]Veterinary Dermatology Referrals, Landbeach, Cambridge UK

David Lloyd (*UK*) opened the workshop by emphasizing the importance and topicality of the subject and its impact on the veterinary profession and treatment of infections over the next decade. He stressed the interactive nature of the session and encouraged discussion from the audience. He gave a brief overview of the structure of the workshop and introduced the speakers.

The Swedish approach to prudent antimicrobial use (K.E. Bergvall)

Kerstin Bergvall (*Sweden*) reported that the emergence of multiresistant bacteria in Sweden triggered the development of a national antibiotic strategy based on directives issued by the government, which include directions regarding animal welfare. The aim is to preserve the future usefulness of antibiotics in both human and animal infectious diseases.

There is a tradition of careful use of antibiotics in Sweden; antibiotics can only be sold through pharmacies and can only be supplied with a prescription from a human physician or a veterinarian after clinical examination of the patient. Prescriptions are registered, allowing monitoring of antibiotic usage over time and by region. The colder climate means that there is a lower incidence of infections, which reduces the need to prescribe antibiotics compared to warmer parts of the world. Until recently the movement of animals abroad has been restricted, although it is now permitted within the European Union (EU). There is a tradition of performing bacterial culture and sensitivity testing, which allows monitoring of susceptibility patterns. There is also an emphasis on disease prevention with hygiene measures and national vaccination programmes, and many diseases are reportable. The use of antibiotics as growth promoters has been banned for some time.

Scandinavian veterinarians have long been aware of the importance of responsible use of antibiotics, dating back to the Proceedings of the Nordic Veterinary Conference 1962, where a contributor spoke of the importance of the penicillins and the need for responsible use by the veterinary profession to preserve their usefulness for the future. The Swedish Strategic Programme for the Rational Use of Antimicrobial Agents and Surveillance of Resistance (STRAMA), a strategy group that receives funding from the Swedish government, monitors antibiotic resistance and the amount of antibiotics prescribed; it issues policy documents on the use of antibiotics and hygiene measures for both human and veterinary healthcare. The antibiotic policy document requires that two criteria should be met for the prescribing of antibiotics: a bacterial infection must be present and the infection cannot be cured without the use of antibiotics.

The other policy of importance in reducing the use of antibiotics is the hygiene policy document. Healthcare personnel are known to transfer bacteria and one of the most important factors in the development of methicillin-resistant *Staphylococcus aureus* (MRSA) in dogs and cats is contact with MRSA-positive humans; repeated courses of antibiotics and being hospitalized are other risk factors. The risk of methicillin-resistant *S. pseudintermedius* (MRSP) infection is twice as common in hospitalized patients compared with outpatients, and 5% of veterinary healthcare workers may be MRSP-positive.[1] To reduce the risk of transmission of infectious organisms the following measures are recommended: wash hands frequently, both before and after handling patients; use alcohol gels; have bare arms below the elbows; clean touch areas such as doorknobs and microscope knobs; autoclave instruments including ear cones, skin scalpel blades and flea combs; and disinfect clipper blades, with a new blade used for each patient.

Information has been disseminated by the media with regard to the use of antibiotics and the risk of development of resistant bacteria so the public is well informed. It is a mandatory topic in elementary schools and consequently there is increased awareness amongst the general public. This helps with discussion with clients in everyday clinical work. The policy documents have changed the behaviour of prescribers. In 2006 there was a peak in antibiotic use in the dog; since then there has been an overall 32% reduction in antibiotic sales, with a 62% reduction in cephalosporins, 44% reduction in amoxicillin/clavulanate, and 39% reduction in fluoroquinolone sales. This reduction of antibiotic usage has not been associated with an increased failure to cure bacterial infections in dogs. Methicillin-resistant infections with MRSA and MRSP are reportable in Sweden. Since 2006, 45 cases of MRSA have been reported in animals, comprising one pig, 18 dogs, 17 horses, five cats and four cattle. Looking at MRSP infections in the dog, 73 cases were reported in 2008, 122 cases in 2009, 100 cases in 2010 and only 53 cases in 2011. Two human diabetic patients have suffered from MRSP infections of leg wounds. Pig holdings have been screened because of the known risk of MRSA carriage; in 2006/7 and 2008 all holdings screened were negative compared to a positive incidence of 27% in other EU states; in 2010 only one pig holding out of 191 screened in Sweden was found to be positive for MRSA. The incidence of death in humans in Sweden due to MRSA is 0.019/1000 inhabitants, compared to 0.08/1000 in the UK (four times higher).

Looking to the future, a global approach is required, as micro-organisms do not respect state borders. Ongoing vigilance of veterinarians, whether or not they as individuals have encountered the problem of bacterial resistance, is important to preserve the usefulness of antibiotics for the future.

Andrew Hillier (*USA*) asked if injectable antibiotics were subject to the same controls as for prescribing antibiotic tablets.

Kerstin Bergvall answered that control and monitoring of the use of injectable antibiotics is not as good, but in hospitalized patients case discussions take place before antibiotic usage, and cephalosporins are rarely used in clinics. She commented that repeated injections of antibiotic are not often used in clinical practice.

Candace Souza (*USA*) asked if there is involvement with the International Network for Action on Antibiotic Resistance (REACT) group monitoring the global use of antibiotics in Sweden.

Kerstin Bergvall answered that personnel at the Swedish Veterinary Institute do have contact with REACT.

Candace Souza then questioned why, with the documented decrease in overall antibiotic usage since 2006, there has been an increase in numbers of cases of MRSP that were seen.

Kerstin Bergvall explained that the increased number of MRSP cases was due to the spread of one particular strain of resistant organisms that originated from a single outbreak, and the dogs that were affected had been treated with several courses of antibiotics.

Kim Boyanowski (*USA*) asked if it was known why lincomycin and clindamycin usage increased over the period from 2005, and if the increased use of clindamycin has been associated with an increase in the amount of resistance to this antibiotic.

Kerstin Bergvall reported that there had been a study that demonstrated that new cases of pyoderma associated with *S. pseudintermedius* were usually sensitive to clindamycin, and isolates from recurrent cases have a 73–80% chance of being susceptible. Therefore, based on these data the recommendation is that clindamycin is a good choice for the treatment of the first episode of pyoderma in a patient. This has contributed to the reduction in the usage of cephalexin, although the increased use of clindamycin is still not as great as the reduction in use of cephalosporins. No increased rates of bacterial resistance to clindamycin (23% in 2010) have been seen as a result of its increased use. First episodes of pyoderma can be treated on an empirical basis without culture, but for patients with repeat infections that have been previously treated with antibiotics, the recommendation is to perform bacterial culture and susceptibility testing before prescribing antibiotics.

David Lloyd introduced the next speaker.

Control of antimicrobial drug use in North America (A. Hillier)

Andrew Hillier (*USA*) stated that there is essentially no control of antimicrobial drug use in the USA. The key piece of legislation, the Animal Medicinal Drug Use Clarification Act of 1994 (AMDUCA) produced by the US Food and Drug Administration (FDA) allows veterinarians to prescribe extra-label uses of certain approved animal drugs and approved human drugs for animals under certain conditions. Extra-label drug use (ELDU) means use of a drug in an animal in a manner that is not in accordance with the approved labelling, including but not limited to: use in species not listed; use for indications not listed; use at dosage levels, frequencies or routes of administration other than stated; and deviation from the labelled withdrawal time based on these different uses. This is limited to circumstances where the health of the animal is threatened or suffering or death may result from failing to treat. Use of drugs for enhancement of food production is prohibited. Only licensed veterinarians may prescribe drugs within a valid veterinary-client-patient relationship, and drug use for animal treatment by laypersons is excluded, except under the supervision of a licensed veterinarian. There are few restrictions on ELDU in non-food-producing animals, compared to food-producing animals. An approved human drug can be considered for use in a non-food-producing animal even when an approved animal drug exists for that species and disease condition. Economic reasons for ELDU of human drugs over an approved animal drug are valid. Generic drugs as well as brand-name drugs are covered by ELDU regulations.

An evaluation of data from the Ohio State University Veterinary Medical Center (OSU-VMC) on antimicrobial drug (AMD) use in dogs prior to admission, recently published in the *Journal of the American Veterinary Medical Association*, found that 55.6% of dogs had received AMDs in the previous 12 months, with beta-lactams being the most commonly administered (72.7%), and of which 57.4% had received cephalexin, 28.1% amoxicillin-clavulanate and 9.5% cefpodoxime.[2] The second most commonly used AMDs were topical aminoglycosides (32.2%), and fluoroquinolones were the third most common (23.1%). Amongst the fluoroquinolones, enrofloxacin had been given to 19.0%, ciprofloxacin to 5.4% and marbofloxacin to 2.9% of the dogs. Of the AMDs administered to dogs prior to admission, 70.1% were approved for use in humans, and thus less than 30% were animal-approved drugs. The most common reason for administration was integumentary disease (51.7%). Further, a pharmacy review of AMD usage at OSU-VMC during 2011 revealed that cefadroxil was dispensed for 14 dogs, cephalexin for 748 dogs, cefovecin for treatment of 27 dogs, cefpodoxime for 105 dogs and amoxicillin-clavulanate for 776 dogs (A. Hillier, personal communication). Although AMD use in food-producing animals is monitored in the USA, there is no central recording of AMD in non-food-producing animals, in contrast to the situation in Sweden.

It is recognized that there is a strong relationship between the emergence of multidrug-resistant (MDR) pathogens and AMD use, that there is now global emergence of methicillin-resistant *S. pseudintermedius* (MRSP), and AMD stewardship practices are a key element in slowing the spread of MDR pathogens. The use of third-generation cephalosporins and fluoroquinolones is a known risk factor for MRSA in humans. According to proposed guidelines for the treatment of staphylococcal bacterial folliculitis in dogs currently being developed by a working group of the International Society of Canine Infectious Diseases, AMDs should not be used empirically and only used on the basis of culture and sensitivity testing. This is in contrast to the manufacturers' labelling and FDA approved indications for these drugs, where they are licensed for use in the treatment of skin wounds and infections. Little has been published about the risk factors for the development of MRSP in dogs, but recent publications have shown these to be AMD usage within the last 30 days in one study,[3] and in the previous 6 months in a second study.[4] An interesting paper recently published[5] looked at two kennels where MRSP had been isolated in 2008. In kennel A the use of AMD was dramatically reduced, and only used under the specific and direct supervision of a veterinarian, whilst in kennel B there was ongoing use of third-generation cephalosporins, fluoroquinolones and macrolides. Two years later six dogs from kennel A and eight dogs from kennel B were screened. No MRSP was isolated from kennel A, but 16 strains of MRSP were isolated from bitches in kennel B. This points to the unrestricted use of AMD as a real risk factor in the emergence of MDR bacterial strains. Guidelines for AMD usage in skin disease are in existence, but it is uncertain if they will be widely disseminated, accepted and followed and how outcomes will be monitored. More data are needed to support these recommendations so that they gain acceptance. Antimicrobial drug use stewardship is one of the key elements in avoidance of emergence of MDR pathogens and the other is infection control, another huge factor that needs to be addressed.

Mark Papich (*USA*) commented that it is impossible to track overall antimicrobial drug usage in non-food-producing animals in the USA.

Svenja Viete (*USA*) highlighted the need to educate and initiate change in the behaviours of general practitioners, particularly more senior colleagues, to discourage use of systemic antibiotics and, when they are necessary, to select first-tier drugs. She commented on the excessive use of antibiotics to 'prevent' secondary bacterial infections in animals with viral infections, particularly in upper respiratory infections in cats, and use of long-acting antibiotic injections to treat cat-bite abscesses. She also made the observation that fluoroquinolone administration is sometimes given at half dose twice daily instead of as labelled.

Andrew Hillier responded that some good points had been made. The importance of demonstrating the presence of infection was emphasized, which is actually not difficult in cutaneous disease. The proposed guidelines for treatment of superficial bacterial folliculitis in dogs include identification and demonstration of infection before selection of appropriate antibiotics. He felt that there is a place for the use of cefovecin, particularly in cats. He said that there is a place for the use of cefpodoxime and fluoroquinolones, but only when the presence of infection is confirmed and no other topical or systemic antibiotics are appropriate, or when these drugs are deemed necessary after taking into account both patient and client considerations.

Deirdre Galbo (*USA*) commented on the need to practise best medicine rather than convenient medicine, and to pick the best drugs rather than the most convenient drugs in veterinary practice. She highlighted the need for education at veterinary schools regarding antibiotic selection behaviours, particularly the tendency to over-use enrofloxacin.

Andrew Hillier agreed that her comments were valid. He emphasized the need for use of topical therapies in cases of superficial folliculitis and to decrease systemic antimicrobial usage. He commented that information about optimal practice for topical therapies is lacking and needs attention and that certainly in the USA veterinarians treating skin infections have become too quick to reach for systemic antimicrobial therapy.

Kerstin Bergvall commented that antibiotic usage in viral diseases may actually not prevent but rather may cause bacterial problems by selecting resistant strains of organisms.

David Lloyd noted that Andrew Hillier's last comments lead appropriately to the next speaker's topic.

Responsible use of topical antimicrobial agents (D.N. Carlotti)

Didier Carlotti (*France*) informed the participants that the French Association of Dermatology Specialists' dermatology study group (GEDAC) has recently published guidelines for the use of antibiotics in the treatment of canine pyoderma. Four categories have been identified: category 1 is antibiotics of choice (cephalexin, amoxicillin-clavulanate, lincosamides); category 2 is antibiotics of restricted use (cefovecin, fluoroquinolones); category 3 is inadvisable antibiotics (nonpotentiated penicillins, tetracyclines, gentamicin); and category 4 is drugs that should never be used in canine pyoderma (mupirocin, rifampicin, imipenem, vancomycin, ticarcillin). At the same time as disseminating these guidelines, the use of topical antimicrobials is being emphasized. Topical therapy includes antibiotics and antiseptics to be used both to treat and control infection, when identified, and also the use of antiseptics to prevent infections. Ointments, creams and gels are good vehicles for antiseptics and antibiotics. Indications for use are localized canine pyoderma and feline acne. Efficacy depends on localization, accessibility and penetration of agent, and susceptibility of the organism. Compliance also plays a role. Many human topical products are available containing various antibiotics, but with variable accessibility and availability, depending on regulations in different countries. Products often contain more than one antibiotic (e.g. polymixin, bacitracin and neomycin) and often are formulated with other agents, particularly corticosteroids, which may be contraindicated in cutaneous infections. Mupirocin and fusidic acid are very effective for the treatment of staphylococcal pyoderma, with high activity against coagulase-positive staphylococci including methicillin-resistant *Staphylococcus pseudintermedius* (MRSP).[6] Mupirocin has good penetration and good tolerance. A publication by Fulham *et al.*[7] showed that mupirocin has high efficacy *in vitro* on canine isolates of *S. pseudintermedius*, including MRSP. There are no clinical studies published regarding its use in dogs, although White *et al.*[8] published an article on the use of mupirocin for feline acne. The current recommendation in France is that because of its importance in human medicine, mupirocin should not be used in animals. Fusidic acid is licensed for veterinary use in Europe. Temporary elimination of *S. pseudintermedius* from cutaneous and mucosal sites in dogs has been demonstrated with this treatment,[9] although published studies regarding its use in clinical infections are lacking. In one study there was significant resistance in MRSP strains.[10] Another paper demonstrated good efficacy of sodium fusidate solution in dogs with superficial pyoderma caused by MRSP.[11] It is a good topical drug for the treatment of localized superficial folliculitis in atopic dogs, and creams can be more convenient than shampoo therapy in such cases. Veterinary combined formulations exist, often including antibiotics, antifungals and glucocorticoids, which have been demonstrated to be helpful for 'hot spots' and more effective than individual agents.[12] However, these products are not indicated in treatment of pyoderma and cutaneous fungal diseases.

Topical therapy is appropriate for cases of otitis externa: ear cleaning with antiseptics is very useful. Antiseptics can have a protective action, and glycotechnology cleaning agents can also be very helpful. Antibiotics are commonly included in otic preparations. Some injectable antibiotic solutions can be used topically in ear canals, but this should only be on the basis of cytological examination of aural exudate and bacterial culture and susceptibility. Although there is debate about the usefulness of sensitivity testing for the selection of antibiotics for topical otic use due to the high concentrations that can be achieved, the speaker felt that it is helpful. *Pseudomonas aeruginosa* can be very difficult to eliminate, but can be treated with topical antibiotic solutions in the ear canals.

Antiseptic creams can be effective for treatment of localized skin infections. Benzoyl peroxide 5% is available as a veterinary product in the USA but is only labelled for human use in Europe, although it may be used according to the prescribing cascade (a provision set out in EU law and transposed into UK legislation, which enables human medicines to be used in animals if a suitable authorized veterinary medicine is not available).[13] A limitation is that it can be irritant. Silver sulfadiazine 1% cream is used on burns in humans and prevents the growth of a wide range of organisms including yeasts. It can be used in dogs with intertrigo, particularly cases of lip-fold pyoderma, although there is increasing resistance of strains of *P. aeruginosa* to the drug and it may not be as useful in the future.

Shampoo therapies decrease the bacterial population on the skin, remove tissue debris and exudate, and can be curative in mild cases of superficial pyoderma. Most often shampoos are used in a supporting role with antibiotics, and will shorten the time to healing and limit relapses. Shampoo therapy should work well in bacterial overgrowth syndrome. The prophylactic efficacies of chlorhexidine, povidone iodine, benzoyl peroxide and ethyl lactate have been demonstrated against staphylococci.[14] Glycotechnology has been demonstrated to block microbial adherence to skin, and inclusion of such compounds in shampoos decreases the adherence of staphylococci and *Pseudomonas* organisms by about 50%.[15,16] A recent review concluded that there is good evidence for the efficacy of chlorhexidine and, to a lesser degree, benzoyl peroxide in canine bacterial skin infections.[17] It is likely that the more frequent use of topical shampoos will reduce the duration and, therefore, the amount of systemic antimicrobial drug usage and may be the only therapy needed for localized cases of pyoderma. They help to normalize the skin surface microenvironment, with an appropriate frequency of application.

David Lloyd commented that sensitivity tests are generally related to systemic therapy and are not related to concentrations achieved for topical therapy unless minimum inhibitory concentrations are performed. He then introduced the final speaker.

Use of antimicrobial combinations in difficult infections (J.S. Weese)

J. Scott Weese (*Canada*) opened his presentation with some observations on spiralling empiricism in respect of drug, particularly antibiotic administration, including the precepts that:

- 'broader is better' – let's kill it all – but this is often not desirable
- 'failure to respond is failure to cover' – if it gets worse it is the clinician's fault, so hit it hard
- 'when in doubt change or add another' – often leads to use of multiple drugs with cross-over and duplication of activity spectra, and if many drugs are used in combination this can lead to a lot of unexpected outcomes
- 'more diseases, more drugs' – if there is a lot going on, let's add more drugs, which may not be appropriate
- 'sickness requires immediate therapy' – may be better to initiate topical therapy whilst waiting for culture and susceptibility results

- 'response implies diagnosis' – a lot of disease gets better in spite of intervention, not just because of therapy
- 'bigger disease, bigger drugs or newer drugs' – a real timely issue with the launch of new products
- 'antibiotics are safe' – not always the case, particularly in respect of bacterial resistance.

The speaker then asked the question, when is the use of antimicrobial combinations appropriate? He stated that combination therapy should not be used in lieu of proper testing, or in the case of a difficult owner, or an expensive animal, or in lieu of rational thought, or if one drug does not work then add another because it cannot hurt. If one is not working, then it may require a switch, but not just the addition of another drug. Use of combination therapy is appropriate in the following circumstances:

- There is a high chance of resistance emerging to a single drug, such as rifampicin. Bacterial mutation leading to resistance to a single drug may happen randomly; double mutation causing resistance to two drugs is highly unlikely so combination therapy makes sense in this situation. Use of rifampicin as monotherapy in methicillin-resistant *Staphylococcus pseudintermedius* (MRSP) infections has shown to be associated with development of rapid emergence of resistance and so single dosing with this drug is not recommended.
- There is unpredictable susceptibility, especially if slow-growing organisms are involved and there is no susceptibility information available, or organisms are difficult to grow, such as some of the mycobacterial species. A broader combination approach may be appropriate rather than a lengthy wait for results, particularly if there is a potentially life-threatening infection such as endocarditis. These situations are different from that of a superficial folliculitis.
- There is synergistic activity between drugs, such as sulphonamides with trimethoprim (TMPS), or the facilitation of activity of aminoglycosides when used in combination with beta-lactam antibiotics against enterococcal organisms.
- Combinations that inhibit bacterial enzymes, such as amoxicillin + clavulanate.
- In polymicrobial infections one drug does not always fit, and two narrow-spectrum drugs may be preferable to one broad-spectrum antibiotic.
- Combinations of antimicrobial drugs may allow a lower effective dose, which is helpful if a drug has potential toxicity issues and dose reduction is desirable.

Potential problems associated with combination therapy include wastefulness, possible increased hazards, effects on the commensal microbiome, increased costs and increased client effort. The latter is more likely to result in poor compliance and administration errors and so is a risk factor for resistance emergence. Combination therapy is more likely to have a broader effect on commensal organisms, and some combinations have antagonistic effects. Very little evidence-based data exist for some of the difficult infections that are encountered, for instance the mycobacterial infections.

David Lloyd opened up the general question and discussion period and started by asking what other antimicrobial drugs can be used in conjunction with rifampicin for MRSP.

Scott Weese responded that this could be problematic, in that there may not be any other drug to which the pathogen is susceptible, and if there are other drug susceptibilities, then the clinician probably should not be using rifampicin. Combination with aminoglycosides or with chloramphenicol might be considered but if there is demonstrable susceptibility then it is difficult to justify the use of rifampicin in combination.

Jared Power (*Canada*) asked if the Swedish government policy bans all prophylactic uses of antibiotics in Sweden.

Kerstin Bergvall responded that the use of antimicrobial drugs immediately preoperatively and for short periods postoperatively is acceptable. She commented on delaying the use of antibiotics whilst waiting for culture and susceptibility testing results; in the case of pyoderma whilst waiting for bacteriology results topical cleansing therapy is initiated. If improvement is seen, it may be appropriate to continue topical therapy without the use of systemic antibiotics. This happens surprisingly often.

Didier Carlotti asked if it was ethical to use rifampicin in animals with pyoderma when it is such an important therapy for humans with mycobacterial infections.

Scott Weese responded that this was a good question, which could be applied to all 'big gun' antibiotics and that it is a discussion that the veterinary profession needs to have. He felt that there was little likelihood of transmission of rifampicin resistance from cutaneous staphylococcal pathogens to mycobacterial organisms, or that treatment of an animal would result in emergence of resistant mycobacteria in that animal that would then infect humans. With drugs such as vancomycin he reported that a restriction policy was in place at Guelph, and as a general rule it was important to be considerate of the use in animals of drugs that are used frequently in humans and are important for human patients with serious infections.

David Lloyd concluded the workshop by thanking the speakers and other contributors to the session.

References

1. Sasaki T, Kikuchi K, Tanaka Y *et al.* Methicillin-resistant *Staphylococcus pseudintermedius* in a veterinary teaching hospital. *J Clin Microbiol* 2007; 45: 1118–1125.
2. Baker SA, Van-Balen J, Lu B *et al.* Antimicrobial drug use in dogs prior to admission to a veterinary teaching hospital. *J Am Vet Med Assoc* 2012; 241: 210–217.
3. Nienhoff U, Kadlec K, Chaberny IF *et al.* Methicillin-resistant Staphylococcus pseudintermedius among dogs admitted to a small animal hospital. *Vet Microbiol* 2011, 150: 191–197.
4. Weese JS, Faires MC, Frank LA *et al.* Factors associated with methicillin-resistant versus methicillin-susceptible *Staphylococcus pseudintermedius* infection in dogs. *J Am Vet Med Assoc* 2012, 240: 1450–1456.

5. Rota A, Milani C, Corro M *et al.* Misuse of antimicrobials and selection of methicillin-resistant *Staphylococcus pseudintermedius* strain in breeding kennels: genetic characterization of bacteria after a two-year interval. *Reprod Dom Anim* 2012; May 3. doi: 10.1111/j.1439-0531.2012.02012.x. [Epub ahead of print.]
6. Loeffler A, Baines SJ, Toleman MS *et al. In vitro* activity of fusidic acid and mupirocin against coagulase-positive staphylococci from pets. *J Antimicrob Chemoth* 2008, 62: 1301–1304.
7. Fulham KS, Lemarie SL, Hosgood G *et al.* In vitro susceptibility testing of meticillin-resistant and meticillin-susceptible staphylococci to mupirocin and novobiocin. *Vet Dermatol* 2011; 22: 88–94.
8. White SD, Bourdeau PB, Blumstein P *et al.* Feline acne and results of treatment with mupirocin in an open clinical trial: 25 cases. *Vet Dermatol* 1997; 8: 157–164.
9. Saijonmaa-Koulumies L, Parsons E, Lloyd DH. Elimination of *Staphylococcus intermedius* in healthy dogs by topical treatment with fusidic acid. *J Small Anim Pract* 1998; 39: 341–347.
10. Meucci V, Vanni M, Guardabassi L *et al.* Evaluation of methicillin resistance in *Staphylococcus intermedius* isolated from dogs. *Vet Res Comm* 2010; 34(Suppl. 1): S79–82.
11. Bardagí M, Ravera I, Abarca ML *et al.* Efficacy of topical 2% sodium fusidate to manage canine superficial bacterial infection caused by multidrug-resistant meticillin-resistant *Staphylococcus*. *Vet Dermatol* 2010; 21: 318.
12. Schroeder H, Swan GE, Berry WL *et al.* Efficacy of a topical antimicrobial-anti-inflammatory combination in the treatment of pyotraumatic dermatitis in dogs. *Vet Dermatol* 1996; 7: 163–170.
13. Veterinary Medicines Directorate. Guidance on the use of Cascade. Veterinary Medicines Guidance Note No. 13, 2011. Available at: http://www.vmd.defra.gov.uk/public/vmr_vmgn.aspx.
14. Kwochka KW, Kowalski J. Prophylactic efficacy of four antibacterial shampoos against *Staphylococcus intermedius* in dogs. *Am J Vet Res* 1991; 52: 115–118.
15. McEwan NA, Rème CA, Gatto H *et al.* Sugar inhibition of adherence by *Staphylococcus intermedius* to canine corneocytes. *Vet Dermatol* 2006; 17: 358.
16. McEwan NA, Rème CA, Gatto H *et al.* Monosaccharide inhibition of adherence by *Pseudomonas aeruginosa* to canine corneocytes. *Vet Dermatol* 2008; 19: 221–225.
17. Mueller RS, Bergvall K, Bensignor E, Bond R. A review of topical therapy for skin infections with bacteria and yeast. *Vet Dermatol* 2012; 23: 330–341.

8.8

Refractory atopic dermatitis therapy

W.S. Rosenkrantz (Chairperson), C.L. Mendelsohn (Secretary)

Animal Dermatology Clinic, Tustin, California, USA

Wayne Rosenkrantz (*USA*) opened the workshop with general comments and an introduction to the topic. He emphasized that this was to be an interactive discussion. Each attendee received a 'clicker' for the Turning Point Technology interactive system generously provided by Pfizer Animal Health. This technology allows for immediate polling of the audience and records the results to stimulate further discussion and for data response collection.

The discussion started with a presentation of a sample case of refractory atopic dermatitis in a 5.5 kg 12-year-old male castrate bichon frise. Overall, Wayne Rosenkrantz had noted that this breed has a tendency to have a higher incidence of refractory canine atopic dermatitis. This patient had a many year history of intense, self-mutilating pruritus. Numerous medications had been tried. The dog had a history of a partial response to glucocorticoids, but had failed two rounds of allergen-specific immunotherapy (ASIT) of adequate duration, and had had numerous elimination diet trials with no response. In the month prior to the referral, he had had a selamectin treatment trial. At presentation, the patient was receiving oral gabapentin 100 mg every 12 hours, phenobarbital 15 mg every 12 hours, and dexamethasone 2 mg twice weekly. The phenobarbital was prescribed by the primary veterinarian in an attempt to deal with what he felt to be a severe psychogenic component. The patient had subsequently been examined by an American College of Veterinary Dermatology (ACVD) diplomate, and gabapentin and dexamethasone were prescribed.

At initial presentation, there was evidence of pedal, groin and facial pruritus and excoriations. There was no overt clinical evidence of infection. Based on the history and clinical signs, refractory atopy was the most likely differential diagnosis, along with a potential of canine adverse food reaction. Also, it was possible that infection and/or bacterial or yeast overgrowth was present even though it could not be appreciated clinically. Additionally it was noted that the dog was depressed and stressed and, therefore, a psychogenic component could not be ruled out.

Cytology did reveal a bacterial component. The plan then was to continue the gabapentin and phenobarbital, but add oral cefpodoxime 50 mg daily and ciclosporin (Atopica®, Novartis Animal Health) 25 mg daily. The dexamethasone was decreased to 1 mg twice weekly and the patient was restarted on an elimination diet of Royal Canin rabbit and potato – previously he had had diet trials with Iams Eukanuba kangaroo and oat (P&G Pet Care) and home-cooked single proteins.

Two months after the initial examination, treatment and diet change, the pruritus and depression were still present, causing distress to the client. At this time, a more aggressive approach was undertaken in an attempt to reduce the pruritus more rapidly. Ketoconazole was added at 50 mg orally once daily. Atopica® was doubled to 25 mg every 12 hours, the phenobarbital was tapered off and dexamethasone 1 mg twice weekly was continued. One month after these changes there was improvement, but the owner was still unable to remove the Elizabethan collar. All therapies and diet were continued and oral clomipramine 25 mg daily was added to help with the potential psychogenic component. Three months after these changes were instituted (6-month follow-up) the dog continued all the medications and restricted diet. He no longer required a protective T-shirt and could use a smaller Elizabethan collar. Clinically the dog had a fuller haircoat and decreased erythema and inflammation in the paws and groin.

This is obviously not a case that specialists would present to general practitioners as an example of how to treat atopic dermatitis, but it does represent the kind of case that specialists may have to deal with. This patient is on multimodal therapy and still not completely controlled! In refractory atopic dermatitis cases dermatologists are often forced to combine therapies; this requires balancing the medications and monitoring for side effects and drug interactions.

Numerous medications are used for atopic dermatitis. There are many that dermatologists use commonly, some that are considered occasionally, some that are rarely tried but should be considered, and some that have been tried and because of lack of efficacy or side effects are no longer used. In Wayne Rosenkrantz's experience, commonly used drugs include: antimicrobials, topical therapies, essential fatty acids (oral and topical), antihistamines, tricyclic antidepressants, ASIT, glucocorticoids and ciclosporin. Occasional drugs considered by Wayne Rosenkrantz include: gabapentin, tacrolimus, nonsteroidal anti-inflammatory drugs (NSAIDs), pentoxifylline and azathioprine as well as autogenous stem cell therapy. Modes of therapy that Wayne Rosenkrantz does not currently have direct experience with but would consider include: herbal therapy and acupuncture, Janus kinase (JAK) inhibitors, folic acid inhibitors, mycophenolate mofetil, tepoxalin, cold laser, monoclonal anti-IgE antibodies and maropitant citrate (Cerenia®, Pfizer). Drugs that Wayne

Rosenkrantz has personally found to be ineffective include misoprostol and interferons. C-kit inhibitors seem to have the potential for side effects (primarily glomerulonephritis) and Wayne Rosenkrantz would avoid those. He emphasized that this is his personal priority list, and that each of the attendees has their own drug selections and their own experiences that they need to draw from.

The discussion then shifted to addressing specific responses to audience polls regarding specific therapies for atopic dermatitis.

Antihistamines: 'What percentage of atopic dermatitis (AD) cases respond to antihistamines?

Ralf Mueller (*Germany*) clarified that this question pertains to use of a single antihistamine as sole therapy for pruritus related to AD. Seventy-eight audience members responded:

- 45% responded that the success rate is <10%
- 51% responded that the success rate is 10–20%
- 4% responded that the success rate is 30–40%
- 0% responded that the success rate is greater than 50%.

Paul Bloom (*USA*) felt that none of the antihistamines work when he uses them and generally he does not prescribe these as sole therapy.

Wayne Rosenkrantz commented they are often recommended and reported as being synergistic with essential fatty acids (EFAs) and also as having a glucocorticoid sparing effect. The literature suggests variable efficacy, and a report by Olivry *et al.* in 2010 stated that there was 'little evidence to recommend' their use.[1] However, a recent survey reported by Dell and Griffin in *Veterinary Dermatology* found that owners reported antihistamines to be 'very' to 'extremely' effective in 33% of the cases when used as sole therapy.[2]

Ralf Mueller commented that when he prescribes hydroxyzine concurrently with chlorpheniramine, the drugs are much more effective than when they are given alone, and that a drug available in Europe contains this combination (Histacalmine®, Virbac). He is completing a randomized clinical trial and his clinical impression is that he is seeing greater than 33% efficacy. The dose, when using the combination product, is about 50% of the regularly recommended dose of each individual drug. However, when he coadministers the two individual drugs, he gives each one at the standard recommended dose for maximum efficacy.

Candace Sousa (*USA*) noted that in her review of the literature, 4% of publications reported success greater than 20%, but there are also reports that placebo versus antihistamines has also had up to a 20% success rate.

Craig Griffin (*USA*) concurred that there are numerous studies that have shown no differences in improvement with antihistamines versus placebo.

Paul Bloom stated that the order in which you perform a sequential antihistamine trial is important. The antihistamine that is tried 'last' is likely used in trying to treat a more refractory case than the antihistamine that was tried first because if the first antihistamine is efficacious owners seldom go on to try other antihistamines.

Kirstin Bergvall (*Sweden*) advised that it is important to pick the cases carefully. If the degree of inflammation is high, and the inflammatory infiltrate is severe, antihistamines will not be efficacious. However, if they are initially used with a drug like a corticosteroid, which can reduce or eliminate inflammation, eventually that same difficult patient may be able to be maintained on single therapy antihistamines.

Wayne Rosenkrantz reported that he no longer recommends antihistamine trials. He has found hydroxyzine to be the most efficacious, and does not use antihistamines as a sole therapy if the case is severe.

Karen Helton-Rhodes (*USA*) asked why the use of hydroxyzine over cetirizine?

Wayne Rosenkrantz replied that his clinical impression has been that hydroxyzine works better.

Ralf Mueller stated that the use of trimeprazine with prednisolone (Temaril P®, Pfizer Animal Health) does indeed allow the use of lower doses of 'pred' and, in his experience, when he uses one to two antihistamines with 'pred' he sees a dramatic decrease in steroid doses and does not see an increase in antihistamine-related side effects. He then asked the audience how many use combinations of antihistamines, and about 50% responded that they do.

Linda Messinger (*USA*) commented that the population a dermatologist sees is skewed because often the cases that present have already failed one or more antihistamines and thus do not represent the general population. A good study would be to evaluate the success of antihistamines on cases in general practice.

Wayne Rosenkrantz reiterated how important it is to pick cases appropriately when antihistamines are going to be used.

Essential fatty acids: 'How do you use EFAs?'

There were 81 responses as follows:

- 7% use oral omega-3 supplements only
- 21% use oral omega-3/6 supplement combinations
- 4% used topical EFAs
- 17% utilize diets that contain EFAs
- 51% utilized a combination of the above.

Wayne Rosenkrantz commented that studies demonstrate marked variable efficacy of EFAs both orally and topically. In the 2010 report by Olivry *et al.* there was 'insufficient evidence to recommend for or against' the use of EFAs.[1] Despite this, EFAs are an easy treatment to add into the allergy management regimen, especially with diets. Some diets have levels as high as, or commonly higher than, supplements. There are numerous references that support this.[3–5] However, there are differences between the diets available in the USA and Europe. EFAs are reported to also be synergistic with antihistamines and have steroid-sparing properties.

Lisbeth Norberg (*Denmark*) noted that in Europe one cannot get the Royal Canin Skin Support® diet that is available in the USA, but there is a diet by Specific called COD-HY that contains hydrolysed salmon and nonhydrolysed rice. This particular diet contains very high levels of omega-3 and omega-6 fatty acids (2.2–2.6%) and provides EFA supplementation during an elimination diet trial. Hill's Prescription Diet j/d® has 3% omega-3 fatty acids and is available in both Europe and the USA.

Wayne Rosenkrantz asked the audience regarding what combinations they use for fatty acid supplementation.

Ralf Mueller answered that there really is no steadfast rule but rather his choice is dictated by the patient and owner.

Craig Griffin agreed, although he noted again that compliance in AD therapy is essential and a diet high in EFAs is likely best because while owners do consistently feed their pets, they do not always give medications and supplements as directed. One of the participants noted that she reaches first for Hill's j/d® diet in Europe. This diet is not only readily available and high in EFAs, but it is easiest to prescribe for animals already on numerous medications so you do not have to add another drug to their regimen.

Pentoxifylline: 'What percentage of AD cases respond to pentoxifylline?'

Sixty attendees responded (**Wayne Rosenkrantz** noted that pentoxifylline is not available everywhere in the world, which is likely the reason for fewer responses):

- 75% felt that the response is seen in fewer than 10% of cases
- 17% reported success 10–20% of the time
- 5% reported success 20–30% of the time
- 2% reported success 30–40% of the time
- 2% reported success 40–50% of the time.

Wayne Rosenkrantz commented that pentoxifylline is a phosphodiesterase inhibitor. There are some reports that suggest it has value in treating AD.[6–9] The literature is highly variable regarding the efficacy. The reported doses range from as low as 10 mg/kg every 12 hours to the more recent dosages of 20–30 mg/kg every 8–12 hours. The more recent reports list as much as a 50% response rate especially when administered in combination with EFAs. In light of the literature, it is interesting that so few of the attendees here noted similar success with pentoxifylline. Perhaps it is best used as a combination drug rather than as monotherapy.

Christine Graham-Mise (*USA*) asked the group what combinations are used with pentoxifylline and at what doses.

Ralf Mueller replied that he uses the coated tablets and that in some small dogs the resulting dose is very high because he does not like to break tablets based on literature recommendations.

Kirstin Bergvall stated there was a report presented at the Finland European College of Veterinary Dermatology meeting in which no difference in bioavailability was noted when the coated tablets were cut.

Craig Griffin recommended 20 mg/kg every 12 hours in combination with dietary EFAs and bathing.

Linda Messinger commented that pentoxifylline has been reported to inhibit collagen synthesis and can cause fragile skin. She saw this in a patient receiving approximately 25 mg/kg every 12 h. When the drug was discontinued the skin returned to normal.

Karen Helton-Rhodes stated that she uses 15 mg/kg every 8–12 hours in combination with antihistamines, and she has never noted cutaneous atrophy.

Ralf Mueller asked the audience whether anyone else had experienced the cutaneous atrophy, and other than Linda Messinger, no one reported seeing that phenomenon.

Wayne Rosenkrantz noted that the primary side effects he has observed are gastrointestinal problems.

Stephen Waisglass (*Canada*) commented that pentoxifylline seems to help most when the problem is ventrally focused – so perhaps when the animal's allergy has a contact component. At the higher doses he does see some panting and gastrointestinal problems. The biggest problem he has with it is that some human pharmacies resist filling the prescription due to the high dose prescribed for dogs.

Wayne Rosenkrantz stated that in his practice it is not used frequently for AD, but it is prescribed at high doses for other conditions such as vasculitis and ischaemic dermatitis, and that he has not experienced problems with the pharmacies.

Guillermina Manigot (*Argentina*) has seen two dogs that had severe vasodilation, erythema and flushing while receiving pentoxifylline. Both of those dogs were also taking enalapril. When pentoxifylline was discontinued, the flushing resolved.

Wayne Rosenkrantz asked the group whether they use brand name pentoxifylline (in the USA – Trental®, Sonofi

Aventis) or generic formulations, and asked if any difference was noted between those two.

Guillermina Manigot stated that she has used both and has not noticed a difference between them.

Christine Rees (*USA*) responded that a pharmacokinetic study was done with patients on 20–30 mg/kg every 12 hours with the brand name drug. Those dogs were then later put on the generic formulation at the end of the study and no difference was noted.

Kim Coyner (*USA*), **Colleen Mendelsohn** (*USA*) and **Rebecca Westermeyer** (*USA*) all reported that they have seen cases in which a decrease in efficacy was noticed in switching from brand name to generic drug, or even from switching generic brands.

Glucocorticoids: 'Which is the favourite steroid to use first?'

Seventy-eight attendees responded:

- 22% use prednisone
- 27% use prednisolone
- 12% use methylprednisolone (although this number may be lower due to lack of availability recently)
- 0% use triamcinolone
- 1% use dexamethasone
- 23% use Temaril P (Pfizer Animal Health)
- 5% use an injection of a steroid followed by an oral steroid.

Wayne Rosenkrantz reported that his experience indicates most practitioners use prednisone or prednisolone as their first choice, and that on occasion just switching to another steroid can provide relief for a patient with relatively lower doses. There is a website based on human therapy guidelines that assists in converting the relative potency of these drugs: http://www.medcalc.com/steroid.html. In 2012 Ganz *et al.* reported ideal doses of triamcinolone and methylprednisolone in cats and showed that oral triamcinolone was approximately 10 times more potent than methylprednisolone.[10] Wayne Rosenkrantz reported that methylprednisolone is often his first choice. He has observed fewer mineralocorticoid side effects, although this observation is based on clinical impressions and has not been well substantiated. Per Wayne Rosenkrantz, Craig Griffin's practice most often uses triamcinolone first. A common dilemma facing practitioners is how to safely convert from the use of one steroid to another.

Craig Griffin confirmed that he uses triamcinolone as his first-choice corticosteroid in patients with extensive scarring, pemphigus or with extensive hyperproliferative tissue reactions in the skin or ears.

Wayne Rosenkrantz discussed the existence of human studies demonstrating triamcinolone's increased effect on inhibiting fibroblasts, which may be why it is noted to be more efficacious in hyperproliferative skin and ear conditions.

Craig Griffin noted that in the cat, triamcinolone is his first choice. His experience is consistent with the Ganz study, showing that it is much more potent and effective in the cat at substantially lower doses.[10]

Candace Sousa reminded attendees that the literature suggests the potency of triamcinolone is really dependent on the formulation and the salt that is with it.

Tim Strauss (*USA*) asked how many of the participants have all the above-mentioned drugs in their pharmacies. About 25% acknowledged that they do carry all of the listed glucocorticoids.

Guillermina Manigot reminded everyone that not all the drugs are available on a worldwide basis. In Argentina, prednisolone, methylprednisolone and Temaril P® are not available.

Gila Zur (*Israel*) mentioned that her favourite steroid has been Temaril P®. She has noted that when she has patients on the same low dose of prednisone, but without trimeprazine, she sees more hepatopathy.

Cynthia Bauer (*USA*) noted that cases referred to her are often not managed well and are already on prednisone. Often, these cases could continue to be maintained with prednisone while adjusting the other therapies. However, she will often change the steroid to methylprednisolone along with the other management changes to appease clients who are frustrated with the therapies the patient is already on and have failed. She is cautious with triamcinolone and dexamethasone and tends to avoid those as first choices.

Wayne Rosenkrantz stated he has been able to decrease the dose substantially when changing from prednisone to methylprednisolone even though the literature reports equal potency. Overall, Wayne Rosenkrantz recommended giving triamcinolone every 72 hours as maintenance to reduce side effects; however, he has also seen cases do well on an every-48 hours basis.

Paul Coward (*UK*) noted that, in his experience, dexamethasone is more clinically effective and he uses twice-weekly oral administration of the injectable dexamethasone sodium phosphate formulation (Dex SP 4 mg/mL; Bimeda-MTC Animal Health, Inc.).

Tiffany Tapp (*USA*) commented that she is not able to get methylprednisolone at all due to severe backorder problems.

Candace Sousa reminded the group that Pfizer's brand name Medrol® is available and is generally less expensive than the generic.

Ciclosporin: 'Do you use the brand name Atopica® versus the generic ciclosporin?'

Seventy-two participants responded:

- 60% always use brand name Atopica®
- 15% always use generic ciclosporin
- 25% start with brand name and then change to generic.

Numerous European participants advised that they cannot get Atopica® in Europe and have to use brand name Neoral® (Novartis).

Paul Coward stated that UK law does not allow the use of generics and they must use brand name by law.

The audience was asked whether any change is noted when generic ciclosporins are used?

Forty-six attendees responded to this question (reflecting only the respondents that actually use generic ciclosporin):

- 41% felt that there is no change when they change to generic
- 59% felt that there is a change in the condition when changing from Atopica® to generic ciclosporin.

Robert Hilton (*Australia*) advised that an additional consideration should be whether there is a difference between generic and compounded formulations. Compounded forms are quite variable with questionable sources of ciclosporin. Umstead *et al.* looked *in vitro* at the different characteristics of compounded ciclosporin sources, noting large variation between the formulations.[11]

Karen Helton-Rhodes asked that if there is no difference in efficacy, why not start with generic for those practitioners who are able to prescribe it?

Joel Griffies (*USA*) believes that some patients do not do as well on generic, but he will start generic if the clients refuse to pay for the brand name.

Rebecca Westermeyer agreed that she always starts with the brand name product and asks for a 2-week commitment from her clients before changing to a generic product.

Christine Graham-Mise commented that for large dogs requiring high doses, such as German shepherd dogs with perianal fistulas, the cost will drive the decision to start with generic.

Jean Greek (*USA*) commented that while the efficacy can be the same, she sees more gastrointestinal problems with the generics, and others agreed with that.

The audience was asked whether there are favourite generic brands, and they did not appear to favour any particular formulations.

Tiffany Tapp commented that in Rhode Island the generics cost the same as the brand name drug. She obtains a compounded formulation from Diamond Back pharmacy and has found their capsules to be much less expensive.

What kind of modification methods are used when the patients don't respond to the usual ciclosporin 5 mg/kg every 24 hour dosing?

Sixty-three responded:

- 14% raise the dose to 5–10 mg/kg every 24 hours
- 14% raise the dose but then divide it every 12 hours
- 41% add ketoconazole
- 30% add other immunosuppressive agents.

The audience was then asked: 'When you use ketoconazole (KTZ) what dosage do you use?'

The majority of the responders use a KTZ dose of 5 mg/kg with ciclosporin administration.

Paul Bloom replied that he uses as high as 7.5 mg/kg.

Wayne Rosenkrantz noted that the 30% who add another immunosuppressive agent most often add steroids, and some said they add azathioprine.

Craig Griffin commented that adding pentoxifylline or antihistamines is a safer alternative.

Wayne Rosenkrantz mentioned a study presented here at the WCVD7 by Gray *et al.*, demonstrating that ciclosporin blood levels were the same between canine patients on ciclosporin 5 mg/kg daily vs ciclosporin 2.5 mg/kg + KTZ 2.5 mg/kg daily.[12] When using higher doses of KTZ it is more common to see increased ciclosporin-related side effects such as hypertrichosis and gingival overgrowth.

Liora Waldman (*Israel*) and **Mitch Song** (*USA*) reported having similar results when itraconazole was used instead of KTZ; they use itraconazole when there is a problem with vomiting.

The audience as a whole did not think that fluconazole would have the same drug-sparing effect on ciclosporin because fluconazole does not have an effect on the same subset of CYP 450.

Stefano Bario (*Italy*) stated that KTZ is not available in Italy and he too has used itraconazole and sometimes tetracycline.

Guillermina Manigot commented that she has used metoclopramide, although there has been a study demonstrating that metoclopramide does not raise ciclosporin levels when the two drugs are combined.

Interferon: 'For those who do not use interferon, why do you not use interferon for atopic dermatitis?'

Fifty-one attendees responded to the question:

- 47% reported that they do not use it due to lack of efficacy
- 27% reported that they do not use it due to its expense
- 25% responded that they do not use it due to lack of availability.

Darin Dell (*USA*) reported that he finds interferon useful in patients that have severe secondary pyoderma or bacterial overgrowth when topical therapy cannot be used.

Lisbeth Norberg commented that she is currently conducting a clinical trial using injectable interferon in dogs that are refractory to other therapies. Preliminary results show that 3/10 of these dogs have some response.

The participants who use interferon were then asked how they use it

There were nine responders:

- 7/9 use low-dose oral every 24 hours or less frequently
- 2/9 responded that they use high-dose injectable 3 times weekly.

Wayne Rosenkrantz commented that there are numerous studies suggesting high efficacy using interferon in treating atopic dermatitis in which low-dose oral interferon had greater success than high-dose injectable interferon.[13–16] However, based on the feedback from this workshop there may be more clinical variability with its success. There are different formulations with numerous protocols reported. The most common formulations include recombinant feline interferon omega (Virbagen Omega®, Virbac Animal Health); recombinant canine interferon gamma (Interdog®, Toray Industries, Inc.); and interferon alpha-2b (Roferon-A®, Roche). In the USA, neither the feline nor canine recombinant formulations are available, so human interferon alpha-2b is used. The lack of veterinary formulations may certainly influence why it is not tried more in atopic dermatitis, with 25% of the polled group stating this reason for not using interferon. Protocols are available in the references mentioned.

Gabapentin: 'How many use the drug and how effective is it?'

Sixty-seven participants responded:

- 61% never used the drug
- 33% found the drug effective in <25% of cases
- 3% found the drug effective in 25–50% of cases
- 3% found the drug effective in 50–75% of cases
- no participants found the drug effective in >75% of the cases.

Wayne Rosenkrantz commented that gabapentin (e.g. Neurontin®, Pfizer) is an anticonvulsant used to treat nerve pain, seizures, mood disorders, anxiety and pruritus. Its efficacy in treating Chiari syndrome in the cavalier King Charles spaniel dog has been reported. There are numerous proposed mechanisms for its use to combat pruritus: inhibition of voltage-dependent calcium channels in the dorsal horn resulting in an increase in gamma-aminobutyric acid (GABA); secondary inhibition of calcitonin gene-related peptide release; and/or modulation of opioid receptors. The dose is generally reported at 4–13 mg/kg every 12 hours but higher doses may be more effective and have been used by some.

Beth McDonald (*Australia*) stated that she uses 20 mg/kg every 12 hours but has not found it to be effective.

Tiffany Tapp commented that she uses 5–15 mg/kg every 12 hours in combination with other therapies and has found that the addition of gabapentin helps about 25% of the time.

Karen Helton-Rhodes stated that she uses 15–20 mg/kg every 8 hours with Allegra® (Sanofi Aventis) and that this seems to be a good combination.

Guillermina Manigot commented that she uses the published dose with about 25% efficacy, whether or not another product is added.

Wayne Rosenkrantz concluded the workshop by informing the participants that due to time constraints they were unable to discuss some of the other medications mentioned at the beginning of the workshop, including azathioprine, c-kit receptor inhibitors (masitinib mesilate), JAK inhibitors, folic acid analogs (methotrexate and aminopterin), maropitant citrate, tepoxalin (Zubrin, MSD Animal Health), mycophenolate, stem cell therapy, cold laser and acupuncture/herbal remedies. In his opinion, the newest group of drugs with great promise for the treatment of canine atopic dermatitis are the JAK inhibitors. The attendees were encouraged to review some of the new data related to these drugs from the WCVD7 proceedings and abstracts. He thanked the attendees for their participation.

References

1. Olivry T, DeBoer DJ, Favrot C et al. Treatment of canine atopic dermatitis: 2010 clinical practice guidelines from the International Task Force on Canine Atopic Dermatitis. *Vet Dermatol* 2010; 21: 233—248.
2. Dell DL, Griffin, CG, Thompson LA, Griffies JD. Owner assessment of therapeutic interventions for canine atopic dermatitis: a long-term retrospective analysis. *Vet Dermatol* 2012; 23: 228–247.
3. Glos K, Linek M, Lowenstein C et al. The efficacy of commercially available veterinary diets recommended for dogs with atopic dermatitis. *Vet Dermatol* 2008; 19: 427–431.
4. Baddaky-Taugbøl B, Vroom MW, Norberg L. A randomized, controlled, double-blinded, multicentre study on the efficacy of a diet rich in fish oil and borage oil in the control of canine atopic dermatitis. *Adv Vet Dermatol* 2006; 5: 173–187.
5. Bensignor E. Usefulness of one hypoallergenic diet in the management of atopic dermatitis in dogs. *Vet Dermatol* 2008; 14: 261–267.
6. Marsella R, Olivry T. The ACVD task force on canine atopic dermatitis (XXII): nonsteroidal anti-inflammatory pharmacotherapy. *Vet Immun Immunopath* 2001; 81: 331–345.

7. Marsella R, Nicklen C. Double-blinded cross-over study on the efficacy of pentoxifylline for canine atopy. *Vet Dermatol* 2000; 11: 255–260.
8. Scott DW, Miller WH. Pentoxifylline in canine dermatology. *Proceedings CVC*, San Diego, 2010.
9. Singh SK, Dimri U, Saxena SK, Jadhav RK. Therapeutic management of canine atopic dermatitis by combination of pentoxifylline and PUFAs. *Vet Pharm Ther* 2010; 3: 495–498.
10. Ganz EC, Griffin CE, Keys DA, Flatgard TA. Evaluation of methylprednisolone and triamcinolone for the induction and maintenance treatment of pruritus in allergic cats: a double-blinded, randomized, prospective study. *Vet Dermatol* 2012; 23: 287–291.
11. Umstead ME, Boothe DM, Cruz-Espindola C *et al.* Accuracy and precision of compounded ciclosporin capsules and solution. *Vet Dermatol* 2012; 23: 431–437.
12. Gray LL, Hillier K, Cole LK *et al.* The effect of ketoconazole on whole blood and skin ciclosporin concentrations in dogs. *Vet Dermatol* 2012; 23 (Suppl. 1): 13.
13. Iwasaki T, Hasegawa A. A randomized comparative clinical trial of recombinant canine interferon-gamma (KT-100) in atopic dogs using antihistamine as control. *Vet Dermatol* 2006; 17: 195–200.
14. Hasegawa A, Sakurai T, Iwasaki T. A placebo-controlled, double-blinded study of recombinant IFN in dogs with atopic dermatitis. *Vet Dermatol* 2004; 15: 55–58.
15. Carlotti DN, Boulet M, Ducret J *et al.* The use of recombinant omega interferon therapy in canine atopic dermatitis: a double-blind controlled study. *Vet Dermatol* 2009; 20: 405–411.
16. Litzlbauer P, Weber K, Mueller RS. Recombinant feline interferon-ω as oral or subcutaneous treatment of canine atopic dermatitis. *Vet Dermatol* 2012; 23 (Suppl. 1): 39.

8.9

Challenges in otitis

A. Burrows[1] (Chairperson), S. Hobi[2] (Secretary), R. Albert[2] (Secretary Assistant)

[1]Murdoch University Veterinary Hospital, Skin, Ear and Allergy Clinic, Western Australia
[2]Small Animal Medicine Clinic, Centre for Clinical Veterinary Medicine, Ludwig Maximilian University, Munich, Germany

Amanda Burrows (*Australia*) opened the meeting and commented that she was delighted to have so many experts in otitis present for this workshop. She began with a short summary, introducing the different speakers and their topics for the afternoon.

Developing an objective clinical score for canine otitis externa (T. Nuttall)

Tim Nuttall (*UK*) outlined a pilot study for the development of a scoring system for the clinical signs of otitis. He explained that a consistent clinical scoring scheme would enable comparison between different studies conducted by different investigators. Two clinical presentations of otitis were evaluated: an erythro-ceruminous form and a suppurative form of otitis externa. Scoring systems that had already been utilized in varying studies or in clinical trials were used and compared: for each ear and for the horizontal and vertical ear canal. The parameters of erythema, oedema, swelling, erosion/ulceration, exudation, pain, odour, tympanic membrane condition, secondary infections and treatment outcome were evaluated.

The study compared different scoring systems including numeric scoring schemes, in which each parameter was assigned a score of 0 to 2, 0 to 3 or 0 to 5; a visual analog scale, an owner pruritus score and an owner pain score. Two centres were involved (located in France and the UK) and 40 ears from 20 healthy dogs and 90 ears from 50 dogs with otitis were analysed. The 0 to 3 scoring system was the most reliable with regard to the parameters erythema, oedema/swelling, erosion/ulceration and exudation. Other parameters, including pain and pruritus, did not correlate with the clinical scores. A maximum total score of 12 for each ear could be achieved using this system. A score of >4 differentiated affected ears from healthy ears (70% sensitivity and 100% specificity) and a score of ≤3 was 99% sensitive for clinical resolution. Tim Nuttall suggested that the presence, but not the number of neutrophils and micro-organisms was found to be additionally useful. He proposed that the next step with the development of this otitis externa scoring system would be the assessment of intra- and inter-observer reliability.

Giovanni Ghibaudo (*Italy*) indicated that it could be challenging to assess some parameters associated with otitis due to significant discharge being present in the external ear canal, and he questioned whether it would be useful to perform ear cleaning before scoring.

Tim Nuttall commented that while it was not always possible to assess all the parameters when the ear contained discharge, ears should not be cleaned before assigning a score because depending on the method used for cleaning, the score of some of the parameters, such as erythema, could be increased by such intervention.

Giovanni Ghibaudo indicated that, in his opinion, dogs with stenotic ear canals could be very difficult to examine and assess and that the scoring system could be invalid for these dogs.

Tim Nuttall indicated that when the horizontal ear canal could not be assessed, the dogs were excluded from the study.

Tim Nuttall posed a question to the audience as to whether they considered the pinnae should be included in the clinical score for this type of scoring system. Several participants indicated this would be worthwhile.

Rod Rosychuk (*USA*) suggested that taking photographs in a blinded fashion could assist in evaluating the efficacy of the scoring system between different investigators.

Tim Nuttall agreed and indicated that further studies were required.

Ekaterina Kuznetsova (*Russia*) questioned whether variation in the quality of a normal otoscope could also influence the score; for example, the colour of the ear canal could vary with the model and lamp. She questioned whether these factors should or could be standardized.

Tim Nuttall agreed that the lamp could influence these parameters but felt it would be difficult to standardize these factors, due not only to the different equipment used in different geographical regions but also to operational factors; for example the strength of the otoscope battery.

The management of *Pseudomonas* otitis (R. Rosychuk)

Rod Rosychuk discussed his approach to *Pseudomonas* otitis, a common entity in his referral practice, with the most common underlying cause being allergy and dogs often having a history of previous antibiotic use. He suggested that *Pseudomonas* otitis should be suspected when several factors are present, including a history of chronic and relapsing infection, severe otitis with ulceration, a yellow to green purulent exudate, and when rod-shaped bacteria are identified on cytological evaluation. *Pseudomonas* can be present as the sole bacterial species but usually (in about 60% of cases) other bacteria, most commonly *Staphylococcus* spp., are also identified.

Important issues when planning management strategies for *Pseudomonas* otitis include *antimicrobial susceptibility* (low for neomycin and enrofloxacin), *ototoxicity* of some preparations (ticarcillin, amikacin, polymixin B, tobramycin), and the *increased risk* of *tympanic membrane perforation* and *otitis media* due to enzyme production (proteases, elastases). A first *empirical treatment* can be initiated (especially when there is no or minimal drug history) because of the higher local concentrations achieved with topical antimicrobial agents. Tromethamine USP disodium EDTA dehydrate (TrizEDTA) can potentiate the action of the selected antibiotic and is useful in combination with topical antimicrobial therapy.

TrizEDTA should be instilled in the external ear as a pre-antibiotic treatment 10 minutes before applying a topical antibiotic (e.g. gentamicin) in an external ear with a *Pseudomonas* otitis if the tympanic membrane is intact and there is no previous history of antimicrobial treatment. Systemic corticosteroids should be administered to decrease the inflammation/swelling of the external ear canal. Rod Rosychuk emphasized the importance of frequent re-evaluation of dogs with *Pseudomonas* otitis and the usefulness of culture and susceptibility testing if rod-shaped bacteria persist. He indicated that there was controversy regarding the interpretation of bacterial culture and susceptibility testing in cases of otitis externa but it was his opinion that the results were often a useful guide for the selection of systemic antimicrobial therapy for otitis media, and for alternative therapy when topical treatment with TrizEDTA failed to resolve infection.

Rod Rosychuk described his typical *Pseudomonas* otitis patient as a dog with a chronic history of having received previous antimicrobial therapy, with profuse exudation in the external ear canal and varying degrees of proliferation and stenosis. He indicated that he usually performs a bacterial culture and sensitivity as part of his diagnostic work-up. As part of the management, an ear flush is useful to remove exudate and micro-organisms and to evaluate the tympanic membrane. There is, however, 'no rush to flush' in his opinion. The ear canal should be 'opened' first by reducing the oedema, swelling, inflammation and stenosis of the external ear canal using either topical and/or systemic corticosteroids (prednisolone: 0.5–1 mg/kg every 24 hours). In severely inflamed and/or proliferative cases doses as high as 1.5–2 mg/kg prednisolone every 24 hours may be used. A CT scan or radiography should be considered if there are signs consistent with concurrent otitis media.

In cases in which the tympanic membrane cannot be evaluated and the integrity of the membrane is unknown, a combination of topical enrofloxacin (22.7 mg/mL) and dexamethasone (4 mg/mL) in a ratio of 1:2 is his topical antimicrobial therapy of choice. When *Malassezia* organisms are additionally present, 1% miconazole can be added to this solution to achieve a ratio of 1:1:2 (enrofloxacin:dexamethasone:miconazole). One millilitre of this combination therapy is administered into the external ear canal twice daily 10 to 20 minutes after pretreatment with TrizEDTA. His choice of a systemic antibiotic prior to obtaining the culture results is typically marbofloxacin (2.5–5 mg/kg every 24 hours) based on one study that showed reasonable bacterial susceptibility.[1]

Rod Rosychuk emphasized the importance of performing regular rechecks every 2–3 weeks to assess patient improvement and owner compliance. In addition, he reiterated the importance of evaluating the patient for an underlying disease. In persistent or refractory cases the most common antimicrobial agents used include topical ciprofloxacin or silver sulfadiazine mixed with water (1:9) every 12 hours. As alternative antimicrobial therapy, Rod Rosychuk suggested that topical ticarcillin can be useful, and although some debate exists as to whether this is safe in the middle ear, it is his opinion that the agent causes minimal problems with ototoxicity. Other alternative antimicrobial agents include ceftazidime or imipenem. If the tympanic membrane is intact, polymixin B, amikacin or tobramycin could also be considered. In resistant cases systemic antimicrobial agents to consider include amikacin, ticarcillin or ceftazidime.

Rod Rosychuk concluded by suggesting that over-treatment of ears affected by *Pseudomonas* otitis is common. He also indicated that many recurrent cases of otitis were due not to antimicrobial resistance, but rather a failure to clean the ears, inadequate duration of treatment, failure to manage the perpetuating or primary factors, or inadequate follow-up.

Alberto Martin (*Mexico*) questioned whether intralesional triamcinolone injections could be useful if topical and systemic corticosteroids were ineffective for the management of external ear canal stenosis.

Rod Rosychuk responded that he had used intralesional triamcinolone in stenotic external ear canals, but in his experience corticosteroid injections were often ineffective and then surgical ear canal ablation was indicated.

Giovanni Ghibaudo questioned whether there was a risk of the development of diabetes mellitus with the use of intralesional triamcinolone.

Rod Rosychuk responded that there was a theoretical risk but that this complication was rare in his experience.

TrizEDTA significantly potentiates the bactericidal activity of silver sulfadiazine against multidrug-resistant *Pseudomonas aeruginosa* associated with chronic otitis (L. Buckley)

Laura Buckley (*UK*) introduced the concept that chronic *Pseudomonas* otitis could be difficult to manage due to its complex pathogenesis and limited topical therapeutic options (as in the presence of a perforated tympanic membrane or multidrug resistance) and ineffective systemic antimicrobial agents. Silver sulfadiazine (Flamazine®, Smith & Nephew Healthcare) is a broad-spectrum antimicrobial agent predominantly used in humans for burn and wound management. It can cause cell membrane damage and inhibit DNA transcription. It is used in *P. aeruginosa* cases due to its beneficial effects on ulcerated otic epithelium and low ototoxicity. TrizEDTA is used as pretreatment but also as a vehicle for antimicrobial agents. It can damage the wall of Gram-negative bacteria and by this mechanism it can potentiate antimicrobial activity. It can also decrease the MIC (minimum inhibitory concentration), at least *in vitro*, for some drugs and may be a good alternative in multidrug-resistant cases.

The aim of the study was to determine the MBC (minimum bactericidal concentration) of silver sulfadiazine with and without the addition of TrizEDTA against multidrug-resistant *P. aeruginosa* isolates from canine otitis. Isolates were obtained from clinical cases (n = 12), identified as multidrug resistant by disc diffusion, grown overnight on SBA (sheep blood agar) and suspended in PBS (phosphate buffered saline) to achieve specific optical density and a consistent number of colony-forming units. The bacterial suspensions were subsequently incubated for 90 minutes, either with silver sulfadiazine alone or with silver sulfadiazine and TrizEDTA. Aliquots were then transferred on SBA and incubated for 18 hours at 37°C, at which time bacterial growth was evaluated.

The results of this study suggest that TrizEDTA has no bactericidal activity alone but significantly reduces the MBC of silver sulfadiazine against multidrug-resistant *P. aeruginosa* isolates. For 11/12 isolates the combination was bactericidal at all tested concentrations. This combination was concluded to be a good option in multidrug-resistant *P. aeruginosa* cases but further studies are indicated to clarify the required contact time, the optimal concentration of the two components and whether the TrizEDTA should be administered prior to or concurrently with the silver sulfadiazine.

Rod Rosychuk asked whether the investigators administered the TrizEDTA separately or whether it was mixed in solution with silver sulfadiazine.

Laura Buckley responded that the TrizEDTA and the silver sulfadiazine were not combined in a mixed solution, but the investigators had considered administering them in combination.

Tim Nuttall indicated that he has also combined TrizEDTA and silver sulfadiazine for treating ear infections.

Rod Rosychuk asked what concentration of silver sulfadiazine was used.

Laura Buckley indicated that the concentration used in the study was the standard commercially available concentration.

Rod Rosychuk commented that in the USA, generic versions of the silver sulfadiazine were available that do not seem to mix easily. He asked Laura Buckley whether she felt this was an issue.

Laura Buckley responded by indicating that in her experience the silver sulfadiazine mixed well with the TrizEDTA.

In vitro antimicrobial activity of *Pseudomonas aeruginosa* isolated from dogs with otitis externa (A. Vercelli)

Antonella Vercelli (*Italy*) outlined the aim of her study, which was to compare the *in vitro* activities of nine antibiotics (amoxicillin/clavulanic acid, cephalexin, enrofloxacin, gentamicin, marbofloxacin, cefadroxil, piperacillin, tobramycin and aztreonam) against strains of *P. aeruginosa* isolated from dogs with recurrent or chronic otitis externa in Italy. Five hundred and fifty ear samples taken by swabs were collected and inoculated onto blood and selective agar. One hundred *P. aeruginosa* strains grown in pure culture were used for the study. Antimicrobial susceptibility was tested by the Kirby–Bauer disc diffusion method. The results of the study showed a high resistance rate to first-line antibiotics such as cephalexin (97%), cefadroxil (95%), amoxicillin/clavulanic acid (93%) and enrofloxacin (51%), but susceptibility to piperacillin (82%), tobramycin (69%), gentamicin (65%) and aztreonam (62%). Antonella Vercelli concluded that veterinarians should always perform a bacterial culture and antimicrobial susceptibility test prior to starting an antibiotic treatment in case of *Pseudomonas* otitis. She recommended that oral corticosteroids be used to relieve pain and inflammation in the interim.

Antonella Vercelli commented that the antimicrobial agent piperacillin was of great interest because it was a drug with activity against several different Gram-negative bacteria and has a synergistic effect with aminoglycoside drugs. Piperacillin (available for use in parenteral and topical forms) and gentamicin (topically) both demonstrate reasonable susceptibility against *Pseudomonas* spp. and have additional synergistic effects that could be clinically useful. Antonella Vercelli mentioned the potential adverse effects that may occur with piperacillin, including drug intolerance (anaphylaxis), and liver and kidney disease. Regular monitoring of liver and kidney parameters is recommended if the drug is given over an extended time period. Currently the use of piperacillin is extra-label in animals, but Antonella Vercelli suggested that it could be considered as a potential veterinary drug for investigation and registration.

Antonella Vercelli acknowledged the limitations of her study, which include the fact that organisms in the external ear canal have been reported to differ from those in the middle ear, with different antibiotic sensitivity patterns. Another limitation is that overall antibiotic sensitivity data are less useful for topical treatment because the concentrations achieved in the ear canal with topical antimicrobial agents are higher than the serum levels used for *in vitro* testing.

Geneviève Marignac (*France*) expressed some concern about the use of unlabelled antibiotics in animals with regard to the potential for development of multidrug-resistant organisms.

Rod Rosychuk agreed and indicated that he found the issue to be a dilemma. He indicated that clinicians should attempt not to use such antibiotics unless there were no other alternative treatment options.

Giovanni Ghibaudo indicated that he had completed several studies *in vitro* and *in vivo* with a combination of TrizEDTA and chlorhexidine and achieved good results. He encouraged clinicians to consider using more antiseptics in the management of otitis externa.

Amanda Burrows asked what concentration of the chlorhexidine was used in these cases.

Giovanni Ghibaudo responded that he was using 0.2% of chlorhexidine in combination with TrizEDTA.

Lynette Cole (*USA*) commented that it was very important to remember the key points regarding the treatment of *Pseudomonas* otitis, which include cleaning the ears, evaluating for the primary disease, and managing the external ear canal stenosis to avoid or at least reduce the use of extra-label antimicrobial therapy.

BAER (brainstem auditory evoked response) testing in practice (S. Paterson)

Sue Paterson (*UK*) discussed several indications for BAER testing including evaluation for congenital sensorineural deafness, certification of puppies and kittens as having normal hearing prior to sale, evaluating adult dogs with conductive hearing loss (cerumen, chronic changes, discharge, otitis media), and evaluating adult dogs with sensorineural deafness (otitis interna, ototoxic medications, presbyacusis). She also indicated that BAER testing is the only method of confirming unilateral hearing loss.

The principle of BAER testing is the acoustic stimulation of an ear with a short pulse (click), which produces a variety of wave forms from different components of the auditory pathway. The response is a series of peaks at about 1 ms (millisecond) with intervals beginning 2 ms after stimulation and lasting in total 10 ms. The different waves refer to different parts of the auditory pathway (*wave 1:* vestibular cochlear nerve segment closest to cochlea; *wave 2:* extramedullary intracranial segment of vestibular cochlear nerve; *wave 3:* dorsal nucleus trapezoid body; *wave 4:* rostral pons; *wave 5:* caudal colliculus).

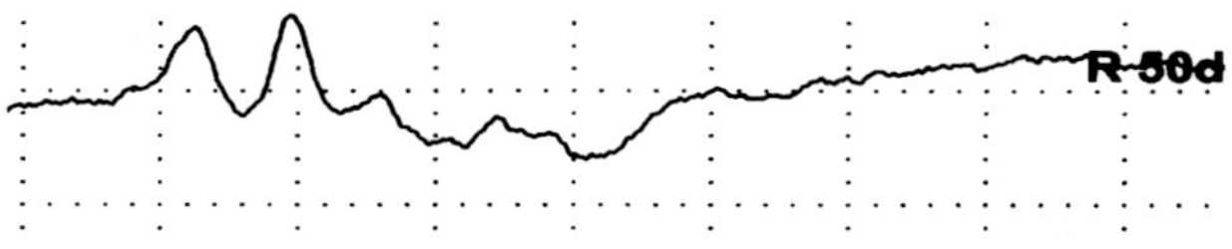

Figure 1. Typical wave form of the brainstem auditory evoked response (BAER) hearing test.

Sue Paterson then reviewed the steps in performing the BAER test. The animal must be calm and relaxed. Three electrodes are placed subdermally into the head region (*recording electrode:* dorsal head; *reference electrode:* front of the tested ear; *ground electrode:* front of the contralateral ear). The electrodes are then connected to a recording system and 'clicks' are delivered. For delivering the sound, headphones instead of ear inserts are preferred. The acoustic signal that results in the best response is a click with a broad frequency spectrum in the region of 2–3 kHz. The intensity of the clicks is calibrated in decibels. The end result is called a BAER trace (Figure 1). When interpreting the results, the point at which the typical five-peak wave form is lost is assessed. Normal dogs have a large peak at 90 dB and the wave becomes flat at 5 dB. Ruptured eardrums can reduce the hearing by 5 dB. Dogs with otitis externa (but not otitis media) rarely have hearing loss beyond 50 dB whereas dogs with otitis externa and otitis media usually have a hearing loss beyond 50 dB. The condition of primary secretory otitis media usually results in a hearing trace lost at 20 to 30 dB.

Study to compare owners' perceptions of their dogs' hearing and brainstem auditory-evoked response findings in 45 dogs (C.L. Ball)

Carly Ball (*UK*) used a questionnaire to assess whether owners were able to determine the degree of hearing impairment of their pet dog with otitis and whether the questionnaire could be used to determine hearing deficits of dogs with otitis when compared to the results of subsequent BAER testing.

A questionnaire with eight questions was sent by postal mail to 45 owners prior to their referral consultation. The first question ascertained whether the dog could hear well and seven additional questions targeted the ability of the dog to hear common noises. When two or more abnormalities were consistently identified by an owner in the questionnaire, hearing deficits were subsequently detected.

A minimal hearing threshold (MHT) was measured for each ear; each ear was assigned a grade and an overall grade was given. The grading system from the World Health Organization for humans was utilized, because there is currently no grading system available for veterinary patients: *grade 0:* no impairment, MHT ≤25 dB; *grade 1:* slight impairment, MHT 26–40 dB; *grade 2:* moderate impairment, MHT 41–60 dB; *grade 3:* severe impairment, MHT 61–80 dB; *grade 4:* profound impairment, MHT ≥81 dB).

With regard to dogs with no measurable hearing loss in both ears detectable by BAER (grade 0), all owners correctly determined absence of hearing impairment in grade 0 cases. Unilateral hearing loss (slight, moderate and severe) was observed in 31.1% of the dogs, and this hearing loss level couldn't be detected by the owners. Bilateral hearing loss was observed in 40% of the tested dogs; grades 2, 3 and 4 of those could be detected by 100% of the owners, whereas only 33% of the owners could detect grade 1 bilateral hearing loss.

In summary, owners were not able to accurately detect unilateral hearing loss in their dogs, and dogs with mild to severe unilateral hearing loss appear to adapt well in their home environment. Owners were able to consistently detect bilateral hearing deficits of grade 2 and higher, consistent with moderate or severe bilateral hearing loss. The questionnaire predicted the detection of bilateral grade 2 and higher hearing deficits, but not unilateral or mild hearing deficits. A larger study is required with more patients in each group to evaluate the sensitivity and specificity of the questionnaire. It is projected that the questionnaire can be adapted to a clinical setting to assist practitioners in the assessment of hearing loss in dogs where practitioners have limited or no access to BAER testing.

Amanda Burrows asked what sort of questions clinicians should be asking owners of dogs with potential unilateral hearing loss to assist in clarifying whether this may be a problem.

Carly Ball responded that her study had not specifically examined that issue, but having owned a dog with unilateral hearing loss, she had observed that by approaching the dog in the home environment from behind and making a loud noise, that the dog would move the head from side-to-side in an attempt to determine the source and the direction of the sound. She stressed that the dog needed to be in a quiet environment, out of sight of the owner, and that a noise stimulus needed to be made from both directions to evaluate whether the dog reacted in a different manner.

Amanda Burrows commented that it seemed as if dogs with unilateral hearing loss lose the ability to locate the direction of the sound, and **Paul Coward** (*UK*) agreed with this, commenting that owners of dogs with unilateral hearing loss mention that when calling their dog while exercising off-lead, the dog has to look around to locate them.

Carly Ball agreed with the comments from Amanda Burrows and Paul Coward.

Myringotomy: when and how to perform; indications and complications (L. Cole)

Lynette Cole defined myringotomy as an incision into the tympanic membrane. Other terminology has been used to describe such an incision, for example myringocentesis, tympanotomy, tympanostomy or paracentesis of the tympanic membrane. The purpose of a myringotomy may be to relieve clinical symptoms, restore hearing, sample fluid or to flush the middle ear. Lynette Cole emphasized that it is important to understand the anatomy of the tympanic membrane and the bulla and associated structures when performing a myringotomy. The dorsal area of the tympanic membrane is the pars flaccida, which is usually flat in the dog. The normal pars flaccida can appear to bulge but this is usually an indication of otitis media in the cavalier King Charles spaniel. The white line with a typical 'C' shape is called the mallear stria and represents the manubrium of the malleus. The ventral part of the tympanic membrane that is transparent and resembles a fish scale is the pars tensa. Lynette Cole then reviewed the site of the myringotomy incision and the structures behind the tympanic membrane. The incision should be performed in the caudo-ventral region of the tympanic membrane, as the rostral and dorsal approach is not safe. There are two important anatomical structures that require noting. The *round window*, located almost opposite to the tympanic membrane serves as the connection to the cochlea of the inner ear, and the *oval window*, located on the dorsal aspect, serves as the connection to the vestibule of the inner ear.

The anatomy of the feline tympanic bulla is different from that of the dog. In cats the bulla is divided by a septum into a small dorso-lateral compartment, containing important structures such as the tympanic membrane, and a larger, air-filled ventro-medial compartment.

Indications for performing a myringotomy after having performed an otic examination and/or imaging include: chronic or recurrent otitis externa with radiographic or computed tomography (CT) changes consistent with middle ear disease; the identification of an abnormal tympanic membrane; neurological signs of otitis media/interna such as facial paralysis; Horner's syndrome; peripheral vestibular signs; and a cavalier King Charles spaniel with suspected primary secretory otitis media.

The technique of myringotomy was reviewed. The medical equipment required includes either a hand-held otoscope with otoscopic cones, a video oto-endoscope or an operating microscope. For flushing irrigation, saline, bowls, syringes and catheters or an external flushing/suction device are required. The incision into the tympanic membrane can be performed using a polypropylene urinary catheter, a myringotomy needle, a cotton-tipped applicator (Calgiswab®, Cardinal Health; Puritan Medical Products), a myringotomy knife or a spinal needle. Complications are more commonly seen in cats than dogs and include neurological signs such as Horner's syndrome, facial paralysis or non-neurological signs such as a nonhealing tympanic membrane. A routine myringotomy incision should heal over 3 to 5 weeks.

Ekaterina Kuznetsova commented that she could not clearly visualize the pars tensa behind the bulging pars flaccida demonstrated in the fourth video otoscopic image.

Lynette Cole responded that it was possible to gently pass a catheter underneath the bulging pars flaccida and aim at the caudo-ventral quadrant with the catheter to penetrate the tympanic membrane. The pars flaccida would deflate subsequent to flushing and suction.

Ekaterina Kuznetsova asked whether there were any medical or surgical management strategies for a dog and cat with a nonhealing tympanic membrane.

Lynette Cole responded that in her opinion, a ruptured tympanic membrane did not translate to a permanent loss of hearing unless there was damage to the auditory nerve. The patient with a perforated tympanic membrane may still be able to hear although it is more difficult to conduct sound waves. The challenge is to thoroughly clean and flush the middle ear and evaluate whether the tympanic membrane will heal in a clean environment. In circumstances where the rupture has persisted for a prolonged period, she indicated that it was common for the tympanic membrane to fail to heal and she was not aware of any useful surgical or medical intervention that was effective in these circumstances. She also mentioned the risk of persistent middle ear infection and whether aggressive ear cleaning by an owner could prevent this complication.

Treatment of primary secretory otitis media (PSOM) with myringotomy in dogs with Chiari-like malformation: 21 dogs (28 bullae) with 24-month follow-up (D. Marino)

Dominic Marino (*USA*) introduced himself as a neurosurgeon with a special interest in Chiari-like malformation (CLM) and a subsequent, indirect interest in primary secretory otitis media (PSOM), which can be associated with Chiari-like malformation. He suggested that the term primary secretory otitis media should be modified. In dogs with PSOM, an accumulation of mucus within the middle ear can be associated with clinical symptoms but it can be asymptomatic and most patients may have mild or no concurrent external ear canal disease. Clinical signs of PSOM are similar to Chiari-like malformation and include pruritus, nystagmus, ataxia, hearing loss and head tilt. Dominic Marino alluded to an important characteristic of the pruritus associated with Chiari-like malformation where dogs tend to 'air guitar' scratch, meaning that these patients scratch but have no contact with the skin.

Briefly, the pathophysiology of PSOM was described. Mucus is normally produced by the epithelium of the middle ear and then transported by cilia via the eustachian tube into the pharynx. In dogs with PSOM there seems to be either a diminished clearance or pressure imbalance resulting in mucus accumulation. Otoscopy, radiography, computerized tomography (CT) or magnetic resonance imaging (MRI) can all be used for the diagnosis of PSOM and/or Chiari-like malformation.

The purpose of his study was to evaluate the effectiveness of myringotomy and flush/aspiration (MFA) in the treatment of PSOM in dogs with Chiari-like malformation. Twenty-one dogs (28 bullae) with PSOM were entered into the study. MRI was performed at the time of diagnosis and then every 6 months for 2 years. MFA was performed in all of the dogs with PSOM. The study revealed that approximately one-third of dogs with CLM had concurrent PSOM. Forty-six percent of cavalier King Charles spaniels with CLM also had PSOM, whereas in other breeds with CLM only approximately 13% had PSOM. Approximately one-third of the dogs with PSOM exhibited no clinical symptoms. The success rate of MFA (judged by clinical signs and MRI) was about 10% after 6 months, 16% after 12 months, 43% after 18 months and 67% after 24 months. The study demonstrated that three to four treatments are required to achieve success in most of these dogs. Dominic Marino also compared CT scan with 3 tesla (3 T) MRI and determined that approximately 25–30% of early cases of PSOM were missed with CT compared to the 3 T MRI. In conclusion, MFA is an effective treatment for PSOM in dogs with CLM (85.7% over 24 months) and multiple MFA treatments are usually necessary.

Lynette Cole asked whether Dominic Marino had worked with eustachian tube stents.

Dominic Marino responded by indicating that he had not. His group was working with a company to develop a stent and evaluating anatomical models to determine how a stent could be placed most successfully.

Lynette Cole asked Dominic Marino whether he flushed out the eustachian tube.

Dominic Marino indicated that he did flush the eustachian tube. He also mentioned that at a recent meeting in Barcelona, a group from Germany had presented a video incorporating a method that employed high-pressure flushing of the mucus plug through the eustachian tube into the nasopharynx. He expressed some concern about the safety of this procedure and advised caution regarding increased pressure levels inside the ear.

Lynette Cole indicated that she was also concerned about these factors. She added that she sometimes observed mucus on the endotracheal tube after removal post-flushing, leading her to conclude that even gentle flushing may result in some mucus being passed through the eustachian tube.

Dominic Marino indicated that the group had claimed no detrimental effect but he was concerned that flushing under pressure could cause adverse effects.

Amanda Burrows asked whether there was any role for tympanostomy tubes in the management of PSOM cases.

Dominic Marino indicated that there were complications with tympanostomy tubes including frequent dislodgement in conjunction with poor drainage of thick mucus via the small tube. He questioned whether a tympanostomy tube was the best way to correct the pressure gradient and expressed the opinion that stenting the eustachian tube was probably more physiological and less intrusive.

Rod Rosychuk asked whether ventral bulla osteotomy with follow-up had been performed on dogs with PSOM.

Dominic Marino responded that as a neurological surgeon he often received cases with Chiari-like malformation with concurrent PSOM that had been missed on diagnostic evaluation. These were often cases that had undergone decompressive surgery but had a persistence of post-operative clinical signs including scratching, and these dogs had undetected PSOM. He encouraged surgeons in these circumstances to consider whether it was a failed surgery or a failed surgical diagnosis.

Paul Coward asked Dominic Marino how often he recorded PSOM exclusively in cavalier dogs that were presented for evaluation of CLM.

Dominic Marino responded that 80–90% of cavalier dogs screened for CLM had some permutation of the disease. Locating cavalier dogs with no evidence of CLM was challenging but PSOM had been detected exclusively in some of these patients. With regard to the Chiari population, he indicated that approximately half of the affected individuals were cavalier dogs and approximately half were other small dog breeds. He indicated he had no explanation as to why cavaliers with CLM and PSOM were over-represented compared to other noncavalier small breed dogs.

Reference

1. Carlotti DN, Guaguere E, Pin D *et al.* Therapy of difficult cases of canine pyoderma with marbofloxacin: a report of 39 dogs. *J Small Anim Pract* 1999; 40: 265–270.

8.10

Allergy testing revisited

R.E.W. Halliwell[1] (Chairperson), S. Gilbert[2] (Secretary)

[1]University of Edinburgh, Edinburgh, UK
[2]Centre Vétérinaire Laval, Québec, Canada

Richard Halliwell (*UK*) acknowledged Veterinary Allergy Reference Laboratory (VARL) for their sponsorship of this workshop, which included seven presentations.

Patch testing and IgE/IgG testing for canine adverse food reactions (R.S. Mueller)

Ralf Mueller (*Germany*) presented a summary of a recently published study that evaluated patch and serology testing for food-specific IgE and IgG in normal dogs and atopic dogs, many of which also had adverse food reactions, as proven via elimination diet trial.[1]

The study included 10 healthy dogs and 23 dogs with atopic dermatitis (AD). Patch and serology testing for allergen-specific IgE and IgG were undertaken for allergens commonly found in dog food including beef, chicken, pork, lamb, turkey, fish (both raw and cooked), wheat, corn and potato. For the patch test, allergens were applied on the lateral thorax under occlusion. Reactions were evaluated at 24, 48 and 72 hours.

Overall, there were 46 positive patch test reactions and 137 negative reactions, with a mean of three reactions for each affected dog. The allergens implicated in each dog's condition were identified by sequential oral single-antigen challenges. There were 29 of 46 true positives and 136 of 137 true negatives. Most reactions were against beef with the majority appearing after 48 hours. The pattern of reaction against the raw or cooked antigen was inconsistent.

For the IgE serology testing, there were 13 positive reactions and 145 negative reactions. Two of 13 were true positives and 117 of 145 were true negatives. For IgG, there were 23 positive reactions and 135 negative reactions. Eight of 23 were true positives and 113/135 were true negatives. Beef was again the most common reaction and there were no reactions to fish, chicken or turkey. Therefore, there were fewer true positive and fewer true negative reactions than in the patch testing.

The negative predictive value (NPV) for serology and patch testing, respectively, ranged from 80.75% to 99.3%, while the positive predictive value (PPV) ranged from 15.4% to 63%. Although the NPV is fairly high, it is important also to look at the positive and negative likelihood ratios (PLR and NLR), as the values depend on the prevalence of the disease in the population. For patch testing, the PLR was 8.8, which increases the probability of a positive result being correct by 40%, while the NLR was 0.04, which halves the probability that a negative result is truly negative. Therefore, the results may not be as good as the NPV and PPV might suggest.

Margreet Vroom (*The Netherlands*) asked if biopsies were taken on positive reactions to ensure these were not irritant reactions.

Ralf Mueller responded that biopsies were not taken, as owners would not have allowed that. However, there were 137 negative reactions of which 136 were true negative, so the chance that they were irritant reactions is unlikely as any irritant reaction would also be seen in the control dogs.

Reliability of intradermal testing in atopic dogs (K. Beale)

Karin Beale (*USA*) presented a study that she had conducted 4 years ago with Gabriel Ferrer-Canals, Jon Plant and Valerie Fadok.[2] Intradermal testing (IDT) is typically considered the gold standard for selection of allergens for allergen-specific immunotherapy (ASIT). However, four other studies have shown no difference in outcome whether ASIT is based on IDT or serum allergy testing. Therefore, the question addressed by their study was 'How reliable is the IDT?'

They assessed this using two parameters: repeatability (consistency of the reading of the duplicates) and reproducibility (between the three investigators). IDTs were performed on 12 atopic dogs using 51 different allergens, and 15 allergens were selected for blinded duplicates by the technician and were injected at the end of the test. The readings were undertaken by three individual investigators in a randomized manner, using a semi-quantitative scale of '0' to '4'.

Agreement was analysed with Cohen's weighted kappa (κw) using a standard linear formula. The investigators assessed repeatability (comparing scores of 15 duplicates by each investigator) and reproducibility (comparing the scores for the same 15 allergens amongst investigators). The Fleiss–Nee–Landis extension of kappa for multiple raters was used to assess the combined reproducibility of the three investigators. A statistical software program (STATSDIRECT) was used for all calculations.

Looking at the three individual investigators, the repeatability was fair with investigators #1 and #2, while it was moderate with investigator #3. Factors that influenced the repeatability were that duplicates were injected at the end of the test, so they were temporally separated. Also, they were injected more ventrally where the skin is thinner.

Reproducibility was done for scores '0' to '4'. Reproducibility was good for '4', fair for '0', '2' and '3', and poor for '1'. One reason for the poor reproducibility for '1' was that one of the investigators did not score reactions of '1'. The juggling of the three investigators to read the tests, while also seeing appointments, led to assessments being done at different times after injections. Therefore, the reliability of IDT was assessed as being fair. Nevertheless, the allergens selected to be included in the ASIT based on the IDT results were almost identical amongst investigators.

Richard Halliwell asked Karen Beale if she does read '1' reactions sometimes, or if she tends to go straight from '0' to '2'.

Karin Beale confirmed that she does not read '1' reactions, which definitely had an effect on the statistics for both the '0' and '1' scores.

Jon Plant (*USA*) commented that because the '1' score was not used by one investigator, the kappa value for the three investigators for the score of '1' was negative, implying that the agreement on '1' was worse than by chance alone. He also mentioned that he was unaware of treatment recommendations when the statistics were done, and thus could not comment on any effect of eliminating all '1' reactions.

Karin Beale confirmed that the results of the IDT were correlated with the history and seasonality of the clinical signs. As all the investigators tended to select allergens for ASIT based upon reactions of '2' or greater, concerns regarding '1' scores was eliminated.

David Robson (*Australia*) asked with respect to the statistics whether different groups were evaluated, for example '0', '1' and '2'. The rationale for this would be that in most cases '0' and '1' reactions would not be included in ASIT vaccines, whereas '2' or more are, irrespective of whether they are '2', '3' or '4'. Using the results in this way might have led to better correlations between the investigators as being more clinically relevant with respect to immunotherapy formulation.

Karin Beale agreed, but said that this was not assessed, although it could have led to a different outcome.

Jon Plant also agreed, but suggested further that it could have been better to just grade reactions as positive or negative.

Ralf Mueller commented that he had done a similar study when working in Melbourne. Although the results differed between investigators, almost identical allergens were included in the ASIT vaccines.

Patrick Hensel (*USA*) asked what the timeframe was between the readings of the tests by the different investigators.

Karin Beale replied that the first investigator read the IDT 8 minutes after completing the test. The goal was to have the second read right after the first, and the third right after the second, but there was sometimes some delay. However, there was never more than 15 minutes between the different readings, and the order of the readings was randomized to minimize any effect.

Richard Halliwell asked whether IDT could still be considered the gold standard.

Jon Plant responded that he did not believe that it could.

Drug interference in intradermal testing and serology: an evidence-based review (M. Saridomichelakis)

Manolis Saridomichelakis (*Greece*) and Thierry Olivry conducted this study for the International Committee on Atopic Diseases of Animals (ICADA) and the results are currently under consideration for publication. The study looked at evidenced-based recommendations for anti-allergic drug withdrawal times before performing intradermal testing (IDT) and allergen-specific IgE serology (ASIS). The authors looked at three Internet databases. In addition, a search was done in the proceedings of the World, American and European Congresses of Veterinary Dermatology. Two different withdrawal times were proposed. The optimal withdrawal times (OWTs), which had no drug interference on the test results, and the minimal withdrawal times (MWTs), which may be associated with a small inhibitory effect that may not affect interpretation of the results.

Results for IDT (based on immediate reactions only)

For antihistamines, there were three studies.[3–5] One comprised 18 dogs with flea allergy dermatitis (FAD), one comprised six normal dogs and one comprised 10 dogs with house dust mite (HDM) reactivity. Two used hydroxyzine and one used cetirizine. Reactants were histamine, flea allergen and HDM allergen. OWT was 1 week and MWT was 2 days.

For oral glucocorticoids, there were five studies.[5–9] One comprised 10 dogs with FAD, one comprised 10 dogs with FAD and 11 dogs with atopic dermatitis (AD), one comprised eight dogs with FAD, one comprised five normal dogs and one comprised 10 dogs with HDM reactivity. Two used prednisone and three used prednisolone. The duration of the glucocorticoid administration was from 3 days to 6 weeks. Reactants were histamine, anti-canine IgE, flea allergen, pollen allergens and HDM allergen. OWT was 21 days and MWT was 7 days.

For injectable glucocorticoids there was only one study,[10] composed of eight dogs with FAD. The study used methylprednisolone acetate, which was administered on two occasions, 1 month apart. The reactant was flea allergen. OWT was unknown, but MWT was 28 days.

For topical glucocorticoids, there were four studies.[11–14] One included 16 normal dogs and seven pruritic dogs, and the other three studies comprised 10 dogs with AD. Three used 0.1% hydrocortisone +/<minus> pramoxine, one used 0.058% hydrocortisone aceponate and one used 0.015% triamcinolone. The duration of the application was from 3 days to 6 weeks. Reactants were histamine and anti-canine IgE. OWT was 2 weeks and MWT was 0 days, especially if the test was not done on the treated side.

For otic glucocorticoids, there were two studies.[15,16] One included eight normal dogs and the second enrolled 20 dogs with atopic dermatitis (AD). The drugs used were 0.088% betamethasone and 0.1% mometasone, which were applied for 2 weeks. Reactants were histamine, anti-canine IgE and environmental allergens. OWT was 14 days and MWT was 0 days.

For ciclosporin there were four studies.[8,17–19] One included six dogs with AD, the second eight dogs with FAD, the third 16 dogs with AD and the fourth involved four dogs sensitized to *Ascaris*. The duration of administration was from 4 to 6 weeks. Reactants were *Ascaris* allergen, flea allergen and environmental allergens. OWT was 0 days.

For tacrolimus, there was one study[20] involving nine dogs with AD. The study used 0.1% tacrolimus applied for 4 weeks. Reactants were histamine, lipopolysaccharide, HD and HDM allergens. OWD was 0 days.

For pentoxifylline there was one study[21] involving 10 dogs with AD treated for 4 weeks. Reactants were HDM allergens. OWD was 0 days.

For ketoconazole, there was one study[22] involving 12 dogs with AD treated for 4 weeks. Reactants were histamine and HDM allergens. OWD was 0 days.

For essential fatty acids there was one study[23] involving 20 dogs with AD treated for up to 118 weeks. Reactants were histamine and environmental allergens. OWD was 0 days.

Results for ASIS

For oral glucocorticoids, there were two studies.[8,24] One included 15 dogs with AD and the other eight dogs with FAD treated with prednisone or prednisolone for 3 to 7 weeks. OWT was 0 days.

For injectable glucocorticoids there was one study[10] involving eight dogs with FAD treated with methylprednisolone acetate two times 1 month apart. OWT was less than 28 days.

For ciclosporin, there were three studies.[8,18,19] One included eight dogs with FAD, another included 16 dogs with AD and the third included four normal dogs. The duration of treatment was 4 to 7 weeks. There was no major influence and OWT was 0 days.

Manolis Saridomichelakis pointed out that this study had several limitations. The main ones were: the small number of studies, which included many abstracts of proceedings; the results apply only to the specific drugs, dosing regimens and duration of administration; and last, but not least, reactivity to histamine is not the same as reactivity to allergens injected intradermally.

Richard Halliwell felt that the histamine wheal will return well before the allergen-induced wheal after withdrawal from corticosteroids, and asked if anybody else shared his feeling.

Ralf Mueller agreed and he also believed that there are differences between allergen groups and that flea and HDM reactivity return quicker than pollen allergen's reactivity.

Manolis Saridomichelakis commented that he had thought of that and therefore he cross-tabulated the data based on the reactant. The outcome was that if IDT reactivity to histamine were excluded, there would be no changes in the OWT. There would only be a change in the MWT for antihistamines. Furthermore, if flea allergen were excluded, there would also be no changes in the results.

Richard Halliwell asked if any of these studies used hydrocortisone aceponate and if there was any difference between that study and studies using other topical corticosteroids.

Manolis Saridomichelakis responded that one study used hydrocortisone aceponate. IDT results were affected for 2 weeks and the untreated side of the thorax was also affected.

Douglas DeBoer (*USA*) commented that when he lectures to general practitioners (GPs), he always says that there isn't really an effect of glucocorticoids on serology results; however, GPs tell him that laboratories ask them to discontinue glucocorticoids for a long time before they can do the test, and he wondered whether anyone from industry could comment.

Don Wassom (*USA*) commented that they did a number of studies on that some years ago at Heska (Fort Collins). The effects of glucocorticoids, whether oral or injectable, on the outcome of IgE serology over time was very minimal. However, in one study, levels of allergen-specific IgE were quantified in some dogs and when those dogs were withdrawn from glucocorticoids the levels of allergen-specific IgE increased. Whether it would have influenced the interpretation of these tests is questionable. However, the fact that allergen-specific IgE tended to increase over time after glucocorticoid withdrawal suggests that steroid withdrawal might be useful.

Manolis Saridomichelakis asked Don Wassom if allergen-specific IgE was measured for perennial allergens (HDM) or for seasonal allergens.

Don Wassom did not remember the details of the study and thought that it might have been done with flea saliva reactivity.

Manolis Saridomichelakis stated that another factor might be time. In studies of long duration, the concentration and exposure to environmental allergens may change and thus it could make a difference, especially for pollen allergens. He added that the good thing here is that all studies assessing the effects of drugs on ASIS were rather short term (no more than 2 months).

Ralf Mueller asked Manolis Saridomichelakis to clarify why this was good.

Manolis Saridomichelakis explained that it is important to bear in mind the short half-life of IgE in serum. Indeed, if environmental allergens are considered, one would not expect the major changes in the exposure and thus in the quantity of allergen-specific IgE in a short-term study that one might find in a long-term study.

Richard Halliwell commented that the half-life of IgE in serum is very short, but it is actually much longer when it is bound to mast cells, namely 2 to 3 weeks.

Manolis Saridomichelakis emphasized that then differences in exposure would have less influence on IDT results than on results of serology testing.

Enzyme coupling methodology and its effects on mab specificity (J. Bexley)

Jennifer Bexley (*UK*) stated that she initially tried to assess two different types of monoclonal antibodies (mab) for canine IgE: mab 5.91 from Bruce Hammerberg (North Carolina) and mab D9 from Doug DeBoer (Wisconsin). The reactivity of both mabs towards canine IgE and the level of cross-reactivity towards canine IgG were checked for validation of the reagents. Both were found suitable. Next, the levels of IgE towards food allergens were compared using mab 5.91 conjugated to biotin and mab D9 conjugated to horseradish peroxidase (HRP). Mab 5.91 biotin seemed to detect meats (beef, pork, lamb) while mab D9 HRP detected some of the cereals. Therefore, it was thought that by combining both mabs, results would be improved by detecting the full range of reactivity. Next, by doing an inhibition study, she checked that the two mabs were not binding the same epitopes of the IgE. The conclusion was that the mabs bind different epitopes. Then, the mabs were conjugated to both biotin and HRP to see which one would be best for the assay. The author was surprised by the results, as when mab D9 was conjugated to HRP, it picked up the cereals, but did not do so when conjugated to biotin. Also, mab 5.91 showed a strong signal to beef when conjugated to biotin, but not when conjugated to HRP, although cereal-specific IgE was detected. Therefore, the reaction seemed to be driven by the conjugate rather than by the mab itself.

To answer this question, the assay was run without including any of the mabs. There was still a signal for the meat and some of the cereals, in some of the sera. The possibility that streptavidin was causing this nonspecific reaction was discarded and it was concluded that it was due to the HRP. Next, reactivity of the two different mabs (D9 and 5.91) was assessed with the same conjugate (biotin) and with streptavidin alkaline phosphatase (AP). There was a slight difference between signals, but the pattern was overall similar. Then, they repeated the same experiment with AP direct conjugate for both mabs, and much of the reactivity was lost. However, mab 5.91 picked up more than mab D9 using the same conjugated label.

The conclusion of the study is that some canine sera had allergen-specific serum components that seem to bind peroxidase to give false positive signals. There were differences in signal between different conjugates of the same mabs and there were differences in signal between mab 5.91 and mab D9 when the same conjugate was used.

Richard Halliwell commented that it appeared that HRP conjugation should be avoided in all assays.

Jennifer Bexley agreed, although she was unsure of the reason.

Ken Lee (*USA*) said that he had demonstrated some years ago that the HRP has a carbohydrate molecule that acts as an epitope that is identical to various carbohydrates that are present on other allergens. The IgG from the serum binds to that epitope on the HRP and also that on the allergen. The HRP activity is not inhibited when IgG binds to it. Therefore, it has nothing to do with the other components in the assay.

Jennifer Bexley asked why it was seen with beef, but not with rice.

Ken Lee explained that it is because the epitope is not present in all allergens and rice does not have that carbohydrate. So, yes, HRP should be eliminated from all assays!

Don Wassom agreed with Ken Lee.

Richard Halliwell commented on the important finding that, when exactly the same conjugates are used (even direct AP), there is some difference in the mab reactivity.

Storage mites and serological reactivity in canine atopic dermatitis (CAD): have we underestimated its importance? (D.L. Wassom)

Don Wassom (*USA*) noted that his data are based on the many *in vitro* IgE tests conducted by Heska Corporation in Fort Collins, Colorado, USA, over the years. He emphasized that improvement in *in vitro* IgE testing is likely to come by improving the allergen extracts that are used in the assays, and that we still do not understand very well the allergens that dogs, cats and horses recognize in the extracts as opposed to humans. Major allergens of house dust mite (HDM) recognized by dogs are der f 15 and der f 18, so they are different from the major allergens recognized by humans. Optimizing the allergen extracts for those components that are recognized by animals is important. Storage mites have some allergens that are unique and not shared by HDM.

Mites are very important as initiators and perpetuators of allergic skin diseases in dogs. A substantial number of allergen-specific immunotherapy (ASIT) prescriptions in the USA and Europe contain mites, and in northern Europe up to 75% of ASIT prescriptions contain mites only.

This raises the question of whether storage mites are the primary source of sensitization rather than HDM in dogs with AD. The rationale for this question is that although HDM are not common in Colorado, Colorado dogs suffer from AD and test positive to HDM. Therefore, if HDM are rare in Colorado, could storage mites account for the mite reactivity? The storage mite *Tyrophagus putrescentiae* can be cultured from opened bags of dog food in Colorado, and *Tyrophagus* and *Dermatophagoides* mites share cross-reacting allergens. Also, there is a subset of dogs that react only to storage mites and not to HDM. This is the origin of the proposition that there are unique allergens associated with storage mites that are not shared by HDM. In fact, in the USA, about 11% of mite-positive ALLERCEPT® tests (Heska) are positive only for *Tyrophagus*. However, in Colorado where HDM are rare, 21% of the animals that test positive for mites are positive only for *Tyrophagus*.

Richard Halliwell asked Don Wassom if he had done any cross-inhibition studies.

Don Wassom responded that he had and that reactivity in sera from animals testing positive to both HDM and storage mites can be inhibited by either antigen. So, there is no question that mites share cross-reacting allergens. Most dogs that test positive to mites have antibodies that cross-inhibit. Usually, dogs that test positive to *Tyrophagus* will test positive to *Dermatophagoides* but a subset of dogs test positive to *Tyrophagus* and negative to *Dermatophagoides*.

Richard Halliwell wondered about *Acarus siro*.

Don Wassom answered that it does usually track with *Tyrophagus* and *Dermatophagoides*. If they are positive to one, they are positive to all of them. They have not identified dogs that test positive for *Acarus* and negative to *Tyrophagus*.

Richard Halliwell asked about cats, as cats recognize different antigens.

Don Wassom said that he does not have enough data to answer that question.

Douglas DeBoer believes that the piece that has always been missing in the whole storage mite story is exposure. Studies showed that open bags of dog food will become contaminated by storage mites, and unopened bags that are then sealed properly after being open do not contain storage mites. These studies looked at the presence of live and dead mites, but not at the protein. Therefore, a study should be done on quantifying storage mite protein to see if unopened bags of dog food contain immunologically detectable storage mite antigens.

Don Wassom commented that the problem is first to identify the storage mite allergens that are relevant to dogs and whether they can survive processing and are able to sensitize via the oral route.

Marie Innera (*Norway*) stated that she sees many dogs with reactions to storage mites only and a poor response to ASIT using *Tyrophagus*. She finds that many of these dogs are springer spaniels, and do not respond to an elimination diet trial with hydrolysed diets but are eventually diagnosed as having food allergy using a home-cooked diet.

Don Wassom commented that there are a lot of dogs that are on ASIT with just *Tyrophagus* immunotherapy based on the test results. He does not know its efficacy although *Tyrophagus* prescriptions that are ordered are usually refilled, suggesting some favourable responses.

Susanne Ahman (*Sweden*) reported that she also sees many dogs being positive only to *Tyrophagus* or *A. siro*. However, she does see a good response to ASIT containing one of these storage mites as the only allergen.

Allan Bell (*New Zealand*) commented on the biology of *Tyrophagus*, which he said was not as dependent on humidity as is HDM. He commented on a New Zealand large animal food company that makes food heavily contaminated with *A. siro*. The company fumigates the food, which seems to lower the level.

Don Wassom answered that it seems to be unusual to find HDM in the dry climate of Colorado. However, storage mites are commonly found suggesting that the requirement of humidity is lower for storage mites than for HDM.

Intradermal testing (IDT) reactivity to dust mites and storage mites in the southeastern USA (P. Hensel)

Patrick Hensel (*USA*) asked, in view of the fact that up to 75% of clinically normal dogs show positive IDT to HDM, whether we were dealing with subclinical hypersensitivity, the use of irritant concentrations for testing, or reactions resulting from cross-reacting allergens.

He reported that he had undertaken two studies[25,26] that were published in *Veterinary Dermatology*. One study conducted with his resident attempted to define the optimal concentrations for skin testing using mite allergens. He believed this should be lower than the commonly used 250 PNU/mL. The next step was to look for ideal intradermal test concentrations. Once the new test concentrations had been selected, they tested dogs with AD using two different test concentrations, the adjusted concentrations (that they believed might be better) and the standard concentrations. Fewer positive reactions were seen with the adjusted test concentrations and their conclusion was that the results may be more reliable.

Using six mites – *Dermatophagoides farinae* (DF), *D. pteronyssinus* (DP), *Acarus siro* (AS), *Lepidoglyphus destructor* (LD), *Tyrophagus putrescentiae* (TP) and *Blomia tropicalis* (BT) – with different adjusted test concentrations, they compared IDT reactivity to these dust mites (DM) in 24 dogs with atopic dermatitis. The test concentrations were: 50 PNU/mL for AS and BT; 75 PNU/mL for

DF, TP and LD; and 200 PNU/mL for DP. Twenty dogs had a positive reaction to DF, 13 dogs to BT, 9 dogs to AS, 8 dogs to DP, 5 dogs to TP and 5 dogs to LD. Nine of 24 dogs had only one reaction, 4 of 24 dogs had two reactions, 4 of 24 dogs had three reactions, 5 of 24 dogs had four reactions, 1 of 24 dogs had five reactions and 1 of 24 dogs had six reactions. Agreement on co-reactivity among the six DM was assessed by a kappa test. Positive and negative agreements/results were assessed. Significant agreement was kappa P-value <0.05. There were many significant agreements between mites; however, the strongest were between DF and BT, BT and AS, AS and TP, and LD and TP ($P < 0.0001$).

In summary, Patrick Hensel concluded that DM are the most common positive reactions and DM hypersensitivity is the most common hypersensitivity in canine atopic dogs. From the results of his study, he believes that test concentrations for mites should be decreased and suggested concentrations of 50 PNU/mL for AS and BT, 75 PNU/mL for DF, TP and LD, and 200 PNU/mL for DP. This should result in fewer false positive reactions. There is strong co-reactivity among different mites and, therefore, cross-reactivity is very likely among DM.

Richard Halliwell commented that he is persuaded that all normal dogs do have HDM-specific IgE. Therefore, he wondered whether when Patrick Hensel uses the reduced concentrations to test with, he might miss the less strong reactions and pick up only the very strong ones. He asked Ken Lee, who works for a company that makes allergen extracts, at what strength he believes that his extracts are irritant.

Ken Lee confirmed that mite allergens are considered irritant over a concentration of 1000 PNU/mL.

Richard Halliwell also mentioned that in the study with Tan Mei Lian[27] in which IDT and serology were done in the same dogs using a sensitive assay, serological reactivity was found in the normal dogs showing positive reactions on the IDT.

Patrick Hensel said he had looked at the correlation between IDT and serology testing and agreed that the results would correlate better if the cut-off value in the serology test were increased. But the question remains as to which test is better, as IDT is not necessarily the gold standard.

Ralf Mueller mentioned that he did a study where he looked at *Tyrophagus* IDT reactivity in normal and atopic dogs with increasing dilutions. He commented that the higher the dilution, the less reaction results but that there was still no difference between the two groups of dogs. Thus, he believes that these results do not seem to support the notion that this is an irritant reaction and that there should be a true cut-off that clearly differentiates the clinically allergic dog from the dog that has a reaction that it is not meaningful.

Richard Halliwell commented that protease from HDM cleaved the CD23 on B-cells deregulating the IgE synthesis thus potentiating the IgE reaction in normal dogs.

Individual allergen vs group testing in IgE serology (K.W. Lee)

As an introduction to his presentation, **Ken Lee** (*USA*) mentioned that he first developed a screening test for high levels of IgE about 30 years ago but over the years, the veterinary profession has moved away from that. However, more recently, he had had some requests to investigate how individual allergens react when they are placed in mixtures in wells. So working at Greer Laboratories, Lenoir, North Carolina, USA, he set out with two objectives. The first was to compare ELISA reactivity of individual allergens and various allergen mixtures. The second objective was to document the utility of a multiple allergen screen in identifying animals possessing allergen-specific IgE in serum.

Wells were coated with individual allergens and with various mixtures of the individual allergens. Six different grasses, trees, weeds and mites were selected, and the mixtures were composed of two, three and six allergens. Two, three and six were selected based on the contribution of each allergen to the mixture (100% for one allergen, 50% for two allergens, 33% for three allergens and 17% for six allergens). Coated wells were evaluated using IgE ELISA on 42 individual sera samples.

A summary of the results they observed with 42 individual samples on each of these mixtures was given and only a few of them were presented. With individual allergens, different responses were seen. However, the average response for the individual allergens was approximately equal to the total mixture of the responses. Each of the components in the mixtures was contributing to the overall response in proportion to the amount that was contained within the mixture. When looking at the response of individual grasses within the group, it was approximately equal to the mixture response. So, what was seen was basically the average of the responses. That held true with the mite mixtures as well as the tree and weed mixtures.

The positive predictive value (PPV) for all individual wells containing mixed allergen was 100%, but the negative predictive value (NPV) was lower and varied from 45% for a tree mixture to 90% for mixed grasses. However, when looking at the summation of the aggregate screen, it was 100% predictive (PPV and NPV). These results were encouraging and induced the author to conduct the second stage of the experiment. Objective 2 was to demonstrate the utility of the multiple allergen screens in identifying animals possessing allergen-specific IgE in serum. Greer ELISAs were done using the regional panels of 48 individual allergens and the screen (four wells coated with taxonomically similar grasses, weeds, trees and mites/fungi). Four hundred and eight clinical sera samples were evaluated as well as control sera on the various panels.

Concordance of results between individual allergens and admixtures of these allergens was assessed and responses that were above 150 ELISA absorbance units (150 EAU, ELISA cut-off point) were considered positive, with anything lower being negative. Overall concordance of results was approximately 90% and ranged from 87.5% for trees to 92.1% for grasses. As would be expected, the greatest discordance was evident for responses that were at or very near the cut-off value of 150 EAU. The overall concordance of results for the mite/ fungi mixture also exceeded 90%, and this compared favourably with the concordance of results evident with the individual mite responses. However, when evaluating the responses to individual mites and fungi, the concordance was severely compromised. Poor concordance of less than 60% resulted because the panel of individual allergens tested for 10 different fungi, and all resulted in negative responses. These results emphasize the importance of defining mixtures using related (taxonomically or antigenically) allergens.

The conclusion of the studies is that composite results from mixed-allergen screens can be used to identify animals that are not reactive to pollen or mite allergens (true negatives). Composite results from mixed-allergen screen can be used to identify animals reactive to pollen and mite allergens (true positives) and provide a basis for further testing to characterize specific reactivity. Further results might be selectively directed from the results observed with the individual wells of the composite screen. However, composite results are not sufficiently discriminatory to provide the basis for selection of allergens to include in an immunotherapeutic regimen.

Richard Halliwell stressed that the validity of the study is based on selection of allergens that are taxonomically from the same family. Also, he wondered what would happen for allergens that are not related (no cross-reactivity/co-sensitization).

Ken Lee replied that some dogs responded only to one or two trees, and when that happens, the reaction to a mixture drops to a very low level. For these dogs he did not find positive reactions when using the mixtures for testing.

Don Wassom emphasized that Ken Lee demonstrated the utility of these screening tests as predictors. On the one hand, if there is a negative screen, the likelihood of a negative test is high and it is not worth running the full panel. It is then less expensive. On the other hand, the likelihood of having a positive test in the face of a positive screen is high. Then, a whole panel should be done to obtain the relevant information necessary to formulate ASIT. Therefore, the screen is helpful in making a decision in terms of submitting a full panel.

Richard Halliwell recalled the letter[28] that Thierry Olivry and Judy published last year in *Veterinary Dermatology*, in which he was using an E-screen from Don Wassom's company. The indoor allergens were very good in terms of positive predictive value, but the outdoor allergens (weeds and trees) were not as good.

Don Wassom commented that the reason for that is that they cannot be all included in a screen. When an animal is positive to one allergen (grass, weed or tree), and that allergen is in the screen, a positive definitive test is likely despite a negative screening test.

Douglas DeBoer has been conducting screening tests for a long time at the University of Wisconsin and stated that they have a potential for use as long as they are not used by themselves to formulate ASIT. Douglas DeBoer's team is using the same principle for IDT based on cluster analysis that they did on their IDT results. They perform a mini-panel of 12 allergens that are very predictive of whether or not the dog would have a positive IDT if tested for all 60 allergens. So, in some cases when the owner is limited financially, screening may be helpful to know if it is worth doing the test with all 60 allergens or not. He believes that the concept of screening with defined numbers of allergens (serology or IDT) needs to be investigated further.

Richard Halliwell commented that they tried the screening tests when he was working at the University of Florida but subsequently returned to using the full screen. However, for financial considerations, the screening tests may be an option that some clients will want to select.

The Chairman thanked all the people who presented and all the people who participated in the discussion.

References

1. Bethlehem S, Bexley, J, Mueller RS. Patch testing and allergen-specific serum IgE and IgG antibodies in the diagnosis of canine adverse food reactions. *Vet Immunol Immunopathol* 2012; 145: 582–589.
2. Ferrer-Canals G, Plant JD, Beale KM *et al.* Reliability of intradermal allergy tests in dogs with atopic dermatitis. *Vet Dermatol* 2009; 20: 228 [abstract].
3. Barbet JL, Halliwell REW. Duration of inhibition of immediate skin test reactivity by hydroxyzine hydrochloride in dogs. *J Am Vet Med Assoc* 1989; 194: 1565–1569.
4. Bizikova P, Papich MG, Olivry T. Hydroxyzine and cetirizine pharmacokinetics and pharmacodynamics after oral and intravenous administration of hydroxyzine to healthy dogs. *Vet Dermatol* 2008; 19: 348–357.
5. Temizel EM, Cihan H, Akhtardanesh B *et al.* Effect of prednisolone and cetirizine on D. farinae and histamine-induced wheal and flare response in healthy dogs. *Tierarztl Prax Ausg Kleintiere Heimtiere* 2011; 39: 25–30.
6. Hickey GJ, Chang CH, Marsilio F *et al.* Effects of prednisone on dermal responses in flea-allergen hypersensitive dogs. *Vet Dermatol* 1993; 4: 71–77.
7. Kunkle G, Hillier A, Beale K *et al.* Steroid effects on intradermal skin testing in sensitized dogs. In: *Proceedings of the American Academy of Veterinary Dermatology & American College of Veterinary Dermatology*. ACVD, Charleston, SC: 1994; 54–55.
8. Clarke K, McCall C, Steffan J *et al.* The effects of ciclosporin A and oral prednisolone on flea allergen specific serum IgE and intradermal tests in experimentally sensitized laboratory beagles. *Vet Dermatol* 2003; 14: 248 [abstract].
9. Pucheu-Haston CM, Shuster D, Olivry T *et al.* A canine model of cutaneous late-phase reactions: Prednisolone inhibition of cellular and cytokine responses. *Immunology* 2006; 117: 177–187.
10. Clarke KB, Bevier DE, Radecki SV *et al.* The effects of corticosteroid treatment on anti-flea saliva IgE, as measured by intradermal

skin test and ELISA, in laboratory beagles with experimentally induced flea allergy dermatitis. *Vet Dermatol* 2000; 11 (Suppl. 1): 50 [abstract].

11. Thomas RC, Logas D, Radosta L *et al.* Effects of a 1% hydrocortisone conditioner on haematological and biochemical parameters, adrenal function testing and cutaneous reactivity to histamine in normal and pruritic dogs. *Vet Dermatol* 1999; 10: 109–116.
12. Rivierre C, Dunston SM, Olivry T. Effects of a 1 per cent hydrocortisone conditioner on the prevention of immediate and late phase reactions in canine skin. *Vet Rec* 2000; 147: 739–742.
13. Bizikova P, Linder KE, Paps JS *et al.* Effect of a novel topical diester glucocorticoid spray on immediate and late phase cutaneous allergic reactions in maltese-beagle atopic dogs: A placebo-controlled study. *Vet Dermatol* 2010; 21: 70–79.
14. Olivry T, Bizikova P, Paps JS. Comparative inhibition of intradermal skin test immediate reactions by topical glucocorticoid-containing sprays in atopic dogs *Vet Dermatol* 2010; 21: 323 [abstract].
15. Ginel PJ, Garrido C, Lucena R. Effects of otic betamethasone on intradermal testing in normal dogs. *Vet Dermatol* 2007; 18: 205–210.
16. Murphy KM, Olivry T. The influence of Mometamax (mometasone furoate) on intradermal test immediate reactions in atopic dogs. *Vet Dermatol* 2009; 20: 226 [abstract].
17. Burton G, Robson D, Bassett R *et al.* A pilot trial on the effect of cyclosporin A on intradermal test reactions in dogs with atopic dermatitis. *Vet Dermatol* 2002; 13: 222 [abstract].
18. Goldman C, Rosser EJ, Petersen A *et al.* Investigation on the effects of ciclosporin (Atopica) on intradermal test reactivity and allergen-specific immunoglobulin (IgE) serology in atopic dogs. *Vet Dermatol* 2010; 21: 393–399.
19. Brazis P, Barandica L, Garcia F *et al.* Dermal microdialysis in the dog: In vivo assessment of the effect of cyclosporin A on cutaneous histamine and prostaglandin D2 release. *Vet Dermatol* 2006; 17: 169–174.
20. Marsella R, Nicklin CF, Saglio S *et al.* Investigation on the effects of topical therapy with 0.1% tacrolimus ointment (Protopic) on intradermal skin test reactivity in atopic dogs. *Vet Dermatol* 2004; 15: 218–224.
21. Marsella R, Nicklin CF. Double-blinded cross-over study on the efficacy of pentoxifylline for canine atopy. *Vet Dermatol* 2000; 11: 255–260.
22. Marsella R, Kunkle GA, Vaughn DM *et al.* Double-blind pilot study on the effects of ketoconazole on intradermal skin test and leukotriene C4 concentration in the skin of atopic dogs. *Vet Dermatol* 1997; 8: 3–10.
23. Bond R, Lloyd DH, Craig M. The effects of essential fatty acid supplementation on intradermal test reactivity in atopic dogs: A preliminary study. *Vet Dermatol* 1993; 4: 191–197.
24. Miller WH, Scott DW, Cayatte SM *et al.* The influence of oral corticosteroids or declining allergen exposure on serologic allergy test results. *Vet Dermatol* 1992; 3: 237–244.
25. Hensel P, Austel M, Medleau L *et al.* Determination of threshold concentrations of allergens and evaluation of two different histamine concentrations in canine intradermal testing. *Vet Dermatol* 2004; 15: 304–308.
26. Bauer CL, Hensel P, Austel M *et al.* Determination of irritant threshold concentrations of six mites through serial dilutions in intradermal testing on healthy clinically non-allergic dogs. *Vet Dermatol* 2009; 20: 227 [abstract].
27. Lian TM, Halliwell REW. Allergen-specific IgE and IgGd antibodies in atopic and normal dogs. *Vet Immunol Immunopathol* 1998; 66: 203–223.
28. Olivry T, Judy P. Evaluation of the agreement between allergen-specific intradermal or IgE serological tests and a point-of-care immunodot assay in dogs with atopic dermatitis. *Vet Dermatol* 2011; 22: 284–285.

8.11

Epidermal barrier function

K. Nishifuji[1] (Chairperson), P. Bizikova[2] (Secretary)

[1]Tokyo University of Agriculture of Technology, Department of Veterinary Medicine, Tokyo, Japan
[2]North Carolina State University, College of Veterinary Medicine, North Carolina, USA

Koji Nishifuji (*Japan*) thanked Sogeval for sponsoring this workshop and expressed his appreciation to all contributing speakers as well as to attendees. He then provided an overview of this workshop on the skin barrier, its structure, function and role in different diseases, particularly in canine atopic dermatitis.

Antimicrobial skin barrier in canine atopic dermatitis: how much do we really know? (D. Santoro)

Domenico Santoro (*USA*) remarked that only a small amount of information about antimicrobial peptides (AMPs) is available in veterinary dermatology compared to human dermatology. He therefore chose to present an overview of current knowledge about AMPs in animals. Antimicrobial peptides are small cationic proteins and, so far, 1500 AMPs have been described in different species. The most studied groups include defensins alpha, beta and theta; the greatest focus is on beta-defensins, cathelicidins and S100 proteins. AMPs are predominantly localized in the epithelia including skin, mucosae, testes and eyes, where they serve as defence mechanisms against environmental pathogens. They are also involved in toxin neutralization, function as chemokines, serve as a bridge between innate and adaptive immunity, and are involved in wound healing and skin colour.

He commented that the audience might be asking 'what is known about beta-defensins and canine atopic dermatitis?' Last year, using a canine atopic dermatitis model, Domenico Santoro and colleagues were able to demonstrate significant increase in mRNA expression of two different beta-defensins (cBD1 and cBD3) as well as cathelicidin in an acute lesional skin of beagles with an experimentally induced atopic dermatitis compared to healthy dogs.[1] However, when the expression was analysed over time, there was decreased expression of these beta-defensins in the lesional skin of the same beagles, although this was not significant. Protein expression measured by a competitive inhibition ELISA on protein extracts from the same dogs showed reduction of measured beta-defensins (cBD3), which was similar to reports from human literature.

Only a couple of studies have addressed the relationship between AMPs and chronic atopic dermatitis. van Damme and colleagues showed decreased expression of cBD103 in skin of dogs with chronic atopic dermatitis compared to healthy control dogs, while cBD1 was increased in affected dogs compared to controls.[2] During this meeting, Domenico Santoro and colleagues presented results from a study that evaluated the expression of AMPs in canine atopic skin using similar conditions as those described in van Damme's study.[3] In this study, the authors demonstrated increased cBD103 mRNA expression in the skin of chronic atopic dermatitis dogs versus healthy controls and also higher cBD103 expression in skin of atopic dogs with skin infection versus atopic dogs without an infection. The opposite findings were obtained for the cBD1-like mRNA expression. At the protein level, no significant differences were seen between atopic and healthy dogs.

For cathelicidin, mRNA expression in the skin of dogs with chronic atopic dermatitis was decreased compared to levels in the skin of healthy dogs – a contrasting finding to that reported for the skin of beagles with an experimentally induced acute atopic dermatitis.[3]

Finally, van Damme *et al.* reported a significant increase in the mRNA levels of S100A7 protein in the lesion and nonlesional skin of atopic dogs compared to healthy controls.[2]

Recently, Torres *et al.* reported the mRNA expression levels of other two AMPs, SKALP and SLPI, which appeared to be decreased in atopic dogs compared to healthy controls.[4]

In summary, although the results are controversial, it appears that the skin of dogs with an acute atopic dermatitis over-expresses some of the AMPs (cBD1-like, cBD3-like, cathelicidin), although data for cBD103 and cBD3 in acute atopic dermatitis are not currently available. Furthermore, older dogs have higher expression of AMPs than young dogs, a feature also reported in humans. In the skin of dogs with chronic atopic dermatitis, mRNA levels of cBD1 were shown to be increased, while cBD103 levels have been shown to be reduced[2] or increased.[3] The difference between these two studies could be explained by a difference in the age of the dogs, localization of the biopsy site, use of topical or systemic antimicrobials, or other factors.[2,3]

Several unanswered questions could be listed. For example, which AMP is critical in protection of the skin against bacteria? Is there an effect of antibiotics and immunomodulatory drugs on the production of these AMPs? Is the correct ratio of AMPs the critical factor protecting the skin from infection?

Koji Nishifuji asked for clarification of whether the expression of cBD1 and cBD3 is increased in acute atopic dermatitis skin lesions while cBD2 expression is not.

Domenico Santoro confirmed that cBD2 expression was not increased.

Koji Nishifuji asked whether there is a difference in the expression of these molecules in relation to the different body areas.

Domenico Santoro replied there probably is, although he was not aware of any published study in animals. In human dermatology, however, it has been demonstrated that there are large differences in the expression of AMPs in different body areas. Higher expression has been shown in areas exposed to the environment (e.g. forehead, palms, feet). Therefore, it is possible that his data could have been different if he had collected samples from other areas such as the interdigital skin.

Koji Nishifuji asked if there is any difference in the function of cBD1, cBD2 and cBD3.

Domenico Santoro answered that this has not yet been determined, although his research group is currently working on experiments that test immunological and antimicrobial functions of different AMPs. The problem is that some AMPs such as cBD1-like, cBD2-like and cBD3-like molecules have very similar, often overlapping amino acid sequences as exemplified by the cBD2/122 group. This makes it difficult to design a unique peptide to test an individual AMP. He is currently working with cBD103 and some other members of the cBD2 group.

Christoph Klinger (*Germany*) asked if Domenico Santoro had any knowledge about different drugs affecting the expression of AMPs, such as the speculation about ciclosporin's positive effect on beta-defensins and maybe cathelicidins.

Domenico Santoro replied that drugs do affect AMPs and that in humans, tacrolimus and ciclosporin have been shown to increase the expression of AMPs, while steroids appear to inhibit the expression of these proteins. Also, stress seems to inhibit the production of AMPs. On the other hand, vitamin D_3 has recently been discussed as a strong stimulator of cathelicidin and human beta-defensin 2 (hBD2) expression. One must be careful, however, as most of the beta-defensins studied in dogs are not true orthologs of those described in humans. The only one is cBD103, which is the ortholog of hBD3. There are studies in progress that look at different drugs and cytokines and their effect on keratinocyte expression of AMPs.

Changes in epidermal ceramides in canine atopic dermatitis (J.S. Yoon)

Ji Seon Yoon (*South Korea*) reviewed the functions of ceramides in the stratum corneum in maintaining the epidermal barrier function. The molecular structure of ceramides consists of sphingosine linked to fatty acids. In the stratum corneum, ceramides are present in extracellular spaces with other lipids. These extracellular lamellar lipids are important contributors to barrier function and maintain skin hydration. If ceramide content is decreased in the stratum corneum, transepidermal water loss as well as penetration of allergens or microbes are increased.

Recently her group reported that the stratum corneum of dogs contains 11 free ceramide classes, a finding similar to that reported in humans. The classes depend on the ceramide composition in which the following molecules play a critical role: sphingosine, dihydrosphingosine, phytosphingosine, 6-hydroxyl-sphingosine, and non-hydroxylated-, alpha-hydroxylated and omega-hydroxylated fatty acids.[5]

Abnormalities of ceramides in the skin of people with atopic dermatitis have been intensely studied. Studies have shown that quantities (μg/mg of protein) of the ceramides EOS (combination of omega-hydroxy fatty acids and sphingosines), EOP (combination of omega-hydroxy fatty acids and phytosphingosines), NP (combination of non-hydroxy fatty acids and phytosphingosines) and NS (combination of non-hydroxy fatty acids and sphingosines) are decreased in humans with atopic dermatitis.

In veterinary medicine, the proportions of ceramides, cholesterol and free fatty acids have been analysed in healthy dogs and dogs with atopic dermatitis.[6] This study demonstrated that the proportion of ceramides in lesional and nonlesional skin of dogs with atopic dermatitis is significantly lower than in healthy controls. Furthermore, Reiter *et al.* reported that the proportion of free extractable ceramides 1 and 9 was lower in nonlesional skin of dogs with atopic dermatitis than in that from breed- and age-matched controls.[6] Meanwhile Ji Seon Yoon's group reported negative correlation between transepidermal water loss (TEWL) and the total fraction of free ceramides in the stratum corneum lipids.[5]

The main goal of Ji Seon Yoon's most recent study was to compare the quantities of ceramide classes in the stratum corneum of dogs with atopic dermatitis and healthy age- and breed-matched dogs.[5] Ten dogs were included in each group. The stratum corneum was collected from the inguinal region using tape-stripping. The lipids from the stratum corneum were extracted with chloroform-methanol treatment. The lipids were then separated using high-performance thin-layer chromatogaphy (HPTLC), which enabled detection of eight ceramide bands. In healthy dogs, there were six strong bands and two weaker bands. These eight bands were assigned as: (i) EOS; (ii) mixture of NDS (combination of non-hydroxy fatty acids and dihydrosphingosine) and NS; (iii) EOP; (iv) NP; (v) EOH (combination of omega-hydroxy fatty acids and 6-hydroxylsphingosines); (vi) mixture of AS (combination of alpha-hydroxy fatty acids and sphingosines) and NH (combination of non-hydroxy fatty acids and 6-hydroxylsphingosines); (vii) AP (combination of alpha-hydroxy fatty acids and phytosphingosines); and (viii) AH (combination of alpha-hydroxy fatty acids and 6-hydroxylsphingosines). The quantities of total ceramides were significantly lower in lesional and nonlesional skin of dogs with atopic dermatitis compared to those in healthy controls. More specifically, quantities of ceramides EOS, EOP, NS+NDS, NP and AS+NH were significantly lower in lesional and nonlesional skin of dogs with atopic dermatitis than in healthy controls.[5] This deficit may lead to impaired barrier function of the skin in dogs with atopic dermatitis.

Ralf Mueller (*Germany*) asked which site(s) were biopsied.

Ji Seon Yoon responded that all samples were taken from an inguinal area.

Catherine Correa (*USA*) asked how samples were normalized to milligrammes of stratum corneum.

Ji Seon Yoon explained that the stratum corneum was put on a filter paper and the weight was measured.

Catherine Correa (*USA*) commented that in people, differences are found in ceramide amounts in lesional versus nonlesional skin. However, Ji Seon Young's group found similar amounts in atopic dog skin regardless of the site. She asked if there are any ideas why dogs with atopic dermatitis are different from humans.

Ji Seon Yoon replied that she does not know.

Catherine Correa asked whether cholesterol and free fatty acids were measured, and if so, whether any differences were found in these two parameters.

Ji Seon Yoon responded that these were not measured in the current study. However, in a previous study they measured proportions of cholesterol and free fatty acids and they did not find any significant differences in cholesterol and free fatty acids between dogs with atopic dermatitis and healthy controls. They were looking at relative amounts and did not compare the actual quantities.

Thierry Olivry (*USA*) commented that his research group has a poster at this meeting of a study performed with Dr Baumer's group (*Germany*) in which ceramides in the stratum corneum were measured before inflammation and after house dust mite-induced inflammation. Samples were taken at the site of inflammation and at a distant (noninflamed) site. The ceramides decreased at the site of the application of house dust mites as well as at the distant site and these changes resolved after the inflammation ceased. So the changes reported in this study are possibly the consequence of the inflammation in these dogs with atopic dermatitis rather than a primary barrier defect.

Koji Nishifuji commented that more studies are definitely needed before we can say whether these findings reflect primary or secondary defects in dogs with atopic dermatitis.

Looking at the stratum corneum barrier function through ichthyosis (E. Guaguere and C. Andre)

Eric Guaguere (*France*) provided an overview of studies on canine ichthyosis and the linkage to the barrier function disruption. There are very few of these studies. In general, ichthyosis represents a heterogeneous group of cornification disorders. Different forms of ichthyosis present clinically with a scaling skin thickening and/or fissures, with an onset at birth. Ichthyosis has been described in humans, dogs, cattle, kudu and llama. A recently published classification of human ichthyoses focuses on clinical signs and its genetic correlates, and it also separates ichthyoses into syndromic and nonsyndromic ichthyoses as well as keratinopathic forms caused by mutations in keratins.[7]

The diversity of the ichthyosis forms and mutations reflects the complex nature of the processes involved in skin barrier formation and function. To date approximately 40 genes have been identified that are involved in human ichthyosis. Excellent recent reviews on this topic can be found in the literature.[7]

Skin barrier dysfunction is caused by abnormalities of the architecture of the extracellular spaces of the stratum corneum – changes that could reflect abnormal lipid metabolism or defects in structural proteins of keratinocytes that impede lipid metabolism. For example, X-linked recessive ichthyosis is caused by mutation of the steroid sulfatase gene (*STS*). The enzyme is localized in cytosol as well as in lamellar bodies, and it is responsible for metabolism of cholesterol sulphate into cholesterol. As a result of this mutation, cholesterol sulphate accumulates in the stratum corneum, which leads to a defect in barrier function and increased permeability of the stratum corneum. Desquamation is dependent on this transformation and accumulation of cholesterol sulphate leads to increase in cornification, cornified envelope production, retention of corneodesmosins and so forth.

At the present time, four genes have been implicated in canine ichthyoses: keratin 10 (*K10*) in Norfolk terriers, transglutaminase 1 (*TGM1*) in Jack Russell terriers, patatin-like phospholipase domain-containing protein 1 (*PNPLA1*) in golden retrievers and *FAM83H* in cavalier King Charles spaniels.[8–11] The effect of these mutations on the skin barrier can be demonstrated by the following examples. A mutation in *K10* in Norfolk terriers leads to altered release of lamellar bodies, decreased exocytosis and reduced amount of intercellular lipid deposits, which are subsequently associated with increased TEWL. A mutation in the *TGM1* gene in (Parson) Jack Russell terriers affects the activity of an enzyme that is critical in the development of cornified envelope. In addition, TGM1 helps to cross-link lipids to the cornified envelope. Hence, a defect in TGM1 function leads to an abnormal formation of cornified envelope accompanied by increased permeability and TEWL. Recently, a lamellar ichthyosis has been described in golden retrievers.[10,12] In these patients, prominent scaling and 'paper' skin have been described.

Catherine Andre (*France*) reported that a new mutation affecting the *PNPLA1* gene has been identified to be the cause of this ichthyosis in golden retrievers.[10] Subsequently, a mutation in the same gene was linked to an ichthyosis in two human families. In these two families, the mutations involved the catalytic domain of the protein, suggesting that these mutations affect the functionality of the protein, which likely results in the clinical signs of disease. In addition, humans with this disease exhibit similar features to those described in affected dogs. Specifically, cholesterol crystals are present in the stratum corneum and abnormal membranes are found in the cytoplasm of keratinocytes. The localization of the mutated PNPLA1 protein was assessed by immunofluorescence and confocal microscopy, which showed that the protein is localized at the lower level of the cornified layer; this was confirmed further by dual immunofluorescence showing a co-localization of the PNPLA1 with filaggrin. As this protein belongs to a group of proteins with lipolytic function, the lipid profiles were also examined. Lipid profiles in human samples demonstrated that triglyceride metabolism was not affected in humans with mutated PNPL1, but possibly this protein could be involved in glycerophospholipid metabolism. Andre's group will continue working on this to further uncover the pathomechanism.

Eric Guaguere commented that management of patients with ichthyosis is complex and focuses on maintaining sufficient hydration, restoring the skin barrier function and removal of scales. Prognoses of different forms of ichthyoses are variable, depending on the type and severity (e.g. ichthyosis of golden retrievers vs ichthyosis of Jack Russell terriers). Keratolytic and keratoplastic shampoos every 2–3 days for a month and then weekly are usually prescribed, although the frequency depends on the severity of the disease. Use of humectants is important. Systemic treatment (e.g. isotretinoin, acitretin) of ichthyosis is restricted to severe cases or cases refractory to topical therapy, and the side effects and cost should be discussed with the owner. Lipid-rich diets constitute an additional management option that is chosen by many owners. However, controlled studies have not been performed to assess the efficacy of any of the above-mentioned treatments.

Koji Nishifuji asked whether the 74 amino acids at the C-terminus of the PNPLA1 contains a critical motif for glycophospholipid enzymatic activity.

Catherine Andre replied that in dogs, the mutation is at the 3′-end, so at the N-terminal. The mutation removes 74 amino acids, so because the protein is not disrupted completely it could still retain some function. There is another PNPLA protein, specifically PNPLA2, and a mutation of this gene will lead to myopathy with several different problems including, for example, heart failure. The gene of this protein also has a mutation towards the C-terminus, an area shown to be important to fix protein to lipid vacuoles. After this fixation, the protein can act as an enzyme.

Changes in the profiles of genes associated with cutaneous barrier function in atopic beagles (R.S. Mueller)

Ralf Mueller (*Germany*) reported that the aim of this study was to identify changes in gene expression in the skin of dogs sensitized to house dust mites (dogs provided by Novartis). For this purpose, the skin tissue was collected from the site of a patch test and from normal skin of sensitized dogs and compared to healthy controls of the same breed in which biopsies were collected from identical sites. Twelve beagles were selected for this study; six were sensitized for *Dermatophagoides farinae* and six were healthy, nonsensitized dogs. Hair was clipped from all dogs 5 days before the experiments, and skin biopsies were collected 1 day before the challenge with the allergen and then again 6 and 24 hours after the allergen challenge. The collected tissues were used for a gene microarray and also histologically assessed for number of inflammatory cells per area. In addition, polymerase chain reaction (PCR) was used to verify the results obtained from the microarray. The microarray data were normalized to minimize the variations caused by multiple external and processing factors.

There was no significant difference between the gene expression profiles of normal and allergic dogs before the challenge. There was a downregulation of genes related to skin barrier function after allergen exposure in the allergic beagles versus normal dogs, in which these genes were slightly upregulated upon the allergen challenge. Nothing significant was observed when saline was used. In contrast, there was an upregulation of genes involved in inflammation in allergic dogs after allergen exposure, while in normal dogs these genes appeared to be downregulated, suggesting that a regulatory component predominates the immune response to the house dust mites.

The next steps should assess whether the DNA data match the actual protein expression and whether the observed changes were only characteristic for sensitized beagles or whether they could be applied to other breeds and natural atopic disease as well.

Overall, these data suggest that allergen exposure in sensitized dogs leads to inflammation and barrier dysfunction. Hence our treatment approach should try to repair both components, and that, at least in these settings, both changes appeared secondary after the challenge.

Rosanna Marsella (*USA*) asked for clarification whether these beagles, which are sensitized against house dust mites, manifest clinical disease compatible with atopic dermatitis.

Ralf Mueller replied that these dogs do have reactions at the site of a patch test, but to his knowledge, a full environmental challenge assessing clinical signs of atopic dermatitis has not been done.

Rosanna Marsella stated that she believes it is important to perform this kind of test on dogs with natural disease to obtain a better idea of which changes are primary versus secondary.

Ralf Mueller agreed that these are valid points, and studies on a large number of dogs of one breed with atopic dermatitis, like those recently performed in Europe and the USA, could provide additional answers. However, models like the one he used do show what changes can be expected just with sensitization with an allergen per se. This allows the assessment of changes in gene expression on the background of, so to speak, a normal genome.

Rosanna Marsella commented that we could potentially breed dogs that are easy to sensitize, collect samples when they are young (compare them to normal breed-/age-matched dogs) and then sensitize them and collect new samples to observe the changes.

Veterinary drugs affecting cutaneous barrier function in dogs (R. Marsella)

Rosanna Marsella (*USA*) stated that she planned to review a few recent studies that focused on skin barrier repair. These studies involved products that are available to veterinary dermatologists, including phytosphingosine- and ceramide-containing products.

The first study with phytosphingosine assessed the ability of this product to repair skin barrier damage in healthy dogs in which tape-stripping had been performed to simulate a barrier disruption. These dogs had 18 squares clipped on both sides of the lateral thorax and half of these spots were damaged by tape-stripping. The damaged and nondamaged areas were then divided into three groups, in which three areas were left untreated, three were treated with a phytosphingosine-containing product and three were treated with a vehicle. The study was performed in a randomized, double-blinded fashion. The treatments were done three times per week using 0.25 mL of solution per site, and TEWL was measured by a closed-chamber device. On the days when the animals were treated, the TEWL measurement was performed immediately before the application of the solutions. The dogs were followed up for 2 weeks.

The tape-stripping significantly increased TEWL. When analysis was focused only at the tape-stripped areas, no significant difference was detected between areas treated with the phytosphingosine-containing product versus the vehicle. The lack of significance could have been due to a positive effect of the vehicle on the skin barrier or because of the high variability of the measurements.

In a subsequent small pilot study, atopic as well as healthy dogs were used to test a product that is not commercially available, composed of phytosphingosine mixed in paraffin. The dogs were divided into groups, each containing one healthy and three atopic dogs. All dogs were housed in the same building. The treated dogs were assessed for the lesion severity using CADESI-3, TEWL was measured, and biopsies were taken for electron microscopy. This study was prospective and blinded. No appreciable improvement of clinical signs was detected. The TEWL was variable among the dogs; in some dogs the TEWL increased further while in some the TEWL remained unchanged. In terms of the microscopic changes, a flattening of the corneocytes was observed in treated animals. The stratum corneum became more compact and an increased number of corneodesmosomes was seen. These changes, however, were seen in the group treated with the phytosphingosine/paraffin compound as well as in the paraffin-only group, although these changes were not as pronounced in the latter group. Healthy dogs did not change much.

No major conclusions could be drawn from this study because of the small sample size and a high variability in some parameters. In the future, Rosanna Marsella's research group would like to conduct another study with the commercially available phytosphingosine product used in the first study, and look at the electron microscopy changes in real patients.

The final study was performed in normal dogs following skin barrier disruption created by tape-stripping. The TEWL was measured as mentioned before. In this particular study, the number of tape strips corresponded to the number needed to double the original TEWL. The dogs were treated with a ceramide-containing product, Allerderm Spot-On® (Virbac), on one area while the other area remained untreated. The treatment was applied in blinded fashion.

No significant improvement in TEWL was detected after a single application of this product on the tape-stripped skin of healthy dogs. It is possible that repeated application of this product is needed to achieve some changes, as was shown in studies looking at the clinical signs. Clearly, this suggests that longer duration studies involving more subjects will be required to assess the efficacy of such products in skin barrier restoration.

Koji Nishifuji concluded the workshop by commenting that although these products may not restore the epidermal barrier as we would wish, they may still help maintain the barrier in better condition and thereby help prevent other diseases.

References

1. Santoro D, Marsella R, Bunick D *et al.* Expression and distribution of canine antimicrobial peptides in the skin of healthy and atopic beagles. *Vet Immunol Immunopathol* 2011; 144: 382–388.
2. van Damme CM, Willemse T, van Dijk A *et al.* Altered cutaneous expression of beta-defensins in dogs with atopic dermatitis. *Mol Immunol* 2009; 46: 2449–2455.
3. Santoro D, Bunic D, Graves T *et al.* Evaluation of canine antimicrobial peptides in infected and non-infected chronic atopic skin. *Vet Dermatol* 2012; 23 (Suppl. 1): 2.
4. Torres S, Lancto C, Koch S *et al.* Comparative expression of antimicrobial peptides in lesional and nonlesional skin of dogs with atopic dermatitis. *Vet Dermatol* 2011; 22: 289.
5. Yoon J, Yoshihara T, Sasaki A *et al.* Alteration of stratum corneum ceramide profiles in spontaneous canine model of atopic dermatitis. *Exp Dermatol* 2011 [Epub ahead of print].
6. Reiter LV, Torres SM, Wertz PW. Characterization and quantification of ceramides in the nonlesional skin of canine patients with atopic dermatitis compared with controls. *Vet Dermatol* 2009; 20: 260–266.

7. Oji V, Tadini G, Akiyama M *et al.* Revised nomenclature and classification of inherited ichthyoses: Results of the first ichthyosis consensus conference in Soreze 2009. *J Am Acad Dermatol* 2010; 63: 607–641.
8. Credille KM, Barnhart KF, Minor JS *et al.* Mild recessive epidermolytic hyperkeratosis associated with a novel keratin 10 donor splice-site mutation in a family of Norfolk terrier dogs. *Br J Dermatol* 2005; 153: 51—58.
9. Credille KM, Minor JS, Barnhart KF *et al.* Transglutaminase 1-deficient recessive lamellar ichthyosis associated with a LINE-1 insertion in jack russell terrier dogs. *Br J Dermatol* 2009; 161: 265–272.
10. Grall A, Guaguere E, Planchais S *et al.* PNPLA1 mutations cause autosomal recessive congenital ichthyosis in golden retriever dogs and humans. *Nat Genet* 2012; 44: 140–147.
11. Forman OP, Penderis J, Hartley C *et al.* Parallel mapping and simultaneous sequencing reveals deletions in BCAN and FAM83H associated with discrete inherited disorders in a domestic dog breed. *PLoS Genet* 2012; 8: e1002462.
12. Cadiergues MC, Patel A, Shearer DH *et al.* Cornification defect in the golden retriever: Clinical, histopathological, ultrastructural and genetic characterisation. *Vet Dermatol* 2008; 19: 120–129.

8.12

The changing faces of parasite control

C. Taylor[1] (Chairperson), K. Glos[2] (Secretary)

[1]Cutaneous Ltd, 10 Ping Tun Village, Sai Kung, Hong Kong
[2]Specialty Clinic Haas & Link, Industriestr. 6, Munich, Germany

Carmel Taylor (*Hong Kong*) gave a brief introduction to the session, pointing out that the session was to be recorded, and acknowledged the support of the sponsor for the session, Merck Animal Health. She mentioned that two new antiparasitical products, Seresto® from Bayer (flumethrin + imidacloprid) and Activyl® (indoxacarb), a proinsecticide by Merck, would be included in the discussions. Carmel Taylor introduced the five discussion topics for the workshop and their contributors.

The use of permethrin spot-on formulations in dogs (M. Kietzmann)

Manfred Kietzmann (Germany) introduced a study he had performed in collaboration with parasitologists evaluating the distribution of permethrin in spot-on formulations and flumethrin incorporated in a collar (Seresto®) over the body surface of dogs, the effects of excipients, and the duration of antiparasitic (repellent) effects. He gave a short introduction on the structure and function of the epidermis. He discussed the three excipients in highly concentrated permethrin formulations: isopropyl myristate, *N*-methylpyrrolidone and propylene glycol with or without methyl ether. An *in vitro* study[1] demonstrated diffusion of permethrin into the deeper layers of the skin, but no significant systemic absorption in dogs (in contrast to cats). Another *in vivo*, cross-over study[2] in beagle dogs looked at the distribution on the body surface, persistence on the skin and the efficacy against Dermacentor reticulatus ticks. In this study, ticks were placed on the dorsal back, close to the treatment area, and on the legs, a site distant from the treatment area. Test formulations were Exspot® (Virbac: permethrin), Preventic® (Virbac: permethrin), Fletic® (permethrin) and Advantix® (Bayer Animal Health: permethrin + imidacloprid). At day 1 all ticks died, and after 2 and 3 weeks, in the face of further infestation, only a few ticks were attached on the legs and backs of the dogs, showing that the permethrin maintained some effectiveness over a 2–3-week period. No significant differences in distribution and efficacy were found between the different products/formulations. Permethrin was distributed rapidly (within 24 hours) over the whole body surface. This distribution was not via the hairs (concentrations in hair are high near treatment area and low at distant sites), but possibly via the horny layer (tape stripping showed a decline in concentration within the stratum corneum over time). This demonstrated the importance of the stratum corneum for the distribution over the body surface. Manfred Kietzmann commented that Seresto® collar from Bayer takes more than 1 day to release its compound flumethrin. He cited preliminary results of another study being performed by a colleague that demonstrated a significantly longer duration of action of the flumethrin (study in progress, currently exceeding 5 months).

Gila Zur (*Israel*) asked about general recommendations for use of flea control products on seborrhoeic dogs with a higher epidermal turnover rate and also for dogs with severe flea allergy.

Manfred Kietzmann replied that the advantage of the permethrin formulations is the repellent effect. In actual parasitoses drugs with immediate onset of action would be needed and, thereafter, permethrin-containing spot-ons or collars could be utilized. He had no data regarding effects of seborrhoea.

Amit Ranjan (*Canada*) asked about the onset of action after application of the Seresto® collar.

Manfred Kietzmann answered that the study found an onset of activity 1 day after application, but shorter periods were not studied. However, there are large variations between individuals. One important factor is the hair coat, as the drug is distributed via the lipophilic horny layer and then via the sebum on the hairs. Therefore, long-haired dogs need more of the compound to get the repellent effect than short-haired breeds.

Luisa Cornegliani (*Italy*) asked about the impact of shampoos used in atopic dogs on the length of action of antiparasitic products.

Manfred Kietzmann replied that more studies would be needed but that in his opinion the time of contact of shampoos with skin is relatively low; however, more frequent administration might be needed. He mentioned studies performed with benzoyl peroxide where no further parasiticide activity was observed after 2–4 weeks, and commented that the flumethrin collar is a good option for animals requiring frequent bathing.

Helena Vaynberg (*USA*) asked whether different recommendations should be made by manufacturers for use of parasiticides on long-haired dogs.

Manfred Kietzmann stated that there is limited information on distribution effects of insecticides in different hair coat types. Further studies would be needed.

The chairperson introduced Richard Malik as the next speaker.

Permethrin intoxication in cats (R. Malik)

Richard Malik (*Australia*) spoke about the pharmacology of permethrin and commented that it is not really known why permethrin is toxic for cats. He described the clinical signs of permethrin toxicity in cats. He pointed out that in many supermarkets, dog and cat ectoparasiticides are next to each other, that many permethrin-containing products have only small warning icons for cats, and there were often no further 'warning icons' once the packet was opened. He mentioned that additionally cat products are often more expensive and, therefore, cat owners might spuriously buy permethrin-containing dog products. He emphasized that no over-the-counter product prominently warns of secondary toxicity due to contact, which can occur through direct contact of cats with dogs, through grooming (licking) of the dog by the companion cat, or through shared brushes or combs. There are no indications of what is the safe period of time that cats should be kept separated from dogs following product application. He then spoke about published data from a survey of veterinarians performed in Australia.[3] Two hundred and fifty-five of the approximately 7000 veterinarians responding reported 207 cases of permethrin intoxications. The study revealed that 750 cats were intoxicated over a 2-year period over all states of Australia. The main sources of intoxication were permethrin spot-on products from supermarkets (146) and pet stores (43), although veterinary products with good labelling additionally caused intoxications. In total, 166 deaths due to intoxication (127) or inability to pay for the treatment (39) occurred. Richard Malik pointed out that those figures are very likely a substantial underestimation of permethrin intoxication in cats, because many cats die before getting to a veterinarian, and many veterinarians had not replied to the survey.

Richard Malik advocates larger and more radical warning labels on permethrin-containing products and limiting distribution of permethrin-containing products to veterinarians only.

Gila Zur asked about the toxicity of permethrin when dogs and cats physically play together.

Richard Malik responded that once the spot-on has dried, most of the permethrin is bound and, therefore, manufacturers advise 8–12 hours of no contact time between dogs and cats immediately following the spot-on application.

Manfred Kietzmann stated that statistics from permethrin-induced deaths or intoxicated cats are available from different countries in Europe. In all countries where the drug is not sold by veterinarians the number of dying or intoxicated cats is significantly higher than in countries where permethrin is available only by prescription. He indicated that all other attempts, including better labelling, have not succeeded in preventing cat deaths.

Richard Malik agreed with this.

The chairperson then introduced Ursula Oberkirchner as the next speaker.

Recent and potential future challenges for veterinary dermatologists arising from 'benign' topical flea preventatives (U. Oberkirchner)

Ursula Oberkirchner (*USA*) presented a study[4] on pemphigus-like reactions in 22 dogs associated with Promeris-Duo®/Promeris® Spot-on Solution for Dogs (Pfizer Animal Health) (metaflumizone + amitraz). She mentioned that in previous safety and efficacy studies of Promeris-Duo®/Promeris® for dogs, problems such as focal skin lesions on the base of the neck and ears in several dogs,[5] and hyperpigmentation, matting of hairs and scales in 6/293 dogs (2%) at application sites were reported.[6] In addition, 1/24 (4%) dogs developed pemphigus foliaceus (PF) at the application site in a demodicosis treatment trial (W. Rosenkrantz, personal communication, 2009). In Oberkirchner's study,[4] dogs were divided into a localized group (lesions at the application site) and a distant group (lesions at the application site and also at a distant site such as ears, nose and/or footpads). In most cases, lesions developed within 14 days of application and the majority of dogs were female large-breed dogs. Lesions developed during use of the first package of Promeris-Duo®/Promeris® for dogs in 50% of the localized group and in 79% of the distant group. Systemic signs were seen in 38% of the localized group (lethargy, pain and lameness) and in 79% of the distant group (lethargy, lameness and fever). Immunosuppressive therapy was prescribed for 38% of the localized group with a duration of 2–14 months (average 8 months), and prescribed for 79% of the distant group with a duration of 1–16 months (average 5 months). She pointed out that some of these dogs may still be on treatment. Complete remission was achieved in 100% and 77% of the localized and distant groups, respectively.

Ursula Oberkirchner discussed whether these reactions were drug-induced or drug-triggered PF. To help determine this, direct (dIF) and indirect (iIF) immunofluorescence was performed. In dIF, skin-fixed antikeratinocyte IgG autoantibodies were found in 14/21 (67%) of the samples: 4/8 (50%) in the localized and 10/13 (77%) in the distant group. Using iIF, 6/14 (43%) samples showed circulating antikeratinocyte IgG autoantibodies: 0/4 (0%) in the localized and 6/10 (60%) in the distant group. This led to the assumption that Promeris-Duo®-associated reactions are likely a contact drug-triggered PF because affected dogs continued to need medical therapy after withdrawal of the Promeris-Duo®.

Ursula Oberkirchner discussed the question of exactly which ingredient in the Promeris-Duo® could have triggered the antibody production and subsequent acantholysis. Could it have been the metaflumizone? In support of this, the European Medicines Agency Scientific Discussion group reported that guinea pigs showed crusting, erythema, scaling and swelling at application sites, and a pharmacokinetic study showed a maximum concentration after 7–14 days (corresponding to the dogs developing skin lesions within 2 weeks after application). Or is it the combination of metaflumizone and amitraz? A study by the European Medicines Agency in guinea pigs with three consecutive topical applications of Promeris-Duo® did not produce a reaction after the first application, but did cause moderate erythema after the second and third applications in at least 20% of guinea pigs. The question remains whether the reaction is caused by the vehicle or the amitraz.

Finally, Ursula Oberkirchner said that another topical flea and tick preventative, Certifect® from Merial, has recently been reported (T. Olivry, personal communication, 2012) to have caused similar skin lesions in dogs. This product contains fipronil, (*S*)-methoprene and amitraz, and has been licensed in Europe and the USA since 2011. Promeris-Duo® and Certifect® both contain amitraz. However, Mitaban® (Pharmacia & Upjohn Company, Inc.) dips containing amitraz have been used for decades without causing PF-like skin lesions. Perhaps there is a dose-related effect; a calculation of the amitraz concentrations for a 26 kg dog showed that Mitaban® (the registered name for the rinse solution in the USA) would be 2 mg/m^2. In contrast, much higher concentrations are contained in Promeris-Duo® (909 mg /m^2) and Certifect® (364 mg /m^2). Further studies are needed.

Richard Malik asked why the Promeris-Duo® is not off the market.

Ursula Oberkirchner answered that Promeris spot-on solution for dogs production has been discontinued in the USA and only products that are still in distributors' inventories are being sold. Promeris® has not been recalled.

Manfred Kietzmann asked about studies of the vehicle alone (of Promeris-Duo®).

Ursula Oberkirchner answered that there are no published studies to the best of her knowledge.

Richard Malik commented that there are other examples of drug-triggered immunological reactions, such as the antifungal 5- fluorocytosine, which can cause toxic epidermal necrolysis in dogs.

The chairperson introduced Masahiko Nagata from Japan as the next speaker.

Resistance of *Sarcoptes* mites to ivermectin (M. Nagata)

Masahiko Nagata (*Japan*) spoke about two cases that had been seen and published by his colleague Yuri Terada in *Veterinary Dermatology* in 2010.[7] Two dogs with scabies were apparently refractory to ivermectin treatment (300 µg/kg orally and then subcutaneously), but had subsequently responded well to fipronil spray. Additionally, the owners were affected and showed pruritic papules on the chest, abdomen and thighs. Living mites were found on the dogs on day 35 of the ivermectin treatment, and their skin condition deteriorated. *In vitro* tests of resistance have not been conducted. A retrospective search in his clinic showed 57 dogs with scabies, treated with orally administered ivermectin (300 µg/kg, three times at 14-day intervals) and the efficacy was 100%. Two human cases with *in vivo* and *in vitro* resistance to ivermectin in Sarcoptes scabiei infestation,[8] and an outbreak of scabies with suspected resistance to ivermectin, in and outside a nursing home, has also been reported.[9] Ivermectin resistance appears to involve efflux pump proteins thought to have a role in the multidrug resistance phenotype seen in some cancers.[10] Alterations in the P-glycoprotein gene structure and/or its transcription have been reported in an ivermectin-resistant sheep nematode, Haemonchus contortus.[11]

Carmel Taylor stated that she had seen a dog with scabies that had not left the owner's apartment for 2 years. The owner worked as a volunteer at an animal shelter where cases of scabies had occurred and the conclusion in this case was that, as scabies mites can live up to 6 days off a host, there was a transmission of the mites by the owner.

Richard Malik commented that in people, scabies-contaminated blankets are a common source of infection. He also stated that two researchers from Australia can perform PCRs and look at the genes of resistant mites.

Ursula Oberkirchner mentioned a case with apparently 'resistant' scabies, in which it was finally determined that the in-contact cat had scabies too, and reinfection of the dog had occurred.

The chairperson lastly introduced Sébastien Viaud as the final speaker.

Clinical experience with the *Leishmania* vaccine (S. Viaud)

Sébastien Viaud (*France*) spoke about Leishmania vaccines, which have been proven to be an efficacious tool to prevent canine leishmaniasis. Purified Leishmania fraction vaccines (Leishmune®, Fort Dodge; Canileish®, Virbac) seem to be the most promising of the four classes of developed vaccines. Vaccination can be started in dogs at 6 months age, and the protocol schedule consists of three injections administered with a 3-week interval between doses. The onset of immunity is within 3–4 weeks after completion of the primary series of three doses. Annual revaccination is needed to maintain immunity. It is recommended to separate the Leishmania vaccine from all other vaccinations by at least 2 weeks. Quantitative serology should be performed before vaccination as the efficacy of the vaccine was established in Leishmania-negative dogs. Side effects after vaccination occurred only in a small percentage of dogs and consisted of general signs such as lethargy, hyperthermia, decreased appetite, vomiting or diarrhoea. Local swelling, with or without pain, was observed to develop at the injection site. No anaphylactic reactions were seen. Expected results from the vaccine are a significant reduction in the number of dogs progressing to symptomatic disease (reportedly a four times lower risk rate), and significant reduction in the number of dogs progressing to active infection (3.6 times lower risk). Sébastien Viaud stated that the development of vaccines changes prevention strategies because now an integrated approach including vaccination and use of insect repellents is recommended.

Richard Malik asked how many people will use the Leishmania vaccine.

Sébastien Viaud answered that it is an expensive and not yet a very well-known vaccine.

Carmel Taylor asked how many people in the audience have experience with the vaccine, and three people raised their hands.

The Chairperson closed the workshop by thanking the speakers for their excellent contributions.

References

1. Lüssenhop J, Stahl J, Wolken S *et al.* Distribution of permethrin in hair and stratum corneum after topical administration of four different formulations in dogs. *J Vet Pharmacol Ther* 2012; 35: 206–208.
2. Lüssenhop J, Bäumer W, Kietzmann M *et al.* Dynamics of distribution and efficacy of different spot-on permethrin formulations in dogs artificially infested with Dermacentor reticulatus. *Parasit Vectors* 2011; 30: 45.
3. Malik R, Ward MP, Seavers A *et al.* Permethrin spot-on intoxication of cats. Literature review and survey of veterinary practitioners in Australia. *Feline Med Surg* 2010; 12: 5–14.
4. Oberkirchner U, Linder KE, Dunston S *et al.* Metaflumizone-amitraz (Promeris)-associated pustular acantholytic dermatitis in 22 dogs: evidence suggests contact drug-triggered pemphigus foliaceus. *Vet Dermatol* 2011; 22: 436–448:
5. DeLay RL, Lacoste E, Mezzasalma T *et al.* Pharmacokinetics of metaflumizone and amitraz in the plasma and hair of dogs following topical application. *Vet Parasitol* 2007; 150: 251–257.
6. Hellmann K, Adler K, Parker L *et al.* Evaluation of the efficacy and safety of a novel formulation of metaflumizone plus amitraz in dogs naturally infested with fleas and ticks in Europe. *Vet Parasitol* 2007; 150: 239–345:
7. Terada Y, Murayama N, Ikemura H *et al.* Sarcoptes scabiei var. canis refractory to ivermectin treatment in two dogs. *Vet Dermatol* 2010; 21; 608–612.
8. Currie BJ, Harumal P, McKinnon M *et al.* First documentation of in vivo and in vitro ivermectin resistance in Sarcoptes scabiei. *Clin Infect Dis* 2004; 39: 8–12.
9. Van den Hoek JA, Van de Weerd JA, Baayen TD *et al.* A persistent problem wit scabies in and outside a nursing home in Amsterdam: indications for resistance to lindane and ivermectin. *Eurosurveillance* 2008; 13: Available at: http://www.eurosurveillance.
org/viewarticle.aspx?articleid=19052. Accessed 2 January 2013.
10. Reed MB, Saliba KJ, Caruana SR *et al.* Pgh1 modulates sensitivity and resistance to multiple antimalarials in Plasmodium falciparum. *Nature* 2000; 403: 906–909.
11. Xu M, Molento M, Blackhall W *et al.* Ivermectin resistance in nematodes may be caused by alteration of P-glycoprotein homolog. *Mol Biochem Parasitol* 1998; 91: 327–335.

8.13

Topical antimicrobial therapy

K. Bergvall[1] (Chairperson), K. Varjonen[2] (Secretary)

[1]Djurakuten i Stockholm, Kungstensgatan 58, 11329 Stockholm, Sweden
[2]Faculty of Veterinary Medicine and Animal Science, Department of Clinical Sciences, Swedish University of Agricultural Sciences, Uppsala, Sweden

---

Kerstin Bergvall (*Sweden*) welcomed everyone to the workshop on topical antimicrobial therapy. The workshop was intended to be an interactive session with four invited speakers followed by a discussion after each subject. The four speakers and their topics were introduced.

Kerstin Bergvall reminded the audience that although bacteria have been around for 3.5 billion years, penicillin was discovered as recently as 1928 by Alexander Fleming. It was only 30 years later that the first report of methicillin-resistant *Staphylococcus aureus* (MRSA) was published. With the emergence of antibiotic resistance, nonantibiotic treatment protocols for infectious diseases have become increasingly interesting and important topics for discussion. The first speaker of the session, Ralf Mueller, was invited to make his presentation.

Antibacterial shampoos – can they relieve/reduce bacterial burden? (R. Mueller)

Ralf Mueller (*Germany*) presented the results of a study, 'Antibacterial activity of hair shafts after shampooing',[1] and some additional work on antimicrobial activity of biocides.

In one study the residual antibacterial activity on keratinocytes of a chlorhexidine and phytosphingosine shampoo was investigated and compared to a shampoo vehicle. Canine keratinocytes were harvested before and after shampooing. The cells were cultured and bacterial growth was compared between the two treatment groups before and after shampooing. No difference was seen between the placebo and active ingredients with regard to the residual antibacterial activity on keratinocytes after shampooing.

Cytological samples from the dogs in the study were taken before shampoo treatment was started and repeated 4 weeks later. Ralf Mueller was unsure whether the dogs were shampooed once or twice weekly. The bacterial count on cytology was reduced significantly in both the placebo (shampoo vehicle) and the active ingredient shampoo treatment groups, indicating that mechanical removal of bacteria by shampooing plays a significant role in the effectiveness of shampoos in treatment of bacterial pyoderma. Ralf Mueller commented that based on this study, any shampoo used properly should reduce bacterial numbers.

Ralf Mueller pointed out that there are many possible problems to consider when evaluating shampoo studies. There are very few randomized controlled studies that look at effects *in vivo*. It is difficult to extrapolate from *in vitro* studies as concentrations of the ingredients on the skin may differ and incubation times may also differ in the clinical settings. Many clinical studies do not have a control group, or they have a control group that is not shampooed and, therefore, underestimates the effects from mechanical actions.

Another study[1] aimed to investigate whether there is a residual antibacterial activity on the hair shaft after shampooing. Previous studies have shown that there are bacterial colonies on the hair shafts as well as the skin surface. Forty-two healthy dogs from the Institute of Physiology at Ludwig-Maximilians University, Munich, Germany, were used in the study. The dogs were beagles, foxhounds and beagle-mixed breed dogs. They were shampooed twice weekly for 2 weeks. A 10-minute shampoo, 10-minute rinsing protocol was used. The following shampoos were evaluated: chlorhexidine 0.8% (Actibac®, Ceva), chlorhexidine 2%/miconazole 2% (Malaseb®, Dermcare), chlorhexidine 3% (Pyohex®, Dermcare), chlorhexidine 4% (Hexocare®, Alfavet), ethyl lactate 10% (Etiderm®, Virbac), benzoyl peroxide 2.5% (Peroxyderm®, Vetoquinol) and a control vehicle (Dermazyme®, Ceva).

The dogs were shampooed twice weekly, four times in total. Two shampoos per dog were used: the right half of the dog was shampooed with one shampoo, the left half of the dog with another shampoo, and a stripe in the middle was left untreated to avoid cross-contamination. One group was treated with ethyl lactate on one side and chlorhexidine/miconazole on the other; one group with 3% chlorhexidine on one side, 2.5% benzoyl peroxide on the other; one group with 3% chlorhexidine and a 3% chlorhexidine conditioner afterwards on one side and 0.8% chlorhexidine on the other side; and one group with 4% chlorhexidine on one side and control on the other side. Hair samples were taken with a clipper from the left and the right sides of the thorax before the first shampoo therapy, after the last shampoo therapy once the dog was dry, and then 2, 4 and 7 days later.

The hair was dried for 10 minutes and then 0.02 g of hair was placed onto agars coated in100 μL of 0.3 McFarland Standard dilution of *Staphylococcus pseudintermedius* (21284) and incubated at 37°C for 24 hours. The inhibition zones were measured by measuring the longitudinal and perpendicular inhibition zones around the hair sample. All samples were done in duplicates. The groups were compared using Kruskal–Wallis and Dunn post-test, $P < 0.05$.

The results of the study were as follows. No inhibition zones were seen before the study. A small inhibition zone was seen around the control group. Ralf Mueller believes this was likely caused by a small bacterial inhibition from the surfactant in the shampoo base. Large inhibition zones were seen around three groups: the Pyohex®, Malaseb® and the 3% chlorhexidine plus conditioner. Smaller inhibition zones were seen in the 0.8% chlorhexidine group, even less in the 4% chlorhexidine, and no inhibition was seen in the ethyl lactate and benzoyl peroxide groups. At day 17 the results were very similar but, at that time there was no residual activity of the base. Large inhibition zones were seen in the Pyohex®, Malaseb® and the 3% chlorhexidine plus conditioner groups, very little inhibition was seen in the remaining two chlorhexidine groups. No inhibition was seen with benzoyl peroxide. Two dogs treated with ethyl lactate had inhibition zones at day 17 but not directly after shampooing. The researchers concluded that there are differences in the residual antibacterial activity depending on the shampoo. The differences are not solely dependent on the concentration of the ingredient because the 2% and 3% chlorhexidine had much higher inhibition zones than the 0.8% and 4% chlorhexidine. This result was found to be compatible with the results of previous *in vitro* studies, including one by Lloyd and Lampert.[2] The different inhibition zones were thought possibly to be due to differences in the diffusion activities of the shampoos. One possible explanation is that some of the ingredients, such as benzoyl peroxide, may not diffuse into the agar and, therefore, no inhibition zone occurs.

Based on the results it was concluded that some shampoos have residual antibacterial activity and others do not, and that the formulation of the shampoo is more important than its concentration of active ingredients. Ralf Mueller pointed out that if you believe the hair shafts play a role in the carriage of bacteria, shampoos that are manufactured to provide residual activity on hairs should be used.

Credit was given to Isabell Kloos, a doctoral student who had performed the study, and all the people involved, the Institute for Nutrition, Institute for Infectious Medicine and Zoonoses, and the dermatology team at the university in Munich.

Paul Bloom (*USA*) asked, what is Pyohex?

Ralf Mueller answered that it is a chlorhexidine 3% shampoo.

Ralf Mueller then asked the audience whether they believe that shampoos can have a residual antibacterial activity. Six people raised their hands. He then asked how many believed hair shafts played a role, and a few people in the audience felt that this was likely.

Ralf Mueller finished his presentation by concluding that much more work was needed in this area. These kinds of studies are a start to determine whether there is a difference between shampoos. Unfortunately, he had found it very difficult to get funding from companies for these kinds of studies, and this study is one of the first shampoo studies funded by a shampoo company, Dermcare. He believes that it should be important for companies that market their products to veterinarians to have their products evaluated, and provide evidence that their products perform according to the claims they make. He hopes for more studies in the future.

Kerstin Bergvall thanked Ralf Mueller for his talk and invited Nobuo Murayama to make his presentation.

Antibacterial shampoos/washing and *staphylococci* (Nobuo Murayama)

Nobuo Murayama (*Japan*) introduced the subject of his talk and presented the results of several studies. He reported that in their hospital they have experienced methicillin-resistant *Staphylococcus pseudintermedius* (MRSP) in two-thirds of cases (113/170).[3] These staphylococci show multidrug resistance including high levels of resistance towards ofloxacin (84.1%), lincomycin (99.2%), clindamycin (92.0%) and minocycline (65.5%). Therefore, alternative treatments, including topical antimicrobial ingredients such as benzoyl peroxide, ethyl lactate and chlorhexidine, need to be considered.

Previous studies have reported clinical improvement of 60–70% with use of benzoyl peroxide in cases of canine superficial pyoderma by two clinical researchers.[4,5] There are some disadvantages with benzoyl peroxide including its antiseborrhoeic effect and propensity to cause irritation. It may thus be difficult to perform frequent shampooing with benzoyl peroxide. In one study with ethyl lactate a 77% clinical improvement of canine superficial pyoderma was reported,[5] but this has not been shown in other studies.

Nobuo Murayama and his team investigated the *in vitro* efficacy of different concentrations of benzoyl peroxide, ethyl lactate and chlorhexidine against *S. pseudintermedius*. In their study a 100 times dilution of benzoyl peroxide showed growth of *S. pseudintermedius* within 15 minutes of contact time. A 500 times dilution of 10% ethyl lactate showed growth of *S. pseudintermedius* within 15 minutes. On the other hand, a 1000 times dilution of 2% chlorhexidine showed no growth of bacteria within 15 minutes. They concluded that chlorhexidine is more effective against *S. pseudintermedius* using a low concentration and a short exposure time compared to benzoyl peroxide and ethyl lactate.

Nobuo Murayama and his team next wanted to compare the clinical efficacy of chlorhexidine to other products. A recently published study by Loeffler *et al.* reported on the clinical efficacy of 3% chlorhexidine gluconate compared to 2.5% benzoyl peroxide.[6] In this study, 70% of cases of pyoderma treated with chlorhexidine showed good clinical improvement whilst 20% of benzoyl peroxide-treated patients showed good clinical improvement.

In their study, Nobuo Murayama and his team compared 2% chlorhexidine acetate and 10% ethyl lactate and looked at resolution of scales, papules/crusts, erythema and pruritus. Treatment was done twice weekly for 1 week. Chlorhexidine significantly improved skin lesions compared to ethyl lactate.[7]

In another study, 2% chlorhexidine acetate and 4% chlorhexidine gluconate were compared. Both showed the same efficacy for canine superficial pyoderma.[8] A 2% chlorhexidine acetate shampoo treatment of canine superficial pyoderma associated with cephalexin-resistant *S. intermedius* group was evaluated. The dogs were shampooed every 2 days for 2 weeks. Seventy-five percent of cases in the study had their lesions resolved or showed clinical improvement.[8]

Nobuo Murayama shared some clinical tips that he recommends to improve success with shampoo therapy. His group compared three different doses of chlorhexidine acetate for treatment efficacy. Group 1 received 57 mL/m^2, group 2 received half the dosage of group 1, and group 3 received one-third of the dosage of group 1. The results showed that groups 1 and 2 showed the same degree of improvement for canine superficial pyoderma. Based on this study, Nobuo Murayama reported that they use a coin measurement when explaining to owners how much shampoo to use. An area of shampoo the size of a Japanese 500 yen coin per two hand-sized areas on the dog's body equals about 29 mL/m^2 as used for group 2 in the study. Coins in other currencies like a quarter US dollar or a 2 euro coin are almost the same size.

The shampoo contact time was then examined. A 1-minute contact time and 10-minute contact time of chlorhexidine were compared and almost the same improvement could be seen for canine superficial pyoderma.

Nobuo Murayama concluded that bathing with high concentrations of chlorhexidine is an effective therapy for canine superficial pyoderma. However, clinical response is not seen in all cases. One possible explanation for the inefficacy of chlorhexidine is the presence of multidrug efflux pumps.These pumps are associated with antimicrobial resistance encoded by antiseptic resistance genes including *qacA, qacB* and *smr*. In humans, *S. aureus* has been shown to have antiseptic resistance genes and this has also been found within equine, bovine and feline staphylococcal strains. Antiseptic resistance genes were not detected in 100 strains of *S. pseudintermedius* from cases of canine superficial pyoderma.

Nobuo Murayama discussed other factors that could cause chlorhexidine to be ineffective. Inefficacy can be caused by organic matter and poor penetration into biofilms. *S. aureus* has recently been shown to produce biofilms. Chlorhexidine treatment of impetigo and furunculosis in humans who have biofilm formation does not show good efficacy. Recently *S. pseudintermedius* has also been shown to produce biofilms. Poor efficacy could also be explained by lack of owner compliance. Nobuo Murayama thanked the audience for their attention.

Kerstin Bergvall thanked Nobuo Murayama for his presentation. She asked whether he would recommend the use of a detergent prior to chlorhexidine to help remove organic matter.

Nobuo Murayama felt that this needs to be investigated. He recommends that owners thoroughly wet the dog with warm water before using chlorhexidine shampoo, but he does not usually recommend the use of degreasers.

Ralf Mueller reported that they usually recommend prebathing dogs prior to use of medicated shampoos that are expensive. There are a couple of shampoos on the market that cost around US$40 a bottle and the owners would not be very compliant if they had to buy a new bottle every week or two. Ralf Mueller feels less shampoo is needed if a detergent is used for the initial lathering.

Kerstin Bergvall thanked the speakers for their answers and invited Lionel Fabriès to the podium.

The *in vitro* antimicrobial activity of a spot-on containing a mixture of essential oils and a plant extract against *Staphylococcus pseudintermedius* and *Malassezia pachydermatis*. (Lionel Fabriès)

Lionel Fabriès (*France*) noted that the prevalence of pyoderma and cutaneous infection is generally considered to be over 25% of the total cases presenting for dermatological consultations, and that multiple clinical lesion types caused by cutaneous infections can be seen. Lionel Fabriès observed that the emergence of multidrug-resistant bacteria, especially of the *Staphylococcus* strains, had been extensively discussed throughout the Congress. He noted that since Drs M. Linek and A. Loeffler published one of the first reports in Europe of MecA multidrug-resistant *S. intermedius* in 12 cases from a veterinary dermatology referral practice in Germany,[9] many more articles have been published in the field. Lionel Fabriès stated that growing antimicrobial resistance is seen, and new strategies for the treatment and control of microbial disease need to be developed. He felt that the use of plant extracts may provide alternatives for treatment, but perhaps also become more important in prevention of infection. Lionel Fabriès and his colleagues had studied a plant-based product containing a mixture of essential oils and a specific plant extract, and evaluated the antimicrobial activity of this product *in vitro*.

The study protocol was described. Different broths were used, Mueller Hinton for *S. pseudintermedius* and modified Dixon growth broth for *Malassezia pachydermatis*. One hundred microlitres of the spot-on test product was added to the first row of the microplate and serial dilutions were made. Subsequently, 100 μL of a tryptone salt dilution at a concentration of 10^8 bacteria/mL or 10^7 yeasts/mL was inoculated into each well. A positive control as well as a negative control of the broth and the test product itself were added. The wells were incubated at 37°C for *S. pseudintermedius* and 32.5°C for *M. pachydermatis*. The minimum inhibitory concentration (MIC) was determined. To find the minimum bactericidal (MBC) or fungicidal (MFC) concentrations, almost the same technique was used except that cultures and subcultures were on agar instead of broth. The MBC and MFC are the lowest concentrations of test product that will kill the respective micro-organisms. The results of the study for *S. pseudintermedius* showed a MIC of between 1/65 536 and 1/32 768 dilution of the product. The positive and negative controls were validated. The MBC of the product for *S. pseudintermedius* was between 1/512 and 1/256. For *Malassezia* the MFC was 1/32 and the MIC was between 1/64 and 1/32 dilution.

Lionel Fabriès observed that the *in vitro* test results show that the test product has strong antibacterial properties and also has anti-*Malassezia* properties. He concluded that the *in vitro* results also show promising efficacy against *S. pseudintermedius* due to the very high dilution, the very low MIC and low MBC seen.

Due to the mixture of different ingredients in the test product, Lionel Fabriès stated that individual activities of any one ingredient could not be interpreted. The plant extract has been proven to have action *in vitro* against the following *S. aureus* strains: (MDR) SA-1199B, EMRSA-15 and 16, SA-1199B, XU212 and RN4220. Some of these strains show high levels of resistance to certain antibiotics, namely fluoroquinolones, tetracycline and macrolides. Lionel Fabriès reported that one of the hypotheses of why the plant extract shows *in vivo* efficacy against bacterial strains resistant to certain antibiotics is that the plant extract has a different mechanism of action compared to the antibiotics. Several of the resistant strains that the plant extract has shown to be effective against have efflux pumps that make it possible for these strains to eject antibiotics. Lionel Fabriès suggested that one possible reason for the efficacy of the plant extract could be that it cannot be ejected by the bacterial efflux pumps and, therefore, kills the bacteria.

Some of the other ingredients in the spot-on product have also been proven to be effective against certain strains of *Staphylococcus*. The product contains several aromatic oils, including carvacol, thymol and eugenol. Lionel Fabriès reported that more studies of the product were planned in the future to further improve the understanding of the individual ingredients, but that the *in vitro* results were considered very promising. He felt the product could be useful in the future in association with conventional antimicrobial therapy such as antibiotics, for the treatment and prevention of pyoderma or *Malassezia* dermatitis in dogs. He reported that further studies as well as an *in vivo* double-blind clinical trial for the spot-on product were starting, and he hoped that he would be able to present great results from these studies before the next World Congress. Lionel Fabriès thanked the audience for their attention.

Kerstin Bergvall thanked Lionel Fabriès for his presentation.

Ralf Mueller also thanked Lionel Fabriès for the presentation and the nice data presented. He asked whether there were any data regarding the product's distribution over the skin and concentrations at distant sites as this is one problem that can occur with spot-on formulations.

Lionel Fabriès answered that these data do not yet exist but that the distribution will need to be studied.

Ralf Mueller suggested the use of a protocol where the product is put on the affected sites.

Lionel Fabriès agreed this should be studied.

Tim Nuttall asked whether it had been calculated if the concentration of the product on the skin, assuming an even distribution over the body surface, matched the MICs and the MBCs that were seen *in vitro*.

Lionel Fabriès answered that this calculation had not yet been done but should be performed.

Kirstin Bergvall asked whether it was known if the product is distributed better if there is a lipid layer left on the skin or if it is better to shampoo before use, which would also mechanically remove some microorganisms?

Lionel Fabriès answered that if the skin is shampooed before application of the product, the lipid layer is removed and the product will not work as well. It can still be effective where applied and a few centimetres around the application site, but a nice diffusion of the product cannot occur as a lipid layer is required for this.

Kirstin Bergvall thanked Lionel Fabriès for the answers and invited Tim Nuttall to make his presentation.

Antimicrobial shampoos: efficacy against staphylococci, *Pseudomonas* and *Malassezia* (Tim Nuttall)

Tim Nuttall (*UK*) presented the results of a study[10] conducted as an undergraduate honours project by a third-year student, Rebecca Young. In his practice, Tim Nuttall uses fewer antibiotics today due to the concerns with resistance. He uses topical biocides and commonly advocates these to help treat skin infection and prevent recurrence, and to prevent contamination of the shampoo bottle. However, he reported that this is not always effective and he has recovered *Pseudomonas* from shampoos and from shampoo bottles.

Tim Nuttall observed that several shampoo studies, both *in vivo* and *in vitro*, have been reported. He noted that benzoyl peroxide traditionally, and certainly during his undergraduate and residency training, was considered a very potent and effective topical antimicrobial product and that ethyl lactate is thought of as less effective. Numerous studies show that chlorhexidine is an effective antimicrobial agent, and Tim Nuttall observed that there are some suggestions that high concentrations may be more effective but he felt Ralf Mueller's study very clearly showed that the formulation of the chlorhexidine seems to be at least as important as the concentration. Tim Nuttall pointed out that chlorhexidine is a difficult molecule to work with; its potency very much depends on whether it is a gluconate or an acetate, and also on the surfactants and other ingredients in the shampoo.

For the current report, seven antimicrobial shampoos were selected and tested against methicillin-sensitive *Staphylococcus pseudintermedius* (MSSP), methicillin-resistant *S. pseudintermedius* (MRSP), *Pseudomonas aeruginosa* (PA), multidrug-resistant *P. aeruginosa* (MDR-PA) and *Malassezia* isolates. While the MDR-PA did not fit the official definition of multidrug-resistant bacteria, these isolates were resistant to both gentamicin and fluoroquinolones. The MRSPs were a kind gift from Luca Guardabassi at the University of Copenhagen.

The shampoos chosen were those available on the UK market that either had some published evidence or implied antimicrobial activity based on the product literature. The products were regarded as broad-spectrum antimicrobials.

Three isolates of each organism were tested. Most of them came from skin infections, except the *Pseudomonas,* which came from cases of otitis. The isolates were cultured in a standard manner, washed in sterile phosphate-buffered saline (PBS), and the suspension was adjusted to optical density (OD 570 nm) of 0.15 (bacteria) and 0.08 (*Malassezia*). This gives a standard number of colony-forming units (approx. 1×10^6 CFU/mL). Doubling dilutions of shampoos was used in the culture plates to give final dilutions of 1:2 to 1:5096 (bacteria) and 1:2 to 1:10 192 (*Malassezia*). Because 100 μL of shampoo was put into the first well and 100 μL of the bacterial suspension was added, concentrations above 1:2 could not be tested. Control wells with 100 μL microbial solution in 100 μL sterile PBS, 100 μL of each shampoo in 100 μL sterile PBS and 200 μL sterile PBS were included. The samples were incubated for 10, 30 and 60 minutes.

Tim Nuttall considered that the 10-minute incubation results were the most interesting because these reflect typical *in vivo* use. Longer exposures were evaluated to see whether this would lead to changes in efficacy. The study was a minimum bactericidal concentration (MBC) study because some of the shampoos were coloured and some were opaque and this prevented measurement of the optical densities in the broth cultures. Aliquots from each well were plated after the incubation period to evaluate the MBC. This is the minimum concentration of the shampoo that completely prevented any microbial growth.

The shampoos used were Malaseb® (Teva Animal Health; 2% chlorhexidine gluconate, 2% miconazole shampoo), Hibiscrub® (Mölnlycke Health Care; 4% chlorhexidine gluconate), Pyoderm® (Virbac Animal Health; 3% chlorhexidine gluconate), Paxcutol® (Virbac Animal Health; 2.5% benzoyl peroxide), Etiderm® (Virbac Animal Health; 10% ethyl lactate), Coatex® medicated (VetPlus; chloroxylenol or PCMX) and Malacetic® (Dechra Veterinary Products; 2% acetic acid, 2% boric acid).

The results showed that the main difference was between the chlorhexidine and the other products: the MBCs for chlorhexidine-containing products were in the range of 1/512 to 1/1024 dilutions whereas the other products were only effective at much higher concentrations (1/2 to 1/4). The Coatex® and the Malacetic® were not effective at all, as bacteria grew in almost all of the wells. Another interesting finding was that there was very little difference, certainly for the chlorhexidine products, between the MSSP and the MRSP, and the PA and the MDR-PA. There were no differences in susceptibility between antibiotic-resistant and -sensitive strains. The MRSPs seemed a bit more susceptible to benzoyl peroxide than the MSSPs, but otherwise, the results were similar.

The benzoyl peroxide and ethyl lactate products were more effective after 60 minutes, when the bacteria were killed at higher dilutions. Tim Nuttall stated that this might be related to the fact that their antimicrobial activity relies on the breakdown products: benzoyl peroxide into peroxide and benzoic acid, and ethyl lactate to lactic acid and ethanol. This may take more time *in vitro* so the actual killing effect in this study may not be accurate and may differ from what happens *in vivo.*

Similar results were seen for PA and MDR-PA isolates: the chlorhexidine-containing products were much more effective than any others. Again, the multidrug-resistant isolates were no less susceptible than the antibiotic-susceptible isolates, and for these organisms longer incubation times did not make any difference in the results.

Three *Malassezia pachydermatis* isolates were used. Other studies have shown that *Malassezia* can be less susceptible to chlorhexidine than bacteria, but the opposite was found in this study. Tim Nuttall thought this may be due to the isolates used. Similar to the results with bacteria, chlorhexidine was more effective than the other products in killing *Malassezia.* While the other products were more efficacious against *Malassezia* than against the bacteria, they were still much less efficacious than the chlorhexidine products.

Chlorhexidine was found to be the most effective topical product with no difference between the different concentrations or products. There might be some synergistic or additive activity between miconazole and chlorhexidine; this has not yet been looked at. Tim Nuttall emphasized that a very important caveat had been put in the conclusions: this study is only applicable to these particular products because chlorhexidine is a very labile molecule, and very difficult to work with when formulating shampoos and washes. The results, therefore, cannot be extrapolated to any other products.

Tim Nuttall had roughly calculated whether the amount of shampoo used by his nurses in clinics would reach the MBCs of the study. He had measured that 20–30 mL/m^2 was a typical volume used during shampooing, delivering approximately 400–1200 mg of chlorhexidine per m^2 body surface area. It therefore seemed that topical therapy was likely to reach the MBCs observed in this study: staphylococci 10–40 μg/mL, *Pseudomonas* 20–80 μg/mL and *Malassezia* 4–20 μg/mL. These calculations are, however, not precise because they compare an area measure with a volume measure.

Chlorhexidine was found to be no less effective against antibiotic-resistant organisms compared to antibiotic-sensitive strains in this study. Murayama *et al.*[8] presented a study using a 2% chlorhexidine acetate shampoo and a 4% chlorhexidine gluconate shampoo, which showed that they were equally effective and cured 5/8 dogs with MRSP skin infections. This shampoo is not on the UK market and was therefore not tested.

Tim Nuttall acknowledged his co-workers Rebecca Young, Laura Buckley and Neil McEwan, and echoed Ralf Mueller's point that it is extremely difficult to obtain funding for these projects because most shampoos and ear cleaners are not registered products. The companies sell them widely and may be reluctant to fund studies that might find the products are not effective. Tim Nuttall encouraged the audience to start asking for evidence when making decisions about which products to stock in their practice and to put pressure on companies to fund this sort of work.

Kerstin Bergvall thanked Tim Nuttall for his presentation.

Margaret Phillips (*USA*) asked if the names for the US equivalents of the specific products used were known.

Tim Nuttall answered that Malaseb® is a Dechra product distributed by Teva Animal Health in the USA. Hibiscrub® is an ICI product in the UK and is actually a surgical hand scrub. They had used it because it is 4% and they wanted to see if there was a difference in efficacy with percentage. It can be quite drying and is not routinely used as a whole body wash. Pyoderm® is a Virbac product; and is called Hexadene® in the USA. It may be marketed by some other names in other countries. Paxcutol®, 2.5% benzoyl peroxide, is a Virbac product. Etiderm®, also a Virbac product, has the same name throughout the world. Coatex® is a VetPlus product, and Tim Nuttall was unsure whether it is available elsewhere. It is a PCMX-containing shampoo but also has other ingredients. Malacetic® was a Dermapet product that is now a Dechra product, and he believed it still has the same name.

Kerstin Bergvall noted that different dosages per area had been recommended to be used. She asked whether a certain amount of shampoo per area was usually recommended to an owner.

Tim Nuttall answered that they usually have their nurses demonstrate the shampooing. He had never watched them do it and could not be sure whether they stated a specific amount. In the study, a bottle of shampoo had been given to the nurses to shampoo a few dogs in the hospital and Tim Nuttall had then measured how much shampoo was used and had done some calculations. The dose was not a specific recommendation, more a reflection of what they were typically using and whether that seemed to fit with the MBCs in the study. Tim Nuttall, however, did like Nobuo Murayama's 2 euro or 500 yen coin amounts because he felt them to be really practical for an owner.

Kerstin Bergvall asked if the dose recommendations should be changed based on hair coat type – short-haired versus long-haired or plush-coated?

Ralf Mueller answered that in the study they did looking at the keratinocytes they doubled the dose in long-haired dogs and chows but he had no scientific basis for this.

Nobuo Murayama felt that a study of the dosage for long- and short-haired dogs should be done, as the differences in efficacy are not known.

Ralf Mueller commented that if he has a long-haired dog with severe pyoderma and the owners allow him to clip it he always recommends it. His clinical impression is it makes the dog easier to bathe.

Nobuo Murayama reiterated that he usually recommends a one coin size area of shampoo per two hand areas. If in 1–2 weeks the dog's condition has not improved he doubles the dosage.

Kerstin Bergvall asked if he thinks he sees a better response with the doubled dose, and Nobuo Murayama answered that he feels that he does.

Nina Shoulberg (*USA*) recalled that about 20 years ago someone looked at benzoyl peroxide versus 2% chlorhexidine versus miconazole in a study. She thought it was a resident study examining the efficacy against bacteria. The take-home message she recalled was that benzoyl peroxide was the strongest shampoo. Several people agreed. Tim Nuttall remembered the same study.

Kerstin Bergvall added that benzoyl peroxide also had been considered to have a hair follicle flushing mechanism and asked if anyone had shown this?

Nina Shoulberg asked how it is that the results of that study differ from the current studies?

Ralf Mueller answered that he thinks there may be other potential explanations. Benzoyl peroxide is extremely degreasing and if the dog has a very greasy pyoderma he thought that the shampoo works really well due to removal of the material. Chlorhexidine might work better in cases with few papules and a dry haircoat. Several contributors discussed the concentrations of the shampoo used in the study.

James Jeffers (*USA*) had recently reviewed the paper in question and thought it was 0.5% chlorhexidine[11] used in that particular study.

Tim Nuttall added that chlorhexidine is not particularly effective if there is biofilm present unless that biofilm is destroyed or mechanically disrupted in some other way. He observed that the problem with *in vivo* studies is that we are dealing with different coat types, seborrhoea, underlying diseases and so on. Large numbers of dogs are required for those studies to get any power, so when a large number of shampoos are tried it becomes a very difficult study to run.

Vanessa Miller (*UK*) commented that there has been a lot of discussion about the value of shampoos for animals with pyoderma, but she had clients that find it very difficult to shampoo their dog. She therefore asked whether anyone had experience with lotions, sprays, other antimicrobials or Malacetic wipes?

Tim Nuttall answered that he uses less of the Malacetic range of products because the shampoo is very poorly effective. A year or two before the shampoo study, Alison Swinney, another honours student in Liverpool, looked at ear cleaners using a similar study design and the Malacetic range performed very poorly there too. Tim Nuttall had not investigated Malacetic sprays and wipes, but he does not use them. He observed that there is a chlorhexidine wipe available, an ICF product in Europe called CLX® wipes, and a Dermapet (now Dechra) product called Triz-Chlor® wipes. Anecdotally using the wipes between bathing on the affected skin seems to be effective but no one has yet done any controlled studies.

Kerstin Bergvall asked whether anybody else is happy using wipes or the chlorhexidine spray that is also available.

Ralf Mueller reported that he has many owners who love the products. Some people greatly prefer wiping the interdigital areas to shampooing. He had no data to support their use.

Tim Nuttall commented that many clients are willing to shampoo once a week and use the wipes or spray between baths and that compliance seems to be better with this protocol rather than asking owners to shampoo two or three times a week.

Richard Meadows (*USA*) reported that there is a product in the USA called Wipe out® (ImmuCell). The ingredient is a bactericidal, antimicrobial, bacteria-produced peptide called nisin. The history of the product goes back to the same period as Alexander Fleming. Nisin has been used as a preservative because it is highly effective against staph.

Richard Meadows had read a study in one of the dairy journals in which the investigators compared chlorhexidine to nisin and found that nisin was superior to the chlorhexidine product. They use the product in the dairy industry on the udder to prevent mastitis. Richard Meadows felt that many people do not want to use the chlorhexidine wipes because they groom their dogs and the dogs get reactions to it very frequently. He felt the nisin wipes do not burn the skin of the pets and hence they are better tolerated. The cost of the wipes is low and they are used twice daily. An abstract was presented a few years ago.[12] Richard Meadows has found the product to be very effective, he had some cases in which the dog still forms collarettes but not many more than three or four, and antibiotics could be avoided.

Tim Nuttall replied that he was not familiar with the product but felt that it was useful information. The aim would be to keep bacterial overgrowth to a minimal level that is not causing harm, and avoid overuse of systemic antimicrobials. He had spoken to medical dermatologists who are quite horrified at the amount of systemic antimicrobials used to treat what they would regard as very minor staphylococcal infections, which could be treated with topical biocides rather than with antibiotics

Kerstin Bergvall asked if anyone used alcogel on their patients. Alcogel is an alcohol and contains skin barrier restoring moisturizer. No one raised their hands.

Tim Nuttall answered that alcohol gels and similar products are really disinfectants.

Kerstin Bergvall commented that she thinks it works very well, and that it is one of her favourites because it does not dry the skin and it seems really efficient. She then asked if anyone uses medical honey.

Tim Nuttall answered that he does, particularly on wounds, especially with MRSP and MRSA. He thought it works very well.

Ralf Mueller answered that he uses it a lot on areas where he used to use Bactoderm® (SmithKline Beecham Pharmaceuticals) or Bactroban® (GlaxoSmithKline).

Kerstin Bergvall observed that there are studies in humans of efficacy.

Tim Nuttall agreed that any product with honey can be effective. He advised that the dog is put in a collar and restraint as they had had a dog that ate a honey-impregnated dressing. The dog had lunged forward and ate it when it was taken out of the package.

Margaret Phillips reported that she frequently uses vinegar.

Tim Nuttall answered that he agrees that vinegar is a useful agent for topical therapy. Ten to fifteen years ago he used diluted vinegar routinely but as the shampoos improved and other topical products became available, he replaced the vinegar. Recently, he has again started using it. He thought the acetic acid as a vinegar rinse is quite effective against the biofilm-forming organisms and his team had used it successfully to treat severe lip fold *Pseudomonas* infections in cocker spaniels and spinones. The spinones have sodden, wet beards that are a reservoir for *Pseudomonas* bacteria. Their owners refuse to trim the beards because then they cannot show the dog. Tim Nuttall had success with using a vinegar rinse after cleansing with a detergent.

James Jeffers asked if anyone uses table sugar as an antibacterial.

Tim Nuttall answered that it should work, simply because of the hypertonicity effect. He had not used it but answered that it is one way the honey dressings work.

Richard Meadows reported that he used sugar 25 years ago with excellent results because it was an absorbent (e.g. in racing greyhounds) but he had not used it for decades.

Tim Nuttall reported that he had used honey on himself after a biking accident. The wounds were packed full of honey with good results.

Marielle St-Laurent (*Canada*) reported that she uses sugar and iodine on horses and feels that it works well and that it stays on the wound nicely.

Lionel Fabriès asked about bleach and whether there was any particular concentration used.

Tim Nuttall answered that he had not used bleach but thought other people have for MRSP. Many participants suggested concentrations varying from 1:8 and 1:10 (0.5–0.05%) dilutions of bleach. A concern about licking was raised.

Richard Meadows reported that he also does dentistry work and that bleach was the standard for many years to disinfect and irrigate the root canal pulp chamber to remove organic material.

Kerstin Bergvall had a question for Ralf Mueller about his recommendation to rinse for 10 minutes after the shampoo. She asked whether he was concerned about causing maceration of the skin with a protocol of first 10 minutes of wetting the coat, then 10 minutes shampoo and then 10 minutes to rinse it off.

Ralf Mueller answered that his clients wash their dogs a maximum of twice weekly and he had never seen a problem with skin maceration from bathing using this interval. He thought more frequent washing would be required to cause a problem with maceration.

Kerstin Bergvall asked whether Ralf Mueller thought it might be more feasible for the owners if you said they could soak the area with a wet sponge, apply the shampoo, take a walk for 15 minutes, then go in and rinse the product off. This was what she recommends.

Ralf Mueller answered that he had not done that for shampoo, only other topicals.

Kerstin Bergvall thanked everybody for contributing to the session and wished them a very good trip home.

References

1. Kloss I, Straubinger RK, Horstmann C, Mueller RS. The residual antibacterial activity of canine hairs after treatment with antibacterial shampoos. *Vet Dermatol* 2012; 23 (Suppl. 1): 31.
2. Lloyd DH, Lamport AI. Activity of chlorhexidine shampoos in vitro against Staphylococcus intermedius, Pseudomonas aeruginosa and Malassezia pachydermatis. *Vet Rec* 1999;144: 536–537.
3. Kawakami T, Shibtat S, Murayama N *et al.* Antimicrobial susceptibility and methicillin resistance in Staphylococcus pseudintermedius and Staphylococcus schleiferi subsp. coagulans isolated from dogs with pyoderma in Japan. *J Vet Med Sci* 2010; 72: 1615–1619.
4. Lloyd H, Reyss-Brion DA. Le peroxide de benzoyle: efficacité clinique et bacteriologique dans le traitement des pyodermites chroniques. *Prat Méd Chir Anim Comp* 1984; 19: 445.
5. Asher F, Maynard L, Laurent J *et al.* Controlled trial of ethyl lactate and benzoyl peroxide shampoos in the management of canine surface pyoderma and superficial pyoderma. *Adv Vet Dermatol* 1990; 1: 375–382.
6. Loeffler A, Cobb MA, Bond R. Comparison of a chlorhexidine and a benzoyl peroxide shampoo as sole treatment in canine superficial pyoderma. *Vet Rec* 2011; 169: 249–253.
7. Nagata M, Terada Y. Efficacy of Nolvasan surgical scrub containing 2% chlorhexidine acetate in topical management of canine superficial pyoderma: a randomized, double-blinded, controlled study. *Jpn J Vet Dermatol* 2006;12: 1–6.
8. Murayama N, Nagata M, Terada Y *et al.* Efficacy of a surgical scrub including 2% chlorhexidine acetate for canine superficial pyoderma. *Vet Dermatol* 2010; 21: 586–592.
9. Loeffler A, Linek M, Moodley A *et al.* First report of multiresistant, mecA-positive Staphylococcus intermedius in Europe: 12 cases from a veterinary dermatology referral clinic in Germany. *Vet Dermatol* 2007; 18: 412–421.
10. Young R, Buckley L, McEwan N, Nuttal T. Comparative in vitro efficacy of antimicrobial shampoos: a pilot study. *Vet Dermatol* 2012; 23: 36–40.
11. Kwochka KW, Kowalski JJ. Prophylactic efficacy of four antibacterial shampoos against *Staphylococcus intermedius* in dogs. *Am J Vet Res* 1991; 52: 115–118.
12. Frank LA. Nisin impregnated wipes for the treatment of canine pyoderma and surface bacterial colonization [abstract]. In: *Proceedings, 24th North American Veterinary Dermatology Forum*, Savanna, GA, 2009; 215.

Index

Page numbers in *italics* denote figures, those in **bold** denote tables.